Current Progress in Respiratory Medicine

Current Progress in Respiratory Medicine

Edited by Miguel Rodriguez

hayle medical

New York

Hayle Medical,
750 Third Avenue, 9th Floor,
New York, NY 10017, USA

Visit us on the World Wide Web at:
www.haylemedical.com

ISBN: 978-1-63241-756-5

The publisher's policy is to use permanent paper from mills that operate a sustainable forestry policy. Furthermore, the publisher ensures that the text paper and cover boards used have met acceptable environmental accreditation standards.

Printed in China.

Cataloging-in-Publication Data

Current progress in respiratory medicine / edited by Miguel Rodriguez.
p. cm.
Includes bibliographical references and index.
ISBN 978-1-63241-756-5
1. Respiratory organs--Diseases. 2. Respiratory organs--Diseases--Diagnosis.
3. Respiratory organs--Diseases--Treatment. 4. Respiratory infections.
I. Rodriguez, Miguel.
RC731 .C87 2019
616.2--dc23

Table of Contents

Preface IX

Chapter 1 **Combined diffusing capacity for nitric oxide and carbon monoxide as predictor of bronchiolitis obliterans syndrome following lung transplantation** 1
Anna Winkler, Kathrin Kahnert, Jürgen Behr, Claus Neurohr, Nikolaus Kneidinger, Rudolf Hatz, Holger Dressel, Thomas Radtke and Rudolf A. Jörres

Chapter 2 **Macrophages: friend or foe in idiopathic pulmonary fibrosis?** 11
Lei Zhang, Yi Wang, Guorao Wu, Weining Xiong, Weikuan Gu and Cong-Yi Wang

Chapter 3 **Impairment of respiratory muscle strength in Berardinelli-Seip congenital lipodystrophy subjects** 21
Jorge Luiz Dantas de Medeiros, Bruno Carneiro Bezerra, Thiago Anderson Brito de Araújo, Aquiles Sales Craveiro Sarmento, Lázaro Batista de Azevedo Medeiros, Lucien Peroni Gualdi, Maria do Socorro Luna Cruz, Thaiza Teixeira Xavier Nobre, Josivan Gomes Lima and Julliane Tamara Araújo de Melo Campos

Chapter 4 **What have we learned from observational studies and clinical trials of mild to moderate COPD?** 32
Miriam Barrecheguren, Cruz González and Marc Miravitlles

Chapter 5 **Elevated serum soluble programmed cell death ligand 1 concentration as a potential marker for poor prognosis in small cell lung cancer patients with chemotherapy** 43
Jianjun Jin, Jiming Si, Yuanhua Liu, Huanqin Wang, Ran Ni and Jing Wang

Chapter 6 **Short and long-term effects of pulmonary rehabilitation in interstitial lung diseases** 52
Silvia Perez-Bogerd, Wim Wuyts, Veronica Barbier, Heleen Demeyer, Alain Van Muylem, Wim Janssens and Thierry Troosters

Chapter 7 **Serum phosphate and phosphate-regulatory hormones in COPD patients** 62
Alexandra Stroda, Vincent Brandenburg, Ayham Daher, Christian Cornelissen, Claudia Goettsch, András Keszei and Michael Dreher

Chapter 8 **The impact of HIV on the prevalence of asthma in Uganda: a general population survey** 69
Bruce J. Kirenga, Levicatus Mugenyi, Corina de Jong, J. Lucian Davis, Winceslaus Katagira, Thys van der Molen, Moses R. Kamya and Marike Boezen

Chapter 9 **PrtA immunization fails to protect against pulmonary and invasive infection by *Streptococcus pneumoniae*** 77
Chen-Fang Hsu, Chen-Hao Hsiao, Shun-Fu Tseng, Jian-Ru Chen, Yu-Jou Liao, Sy-Jou Chen, Chin-Sheng Lin, Huey-Kang Sytwu and Yi-Ping Chuang

Chapter 10 **Efficacy and effectiveness of Ceftaroline Fosamil in patients with pneumonia** 90
Giovanni Sotgiu, Stefano Aliberti, Andrea Gramegna, Marco Mantero, Marta Di Pasquale, Federica Trogu, Laura Saderi and Francesco Blasi

Chapter 11 **From blood to lung tissue: effect of cigarette smoke on DNA methylation and lung function** 103
Maaike de Vries, Diana A van der Plaat, Ivana Nedeljkovic, Rikst Nynke Verkaik-Schakel, Wierd Kooistra, Najaf Amin, Cornelia M van Duijn, Corry-Anke Brandsma, Cleo C van Diemen, Judith M Vonk and H Marike Boezen

Chapter 12 **The utility of biomarkers in diagnosis of aspirin exacerbated respiratory disease** 112
Suzy A. A. Comhair, Grazyna Bochenek, Sara Baicker-McKee, Zeneng Wang, Tomasz Stachura, Marek Sanak, Jeffrey P. Hammel, Stanley L. Hazen, Serpil C. Erzurum and Ewa Nizankowska-Mogilnicka

Chapter 13 **Efficacy and safety of nintedanib in advanced idiopathic pulmonary fibrosis** 119
Hee-Young Yoon, Sojung Park, Dong Soon Kim and Jin Woo Song

Chapter 14 **Modulation of airway hyperresponsiveness by rhinovirus exposure** 130
Dennis Lo, Joshua L. Kennedy, Richard C. Kurten, Reynold A. Panettieri Jr and Cynthia J. Koziol-White

Chapter 15 **Therapeutic potential of products derived from mesenchymal stem/stromal cells in pulmonary disease** 141
Arezoo Mohammadipoor, Ben Antebi, Andriy I. Batchinsky and Leopoldo C. Cancio

Chapter 16 **Heterogeneous burden of lung disease in smokers with borderline airflow obstruction** 155
Cheryl S. Pirozzi, Tian Gu, Pedro M. Quibrera, Elizabeth E. Carretta, MeiLan K. Han, Susan Murray, Christopher B. Cooper, Donald P. Tashkin, Eric C. Kleerup, Igor Barjaktarevic, Eric A. Hoffman, Carlos H. Martinez, Stephanie A. Christenson, Nadia N. Hansel, R. Graham Barr, Eugene R. Bleecker, Victor E. Ortega, Fernando J. Martinez, Richard E. Kanner and Robert Paine III

Chapter 17 **Association of lung function with cardiovascular risk: a cohort study** 165
Bin Wang, Yun Zhou, Lili Xiao, Yanjun Guo, Jixuan Ma, Min Zhou, Tingming Shi, Aijun Tan, Jing Yuan and Weihong Chen

Chapter 18 **Serum AGE/RAGEs as potential biomarker in idiopathic pulmonary fibrosis** 173
Carlos Machahua, Ana Montes-Worboys, Lurdes Planas-Cerezales, Raquel Buendia-Flores, Maria Molina-Molina and Vanesa Vicens-Zygmunt

Chapter 19 **MUC1 deficiency mediates corticosteroid resistance in chronic obstructive pulmonary disease** 182
Javier Milara, Lucía Díaz-Platas, Sonia Contreras, Pilar Ribera, Inés Roger, Beatriz Ballester, Paula Montero, Ángel Cogolludo, Esteban Morcillo and Julio Cortijo

Chapter 20 **Primary immunodeficiency diseases in lung disease: warning signs, diagnosis and management** 200
Pere Soler-Palacín, Javier de Gracia, Luis Ignacio González-Granado, Carlos Martín, Carlos Rodríguez-Gallego and Silvia Sánchez-Ramón

Chapter 21 **Role of SOD3 in silica-related lung fibrosis and pulmonary vascular remodeling** ... 213
Igor N. Zelko, Jianxin Zhu and Jesse Roman

Chapter 22 **Alterations in VASP phosphorylation and profilin1 and cofilin1 expression in hyperoxic lung injury and BPD** ... 227
Mehboob Ali, Kathryn Heyob, Trent E. Tipple, Gloria S. Pryhuber and Lynette K. Rogers

Permissions

List of Contributors

Index

Preface

This book has been a concerted effort by a group of academicians, researchers and scientists, who have contributed their research works for the realization of the book. This book has materialized in the wake of emerging advancements and innovations in this field. Therefore, the need of the hour was to compile all the required researches and disseminate the knowledge to a broad spectrum of people comprising of students, researchers and specialists of the field.

Respiratory medicine, widely known as pulmonology, is a field of medicine concerned with diseases related to the respiratory tract. The human respiratory tract is that part of the respiratory system which is involved with respiration. Respiratory medicine is a branch of internal medicine. A specialist in this field is called a respiratory therapist. Such doctors deal with chest conditions, including asthma, pneumonia and tuberculosis. Interventional pulmonology is a new sub-speciality, which falls under the domain of respiratory medicine. It is concerned with the use of minimally invasive endoscopic procedures for diagnosing and treating respiratory diseases. Pleuroscopy and bronchoscopy are two therapeutic procedures used in interventional pulmonology. This book unfolds the innovative aspects of respiratory medicine which will be crucial for the progress of this field in the future. It elucidates new techniques and their applications in a multidisciplinary manner. As this field is emerging at a rapid pace, the contents of this book will help the readers understand the modern concepts and applications of the subject.

At the end of the preface, I would like to thank the authors for their brilliant chapters and the publisher for guiding us all-through the making of the book till its final stage. Also, I would like to thank my family for providing the support and encouragement throughout my academic career and research projects.

Editor

1

Combined diffusing capacity for nitric oxide and carbon monoxide as predictor of bronchiolitis obliterans syndrome following lung transplantation

Anna Winkler[1†], Kathrin Kahnert[2*†], Jürgen Behr[2], Claus Neurohr[3], Nikolaus Kneidinger[2], Rudolf Hatz[4], Holger Dressel[5,6], Thomas Radtke[5,6] and Rudolf A. Jörres[1]

Abstract

Background: There is a need for non-invasive parameters that are sensitive to the development of the bronchiolitis obliterans syndrome (BOS) in lung transplantation (LTx) patients. We studied whether the pulmonary diffusing capacity for inhaled nitric oxide is capable of detecting BOS stages.

Methods: Sixty-one LTx patients were included into this cross-sectional study (19/29/7/3/3 in BOS stages 0/0-p/1/2/3). For analysis stages 0/0-p versus 1/2/3 ("BOS binary-early"), and stages 0/0-p/1 versus 2/3 ("BOS binary-late") were summarized. Measurements of the combined diffusing capacity for nitric oxide (DLNO) and carbon monoxide (DLCO) were compared with spirometry and bodyplethysmography, and their relative importance was evaluated by discriminant analysis.

Results: Regarding the recognition of "BOS binary-early", among spirometric parameters forced expiratory volume in 1 s (FEV_1) was best, among bodyplethysmographic parameters airway resistance, and among diffusing parameters DLNO. Regarding "BOS binary-late", DLNO was inferior to bodyplethysmographic parameters.

Conclusion: Although the study comprised only measurements at a single time point and no follow-up, DLNO outperformed FEV_1, the time course of which is used in detecting BOS. Together with its pathophysiological plausibility, this result suggests that the measurement of DLNO, possibly over time, could be an easily applicable tool for the monitoring of LTx patients and should be evaluated in larger studies.

Keywords: Lung transplantation, Diffusing capacity, Bronchiolitis obliterans syndrome

Background

Lung transplantation (LTx) is an established therapeutic option to increase survival rates and improve quality of life in selected end-stage lung disease patients [1]. Despite increased survival rates, lung transplant recipients still have a poor prognosis compared with other organ transplant patients [1]. Long-term survival is limited by the occurrence of chronic lung allograft dysfunction (CLAD), an umbrella term used to describe various pathophysiological processes affecting the allograft [2], among them bronchiolitis obliterans syndrome (BOS), the most common form of CLAD, and less frequently restrictive allograft syndrome (RAS), and/or a combination of the two [3]. As the detection of BOS enables immediate therapeutic intervention, early diagnosis is essential.

The main clinical finding of BOS is an irreversible airway obstruction with a persistent (≥3 weeks) reduction of forced expiratory volume in 1 s (FEV_1) [4], without evidence of acute infection, acute cellular and/or antibody-mediated rejection and other factors [5, 6]. The classification covers BOS-0 (no BOS), BOS-0-p (potential BOS), and BOS 1–3, based on increasing airway obstruction (FEV_1) compared with the best-ever

* Correspondence: kathrin.kahnert@med.uni-muenchen.de
†Anna Winkler and Kathrin Kahnert contributed equally to this work.
[2]Department of Internal Medicine V, University of Munich (LMU), Comprehensive Pneumology Center, Member of the German Center for Lung Research (DZL), Ziemssenstr. 1, 80336 Munich, Germany
Full list of author information is available at the end of the article

value post-transplantation. Moreover, a reduction in the mean forced expiratory flow during the middle half of forced vital capacity (FEF_{25-75}) is used as an early marker [4, 7]. FEV_1 is an easily measurable but non-specific parameter, which is unlikely to fully reflect the situation in the lung periphery, where BOS originates [8]. The fact that BOS is characterized by an abnormal remodelling of terminal bronchioles, leading to airflow limitation of the small airways [9], raises the question whether other lung parameters could provide more detailed information. It is known that total lung capacity (TLC) and the ratio of TLC and residual volume (RV) are predictors of CLAD and can help to identify high-risk patients [10]. Prior investigations from our group demonstrated that elevated levels of exhaled nitric oxide (FeNO) could predict the development of BOS in LTx patients and also could be an early marker of deterioration in patients with or without pre-existing functional impairment [11]. The data also showed that a marked increase in follow-up FeNO measurements could identify patients at risk for an unfavourable course, whereas stable LTx recipients showed a significantly lower individual variation in FeNO values [11]. Cameli et al. [12] investigated the role of exhaled NO (eNO) and carbon monoxide (eCO) as markers of pulmonary inflammation associated with acute graft rejection and lung infection in LTx patients and found higher values of FeNO and in particular a higher alveolar concentration of nitric oxide ($Calv_{NO}$) in LTx patients with BOS compared to non-BOS patients [12]. This indicates that alveolar markers might be suitable for detecting BOS, as airway inflammation and remodelling of the small airways in LTx patients with BOS could be associated with alveolar changes such as elevated levels of peripheral eNO and $Calv_{NO}$ [12]. Thus, gas-exchange parameters are also candidates for detecting the malfunction of peripheral structural changes. For this purpose the differentiation from a capillary disorder would be helpful, and this task could be performed by the diffusing capacity for nitric oxide (DLNO), especially in combination with that for carbon monoxide (DLCO). This combination has been evaluated in various lung diseases but is not yet part of clinical routine [13, 14].

The comparison of DLNO and DLCO allows for the differentiation of lung components affected by the lung disease, since the affinity for NO to hemoglobin is much higher compared with that of CO [15]. Therefore, NO uptake is largely unaffected by pulmonary capillary blood volume (Vcap), in contrast with CO [16, 17], while the diffusion resistance (membrane factor, DMCO) is similar for both gases. DLNO can therefore be used to assess the membrane factor, and in combination with DLCO the Vcap. This allows for the differentiation between a thickened alveolar capillary membrane and reduced blood flow which is not possible by DLCO alone [18]. In case of membrane thickening both DLCO and DLNO would be affected, but DLNO stronger, while in case of a reduced alveolar volume (V_A) or a reduced Vcap, DLCO would decrease more than DLNO [19]. Although BOS has an obstructive component, it could also be associated with a transport disorder of the alveolar membrane.

Based on these considerations, the aim of this investigation was to reveal whether the non-invasive measurement of DLNO and DLCO is capable of an early detection of BOS in LTx recipients.

Methods

Study population

This cross-sectional study was performed at the Department of Internal Medicine V and the Institute and Outpatient Clinic for Occupational, Social and Environmental Medicine at the Ludwig Maximilian University of Munich, Germany. The cohort was recruited through the outpatient and inpatient sectors. A patient was enrolled in the cohort if he or she fulfilled the following inclusion criteria: (a) the patient was the recipient of a LTx performed at the study center, and (b) the patient expressed his or her willingness to participate in individually planned follow-up assessments; and if the patient did not fulfill any of the following exclusion criteria: (a) acute infections, (b) high levels of physical exertion or food intake prior to the measurements, (c) nicotine abuse on the day of measurements, or (d) physical impairment resulting in an inability to perform two valid and reproducible DLNO-DLCO measurements [13]. All assessments were approved by the local ethics committee (Ludwig Maximilian University of Munich, Germany) and all patients gave their written informed consent.

Assessments

Patients underwent a panel of assessments in order to collect clinical characteristics and functional status. The following parameters were recorded: height, weight, date of birth, lung disease which led to LTx, date of transplantation, type of transplantation (single LTx (SLTx), bilateral LTx (BLTx)), BOS stage, allergies, past medication, date of last food intake, acute respiratory infections, and smoking history.

Measurements combined diffusing capacity (DLNO-DLCO)

Simultaneous measurements of DLNO, DLCO and V_A were performed using the single-breath method (MasterScreen™ PFT Pro, Jaeger, CareFusion, Hoechberg, Germany). Although the study was performed prior to the recommendations of the American Thoracic Society and European Respiratory Society, [20] the study was in accordance with their standards. After careful instruction, patients performed three measurements at a breath-hold time of 8 s [21, 22] with at least five-minute resting intervals in between maneuvers to assure elimination of the test gas from the lungs. Incorrect measurements were repeated, to gain at least two plausible measurements, the mean of which was included in the further analyses. Using a breath-hold time of 8 s, excellent test-retest reliability has been reported for combined DLNO-DLCO measurements in patients with cystic fibrosis [21]. The test gas comprised a mixture of 0.28% carbon monoxide (CO), 600 mg/m^3 nitric oxide (NO) and 9.5% helium. Again, the measurements of V_A, DLCO and DLNO satisfied the technical standards proposed by Zavorsky et al. [23], although the study was performed prior to publication of these recommendations. The transfer coefficients for nitric oxide (KNO) and carbon monoxide (KCO) were calculated by dividing DLNO and DLCO through V_A, while the alveolar-capillary membrane diffusing capacity for carbon monoxide (DMCO) and Vcap were derived as proposed [13]. Percent predicted values for DLNO and DLCO were calculated according to Zavorsky et al. [23] based on previous work by Roughton et al. [24] and Guènard et al. [16], and DLCO was adjusted for hemoglobin [13, 17, 18].

In addition to DLNO and DLCO, conventional parameters of spirometry and bodyplethysmography were collected [25, 26]. For analysis the forced expiratory volume in 1 s (FEV_1) and forced vital capacity (FVC) were used, as well as intrathoracic gas volume (ITGV), residual volume (RV), total lung capacity (TLC), airway resistance (Raw) and specific airway resistance (sRaw). Percent predicted values for spirometry and bodyplethysmography were taken from the Global Lung Initiative [27], or the European Coal and Steel Community (ECCS) [28], respectively. Furthermore, routine laboratory parameters including hemoglobin, sodium, potassium, creatinine and CRP values were collected.

Statistical analysis

For data description, mean values and standard deviations (SD) were used. Comparisons between groups were performed using non-parametric tests, especially the Mann-Whitney-U test and the Kruskal-Wallis test, as well as chi-squared statistics for categorical data. To evaluate the value of the combined diffusing capacity for BOS recognition, patients were grouped into binary categories according to their BOS-stage. For the purpose of early diagnosis ("BOS binary-early"), stages 0 and 0-p were combined and compared with stages 1–3. To reveal whether it was possible to differentiate an initial diagnosis from progression, stages 0, 0-p and 1 were combined versus the combination of stages 2 and 3; this classification was termed "BOS-binary-late". The relationship between BOS groups and predictors was analyzed by means of linear discriminant analysis in order to identify the best parameters to differentiate between the respective groups. We used an approach with forward selection. The results were checked by logistic regression analyses performed in an analogous manner. The level of statistical significance (alpha) was set at 0.05 for all analyses. Statistical analyses were performed with SPSS Statistics 23 (IBM Corp., Armonk, NY, USA).

Results

Patient population

Sixty-four patients were screened for the study. Three patients were excluded because they were not capable of performing valid diffusing capacity measurements. Therefore, 61 patients (29 males, 32 females; mean ± SD age 50.8 ± 13.7 years) were included in the analysis. BLTx had been performed in 19/23 male/female patients. SLTx and BLTx patients showed no significant differences in anthropometric characteristics and the time between LTx and measurements, while BLTx patients were younger (45.8 ± 13.0 years, $p < 0.001$) than SLTx patients (61.8 ± 7.5 years).

BOS stages and pre-existing conditions

Idiopathic lung fibrosis (IPF) was the reason for transplantation in 22 patients. Following the official American Thoracic Society Statement, IPF was defined as chronic, progressive fibrosing interstitial pneumonia of unknown cause occurring primarily in adults, limited to the lungs, with radiological signs and/or histopathologic patterns consistent with usual interstitial pneumonia [29]. Further reasons for transplantation were COPD with emphysema in 16 patients (2 with alpha-1-antitrypsine deficiency), cystic fibrosis in 11 patients, three patients suffered from sarcoidosis, while the remaining 9 patients formed a heterogeneous group of diagnoses, including systemic lupus erythematosis, lymphangioleiomyomatosis, silicosis, Kartagener syndrome, or hypersensitivity pneumonitis alveolitis. There was no significant association between BOS-stages and the pre-existing lung disease.

BOS stages and patients' characteristics

The average interval between LTx and time of measurement was 4.3 ± 3.7 years. Nineteen patients were diagnosed as BOS-0, 29 patients as BOS 0-p, 7 as BOS 1, 2 as BOS 2, and 3 as BOS 3 (Table 1). There were no significant differences for age and BMI (Table 1) between BOS stages, when using the full classification or the binary groups. There was a significant difference in the number of years after LTx ($p = 0.001$), with the shortest period of time in BOS 0 and the longest in BOS 3There were no significant differences in the laboratory parameters hemoglobin, creatinine, CRP, sodium and potassium across the BOS-stages.

Table 1 BMI and age versus BOS stages

Parameter	BOS	N	Mean ± SD
Age (y)	0	19	47.4 ± 15.1
	0-p	29	50.8 ± 12.6
	1	7	60.4 ± 10.9
	2	3	46.7 ± 21.6
	3	3	53.7 ± 9.3
	Total	61	50.8 ± 13.7
BMI (kg/m^2)	0	19	22.3 ± 3.9
	0-p	29	24.3 ± 4.7
	1	7	22.9 ± 3.9
	2	3	23.9 ± 3.3
	3	3	21.5 ± 7.6
	Total	61	23.4 ± 4.4

The table shows mean values and standard deviations for age and body mass index (BMI) across the different BOS stages

BOS stages, lung function and combined DLNO-DLCO

Pulmonary function characteristics for all patients ($n = 61$) are shown in Tables 2 and 3. Increasing BOS stages were significantly associated with higher values of Raw and sRAw, and with lower values of FEV_1 and FEV_1/FVC ($p < 0.05$ each); RV/TLC and ITGV/TLC were borderline to non-significant ($p = 0.055$ each). Higher BOS stages were also significantly linked to lower values of DLCO, DLNO, and DMCO (p < 0.05 each). The discrimination capability of DLNO % predicted versus FEV_1% predicted is shown in Fig. 1.

Recognition of early BOS

The comparison of pulmonary function parameters between the two groups BOS 0/0-p and BOS 1–3 (BOS binary-early) showed lower values of FEV_1 and higher values of RV/TLC (Mann-Whitney-U test, $p < 0.05$ each). When comparing diffusing capacity parameters between groups, DLCO, DLNO, V_A and DMCO turned out to be significantly reduced in the BOS 1–3 group, either regarding the absolute or % predicted values (Mann-Whitney-U test, $p < 0.05$). The individual data for FEV_1 and DLNO are shown in Fig. 2.

In a discriminant analysis using the spirometric parameters only, FEV_1% predicted was identified as the major variable separating the two BOS groups "BOS binary-early" (specificity 60.4%, sensitivity 61.5%, positive predictive value 60.7%). It should be noted that the numbers of patients in both groups were unbalanced ($n = 48$ versus $n = 13$), and that sensitivity and specificity were low. Likewise, when performing the analysis with bodyplethysmographic parameters only, Raw was the only significant variable discriminating between the two BOS groups (specificity 70.8%; sensitivity 46.2%, positive predictive value 65.5%). When repeating the discriminant analysis with data from both spirometry and bodyplethysmography, Raw again remained as major variable separating the two groups "BOS binary-early", thus the combination of data had no additive value.

When the analysis was performed with all directly measured and derived parameters of the combined diffusing capacity, DLNO % predicted remained as only significant variable separating the two groups "BOS binary-early" (specificity 64.6%, sensitivity 69.2%, positive predictive value 65.6%). Since the combined measurement allows for the separation of membrane factor and Vcap, in a separate analysis only the derived parameters were tested, which revealed the membrane factor DMCO % predicted as only significant variable for "BOS binary-early" (positive predictive value 60.7%); Vcap played no role. As DMCO depends on DLNO, this result is plausible.

Finally, to compare the predictive value between the three lung function domains described above, a discriminant analysis with the best parameters from each; i.e., FEV_1, DLNO or DMCO (each in % predicted), and Raw was performed. In this analysis DLNO % predicted was the dominant and only significant variable discriminating between no BOS and "BOS binary-early" (positive predictive value as above: 65.6%). This finding demonstrated that DLNO carried more information than spirometry and bodyplethysmography in the detection of early BOS stages, even though the specificity was low. All of the above results were confirmed by logistic regression analysis.

Recognition of advanced BOS stages

To analyze advanced BOS stages, patients were grouped into BOS 0–1 versus BOS 2–3, although this grouping led to an even greater imbalance of group sizes ($n = 55$ versus $n = 6$). In a discriminant analysis using only spirometric parameters, most of them were significant in separating the two groups "BOS binary-late". FEV_1 and FEV_1/FVC, both in % predicted, achieved the strongest separation, whereas FVC % predicted was not significant. The positive predictive value of 82.0%, with high specificity (85.5%) but low sensitivity (50.0%) indicated a bias due to the unbalanced group sizes. When performing the analysis with bodyplethysmographic parameters only, all parameters except for TLC % predicted were significant in discriminating between the two BOS groups, with Raw and sRaw as most informative parameters ($p < 0.001$ each; sRaw: specificity 90.9%, sensitivity 66.7%, positive predictive value 88.5%). To evaluate the role of the other bodyplethysmographic parameters, the analysis was repeated without Raw and sRaw. ITGV/TLC % predicted was the only remaining significant variable (specificity 76.4%, sensitivity 66.7%, positive predictive value 75.4%), while the RV/TLC ratio was inferior

Table 2 Parameters of spirometry and bodyplethysmography versus BOS stages

	BOS	*N*	Mean ± SD	*p*-value
FEV_1% predicted	0	19	73.1 ± 20.3	0.004
	0-p	29	67.4 ± 16.8	
	1	7	64.9 ± 8.2	
	2	3	62.0 ± 5.0	
	3	3	29.5 ± 9.9	
FVC % predicted	0	19	74.7 ± 18.0	0.045
	0-p	29	77.9 ± 17.3	
	1	7	72.2 ± 15.4	
	2	3	84.6 ± 12.2	
	3	3	46.6 ± 10.2	
FEV_1/FVC % predicted	0	19	97.9 ± 15.3	0.002
	0-p	29	86.9 ± 14.8	
	1	7	92.6 ± 20.3	
	2	3	73.7 ± 11.5	
	3	3	62.2 ± 11.7	
TLC % predicted	0	19	88.4 ± 21.8	0.576
	0-p	29	110.1 ± 18.4	
	1	7	82.2 ± 30.5	
	2	3	107.2 ± 26.9	
	3	3	82.7 ± 3.1	
ITGV % predicted	0	19	102.9 ± 35.0	0.140
	0-p	29	100.1 ± 31.7	
	1	7	89.8 ± 39.3	
	2	3	146.4 ± 52.5	
	3	3	124.3 ± 15.4	
RV % predicted	0	19	108.8 ± 49.1	0.233
	0-p	29	119.9 ± 54.7	
	1	7	139.7 ± 83.0	
	2	3	75.7 ± 31.3	
	3	3	65.7 ± 12.6	
RV/TLC % predicted	0	19	118.1 ± 31.5	0.014
	0-p	29	107.9 ± 33.1	
	1	7	106.9 ± 27.0	
	2	3	131.9 ± 29.8	
	3	3	175.0 ± 24.4	
Raw ($kPa*s*l^{-1}$)	0	19	0.27 ± 0.11	< 0.001
	0-p	29	0.31 ± 0.10	
	1	7	0.27 ± 0.09	
	2	3	0.39 ± 0.11	
	3	3	0.80 ± 0.19	
sRaw (kPa*s)	0	19	0.99 ± 0.65	< 0.001
	0-p	29	1.12 ± 0.52	
	1	7	0.84 ± 0.36	
	2	3	1.85 ± 1.06	
	3	3	3.56 ± 1.17	

The table shows mean values and standard deviations. The comparisons between groups were performed by ANOVA. *FEV_1* forced expiratory volume in one second, *FVC* forced vital capacity, *ITGV* intrathoracic gas volume, *TLC* total lung capacity, *RV* residual volume, *Raw*, airway resistance, *sRaw* specific airway resistance

to this. The discrimination capability of RV/TLC ratio versus DLNO % predicted is shown in Fig. 3. The discriminant analysis using only parameters of diffusing capacity except DLNO/DLCO ratio and DMCO/Vcap showed that KNO, KCO and DMCO/VA, each in % predicted, were significant in separating the two BOS groups. The addition of the DLNO/DLCO ratio and DMCO/Vcap in the discriminant analysis revealed DLNO/DLCO ratio as only remaining variable significantly separating the "BOS binary-late" groups (specificity 74.5%, sensitivity 66.7%, positive predictive value 73.8%). The results given above were confirmed by logistic regression analysis.

Discussion

This study revealed that the diffusing capacity of the lung for NO allows the early detection of BOS in patients following BLTx but has no additional value for patients following SLTx.. Compared to a panel of conventional lung function measures DLNO was the parameter with the highest reliability in the detection of early BOS stages. By contrast, we were not able to show an additional value of DLNO for the detection of advanced BOS stages within the limits of a very small number of patients with advanced BOS stages.

The study population was comprised of 61 patients with well-balanced gender distribution, and the proportion of SLTx and BLTx patients ($n = 19$ versus 42) was in accordance with the international practice favoring BLTx [1]. The only statistically significant difference between SLTx and BLTx patients was age, due to the fact that SLTx was mainly performed in patients with emphysema, whereas BLTx was mostly chosen in younger patients with cystic fibrosis, in line with international data [1, 30]. Thus, the study population can be regarded as representative.

Regarding the early diagnosis of BOS, discriminant analyses identified FEV_1% predicted, Raw and DLNO % predicted as the parameters from spirometry, bodyplethysmography and combined NO-CO diffusing capacity, respectively, which could best differentiate between both groups. In the competition of these parameters, DLNO % predicted outperformed the other two parameters which

Table 3 Parameters of diffusing capacity versus BOS stages

	BOS	*N*	Mean ± SD	*p*-value
DLCO % predicted	0	19	52.0 ± 13.8	0.018
	0-p	29	58.0 ± 12.5	
	1	7	44.3 ± 12.1	
	2	3	63.8 ± 18.3	
	3	3	37.9 ± 14.9	
KCO % predicted	0	19	75.8 ± 13.2	0.439
	0-p	29	84.1 ± 15.0	
	1	7	77.7 ± 13.7	
	2	3	87.0 ± 38.9	
	3	3	77.3 ± 25.8	
DLNO % predicted	0	19	44.1 ± 11.8	0.002
	0-p	29	47.9 ± 11.0	
	1	7	35.3 ± 10.2	
	2	3	48.8 ± 7.1	
	3	3	22.8 ± 2.2	
KNO % predicted	0	19	66.0 ± 11.1	0.014
	0-p	29	70.5 ± 9.1	
	1	7	62.9 ± 12.4	
	2	3	65.7 ± 19.2	
	3	3	48.4 ± 4.2	
DMCO % predicted	0	19	34.0 ± 10.6	0.004
	0-p	29	37.3 ± 11.0	
	1	7	27.4 ± 9.5	
	2	3	39.6 ± 5.6	
	3	3	14.7 ± 0.7	
V_A % predicted	0	19	67.5 ± 14.7	0.056
	0-p	29	67.4 ± 14.1	
	1	7	55.7 ± 16.7	
	2	3	71.2 ± 13.0	
	3	3	46.5 ± 6.4	
Vcap % predicted	0	19	69.2 ± 18.9	0.290
	0-p	29	75.0 ± 21.4	
	1	7	58.2 ± 14.5	
	2	3	75.6 ± 22.8	
	3	3	93.9 ± 82.6	
Vcap/V_A % predicted	0	19	106.7 ± 25.6	0.031
	0-p	29	116.5 ± 36.5	
	1	7	111.1 ± 29.4	
	2	3	115.4 ± 56.5	
	3	3	201.9 ± 167.0	
DMCO/V_A % predicted	0	19	52.8 ± 13.1	0.044
	0-p	29	57.3 ± 12.0	
	1	7	51.9 ± 14.7	
	2	3	59.3 ± 21.7	
	3	3	33.1 ± 3.1	

The table shows mean values and standard deviations. The comparisons between groups were performed by ANOVA. *DLCO* diffusing capacity for carbon monoxide, *DMCO* alveolar-capillary membrane diffusing capacity for carbon monoxide, *DLNO* diffusing capacity for nitric oxide, *KCO* transfer factor for carbon monoxide, *KNO* transfer factor for nitric oxide; V_A alveolar volume, *Vcap* pulmonary capillary blood volume

yielded no additional information. Therefore, in line with our hypothesis, DLNO carried substantial information regarding the detection of early BOS stages. The major pathophysiological changes leading to BOS include inflammation, repetitive injury of airway epithelia, fibrotic changes and airway remodelling [9]; thus, it is reasonable to expect an impact on pulmonary function due to the resulting membrane thickening, which should be reflected in changes of DLNO. BOS histopathology is in the early stages characterized by inflammation and fibrosis of the airway with sparing of the surrounding alveoli. Still, this raises the possibility that the gas transport to and within the alveoli is affected, which could be detected by a highly sensitive method assessing gas uptake without major interference with factors arising from the pulmonary capillaries. In our study we tested whether DLNO could achieve this task, as a sort of indirect test of peripheral airway dysfunction.

In diagnosing advanced BOS stages the results were different, and FEV_1 and FEV_1/FVC, each in % predicted, emerged as most informative parameters. This is reasonable insofar as FEV_1 is used for the definition of these BOS stages. From bodyplethysmography, sRaw and ITGV/TLC were informative, while in the combined diffusing capacity the DLNO/DLCO ratio remained as sole differentiating variable. When comparing these parameters to determine their relative predictive value, FEV_1/VC and ITGV/TLC remained informative, while the combined DLNO-DLCO carried no additional value. To facilitate the comparison with the literature [10], instead of ITGV/TLC the ratio RV/TLC was also tested, leading to similar results.

In the evaluation of all results, the inhomogeneous group sizes must be considered. The group "BOS-binary-late" was comprised of 6 versus 55 patients, whereas in the group "BOS-binary-early" the relationship was more favourable with 13 versus 48 patients. Although the analysis of the advanced stages was heavily handicapped by the unbalanced group sizes, the results are consistent with known data regarding RV/TLC [10], possibly indicating that the relative unimportance of DLNO in this condition was a valid result.

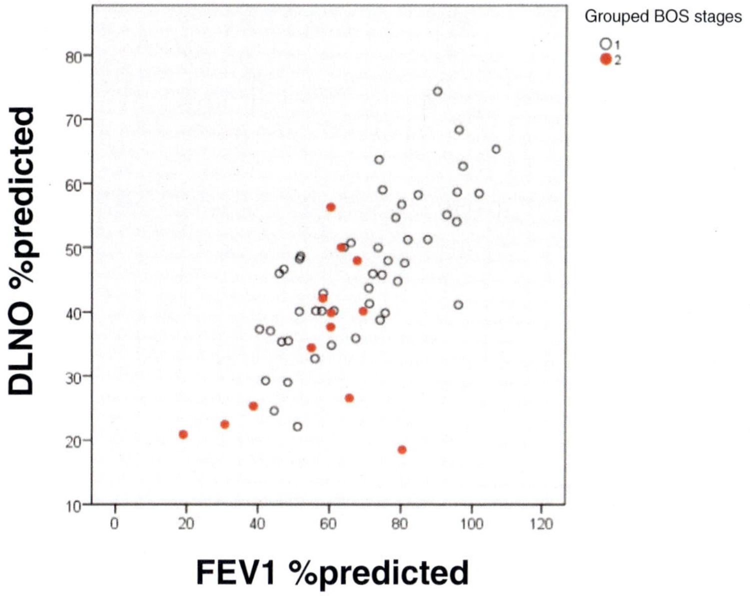

Fig. 1 Detection of early BOS. Discrimination capability of DLNO %predicted versus FEV1%predicted in the detection of early BOS. 1 = BOS 0/0-p, 2 = BOS 1/2/3

Thus far, the combined DLNO-DLCO has not been investigated in patients post LTx for the detection of BOS. Regarding the early diagnosis DLNO was superior to all other lung function parameters under study, confirming our hypothesis that DLNO is especially sensitive to changes in peripheral airways which are common in early stages of BOS. This is remarkable because the definition of BOS is based not on single measurements but on the individual time course of spirometric measurements, while we performed only single measurements expressed

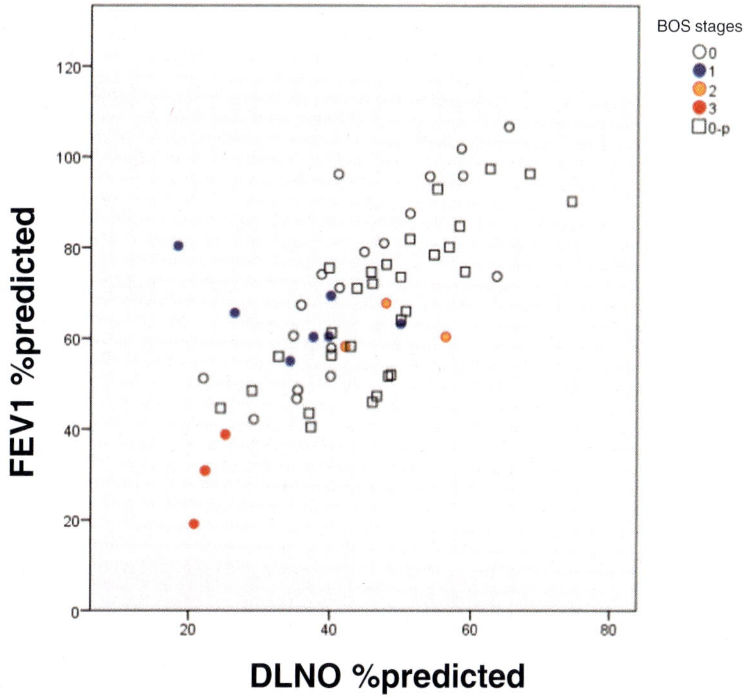

Fig. 2 Detection of BOS. Discrimination capability of DLNO %predicted versus FEV1%predicted. In this figure the five different BOS categories are indicated separately

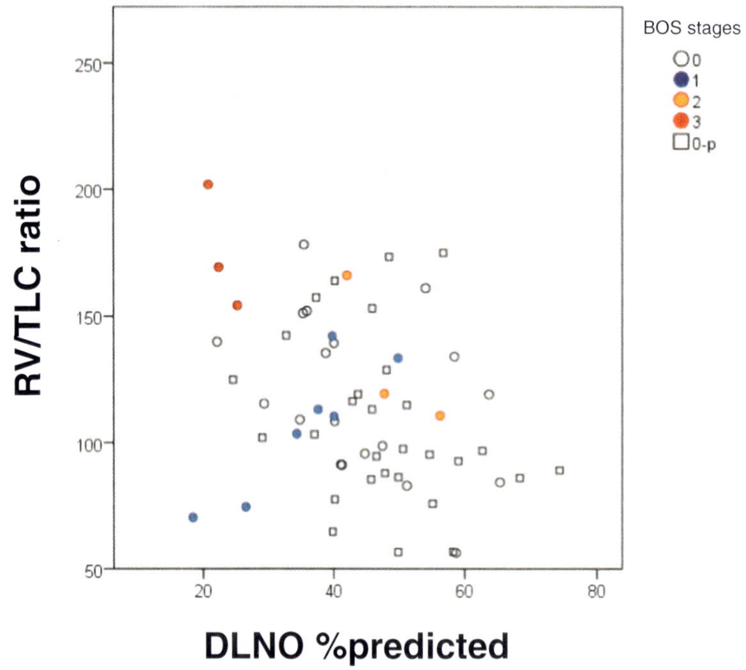

Fig. 3 Detection of BOS. Discrimination capability of RV/TLC ratio versus DLNO % predicted. In this figure the five different BOS categories are indicated separately

as % predicted. The fact that DLNO was superior even to FEV_1 used in the definition of BOS is a hint that the sensitivity of DLNO could be even greater when used in individual follow-up measurements. In eight patients, repeated measurements were available at an average time interval of 99 days, demonstrating good reproducibility, but no incident BOS cases occurred during this time period.

As expected, FEV_1 showed a significant capability of discrimination between BOS stages, as well as RV/TLC, Raw and sRaw, but only if the combined DLNO-DLCO was not included. Former investigations revealed that a high RV/TLC ratio, as indicator of hyperinflation and air trapping, predicts survival in patients with CLAD [10]. In our study the RV/TLC ratio was also significantly higher in patients with BOS 2–3 as well as in BOS 1–3, compared to the other BOS stages. Despite this, the ratio was inferior to DLNO in the detection of early BOS. Regarding advanced BOS stages the results for RV/TLC were in line with a previous publication from our group [10].

The measurement of DLNO-DLCO was performed before the publication of the European Respiratory Society (ERS) technical standards document for the single-breath CO and NO diffusing capacity [20, 13]. Therefore, the procedure of measurements followed previous approaches published by van der Lee et al. [31] and Dressel et al. [21]. Irrespective of this, the measurements were in accordance with recent recommendations for single-breath DLCO [20, 32] as well as DLNO [13], taking into account that breath-hold time was within the range, in which diffusing capacity is not markedly affected by different breath-hold times [33].

The combined DLNO-DLCO allows the non-invasive discrimination between alterations of gas uptake resulting from lung parenchyma versus pulmonary capillary circulation. This capability has proved useful in different diseases such as heart failure [34], liver cirrhosis [35], pulmonary arterial hypertension [17, 36], chronic obstructive pulmonary disease [37], cystic fibrosis [22] and stem cell transplantation [38]. In the present study, we could extend this range to lung transplant recipients. Apparently, early structural and/or inflammatory changes in the lung of patients with BOS deteriorate alveolar gas uptake as measurable by DLNO, whereas DLCO, being more dependent on Vcap, seems less affected.

Additional analyses revealed that DLNO had no value in recognizing "early BOS" in single-lung transplant patients, whereas it still showed a significant difference in double-lung transplant patients (Mann-Whitney-U test, $p = 0.002$). This might indicate differences arising from the different clinical background which led to either single or double transplantation. Even more likely is that in single-lung transplant patients the remaining lung still affected from the background disease dominates the test results thereby preventing the use of DLNO.

Limitations and strengths

The major limitation of our analysis was the small study cohort; in particular, the low number of patients with advanced BOS stages. Moreover, the sample size was not sufficient to find out whether DLNO is even of value in discriminating between BOS 0 and 0-p; individual follow-up measurements may be necessary for this. Nevertheless, at least the result for the early detection of BOS appears plausible enough to motivate larger, multi-center follow-up studies. This appears feasible, as the measurement of the combined diffusing capacity is standardized, can be performed simultaneously with the DLCO measurement and does not require specific cooperation or expertise. In light of the poor prognosis of LTx patients, any additional non-invasive parameter that could help in disease monitoring is highly appreciated. As BOS causes changes in the lung periphery, parameters targeting this part of the lung are particularly promising, and among these DLNO appears to be a prime candidate, at least in patients with double-lung transplants.

Abbreviations

ANOVA: Analysis of variance; BLTx: Bilateral LTx; BOS: Bronchiolitis obliterans syndrome; CLAD: Chronic lung allograft dysfunction; CO: Carbon monoxide; DLCO: Carbon monoxide; DLNO: Diffusing capacity for nitric oxide; DMCO: Diffusion resistance, membrane factor; FEF_{25-75}: Middle half of forced vital capacity; FEV_1: Forced expiratory volume in 1 s; FVC: Forced vital capacity; ITGV: Intrathoracic gas volume; KCO: Transfer coefficients for carbon monoxide; KNO: Transfer coefficients for nitric oxide; LTx: Lung transplantation; NO: Nitric oxide; RAS: Restrictive allograft syndrome; Raw: Airway resistance; RV: Residual volume; SD: Standard deviations; SLTx: Single LTx; sRaw: Specific airway resistance; TLC: Total lung capacity; V_A: Alveolar volume; Vcap: Pulmonary capillary blood volume

Acknowledgements

We thank Professor Rudolf Maria Huber for ongoing support during this project.

Authors' contributions

AW and KK were involved in the conception of the study, analyzing and interpreting the data, statistical analysis, conceptualizing and drafting of the manuscript, approved the final submitted version, and agreed to be accountable for all aspects of the work. JB was involved in the interpretation of the data from this analysis and drafting of the manuscript, approved the final submitted version, and agreed to be accountable for all aspects of the work. CN contributed to the overall design of COSYCONET, to the interpretation of the data from this analysis, to the development and critical revision of the manuscript, approved the final submitted version, and agreed to be accountable for all aspects of the work. NK was involved in the interpretation of the data from this analysis, took part in the discussion and critical revision of this manuscript, approved the final submitted version, and agreed to be accountable for all aspects of the work. RH was involved in the interpretation of the data from this analysis, took part in the discussion and critical revision of this manuscript, approved the final submitted version, and agreed to be accountable for all aspects of the work. HD was involved in the interpretation of the data from this analysis, took part in the discussion and critical revision of this manuscript, approved the final submitted version, and agreed to be accountable for all aspects of the work. TR was involved in the interpretation of the data from this analysis and drafting of the manuscript, approved the final submitted version, and agreed to be accountable for all aspects of the work. RAJ was involved in the design and set-up of the study, as well as quality control, statistical analysis and conceptualizing and drafting of the manuscript, approved the final submitted version, and agreed to be accountable for all aspects of the work.

Competing interests

The authors declare that they have no competing interests.

Author details

[1]Institute and Outpatient Clinic for Occupational, Social and Environmental Medicine, Comprehensive Pneumology Center Munich (CPC-M), Ludwig-Maximilians-Universität München, Munich, Germany. [2]Department of Internal Medicine V, University of Munich (LMU), Comprehensive Pneumology Center, Member of the German Center for Lung Research (DZL), Ziemssenstr. 1, 80336 Munich, Germany. [3]Robert-Bosch-Hospital, Klinik Schillerhöhe, Gerlingen, Germany. [4]Department of Thoracic Surgery, University of Munich (LMU), Munich, Germany. [5]Epidemiology, Biostatistics and Prevention Institute, University of Zurich, Zurich, Switzerland. [6]Division of Occupational and Environmental Medicine, University of Zurich and University Hospital Zurich, Zurich, Switzerland.

References

1. Chambers DC, Yusen RD, Cherikh WS, Goldfarb SB, Kucheryavaya AY, Khusch K, Levvey BJ, Lund LH, Meiser B, Rossano JW, et al. The Registry of the International Society for Heart and Lung Transplantation: Thirty-fourth Adult Lung And Heart-Lung Transplantation Report-2017; Focus Theme: Allograft ischemic time. J Heart Lung Transplant. 2017;36(10):1047–59.
2. Yusen RD, Edwards LB, Kucheryavaya AY, Benden C, Dipchand AI, Goldfarb SB, Levvey BJ, Lund LH, Meiser B, Rossano JW, et al. The Registry of the International Society for Heart and Lung Transplantation: Thirty-second Official Adult Lung and Heart-Lung Transplantation Report--2015; Focus Theme: Early Graft Failure. J Heart Lung Transplant. 2015;34(10):1264–77.
3. Royer PJ, Olivera-Botello G, Koutsokera A, Aubert JD, Bernasconi E, Tissot A, Pison C, Nicod L, Boissel JP, Magnan A, et al. Chronic Lung Allograft Dysfunction: A Systematic Review of Mechanisms. Transplantation. 2016; 100(9):1803–14.
4. Hayes D Jr. A review of bronchiolitis obliterans syndrome and therapeutic strategies. J Cardiothorac Surg. 2011;6:92.
5. Levine DJ, Glanville AR, Aboyoun C, Belperio J, Benden C, Berry GJ, Hachem R, Hayes D, Jr., Neil D, Reinsmoen NL et al.: Antibody-mediated rejection of the lung: A consensus report of the International Society for Heart and Lung Transplantation. J Heart Lung Transplant 2016, 35(4):397–406.
6. Sato M, Waddell TK, Wagnetz U, Roberts HC, Hwang DM, Haroon A, Wagnetz D, Chaparro C, Singer LG, Hutcheon MA, et al. Restrictive allograft syndrome (RAS): a novel form of chronic lung allograft dysfunction. J Heart Lung Transplant. 2011;30(7):735–42.
7. Estenne M, Maurer JR, Boehler A, Egan JJ, Frost A, Hertz M, Mallory GB, Snell GI, Yousem S. Bronchiolitis obliterans syndrome 2001: an update of the diagnostic criteria. J Heart Lung Transplant. 2002;21(3):297–310.
8. Yousem SA, Duncan SR, Griffith BP. Interstitial and airspace granulation tissue reactions in lung transplant recipients. Am J Surg Pathol. 1992; 16(9):877–84.
9. Verleden SE, Sacreas A, Vos R, Vanaudenaerde BM, Verleden GM. Advances in Understanding Bronchiolitis Obliterans After Lung Transplantation. Chest. 2016;150(1):219–25.
10. Kneidinger N, Milger K, Janitza S, Ceelen F, Leuschner G, Dinkel J, Konigshoff M, Weig T, Schramm R, Winter H et al.: Lung volumes predict survival in patients with chronic lung allograft dysfunction. Eur Respir J 2017, 49(4).
11. Neurohr C, Huppmann P, Leuschner S, von Wulffen W, Meis T, Leuchte H, Ihle F, Zimmermann G, Baezner C, Hatz R, et al. Usefulness of exhaled nitric oxide to guide risk stratification for bronchiolitis obliterans syndrome after lung transplantation. Am J Transplant. 2011;11(1):129–37.
12. Cameli P, Bargagli E, Fossi A, Bennett D, Voltolini L, Refini RM, Gotti G, Rottoli P. Exhaled nitric oxide and carbon monoxide in lung transplanted patients. Respir Med. 2015;109(9):1224–9.
13. Zavorsky GS, Hsia CC, Hughes JM, Borland CD, Guenard H, van der Lee I, Steenbruggen I, Naeije R, Cao J, Dinh-Xuan AT. Standardisation and application of the single-breath determination of nitric oxide uptake in the lung. Eur Respir J. 2017:49(2).

14. Nyilas S, Carlens J, Price T, Singer F, Muller C, Hansen G, Warnecke G, Latzin P, Schwerk N. Multiple breath washout in pediatric patients after lung transplantation. Am J Transplant. 2018;18(1):145–53.
15. Gibson QH, Roughton FJ. The kinetics and equilibria of the reactions of nitric oxide with sheep haemoglobin. J Physiol. 1957;136(3):507–24.
16. Guenard H, Varene N, Vaida P. Determination of lung capillary blood volume and membrane diffusing capacity in man by the measurements of NO and CO transfer. Respir Physiol. 1987;70(1):113–20.
17. Borland C, Bottrill F, Jones A, Sparkes C, Vuylsteke A. The significant blood resistance to lung nitric oxide transfer lies within the red cell. J Appl Physiol (1985). 2014;116(1):32–41.
18. van der Lee I, Zanen P, Biesma DH, van den Bosch JM. The effect of red cell transfusion on nitric oxide diffusing capacity. Respiration. 2005;72(5):512–6.
19. Hughes JM, van der Lee I. The TL,NO/TL,CO ratio in pulmonary function test interpretation. Eur Respir J. 2013;41(2):453–61.
20. Graham BL, Brusasco V, Burgos F, Cooper BG, Jensen R, Kendrick A, MacIntyre NR, Thompson BR, Wanger J. Executive Summary: 2017 ERS/ATS standards for single-breath carbon monoxide uptake in the lung. Eur Respir J. 2017;49(1). https://doi.org/10.1183/13993003.00016-2016.
21. Dressel H, Filser L, Fischer R, de la Motte D, Steinhaeusser W, Huber RM, Nowak D, Jorres RA. Lung diffusing capacity for nitric oxide and carbon monoxide: dependence on breath-hold time. Chest. 2008;133(5):1149–54.
22. Dressel H, Filser L, Fischer R, Marten K, Muller-Lisse U, de la Motte D, Nowak D, Huber RM, Jorres RA. Lung diffusing capacity for nitric oxide and carbon monoxide in relation to morphological changes as assessed by computed tomography in patients with cystic fibrosis. BMC Pulm Med. 2009;9:30.
23. Zavorsky GS. Nitric oxide uptake in the lung: It is about time that clinicians use this test routinely. Respir Physiol Neurobiol. 2017;241:1–2.
24. Roughton FJ, Forster RE. Relative importance of diffusion and chemical reaction rates in determining rate of exchange of gases in the human lung, with special reference to true diffusing capacity of pulmonary membrane and volume of blood in the lung capillaries. J Appl Physiol. 1957;11(2):290–302.
25. Criee CP, Sorichter S, Smith HJ, Kardos P, Merget R, Heise D, Berdel D, Kohler D, Magnussen H, Marek W, et al. Body plethysmography--its principles and clinical use. Respir Med. 2011;105(7):959–71.
26. Miller MR, Hankinson J, Brusasco V, Burgos F, Casaburi R, Coates A, Crapo R, Enright P, van der Grinten CP, Gustafsson P et al: Standardisation of spirometry. Eur Respir J 2005, 26(2):319–338.
27. Quanjer PH, Stanojevic S, Cole TJ, Baur X, Hall GL, Culver BH, Enright PL, Hankinson JL, Ip MS, Zheng J, et al. Multi-ethnic reference values for spirometry for the 3–95-yr age range: the global lung function 2012 equations. Eur Respir J. 2012;40(6):1324–43.
28. Quanjer PH, Tammeling GJ, Cotes JE, Pedersen OF, Peslin R, Yernault JC. Lung volumes and forced ventilatory flows. Eur Respir J. 1993;6(Suppl 16):5–40.
29. Raghu G, Collard HR, Egan JJ, Martinez FJ, Behr J, Brown KK, Colby TV, Cordier JF, Flaherty KR, Lasky JA, et al. An official ATS/ERS/JRS/ALAT statement: idiopathic pulmonary fibrosis: evidence-based guidelines for diagnosis and management. Am J Respir Crit Care Med. 2011; 183(6):788–824.
30. Schuba B, Scheklinski M, von Dossow V, Schneider C, Preissler G, Kneidinger N, Neurohr C, Michel S, Hagl C, Schramm R: Five-year experience using the Lung Allocation Score: the Munich Lung Transplant Group. Eur J Cardiothorac Surg 201854(2):328-333.
31. van der Lee I, van Es HW, Noordmans HJ, van den Bosch JM, Zanen P. Alveolar volume determined by single-breath helium dilution correlates with the high-resolution computed tomography-derived nonemphysematous lung volume. Respiration. 2006;73(4):468–73.
32. Stanojevic S, Graham BL, Cooper BG, Thompson BR, Carter KW, Francis RW, Hall GL. Global Lung Function Initiative Twg, Global Lung Function Initiative T: Official ERS technical standards: Global Lung Function Initiative reference values for the carbon monoxide transfer factor for Caucasians. Eur Respir J. 2017;50(3):139-43.
33. Radtke T, Benden C, Maggi-Beba M, Kriemler S, van der Lee I, Dressel H. Intra-session and inter-session variability of nitric oxide pulmonary diffusing capacity in adults with cystic fibrosis. Respir Physiol Neurobiol. 2017;246:33–8.
34. Magini A, Apostolo A, Salvioni E, Italiano G, Veglia F, Agostoni P. Alveolar-capillary membrane diffusion measurement by nitric oxide inhalation in heart failure. Eur J Prev Cardiol. 2015;22(2):206–12.
35. Degano B, Mittaine M, Guenard H, Rami J, Garcia G, Kamar N, Bureau C, Peron JM, Rostaing L, Riviere D. Nitric oxide and carbon monoxide lung transfer in patients with advanced liver cirrhosis. J Appl Physiol (1985). 2009; 107(1):139–43.
36. Farha S, Laskowski D, George D, Park MM, Tang WH, Dweik RA, Erzurum SC. Loss of alveolar membrane diffusing capacity and pulmonary capillary blood volume in pulmonary arterial hypertension. Respir Res. 2013;14:6.
37. van der Lee I, Gietema HA, Zanen P, van Klaveren RJ, Prokop M, Lammers JW, van den Bosch JM. Nitric oxide diffusing capacity versus spirometry in the early diagnosis of emphysema in smokers. Respir Med. 2009;103(12):1892–7.
38. Le Bourgeois A, Malard F, Chevallier P, Urbistandoy G, Guillaume T, Delaunay J, Peterlin P, Lemarchand P, Germaud P, Mohty M, et al. Impact of pre-transplant diffusion lung capacity for nitric oxide (DLNO) and of DLNO/pre-transplant diffusion lung capacity for carbon monoxide (DLNO/DLCO) ratio on pulmonary outcomes in adults receiving allogeneic stem cell transplantation for hematological diseases. Bone Marrow Transplant. 2016; 51(4):589–92.

2

Macrophages: friend or foe in idiopathic pulmonary fibrosis?

Lei Zhang[1], Yi Wang[1], Guorao Wu[1], Weining Xiong[1], Weikuan Gu[2] and Cong-Yi Wang[1*]

Abstract

Idiopathic pulmonary fibrosis (IPF) is a prototype of lethal, chronic, progressive interstitial lung disease of unknown etiology. Over the past decade, macrophage has been recognized to play a significant role in IPF pathogenesis. Depending on the local microenvironments, macrophages can be polarized to either classically activated (M1) or alternatively activated (M2) phenotypes. In general, M1 macrophages are responsible for wound healing after alveolar epithelial injury, while M2 macrophages are designated to resolve wound healing processes or terminate inflammatory responses in the lung. IPF is a pathological consequence resulted from altered wound healing in response to persistent lung injury. In this review, we intend to summarize the current state of knowledge regarding the process of macrophage polarization and its mediators in the pathogenesis of pulmonary fibrosis. Our goal is to update the understanding of the mechanisms underlying the initiation and progression of IPF, and by which, we expect to provide help for developing effective therapeutic strategies in clinical settings.

Keywords: IPF, Macrophage polarization, Classically activated (M1) macrophages, Alternatively activated (M2) macrophages, Therapeutic strategies

Background

Idiopathic pulmonary fibrosis (IPF) is the most common fibrosing lung disease with poor prognosis and no effective treatment. It is characterized by the development of excessive extracellular matrix deposition, leading to decreased static lung compliance, disrupted gas exchange, and ultimately, respiratory failure and death [1–4]. The median survival time for IPF patients is approximately 3 years after the initial diagnosis [5, 6]. Notably, the incidence of IPF rises dramatically with age and is estimated to be 3–9 cases per 100,000 people in Europe and North America [7, 8], which is slightly higher than that in Asia and South America.

It is believed that IPF is resulted from a complex interaction between multiple genetic and non-genetic risk factors (e.g., cigarette smoking and infection). However, the relative contribution of genetic and non-genetic risk factors is likely to vary among individuals [9]. Past genetic studies in familial and sporadic IPF patients have characterized that the surfactant-associated genes (*surfactant protein C, SFTPC*; *surfactant protein A2, SFTPA2*; and *ATP binding cassette member A3, ABCA3*) [10, 11] and the telomerase-related genes (telomerase reverse transcriptase, *TERT*; *telomerase RNA component, TERC*; and *regulator of telomere elongation helicase 1, RTEL1*) [12] are associated with IPF susceptibility. More recently, two large genome-wide association studies (GWASs) conducted in patients with sporadic and familiar IPF not only confirmed known associations with TERC, TERT, and mucin 5B gene (MUC5B), but also identified novel risk genes such as the *toll interacting protein* (*TOLLIP*) and the *signal peptide peptidase like 2C* (*SPPL2C*) [13, 14]. Of note, excess matrix accumulation is thought to be an important part in the pathological process of IPF, and its related proteins such as matrix metalloproteinase 1 (MMP1) and matrix metalloproteinase 19 (MMP19) that are strongly upregulated in IPF are proposed to be potential peripheral blood biomarkers [15, 16]. In support of this notion, a frameshift deletion (c.988delG, p.A330fs) in MMP1 and a nonsense mutation (c.T1155A, p.Y385X) in MMP19 were characterized in IPF patients [17]. Although these discoveries are exciting, how non-genetic factors trigger those

* Correspondence: wangcy@tjh.tjmu.edu.cn
[1]The Center for Biomedical Research, Key Laboratory of Organ Transplantation, Ministry of Education and Ministry of Health, Tongji Hospital, Tongji Medical College, Huazhong University of Science and Technology, 1095 Jiefang Avenue, Wuhan 430030, China
Full list of author information is available at the end of the article

genetic predisposed individuals to initiate IPF process is unfortunately remained poorly understood, which is not our focus in the current review and will be reviewed elsewhere.

Monocytes/macrophages, which originate from progenitors in the bone marrow, circulate in the peripheral blood or migrate into different tissues and constitute the foremost controllers of both innate and acquired immunity [18, 19]. In general, circulating monocytes leave the blood and migrate into tissues, where they differentiate into macrophages following exposure to different stimuli, including local growth factors, cytokines and microbial debris [20, 21]. Macrophages are critical to antigen removal by phagocytosis and the clearance of microbes, apoptotic cells and neoplastic cells [22, 23]. Furthermore, in activated immune responses, macrophages are an extremely heterogeneous population, exerting a combination of pro-inflammatory and anti-inflammatory functions [20, 24]. Typically, macrophages that mainly produce pro-inflammatory cytokines are called classically activated macrophages (M1), which can be activated either by IFN-γ or lipopolysaccharide (LPS). In contrast, macrophages that attenuate inflammation and encourage wound repair are referred to as alternatively activated macrophages (M2), which can be activated by IL-4 or IL-13 [25]. It is believed that enhanced macrophage M2 program is associated with fibrotic remodeling of internal organs, including the heart, kidneys, liver, gastrointestinal tract and lungs [26]. Therefore, in this review, we mainly discuss the current state of knowledge regarding the process of macrophage polarization and its mediators in the pathogenesis of pulmonary fibrosis. Our goal is to update the understanding of the mechanisms underlying the initiation and progression of IPF, and by which, we expect to provide help for developing effective therapeutic strategies in clinical settings.

Origin of macrophages

Macrophages are small populations of leukocytes that play an important role in the cross-talk between innate and adaptive immunity [27]. As early as 1893, Metchnikoff first described the term "phagocytes" when he used a rose thorn to challenge a starfish [28]. He classified the phagocytes into macrophages (macro = big, phage = eater) and microphages (now better known as neutrophils), which promoted the development of a theory of phagocytosis [29, 30]. In the 1960s, several studies proposed that macrophages were solely derived from the terminal differentiation of circulating monocytes [31–33]. However, this theory has been refuted by the recent discoveries that most adult tissue-resident macrophages are seeded before birth, stem from the embryonal yolk sac and fetal liver, possess a self-renewing capacity and are maintained independent of circulating monocytes [27, 34]. In addition, the function of macrophages varies significantly based on their anatomical location, functional phenotype, morphology, as well as their gene expression profile, such as the alveolar macrophages, adipose tissue macrophages, Kupffer cells in the liver, and microglia cells in the central nervous system [26, 35].

Pulmonary macrophages

Pulmonary macrophage populations are classified into two main categories: alveolar macrophages (AMs), which strategically reside in the alveoli, and interstitial macrophages (IMs), which are located within the lung parenchymal tissue [36, 37]. Given the fact that previous studies in macrophages were conducted in animals or human mononuclear phagocytes from blood and small tissue resections around tumors, Desch and colleagues recently collected pulmonary mononuclear phagocytes from fully intact non-diseased human lungs and identified five extravascular macrophage phagocytes based on phenotype, location, and gene expression, supporting the growing approval of myeloid cell diversity in tissues [38]. It is now clear that AMs colonize the lung tissues shortly after birth and display remarkable self-renewal properties independent of blood monocyte input in the steady-state [39–41]. In contrast, IMs are less well studied. Scott et al. demonstrated that the IM compartment contains cells derived from both yolk-sac macrophages and bone marrow-derived monocytes (BMDMs) [42]. However, the contribution of BMDMs to this population is still under investigation. Functionally, AMs are the chief effector cells of immune responses and have both proinflammatory and anti-inflammatory properties, whereas IMs play a major role in maintaining immune homeostasis in the respiratory tract and inducing immune tolerance to harmless antigens [43, 44]. Currently, a growing body of evidence supports a role for both AMs and IMs in the pathogenesis of pulmonary fibrosis.

Macrophage polarization in IPF

Macrophages are remarkable plastic cells that can transform from one phenotype to another [42, 45]. Macrophage polarization is a dynamic process whereby macrophages manifest different functional phenotypes in response to micro-environmental stimuli and signals [25]. As the most abundant immune cells in the lungs (approximately 70% of the immune cells), macrophages play a vital role in airway remodeling in pulmonary fibrosis [43]. Beyond the AM/IM macrophage subtype delineation, pulmonary macrophages as aforementioned, can be characterized as classically activated macrophages (also termed M1) or alternatively activated macrophages (M2) [46] (Fig. 1). These macrophage subtypes differ in the expression of their cell surface markers, production of specific factors, and biological activities. Both M1 and M2 macrophages have been noted

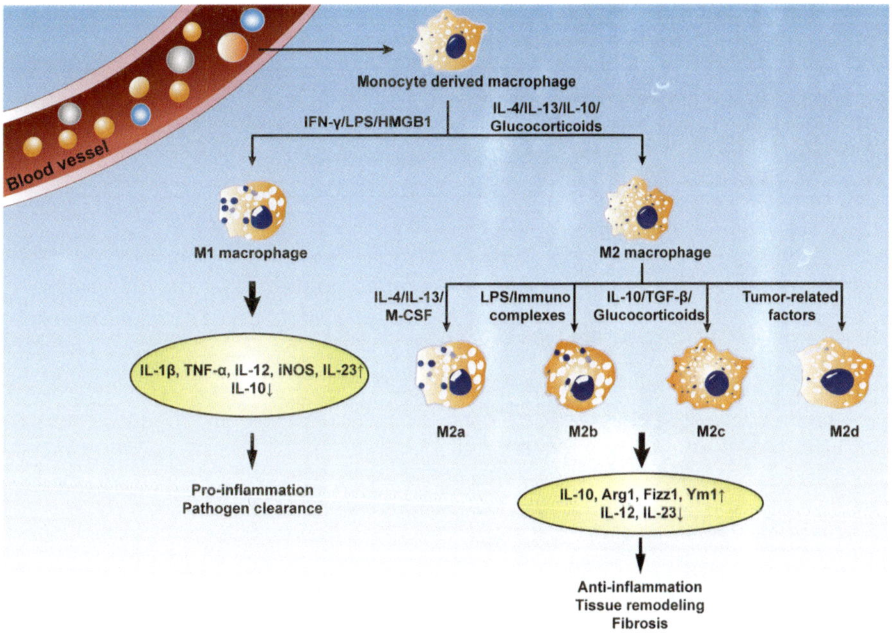

Fig. 1 Schematic diagram of macrophage subtypes. The M1 subtype is generally considered to be proinflammatory. The M2a subtype is induced by IL-4 and IL-13, which are critical mediators of allergic inflammation. The M2b and M2c subtypes predominately participate in tissue remodeling and fibrosis. BV, blood vessel; M0, monocyte; LPS, lipopolysaccharide; IL, interleukin

to be involved in the pathogenesis of pulmonary fibrosis, which will be discussed in detail in the following sections.

Classically activated macrophages (M1) and IPF

M1 macrophages contribute to the host defense against pathogens by generating reactive nitric oxide (NO) via inducible nitric oxide synthase (iNOS) and releasing proinflammatory cytokines and chemokines such as IL-1β, IL-12, IL-23, CCL2 and TNF-α [47, 48]. Phenotypically, this cell type is characterized by the expression of high levels of CD80, TLR4, MHCII and CD86 [25, 49]. Therefore, M1 macrophages have robust anti-microbial and anti-tumor activities, mediate tissue damage and initiate inflammatory responses. Potent inducers such as LPS, IFN-γ, and granulocyte-macrophage colony-stimulating factor (GM-CSF), stimulate the generation of M1 macrophages, from either naïve M0 or polarized M2 macrophages [50]. Other endogenous alarmins such as oxidized low-density lipoprotein, fatty acids, caveolin-1 (Cav-1), and high-mobility group box 1 (HMGB1), are also found to induce M1 biased macrophage polarization [51–54]. Nevertheless, it still remains unknown whether they exert similar effects on pulmonary fibrosis. Of importantly note, there is evidence that the polarized M1 macrophages can be switched back to the M0 state in a cytokine-deficient medium for 12 days or re-differentiated into another cell phenotype after culture in an alternative polarizing medium [55].

In the current paradigm of IPF pathogenesis, pulmonary fibrosis progresses as a final pathological outcome of aberrant wound healing responses to persistent lung injury. Pulmonary cellular damage caused by environmental particulates, infection or mechanical damage, often result in the disruption of normal lung architecture, initiating a wound healing response [56]. At the early inflammatory stages, acute lung injury promotes an M1 phenotype under the control of transcription factor interferon regulatory factor 5 (IRF-5) with expression of high levels of iNOS and proinflammatory cytokines,- which is associated with Th1 immune responses and responds to IFN-γ and toll-like receptor (TLR) ligands to maximize cytotoxic activity [57–59]. However, sustained inflammatory responses would serve as a trigger to initiate fibrotic responses in the lung. Indeed, during the course of aberrant wound healing processes, there is an early and sustained enrichment in the numbers of exudate macrophages (ExM) and their precursors, the Ly-6C^{high} monocytes [60, 61]. For example, targeted type II alveolar epithelial cell (AEC II) injury induces a modest inflammatory response that is nonetheless significantly enriched for alternatively activated and profibrotic ExM and Ly-6C^{high} monocytes. The accumulation of these nonresident cells and the development of pulmonary fibrosis in response to targeted alveolar injury is CCR2 dependent, thereby implicating ExM and Ly-6C^{high} monocytes and the CCR2/CCR2-ligand axis as potential therapeutic targets to treat or prevent fibrotic lung disease [62].

Generally, the LPS/TLR4 pathway has been considered one of the major pathways in M1 macrophage polarization 63]]. For example, the LPS/TLR4 pathway activates NF-kB and IRF3 and promotes the secretion of proinflammatory cytokines (e.g., IL-6 and TNF-α) to exacerbate macrophage M1 polarization [64]. This was further supported by studies showing that the LPS/TLR4 activates STAT1 to induce M1 polarization in an MyD88-independent fashion [65]. Interestingly, deletion of both TLR2 and TLR4 increased the susceptibility to bleomycin- and radiation-induced pulmonary fibrosis [66, 67]. Similarly, IL-1R–associated kinase-M (IRAK-M), an MyD88-dependent inhibitor of TLR signaling, suppresses deleterious inflammation but may paradoxically promote fibrogenesis, where IRAK-M was noted to promote macrophage M2 program in the setting of bleomycin-induced lung injury, which drives lung fibrogenesis in an IL-13–dependent fashion [68]. Furthermore, during the evolution of radiation-induced pulmonary fibrosis, patients manifested enhanced mRNA and protein expression of iNOS within the radiation pneumonic stage, whereas the high levels of arginase 1 (Arg 1) expression occurred within the radiation-induced fibrotic phase [69]. Intriguingly, macrophage inflammatory protein-1α (MIP-1α, also known as CCL3) arises mainly from M1, while its chemotactic affinity toward M2 is stronger than it is for M1. The interaction between MIP-1α and macrophages in different activated states may play a crucial role in regulating the transition from radiation pneumonitis to radiation pulmonary fibrosis [70]. It was also noted that TLR2 was elevated in IPF patients [71], and pharmacologic inhibition of TLR2 protected mice from bleomycin induced lung injury and fibrosis [72]. Similarly, mice with macrophage specific deletion of *IRF-5* manifested fibrotic responses in adipose tissue following high-fat diet induction [73]. Collectively, those data indicate that M1 macrophage plays an essential role for wound repair, but it may also serve as a double edged sword to either trigger or prevent fibrotic responses. Nevertheless, the exact extracellular microenvironments relevant to its functional direction (e.g., in favor or against fibrotic responses) are yet to be elucidated.

Alternatively activated macrophages (M2) and IPF

M2 macrophages could be induced by a broad array of mediators such as IL-4, IL-13, TGF-β, and IL-10, and are implicated in the aberrant wound-healing cascade during fibrosis [74]. Depending upon the specific stimulators, M2 macrophages are further subdivided into 3 subgroups, namely, M2a, M2b, and M2c [23, 45]. The M2a subtype is induced by IL-4, IL-13, fungal and helminthic infections. M2b is elicited by IL-1 receptor ligands, immune complexes, and LPS, whereas M2c is activated by IL-10, TGF-β1, and glucocorticoids. More recently, an additional M2 subset, the M2d macrophage, was identified designated by the reduced secretion of IL-12 and enhanced release of IL-10 [75] (Fig. 1). However, there is no unique surface marker to distinguish each subset of M2 macrophages, and they are characterized by low levels of MHCII, CD86, and iNOS2 but high levels of arginase-1, the family proteins chitinase-like Ym1/2 and Fizz1/RELM-α (found in inflammatory zone 1) [76, 77], and cell surface receptors such as macrophage mannose receptor, also called CD206. Analysis of over 72 non-diseased human lungs consistently indicated that CD206 is exclusively expressed on alveolar macrophages rather than on cells found in blood or in the intravascular compartment of the lung [38], which exerts an important function in the phagocytosis of M2 cells via increasing efferocytosis of invading pathogens and apoptotic cells [78]. In addition, recent studies have indicated that transcription factors and other intracellular proteins, such as tuberous sclerosis complex 1 (TSC1) [79], stress-responsive activating transcription factor 7 (ATF 7) [80], STIP1 homology and U-Box containing protein 1 (STUB1) [81], ten eleven translocation (Tet) methylcytosine dioxygenase (Tet2) [82], microRNA (MiR-511) [83], interferon regulatory factor 4 (IRF4) [84], peroxisome proliferator-activated receptor gamma (PPARγ) [85], and Krueppel-like factor 4 (KLF-4) [86] are also involved in the polarization of M2 macrophages.

During the course of IPF development and progression, the predominant infiltration of M2 macrophages in the areas of lung fibrosis acts as a vital regulator of fibrogenesis [58, 87, 88]. Generally, excessive M2-associated and Th2-driven responses are an important part of many fibrotic diseases [58, 89]. For example, alveolar M2 macrophages, which are located close in proximity to sites of pulmonary injury undergoing repair, release CCL18 to stimulate fibroblast producing collagen. On the other hand, the proximate M2 macrophages bind to collagen type I via β2-integrins and scavenger receptors, thereby further increasing their CCL18 production, which creates a self-perpetuating vicious cycle of augmented, continuous M2 macrophage activation and excessive collagen production by lung fibroblasts [90]. Indeed, upon activation, M2 macrophages can produce profibrotic mediators such as TGF-β and PDGF to induce continuous fibroblast activation and to promote myofibroblast proliferation. Similarly, IL-10 generates a Th2 microenvironment in favor of bleomycin- or helminth-induced lung fibrosis [91–93], which involves fibrocyte recruitment and M2 macrophage activation likely through the CCL2/CCR2 axis [94], leading to excessive extracellular matrix (ECM) deposition along with distorted lung tissue architecture, and ultimately resulting in pulmonary fibrosis and respiratory failure [95], although the underlying mechanisms are yet to be fully established.

In addition to Th2 cells, eosinophils, innate lymphoid type 2 cells (ILC2s), $CD4^+CD25^+$ regulatory T cells (Tregs), and mesenchymal stromal cells (MSCs) were recently reported to drive the polarization of M2 macrophages [96–99]. For example, mice infused with syngeneic $CD4^+CD25^+$ Treg cells have an increased population of $CD206^+$ peritoneal macrophages, with low levels of CD80 and MHCII [100]. Interestingly, Tregs lack of *Tim-3* are noted to repress the expression of p-STAT3, thereby attenuating the induction of M2 macrophages in acute respiratory distress syndrome (ARDS)-associated pulmonary fibroproliferation [101]. Similarly, natural killer T cells (NKTs), a subset of T lymphocytes expressing membrane receptors from both T and NK lineages [102], can mediate a protective effect against fibrosis by inhibiting a Th2 response and preventing M2 macrophage polarization [103] in the bleomycin animal model.

It has been well known that IL-4 is the major inducer for macrophage M2 program by activating its two major downstream signals, JAK1/STAT6 and PI3K/AKT [88, 104]. Indeed, Guo et al. reported that elevated Gab1 and Gab2 regulate IL-4-induced macrophage polarization in bleomycin-induced fibrotic lungs, with Gab1 positively regulating AKT signaling and Gab2 positively regulating STAT6 signaling [105]. Similarly, Kral et al. noted that myeloid *PTEN* deficiency mice following bleomycin induction manifest sustained PI3K activation to enhance macrophage M2 program, leading to increased morbidity and decreased survival, although these mice exhibit impaired recruitment function [106]. Furthermore, deficiency of *shp2*, a ubiquitously expressed cytoplasmic tyrosine phosphatase, increases the sensitivity to chitin-induced M2 macrophage polarization and bleomycin-induced pulmonary fibrosis by enhancing IL-4–induced JAK1/STAT6 signaling [107]. Other than cytokines, altered adenosine metabolism was also noted to regulate macrophage M2 program. Adenosine is generated in response to cellular stress and damage, and extracellular accumulation of adenosine and subsequent activation of its receptor, ADORA2B, polarizes macrophages to a fibrotic phenotype. Therefore, mice with macrophage specific deletion of *ADORA2B* are protected from bleomycin-induced lung injury and fibrosis [108]. It was further noted that hypoxia-inducible factor 1-α (HIF-1α) enhances ADORA2B expression to regulates M2 macrophage differentiation and production of profibrotic mediators [109].

It is noteworthy that mitochondrial oxidative stress and mitochondrial turnover in alveolar macrophages are directly linked to pulmonary fibrosis [110–112], although the exact molecular mechanisms that modulate mitochondrial dynamics are currently not known. The mitochondrial calcium uniporter (MCU) is a highly selective ion channel to transport Ca^{2+} into the mitochondrial matrix for modulation of cellular metabolism [113, 114]. MCU was recently found to polarize macrophages to a profibrotic phenotype after exposure to asbestos by regulating ATP production [115]. Similarly, mitochondrial Cu,Zn-SOD accelerates the development of pulmonary fibrosis by inducing early and sustained alternative activation of macrophages through redox regulation of the Jumonji domain-containing protein 3 (Jmjd3) [116, 117]. Collectively, these data provided convincing evidence that mitochondrial stress also regulates macrophage M2 program implicated in the pathogenesis of pulmonary fibrosis.

Interestingly, there is compelling evidence that endoplasmic reticulum (ER) stress modulates the activation of M2 macrophages [118, 119]. During the past few years, our laboratory has been focused on the effect of ER stress on fibrogenesis. We first demonstrated evidence that pulmonary fibrosis manifests altered C/EBP homologous protein (CHOP) expression and ER stress in both IPF patients and animals with bleomycin-induced pulmonary fibrosis. In consistent with these observations, mice deficient in *Chop* were protected from bleomycin-induced lung injury and fibrosis. Specifically, the loss of *Chop* significantly attenuated TGF-β production along with reduced M2 macrophage infiltration in the lung following bleomycin induction. Mechanistic studies revealed that *Chop* deficiency suppressed the M2 program in macrophages, which then attenuated TGF-β secretion. The loss of *Chop* enhanced the expression of SOCS1 and SOCS3, thereby inhibiting STAT6/PPARγ signaling that is essential for macrophage M2 program [87]. Similarly, an ovalbumin (OVA)-induced allergic airway inflammatory model revealed that Chop regulates STAT6 phosphorylation, thereby enhancing the expression of mouse transcription factor EC (Tfec), which then transcribes IL-4 receptor a (IL-4Ra) expression to promote M2 program in macrophages [120]. Taken together, those data provide novel insights into the role of ER stress in modulating macrophage M2 program implicated in the pathogenesis of pulmonary fibrosis.

Conclusion

Lung M1 and M2 macrophages are distinct cell subtypes and are both involved in the pathogenesis of pulmonary fibrosis. M1 macrophages express high levels of proinflammatory cytokines, while M2 macrophages express high levels of Th2-type cytokines. Owing to their different cytokine expression profiles, M1 and M2 macrophages play different roles in the pathogenesis of pulmonary fibrosis. Generally, M1 macrophages are responsible for wound healing after alveolar epithelial injury, while M2 macrophages are designated to resolve wound healing processes or terminate inflammatory responses in the lung. IPF is a pathological consequence resulted from altered wound healing in response to persistent lung injury.

A variety of regulatory cytokines, chemokines, mediators, and immune-regulatory cells affect polarization and chemotaxis of the lung macrophages (Fig. 2). These mediators interplay and influence disease duration and severity through altered polarization of M1 and M2 cells. Therefore, strategies aimed at modulation of lung macrophage phenotypes may have great potential for prevention and treatment of pulmonary fibrosis in clinical settings.

As noted above, IPF is a hard-to-diagnose fatal interstitial lung disease with a poor response to traditional therapies. Therefore, the development of reliable and fast diagnostic techniques and effective therapies is highly

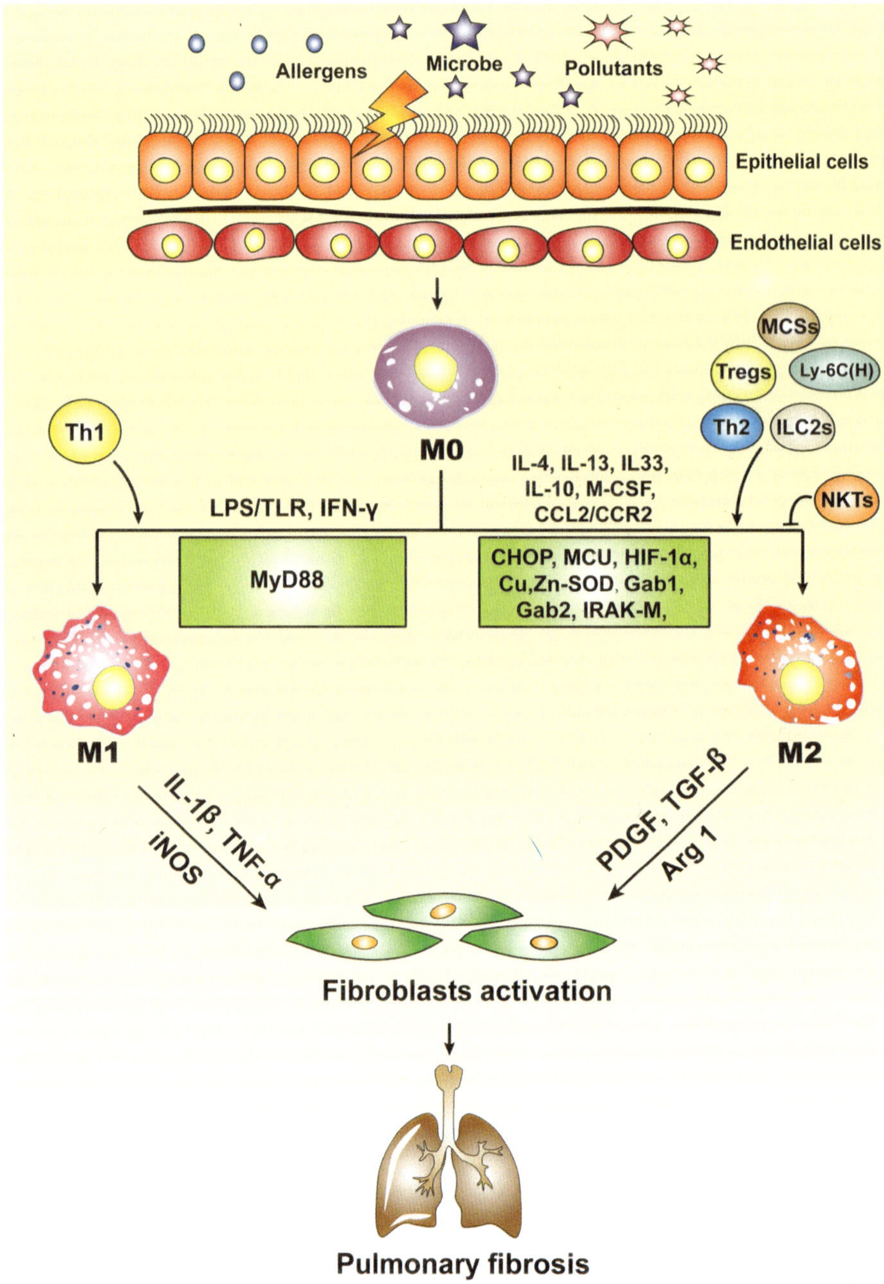

Fig. 2 Macrophages in the pathogenesis of pulmonary fibrosis. This schematic diagram demonstrates the mediators for modulation of macrophage subtypes and how macrophages contribute to IPF initiation and progression. M1 macrophages play an essential role for wound healing after alveolar epithelial injury, while M2 macrophages are require to resolve inflammatory responses in the lung, and IPF is a pathological outcome resulted from altered wound healing in response to persistent lung injury. Ly-6C (H), Ly-6C^{high} monocytes; MCS, mesenchymal stem cells; ILC2s, lymphoid type 2 cells; NKTs, natural killer T cells; MCU, mitochondrial calcium uniporter; CHOP, C/EBP homologous protein; IRAK-M, IL-1R–associated kinase-M; Arg 1, arginase 1; iNOS, inducible nitric oxide synthase

desirable, while targeting the activation and recruitment of M2 macrophages could be a viable therapeutic strategy. Indeed, pirfenidone, one of the two currently US Food and Drug Administration (FDA) approved drugs (pirfenidone and nintedanib) for treatment of human IPF, exerts its anti-fibrotic property in part by suppressing TGF-β expression relevant to macrophage M2 polarization and fibroblast activation [121]. Moreover, neotuberostemonine (NTS), one of the traditional Chinese medicines included in all versions of the Chinese Pharmacopoeia, can effectively attenuate BLM-induced lung fibrosis via suppressing the recruitment and polarization of M2 macrophages [122]. Intriguingly, Ji et al. demonstrated that mineralocorticoid receptor (MR) antagonism by liposome-encapsulated spironolactone (Lipo-SP) could alleviate bleomycin-induced acute pulmonary injury and fibrosis, partially by reducing circulating inflammatory $Ly6C^{high}$ monocyte expansion and repressing alternatively activated mononuclear phagocytes in the alveolar compartment [123, 124].

Although therapies for IPF include a variety of drugs and non-pharmacological interventions, there is still a pressing need for new therapeutic approaches as current therapies are unable to effectively attenuate disease progression or reverse lung fibrosis. Despite past extensive studies, many questions remain unsolved regarding the exact mechanisms of manipulating the balance of M1/M2 phenotype in IPF pathogenesis. Future studies aimed at dissecting the interplay between macrophages and fibroblasts and how macrophages create an extracellular milieu in favor of fibroblast activation and myofibroblast proliferation, would be crucial for developing effective therapies against IPF and other fibrotic diseases.

Abbreviations

ABCA3: ATP binding cassette member A3; AEC II: Type II alveolar epithelial cell; AMs: Alveolar macrophages; ARDS: Acute respiratory distress syndrome; Arg 1: Arginase 1; ATF 7: Activating transcription factor 7; BMDMs: Bone marrow-derived monocytes; Cav-1: Caveolin-1; CHOP: C/EBP homologous protein; ECM: Excessive extracellular matrix; ER: Endoplasmic reticulum; ExM: Exudate macrophages; FDA: Food and drug administration; Fizz1/RELM-α: Found in inflammatory zone 1; GM-CSF: Granulocyte-macrophage colony-stimulating factor; GWASs: Genome-wide association studies; HIF-1α: Hypoxia-inducible factor 1-α; HMGB1: High-mobility group box 1; IL-4Rа: IL-4 receptor a; ILC2s: Innate lymphoid type 2 cells; IMs: Interstitial macrophages; iNOS: Inducible nitric oxide synthase; IPF: Idiopathic pulmonary fibrosis; IRAK-M: IL-1R–associated kinase-M; IRF4: Interferon regulatory factor 4; IRF-5: Interferon regulatory factor 5; Jmjd3: Jumonji domain-containing protein 3; KLF-4: Krueppel-like factor 4; Lipo-SP: liposome-encapsulated spironolactone; LPS: Lipopolysaccharide; M1: Classically activated macrophages; M2: Alternatively activated macrophages; MCU: Mitochondrial calcium uniporter; MIP-1α: Macrophage inflammatory protein-1α; MMP1: Matrix metalloproteinase 1; MMP19: Matrix metalloproteinase 19; MR: mineralocorticoid receptor; MSCs: Mesenchymal stem cells; MUC5B: Mucin 5B gene; NKTs: Natural killer T cells; NO: Nitric oxide; NTS: Neotuberostemonine; PPARγ: Peroxisome proliferator-activated receptor gamma; RTEL1: Regulator of telomere elongation helicase 1; SFTPA2: Surfactant protein A2; SFTPC: Surfactant protein C; SPPL2C: Signal peptide peptidase like 2C; STUB1: STIP1 homology and U-Box containing protein 1; TERC: Telomerase RNA component; TERT: Telomerase reverse transcriptase; Tet: Ten eleven translocation; Tet2: Ten eleven translocation methylcytosine dioxygenase; Tfec: Transcription factor EC; TLR: Toll-like receptor; TOLLIP: Toll interacting protein; Tregs: Regulatory T cells; TSC1: Tuberous sclerosis complex 1

Acknowledgments

Our research was supported by the Natural Science Foundation of China (81530024, 9174920038 and 81770823), the Ministry of Science and Technology (2017ZX09304022 and 2016YFC1305002), the Department of Science and Technology of Hubei State (2017ACA096), and the Integrated Innovative Team for Major Human Disease Programs of Tongji Medical College, Huazhong University of Science and Technology.

Authors' contributions

CYW contributed to the conception and edition of the manuscript. LZ, YW, GW, WX and WG drafted the manuscript. All authors reviewed the manuscript critically and approved the final version.

Competing interests

The authors declare that they have no competing interests.

Author details

[1]The Center for Biomedical Research, Key Laboratory of Organ Transplantation, Ministry of Education and Ministry of Health, Tongji Hospital, Tongji Medical College, Huazhong University of Science and Technology, 1095 Jiefang Avenue, Wuhan 430030, China. [2]Departments of Orthopaedic Surgery-Campbell Clinic, and Pathology, University of Tennessee Health Science Center (UTHSC), Memphis, TN 38163, USA.

References

1. Richeldi L, Collard HR, Jones MG. Idiopathic pulmonary fibrosis. Lancet. 2017;389:1941–52.
2. Wilson MS, Wynn TA. Pulmonary fibrosis: pathogenesis, etiology and regulation. Mucosal Immunol. 2009;2:103–21.
3. Helling BA, Yang IV. Epigenetics in lung fibrosis: from pathobiology to treatment perspective. Curr Opin Pulm Med. 2015;21:454–62.
4. Hewlett JC, Kropski JA, Blackwell TS. Idiopathic pulmonary fibrosis: epithelial-mesenchymal interactions and emerging therapeutic targets. Matrix Biol. 2018.
5. Zhang L, Wang Y, Pandupuspitasari NS, Wu G, Xiang X, Gong Q, Xiong W, Wang CY, Yang P, Ren B. Endoplasmic reticulum stress, a new wrestler, in the pathogenesis of idiopathic pulmonary fibrosis. Am J Transl Res. 2017;9:722–35.
6. Kropski JA, Lawson WE, Young LR, Blackwell TS. Genetic studies provide clues on the pathogenesis of idiopathic pulmonary fibrosis. Dis Model Mech. 2013;6:9–17.
7. Hutchinson J, Fogarty A, Hubbard R, McKeever T. Global incidence and mortality of idiopathic pulmonary fibrosis: a systematic review. Eur Respir J. 2015;46:795–806.
8. Hopkins RB, Burke N, Fell C, Dion G, Kolb M. Epidemiology and survival of idiopathic pulmonary fibrosis from national data in Canada. Eur Respir J. 2016;48:187–95.
9. Evans CM, Fingerlin TE, Schwarz MI, Lynch D, Kurche J, Warg L, Yang IV, Schwartz DA. Idiopathic pulmonary fibrosis: a genetic disease that involves Mucociliary dysfunction of the peripheral airways. Physiol Rev. 2016;96:1567–91.
10. Lawson WE, Grant SW, Ambrosini V, Womble KE, Dawson EP, Lane KB, Markin C, Renzoni E, Lympany P, Thomas AQ, et al. Genetic mutations in

surfactant protein C are a rare cause of sporadic cases of IPF. Thorax. 2004; 59:977–80.

11. Wang Y, Kuan PJ, Xing C, Cronkhite JT, Torres F, Rosenblatt RL, DiMaio JM, Kinch LN, Grishin NV, Garcia CK. Genetic defects in surfactant protein A2 are associated with pulmonary fibrosis and lung cancer. Am J Hum Genet. 2009;84:52–9.
12. Diaz de Leon A, Cronkhite JT, Katzenstein AL, Godwin JD, Raghu G, Glazer CS, Rosenblatt RL, Girod CE, Garrity ER, Xing C, Garcia CK. Telomere lengths, pulmonary fibrosis and telomerase (TERT) mutations. PLoS One. 2010;5: e10680.
13. Fingerlin TE, Murphy E, Zhang W, Peljto AL, Brown KK, Steele MP, Loyd JE, Cosgrove GP, Lynch D, Groshong S, et al. Genome-wide association study identifies multiple susceptibility loci for pulmonary fibrosis. Nat Genet. 2013; 45:613–20.
14. Noth I, Zhang Y, Ma SF, Flores C, Barber M, Huang Y, Broderick SM, Wade MS, Hysi P, Scuirba J, et al. Genetic variants associated with idiopathic pulmonary fibrosis susceptibility and mortality: a genome-wide association study. Lancet Respir Med. 2013;1:309–17.
15. Rosas IO, Richards TJ, Konishi K, Zhang Y, Gibson K, Lokshin AE, Lindell KO, Cisneros J, Macdonald SD, Pardo A, et al. MMP1 and MMP7 as potential peripheral blood biomarkers in idiopathic pulmonary fibrosis. PLoS Med. 2008;5:e93.
16. Yu G, Kovkarova-Naumovski E, Jara P, Parwani A, Kass D, Ruiz V, Lopez-Otin C, Rosas IO, Gibson KF, Cabrera S, et al. Matrix metalloproteinase-19 is a key regulator of lung fibrosis in mice and humans. Am J Respir Crit Care Med. 2012;186:752–62.
17. Deng Y, Li Z, Liu J, Wang Z, Cao Y, Mou Y, Fu B, Mo B, Wei J, Cheng Z, et al. Targeted resequencing reveals genetic risks in patients with sporadic idiopathic pulmonary fibrosis. Hum Mutat. 2018;39:1238–1245.
18. Saha S, Shalova IN, Biswas SK. Metabolic regulation of macrophage phenotype and function. Immunol Rev. 2017;280:102–11.
19. Ginhoux F, Guilliams M, Naik SH. Editorial: dendritic cell and macrophage nomenclature and classification. Front Immunol. 2016;7:168.
20. Sica A, Mantovani A. Macrophage plasticity and polarization: in vivo veritas. J Clin Invest. 2012;122:787–95.
21. Arora S, Dev K, Agarwal B, Das P, Syed MA. Macrophages: their role, activation and polarization in pulmonary diseases. Immunobiology. 2018; 223:383–96.
22. Biswas SK, Mantovani A. Macrophage plasticity and interaction with lymphocyte subsets: cancer as a paradigm. Nat Immunol. 2010;11:889–96.
23. Mantovani A, Biswas SK, Galdiero MR, Sica A, Locati M. Macrophage plasticity and polarization in tissue repair and remodelling. J Pathol. 2013; 229:176–85.
24. Murray PJ, Allen JE, Biswas SK, Fisher EA, Gilroy DW, Goerdt S, Gordon S, Hamilton JA, Ivashkiv LB, Lawrence T, et al. Macrophage activation and polarization: nomenclature and experimental guidelines. Immunity. 2014; 41:14–20.
25. Murray PJ. Macrophage polarization. Annu Rev Physiol. 2017;79:541–66.
26. Hashimoto D, Chow A, Noizat C, Teo P, Beasley MB, Leboeuf M, Becker CD, See P, Price J, Lucas D, et al. Tissue-resident macrophages self-maintain locally throughout adult life with minimal contribution from circulating monocytes. Immunity. 2013;38:792–804.
27. Epelman S, Lavine KJ, Randolph GJ. Origin and functions of tissue macrophages. Immunity. 2014;41:21–35.
28. Gordon S. Elie Metchnikoff: father of natural immunity. Eur J Immunol. 2008; 38:3257–64.
29. Divangahi M, King IL, Pernet E. Alveolar macrophages and type I IFN in airway homeostasis and immunity. Trends Immunol. 2015;36:307–14.
30. Stefater JA 3rd, Ren S, Lang RA, Duffield JS. Metchnikoff's policemen: macrophages in development, homeostasis and regeneration. Trends Mol Med. 2011;17:743–52.
31. van Furth R, Cohn ZA, Hirsch JG, Humphrey JH, Spector WG, Langevoort HL. The mononuclear phagocyte system: a new classification of macrophages, monocytes, and their precursor cells. Bull World Health Organ. 1972;46: 845–52.
32. Marchesi VT, Florey HW. Electron micrographic observations on the emigration of leucocytes. Q J Exp Physiol Cogn Med Sci. 1960;45:343–8.
33. Volkman A, Gowans JL. The origin of macrophages from bone marrow in the rat. Br J Exp Pathol. 1965;46:62–70.
34. Yona S, Kim KW, Wolf Y, Mildner A, Varol D, Breker M, Strauss-Ayali D, Viukov S, Guilliams M, Misharin A, et al. Fate mapping reveals origins and dynamics of monocytes and tissue macrophages under homeostasis. Immunity. 2013; 38:79–91.
35. Wynn TA, Chawla A, Pollard JW. Macrophage biology in development, homeostasis and disease. Nature. 2013;496:445–55.
36. Guilliams M, De Kleer I, Henri S, Post S, Vanhoutte L, De Prijck S, Deswarte K, Malissen B, Hammad H, Lambrecht BN. Alveolar macrophages develop from fetal monocytes that differentiate into long-lived cells in the first week of life via GM-CSF. J Exp Med. 2013;210:1977–92.
37. Bedoret D, Wallemacq H, Marichal T, Desmet C, Quesada Calvo F, Henry E, Closset R, Dewals B, Thielen C, Gustin P, et al. Lung interstitial macrophages alter dendritic cell functions to prevent airway allergy in mice. J Clin Invest. 2009;119:3723–38.
38. Desch AN, Gibbings SL, Goyal R, Kolde R, Bednarek J, Bruno T, Slansky JE, Jacobelli J, Mason R, Ito Y, et al. Flow cytometric analysis of mononuclear phagocytes in nondiseased human lung and lung-draining lymph nodes. Am J Respir Crit Care Med. 2016;193:614–26.
39. Byrne AJ, Maher TM, Lloyd CM. Pulmonary macrophages: a new therapeutic pathway in Fibrosing lung disease? Trends Mol Med. 2016;22:303–16.
40. Van den Bossche J, Malissen B, Mantovani A, De Baetselier P, Van Ginderachter JA. Regulation and function of the E-cadherin/catenin complex in cells of the monocyte-macrophage lineage and DCs. Blood. 2012;119:1623–33.
41. Misharin AV, Morales-Nebreda L, Reyfman PA, Cuda CM, Walter JM, McQuattie-Pimentel AC, Chen CI, Anekalla KR, Joshi N, Williams KJN, et al. Monocyte-derived alveolar macrophages drive lung fibrosis and persist in the lung over the life span. J Exp Med. 2017;214:2387–404.
42. Scott CL, Henri S, Guilliams M. Mononuclear phagocytes of the intestine, the skin, and the lung. Immunol Rev. 2014;262:9–24.
43. Cai Y, Sugimoto C, Arainga M, Alvarez X, Didier ES, Kuroda MJ. In vivo characterization of alveolar and interstitial lung macrophages in rhesus macaques: implications for understanding lung disease in humans. J Immunol. 2014;192:2821–9.
44. Ji WJ, Ma YQ, Zhou X, Zhang YD, Lu RY, Sun HY, Guo ZZ, Zhang Z, Li YM, Wei LQ. Temporal and spatial characterization of mononuclear phagocytes in circulating, lung alveolar and interstitial compartments in a mouse model of bleomycin-induced pulmonary injury. J Immunol Methods. 2014;403:7–16.
45. Mantovani A, Sica A, Sozzani S, Allavena P, Vecchi A, Locati M. The chemokine system in diverse forms of macrophage activation and polarization. Trends Immunol. 2004;25:677–86.
46. Locati M, Mantovani A, Sica A. Macrophage activation and polarization as an adaptive component of innate immunity. Adv Immunol. 2013;120: 163–84.
47. Saradna A, Do DC, Kumar S, Fu QL, Gao P. Macrophage polarization and allergic asthma. Transl Res. 2018;191:1–14.
48. Murray PJ, Wynn TA. Obstacles and opportunities for understanding macrophage polarization. J Leukoc Biol. 2011;89:557–63.
49. Wang N, Liang H, Zen K. Molecular mechanisms that influence the macrophage m1-m2 polarization balance. Front Immunol. 2014;5:614.
50. Sierra-Filardi E, Vega MA, Sanchez-Mateos P, Corbi AL, Puig-Kroger A. Heme Oxygenase-1 expression in M-CSF-polarized M2 macrophages contributes to LPS-induced IL-10 release. Immunobiology. 2010;215:788–95.
51. van Tits LJ, Stienstra R, van Lent PL, Netea MG, Joosten LA, Stalenhoef AF. Oxidized LDL enhances pro-inflammatory responses of alternatively activated M2 macrophages: a crucial role for Kruppel-like factor 2. Atherosclerosis. 2011;214:345–9.
52. Tian S, Zhang L, Tang J, Guo X, Dong K, Chen SY. HMGB1 exacerbates renal tubulointerstitial fibrosis through facilitating M1 macrophage phenotype at the early stage of obstructive injury. Am J Physiol Renal Physiol. 2015;308: F69–75.
53. Shivshankar P, Halade GV, Calhoun C, Escobar GP, Mehr AJ, Jimenez F, Martinez C, Bhatnagar H, Mjaatvedt CH, Lindsey ML, Le Saux CJ. Caveolin-1 deletion exacerbates cardiac interstitial fibrosis by promoting M2 macrophage activation in mice after myocardial infarction. J Mol Cell Cardiol. 2014;76:84–93.
54. Nomura M, Liu J, Rovira II, Gonzalez-Hurtado E, Lee J, Wolfgang MJ, Finkel T. Fatty acid oxidation in macrophage polarization. Nat Immunol. 2016;17:216–7.
55. Tarique AA, Logan J, Thomas E, Holt PG, Sly PD, Fantino E. Phenotypic, functional, and plasticity features of classical and alternatively activated human macrophages. Am J Respir Cell Mol Biol. 2015;53:676–88.
56. Burgy O, Konigshoff M. The WNT signaling pathways in wound healing and fibrosis. Matrix Biol. 2018;68-69:67–80.

57. Richards CD. Innate immune cytokines, fibroblast phenotypes, and regulation of extracellular matrix in lung. J Interf Cytokine Res. 2017;37:52–61.
58. Wynn TA, Vannella KM. Macrophages in tissue repair, regeneration, and fibrosis. Immunity. 2016;44:450–62.
59. Weiss M, Byrne AJ, Blazek K, Saliba DG, Pease JE, Perocheau D, Feldmann M, Udalova IA. IRF5 controls both acute and chronic inflammation. Proc Natl Acad Sci U S A. 2015;112:11001–6.
60. Xiang GA, Zhang YD, Su CC, Ma YQ, Li YM, Zhou X, Wei LQ, Ji WJ. Dynamic changes of mononuclear phagocytes in circulating, pulmonary alveolar and interstitial compartments in a mouse model of experimental silicosis. Inhal Toxicol. 2016;28:393–402.
61. Gibbons MA, MacKinnon AC, Ramachandran P, Dhaliwal K, Duffin R, Phythian-Adams AT, van Rooijen N, Haslett C, Howie SE, Simpson AJ, et al. Ly6Chi monocytes direct alternatively activated profibrotic macrophage regulation of lung fibrosis. Am J Respir Crit Care Med. 2011;184:569–81.
62. Osterholzer JJ, Olszewski MA, Murdock BJ, Chen GH, Erb-Downward JR, Subbotina N, Browning K, Lin Y, Morey RE, Dayrit JK, et al. Implicating exudate macrophages and Ly-6C(high) monocytes in CCR2-dependent lung fibrosis following gene-targeted alveolar injury. J Immunol. 2013;190:3447–57.
63. Sica A, Erreni M, Allavena P, Porta C. Macrophage polarization in pathology. Cell Mol Life Sci. 2015;72:4111–26.
64. Mills CD, Ley K. M1 and M2 macrophages: the chicken and the egg of immunity. J Innate Immun. 2014;6:716–26.
65. Toshchakov V, Jones BW, Lentschat A, Silva A, Perera PY, Thomas K, Cody MJ, Zhang S, Williams BR, Major J, et al. TLR2 and TLR4 agonists stimulate unique repertoires of host resistance genes in murine macrophages: interferon-beta-dependent signaling in TLR4-mediated responses. J Endotoxin Res. 2003;9:169–75.
66. Jiang D, Liang J, Fan J, Yu S, Chen S, Luo Y, Prestwich GD, Mascarenhas MM, Garg HG, Quinn DA, et al. Regulation of lung injury and repair by toll-like receptors and hyaluronan. Nat Med. 2005;11:1173–9.
67. Paun A, Fox J, Balloy V, Chignard M, Qureshi ST, Haston CK. Combined Tlr2 and Tlr4 deficiency increases radiation-induced pulmonary fibrosis in mice. Int J Radiat Oncol Biol Phys. 2010;77:1198–205.
68. Ballinger MN, Newstead MW, Zeng X, Bhan U, Mo XM, Kunkel SL, Moore BB, Flavell R, Christman JW, Standiford TJ. IRAK-M promotes alternative macrophage activation and fibroproliferation in bleomycin-induced lung injury. J Immunol. 2015;194:1894–904.
69. Zhang H, Han G, Liu H, Chen J, Ji X, Zhou F, Zhou Y, Xie C. The development of classically and alternatively activated macrophages has different effects on the varied stages of radiation-induced pulmonary injury in mice. J Radiat Res. 2011;52:717–26.
70. He Z, Zhang H, Yang C, Zhou Y, Zhou Y, Han G, Xia L, Ouyang W, Zhou F, Zhou Y, Xie C. The interaction between different types of activated RAW 264.7 cells and macrophage inflammatory protein-1 alpha. Radiat Oncol. 2011;6:86.
71. Samara KD, Antoniou KM, Karagiannis K, Margaritopoulos G, Lasithiotaki I, Koutala E, Siafakas NM. Expression profiles of toll-like receptors in non-small cell lung cancer and idiopathic pulmonary fibrosis. Int J Oncol. 2012;40: 1397–404.
72. Liu HZ, Yang HZ, Mi S, Cui B, Hua F, Hu ZW. Toll like receptor 2 mediates bleomycin-induced acute lung injury, inflammation and fibrosis in mice. Yao Xue Xue Bao. 2010;45:976–86.
73. Dalmas E, Toubal A, Alzaid F, Blazek K, Eames HL, Lebozec K, Pini M, Hainault I, Montastier E, Denis RG, et al. Irf5 deficiency in macrophages promotes beneficial adipose tissue expansion and insulin sensitivity during obesity. Nat Med. 2015;21:610–8.
74. Zhong B, Yang X, Sun Q, Liu L, Lan X, Tian J, He Q, Hou W, Liu H, Jiang C, et al. Pdcd4 modulates markers of macrophage alternative activation and airway remodeling in antigen-induced pulmonary inflammation. J Leukoc Biol. 2014;96:1065–75.
75. Wang Q, Ni H, Lan L, Wei X, Xiang R, Wang Y. Fra-1 protooncogene regulates IL-6 expression in macrophages and promotes the generation of M2d macrophages. Cell Res. 2010;20:701–12.
76. Raes G, De Baetselier P, Noel W, Beschin A, Brombacher F, Hassanzadeh Gh G. Differential expression of FIZZ1 and Ym1 in alternatively versus classically activated macrophages. J Leukoc Biol. 2002;71:597–602.
77. Raes G, Noel W, Beschin A, Brys L, de Baetselier P, Hassanzadeh GH. FIZZ1 and Ym as tools to discriminate between differentially activated macrophages. Dev Immunol. 2002;9:151–9.
78. Hong JY, Chung Y, Steenrod J, Chen Q, Lei J, Comstock AT, Goldsmith AM, Bentley JK, Sajjan US, Hershenson MB. Macrophage activation state determines the response to rhinovirus infection in a mouse model of allergic asthma. Respir Res. 2014;15:63.
79. Zhu L, Yang T, Li L, Sun L, Hou Y, Hu X, Zhang L, Tian H, Zhao Q, Peng J, et al. TSC1 controls macrophage polarization to prevent inflammatory disease. Nat Commun. 2014;5:4696.
80. Yoshida K, Maekawa T, Zhu Y, Renard-Guillet C, Chatton B, Inoue K, Uchiyama T, Ishibashi K, Yamada T, Ohno N, et al. The transcription factor ATF7 mediates lipopolysaccharide-induced epigenetic changes in macrophages involved in innate immunological memory. Nat Immunol. 2015;16:1034–43.
81. Wei Q, Sha Y, Bhattacharya A, Abdel Fattah E, Bonilla D, Jyothula SS, Pandit L, Khurana Hershey GK, Eissa NT. Regulation of IL-4 receptor signaling by STUB1 in lung inflammation. Am J Respir Crit Care Med. 2014;189:16–29.
82. Zhang Q, Zhao K, Shen Q, Han Y, Gu Y, Li X, Zhao D, Liu Y, Wang C, Zhang X, et al. Tet2 is required to resolve inflammation by recruiting Hdac2 to specifically repress IL-6. Nature. 2015;525:389–93.
83. Karo-Atar D, Itan M, Pasmanik-Chor M, Munitz A. MicroRNA profiling reveals opposing expression patterns for miR-511 in alternatively and classically activated macrophages. J Asthma. 2015;52:545–53.
84. Satoh T, Takeuchi O, Vandenbon A, Yasuda K, Tanaka Y, Kumagai Y, Miyake T, Matsushita K, Okazaki T, Saitoh T, et al. The Jmjd3-Irf4 axis regulates M2 macrophage polarization and host responses against helminth infection. Nat Immunol. 2010;11:936–44.
85. Chang HY, Lee HN, Kim W, Surh YJ. Docosahexaenoic acid induces M2 macrophage polarization through peroxisome proliferator-activated receptor gamma activation. Life Sci. 2015;120:39–47.
86. Liao X, Sharma N, Kapadia F, Zhou G, Lu Y, Hong H, Paruchuri K, Mahabeleshwar GH, Dalmas E, Venteclef N, et al. Kruppel-like factor 4 regulates macrophage polarization. J Clin Invest. 2011;121:2736–49.
87. Yao Y, Wang Y, Zhang Z, He L, Zhu J, Zhang M, He X, Cheng Z, Ao Q, Cao Y, et al. Chop deficiency protects mice against bleomycin-induced pulmonary fibrosis by attenuating M2 macrophage production. Mol Ther. 2016;24:915–25.
88. Van Dyken SJ, Locksley RM. Interleukin-4- and interleukin-13-mediated alternatively activated macrophages: roles in homeostasis and disease. Annu Rev Immunol. 2013;31:317–43.
89. Duffield JS, Lupher M, Thannickal VJ, Wynn TA. Host responses in tissue repair and fibrosis. Annu Rev Pathol. 2013;8:241–76.
90. Prasse A, Pechkovsky DV, Toews GB, Jungraithmayr W, Kollert F, Goldmann T, Vollmer E, Muller-Quernheim J, Zissel G. A vicious circle of alveolar macrophages and fibroblasts perpetuates pulmonary fibrosis via CCL18. Am J Respir Crit Care Med. 2006;173:781–92.
91. Joshi AD, Raymond T, Coelho AL, Kunkel SL, Hogaboam CM. A systemic granulomatous response to Schistosoma mansoni eggs alters responsiveness of bone-marrow-derived macrophages to toll-like receptor agonists. J Leukoc Biol. 2008;83:314–24.
92. Liu T, Jin H, Ullenbruch M, Hu B, Hashimoto N, Moore B, McKenzie A, Lukacs NW, Phan SH. Regulation of found in inflammatory zone 1 expression in bleomycin-induced lung fibrosis: role of IL-4/IL-13 and mediation via STAT-6. J Immunol. 2004;173:3425–31.
93. Sandler NG, Mentink-Kane MM, Cheever AW, Wynn TA. Global gene expression profiles during acute pathogen-induced pulmonary inflammation reveal divergent roles for Th1 and Th2 responses in tissue repair. J Immunol. 2003;171:3655–67.
94. Sun L, Louie MC, Vannella KM, Wilke CA, LeVine AM, Moore BB, Shanley TP. New concepts of IL-10-induced lung fibrosis: fibrocyte recruitment and M2 activation in a CCL2/CCR2 axis. Am J Physiol Lung Cell Mol Physiol. 2011; 300:L341–53.
95. Song E, Ouyang N, Horbelt M, Antus B, Wang M, Exton MS. Influence of alternatively and classically activated macrophages on fibrogenic activities of human fibroblasts. Cell Immunol. 2000;204:19–28.
96. Tiemessen MM, Jagger AL, Evans HG, van Herwijnen MJ, John S, Taams LS. CD4+CD25+Foxp3+ regulatory T cells induce alternative activation of human monocytes/macrophages. Proc Natl Acad Sci U S A. 2007;104:19446–51.
97. Wu D, Molofsky AB, Liang HE, Ricardo-Gonzalez RR, Jouihan HA, Bando JK, Chawla A, Locksley RM. Eosinophils sustain adipose alternatively activated macrophages associated with glucose homeostasis. Science. 2011;332:243–7.
98. Molofsky AB, Nussbaum JC, Liang HE, Van Dyken SJ, Cheng LE, Mohapatra A, Chawla A, Locksley RM. Innate lymphoid type 2 cells sustain visceral

adipose tissue eosinophils and alternatively activated macrophages. J Exp Med. 2013;210:535–49.
99. Morrison TJ, Jackson MV, Cunningham EK, Kissenpfennig A, McAuley DF, O'Kane CM, Krasnodembskaya AD. Mesenchymal stromal cells modulate macrophages in clinically relevant lung injury models by extracellular vesicle mitochondrial transfer. Am J Respir Crit Care Med. 2017;196:1275–86.
100. Liu G, Ma H, Qiu L, Li L, Cao Y, Ma J, Zhao Y. Phenotypic and functional switch of macrophages induced by regulatory CD4+CD25+ T cells in mice. Immunol Cell Biol. 2011;89:130–42.
101. Liu X, Jiang S, Zhang Q, Xu S, Bao X, Cao W, Bai J, Tang L. Tim-3 regulates Tregs' ability to resolve the inflammation and proliferation of acute lung injury by modulating macrophages polarization. Shock. 2017.
102. Van Kaer L, Parekh VV, Wu L. Invariant natural killer T cells: bridging innate and adaptive immunity. Cell Tissue Res. 2011;343:43–55.
103. Grabarz F, Aguiar CF, Correa-Costa M, Braga TT, Hyane MI, Andrade-Oliveira V, Landgraf MA, Camara NOS. Protective role of NKT cells and macrophage M2-driven phenotype in bleomycin-induced pulmonary fibrosis. Inflammopharmacology. 2018;26:491–504.
104. Wills-Karp M, Finkelman FD. Untangling the complex web of IL-4- and IL-13-mediated signaling pathways. Sci Signal. 2008;1:pe55.
105. Guo X, Li T, Xu Y, Xu X, Zhu Z, Zhang Y, Xu J, Xu K, Cheng H, Zhang X, Ke Y. Increased levels of Gab1 and Gab2 adaptor proteins skew interleukin-4 (IL-4) signaling toward M2 macrophage-driven pulmonary fibrosis in mice. J Biol Chem. 2017;292:14003–15.
106. Kral JB, Kuttke M, Schrottmaier WC, Birnecker B, Warszawska J, Wernig C, Paar H, Salzmann M, Sahin E, Brunner JS, et al. Sustained PI3K activation exacerbates BLM-induced lung fibrosis via activation of pro-inflammatory and pro-fibrotic pathways. Sci Rep. 2016;6:23034.
107. Tao B, Jin W, Xu J, Liang Z, Yao J, Zhang Y, Wang K, Cheng H, Zhang X, Ke Y. Myeloid-specific disruption of tyrosine phosphatase Shp2 promotes alternative activation of macrophages and predisposes mice to pulmonary fibrosis. J Immunol. 2014;193:2801–11.
108. Karmouty-Quintana H, Philip K, Acero LF, Chen NY, Weng T, Molina JG, Luo F, Davies J, Le NB, Bunge I, et al. Deletion of ADORA2B from myeloid cells dampens lung fibrosis and pulmonary hypertension. FASEB J. 2015;29:50–60.
109. Philip K, Mills TW, Davies J, Chen NY, Karmouty-Quintana H, Luo F, Molina JG, Amione-Guerra J, Sinha N, Guha A, et al. HIF1A up-regulates the ADORA2B receptor on alternatively activated macrophages and contributes to pulmonary fibrosis. FASEB J. 2017;31:4745–58.
110. Larson-Casey JL, Deshane JS, Ryan AJ, Thannickal VJ, Carter AB. Macrophage Akt1 kinase-mediated Mitophagy modulates apoptosis resistance and pulmonary fibrosis. Immunity. 2016;44:582–96.
111. Osborn-Heaford HL, Murthy S, Gu L, Larson-Casey JL, Ryan AJ, Shi L, Glogauer M, Neighbors JD, Hohl R, Carter AB. Targeting the isoprenoid pathway to abrogate progression of pulmonary fibrosis. Free Radic Biol Med. 2015;86:47–56.
112. Osborn-Heaford HL, Ryan AJ, Murthy S, Racila AM, He C, Sieren JC, Spitz DR, Carter AB. Mitochondrial Rac1 GTPase import and electron transfer from cytochrome c are required for pulmonary fibrosis. J Biol Chem. 2012;287:3301–12.
113. Kirichok Y, Krapivinsky G, Clapham DE. The mitochondrial calcium uniporter is a highly selective ion channel. Nature. 2004;427:360–4.
114. Patron M, Raffaello A, Granatiero V, Tosatto A, Merli G, De Stefani D, Wright L, Pallafacchina G, Terrin A, Mammucari C, Rizzuto R. The mitochondrial calcium uniporter (MCU): molecular identity and physiological roles. J Biol Chem. 2013;288:10750–8.
115. Gu L, Larson-Casey JL, Carter AB. Macrophages utilize the mitochondrial calcium uniporter for profibrotic polarization. FASEB J. 2017;31:3072–83.
116. He C, Ryan AJ, Murthy S, Carter AB. Accelerated development of pulmonary fibrosis via Cu,Zn-superoxide dismutase-induced alternative activation of macrophages. J Biol Chem. 2013;288:20745–57.
117. He C, Larson-Casey JL, Gu L, Ryan AJ, Murthy S, Carter AB. Cu,Zn-Superoxide Dismutase-Mediated Redox Regulation of Jumonji Domain Containing 3 Modulates Macrophage Polarization and Pulmonary Fibrosis. Am J Respir Cell Mol Biol. 2016;55:58–71.
118. Oh J, Riek AE, Weng S, Petty M, Kim D, Colonna M, Cella M, Bernal-Mizrachi C. Endoplasmic reticulum stress controls M2 macrophage differentiation and foam cell formation. J Biol Chem. 2012;287:11629–41.
119. Burman A, Tanjore H, Blackwell TS. Endoplasmic reticulum stress in pulmonary fibrosis. Matrix Biol. 2018;68-69:355–65.
120. Wang Y, Zhu J, Zhang L, Zhang Z, He L, Mou Y, Deng Y, Cao Y, Yang P, Su Y, et al. Role of C/EBP homologous protein and endoplasmic reticulum stress in asthma exacerbation by regulating the IL-4/signal transducer and activator of transcription 6/transcription factor EC/IL-4 receptor alpha positive feedback loop in M2 macrophages. J Allergy Clin Immunol. 2017; 140:1550–61. e1558
121. Inomata M, Kamio K, Azuma A, Matsuda K, Kokuho N, Miura Y, Hayashi H, Nei T, Fujita K, Saito Y, Gemma A. Pirfenidone inhibits fibrocyte accumulation in the lungs in bleomycin-induced murine pulmonary fibrosis. Respir Res. 2014;15:16.
122. Xiang J, Cheng S, Feng T, Wu Y, Xie W, Zhang M, Xu X, Zhang C. Neotuberostemonine attenuates bleomycin-induced pulmonary fibrosis by suppressing the recruitment and activation of macrophages. Int Immunopharmacol. 2016;36:158–64.
123. Ji WJ, Ma YQ, Zhou X, Zhang YD, Lu RY, Guo ZZ, Sun HY, Hu DC, Yang GH, Li YM, Wei LQ. Spironolactone attenuates bleomycin-induced pulmonary injury partially via modulating mononuclear phagocyte phenotype switching in circulating and alveolar compartments. PLoS One. 2013;8: e81090.
124. Ji WJ, Ma YQ, Zhang X, Zhang L, Zhang YD, Su CC, Xiang GA, Zhang MP, Lin ZC, Wei LQ, et al. Inflammatory monocyte/macrophage modulation by liposome-entrapped spironolactone ameliorates acute lung injury in mice. Nanomedicine (Lond). 2016;11:1393–406.

3

Impairment of respiratory muscle strength in Berardinelli-Seip congenital lipodystrophy subjects

Jorge Luiz Dantas de Medeiros[1], Bruno Carneiro Bezerra[1], Thiago Anderson Brito de Araújo[1], Aquiles Sales Craveiro Sarmento[2], Lázaro Batista de Azevedo Medeiros[2], Lucien Peroni Gualdi[1], Maria do Socorro Luna Cruz[1], Thaiza Teixeira Xavier Nobre[1], Josivan Gomes Lima[3] and Julliane Tamara Araújo de Melo Campos[1,2*]

Abstract

Background: Berardinelli-Seip Congenital Generalized Lipodystrophy (BSCL) is an ultra-rare metabolic disease characterized by hypertriglyceridemia, hyperinsulinemia, hyperglycemia, hypoleptinemia, and diabetes mellitus. Although cardiovascular disturbances have been observed in BSCL patients, there are no studies regarding the Respiratory Muscle Strength (RMS) in this type of lipodystrophy. This study aimed to evaluate RMS in BSCL subjects compared with healthy subjects.

Methods: Eleven individuals with BSCL and 11 healthy subjects matched for age and gender were included in this study. The Maximum Inspiratory Pressure (MIP), Maximum Expiratory Pressure (MEP), and Peripheral Muscle Strength (PMS) were measured for three consecutive years. BSCL subjects were compared to healthy individuals for MIP, MEP, and PMS. Correlations between PMS and MIP were also analyzed. The genetic diagnosis was performed, and sociodemographic and anthropometric data were also collected.

Results: BSCL subjects showed significantly lower values for MIP and MEP ($p < 0.0001$ and $p = 0.0002$, respectively) in comparison to healthy subjects, but no changes in handgrip strength ($p = 0.15$). Additionally, we did not observe changes in MIP, MEP, and PMS two years after the first analysis, showing maintenance of respiratory dysfunction in BSCL subjects ($p = 0.05$; $p = 0.45$; $p = 0.99$). PMS and MIP were not correlated in these subjects ($r = 0.56$; $p = 0.18$).

Conclusion: BSCL subjects showed lower respiratory muscle strength when compared with healthy subjects; however, PMS was not altered. These findings were maintained at similar levels during the two years of evaluation. Our data reveal the first association of BSCL with the development of respiratory muscle weakness.

Keywords: Lipodystrophy, MIP, MEP, PMS, Metreleptin

Background

Berardinelli-Seip Congenital Lipodystrophy (BSCL) is a rare genetic disease characterized by the absence of adipose tissue that contributes to the impairment of glucose and lipid metabolism [1, 2]. At the metabolic level, BSCL patients present dyslipidemia, hyperinsulinemia, disrupted carbohydrate metabolism, insulin resistance, diabetes mellitus (DM), hepatosplenomegaly, hepatic steatosis, acanthosis nigricans, low levels of leptin and adiponectin, decreased levels of high-density lipoprotein (HDL), and hypertriglyceridemia [2, 3]. The phenotype of BSCL patients is typical, revealing acromegaloid facies, prognathism, prominent musculature, hypertrophic cardiomyopathy, umbilical protrusion, acanthosis nigricans, and other clinical features [1–5].

Worldwide prevalence of BSCL has been estimated in 1:10,000,000 live births, with approximately 500 cases around the world [6, 7]. In Brazil, a high prevalence of

* Correspondence: tamara_bio@yahoo.com.br
[1]Faculdade de Ciências da Saúde do Trairi, Universidade Federal do Rio Grande do Norte, Santa Cruz, RN, Brazil
[2]Laboratório de Biologia Molecular e Genômica, Departamento de Biologia Celular e Genética, Centro de Biociências, Universidade Federal do Rio Grande do Norte, Natal, RN, Brazil
Full list of author information is available at the end of the article

BSCL was found in the Rio Grande do Norte (RN) state, in the Northeast region (3 in 100,000), with 103 cases described [7]. Clinical, laboratory and genetic data for BSCL patients from RN were reported by Lima et al. [3]. Genetic data were also reported by Medeiros et al. [7]. Recently, our research group analyzed the leading causes of death in BSCL patients from RN. We found that many of our patients died due to infections, mainly pulmonary [8].

It is well known that maximal respiratory pressure impairment leads to ventilatory inefficiency. Besides the ventilatory importance, inspiratory and expiratory muscles are also important in maintaining upper airway patency [9]. Studies have shown that several chronic conditions may lead to respiratory muscle weakness (RMW). Inspiratory muscle strength is decreased in 30–50% of patients with chronic heart failure [10, 11], and is also associated with autonomic cardiovascular dysfunction in type 2 diabetic patients [12]. Additionally, RMW was also found in type 2 diabetic patients [13]. Considering the metabolic, cardiovascular, and cognitive complications related to BSCL subjects worldwide [5, 14–16], the abnormal cardiovascular autonomic modulation shown by BSCL subjects from RN [4, 5], as well as the lack of studies investigating respiratory maximal pressures in these subjects, the aim of this research was to evaluate the respiratory and peripheric muscle strength in BSCL subjects compared to healthy subjects.

Methods

Study design and data collection

This cross-sectional and longitudinal study was conducted from November 2015 to December 2017. The size sample was not precisely calculated. Eleven BSCL subjects from Seridó of RN were recruited in 2015 by *ASPOSBERN* (*Associação de Pais e Pessoas com a Síndrome de Berardinelli do Estado do Rio Grande do Norte*), a non-profit organization aiming to improve the life quality of BSCL subjects and their families. This organization performs an important role in the management of BSCL subjects diagnosed by qualified physicians and researchers from the Brazilian Research Group for Studies about the Genetics and Morphophysiological Features of Berardinelli-Seip Lipodystrophy [7]. Four BSCL individuals of our study were lost to follow-up: one had died (subject 9) and three did not participate in the 2016 and 2017 data collection (subjects 2, 6, and 11). However, the participant number was considered high since BSCL is an ultra-rare disease with approximately 500 cases described worldwide [3] and the RN state has the highest prevalence documented for this disease [7]. Subjects included in the study participated in a one-day standard physical therapy program during the Annual Meeting of ASPOSBERN held in 2015 to 2017. Inclusion criteria were to be genetically and/or clinically diagnosed with BSCL, to be older than 18 years-old, to be able to understand the tests, and to sign the Written Informed Consent Form (WICF). We excluded subjects who had previously had respiratory diseases or who did not understand how to perform the test. Healthy individuals matched for age and gender were recruited in the Clínica Escola de Fisioterapia, da Faculdade de Ciências da Saúde do Trairi, campus da Universidade Federal do Rio Grande do Norte (UFRN), during February 2016. Inclusion and exclusion criteria were the same as those for BSCL subjects, except for BSCL diagnosis. Table 1 summarizes the clinical, metabolic, and genetic features of BSCL subjects. These data for all BSCL patients from RN were previously described by Lima et al. [3] and Medeiros et al. [7]. Sociodemographic and anthropometrical data were also collected. Participants were also asked about the time after BSCL diagnosis and their practice and weekly frequency of physical activities, according to the International Physical Activity Questionnaire (IPAQ), by using the 8-question short version [17–19]. Table 3 summarizes the physical activity profile of BSCL subjects among the three annual evaluations. Some BSCL patients started the use of metreleptin replacement to treat complications of leptin deficiency, such as insulin resistance, diabetes, and/or hypertriglyceridemia. The metreleptin replacement therapy was performed according to Musso and co-workers [20].

Biochemical measurements in plasma

The measurement of glucose, triglycerides and total cholesterol was performed following the instructions from the Labtest protocols (Lagoa Santa, Brazil) and LABMAX PLENNO equipment (LABTEST, Lagoa Santa, Brazil) [21]. Glucose was determined by end-point method of glucose oxidase and with the measurement of absorbance in 505 nm. Triglycerides was determined by enzymatic method by end-point and with the measurement of absorbance in 505 nm. Total cholesterol was also determined by enzymatic method by end-point and with the measurement of absorbance in 500 nm.

Maximum respiratory pressure measurement

We assessed respiratory muscle strength by measuring Maximum Inspiratory Pressure (MIP) and Maximum Expiratory Pressure (MEP) using an analogic manuvacuometer (MV 300®, WIKA +/− 300 cmH_2O) attached to an unidirectional valve connected to a paper mouthpiece. Subjects were in sitting position with a nose clip in place to prevent nasal air leakage. The MIP and MEP pressures were measured according to *American Thoracic Society* and *European Respiratory Society* (ATS/ERS) [22]. The maximal pressure was maintained for at least 1 second, and 3 to 5 maneuvers were performed [23].

Table 1 Clinical and genetic data of BSCL subjects

Case	Gender/Age (Years)	Comorbidities	Mutated gene	Drugs	Metreleptin use (since year)	RMW (Yes/No)	PMW (Yes/No)
1	♀ / 21	DM, HT, SH	*AGPAT2*	ISL	*Yes (2016)*	*Yes*	No
2[a]	♀ / 22	DM, HT, HT, SH	*BSCL2*	ISL, RMP	–	*Yes*	No
3	♂ / 24	DM, HT	*BSCL2*	MTF, HCT, SXG, CPF, RMP	*Yes (2016)*	*Yes*	No
4	♀ / 28	DM, AH, HT, SH	*BSCL2*	ISL	*Yes (2017)*	*Yes*	No
5	♂ / 29	DM, AH, HT, SH	*BSCL2*	ISL, SXG, MTF, RMP	*Yes (2016)*	*Yes*	No
6[a]	♀ / 29	DM, HT, SH	*BSCL2*	ISL	–	*Yes*	No
7	♂ / 31	DM, HT	*BSCL2*	MTF, SVT	–	Yes	No
8[b]	♂ / 36	DM, AH, HT	*BSCL2*	NA	–	*Yes*	No
9[a]	♀ / 39	DM, AH, HT, KF	*BSCL2*	ISL	–	*Yes*	No
10	♀ / 43	DM, HT	*BSCL2*	ISL	–	*Yes*	No
11[a]	♀ / 44	DM, AH, HT	*BSCL2*	ISL, MTF, ATN, HCT	–	Yes	No

DM diabetes mellitus, *AH* arterial hypertension, *HT* hypertriglyceridemia, *SH* steatohepatitis, *KF* kidney failure, *RMW* Respiratory Muscle Weakness, *MTF* Metformin, *HCT* Hydrochlorothiazide, *SXG* Saxagliptin, *CPF* Ciprofibrate, *RMP* Ramipril, *ISL* Insulin, *SVT* Sinvastatin, *ATN* Atenolol
[a]Subjects that participated in 2015 but were lost to follow-up in 2016–2017. [b]BSCL subject that declared to be a smoker

Reference values standardized for the studied population were used [24].

We evaluated both respiratory pressures at three time-points: 2015, 2016, and 2017. The respiratory muscle weakness (RMW) state was defined as having MIP and/or MEP values lower than 70% of predictive values, as previously described. Therefore, healthy subjects with predicted values lower than 70% were considered unsuitable and, therefore, were excluded [25–27]. Results are shown in percentage of predicted (%) values.

Peripheral muscle strength measurement

Peripheral muscle strength was measured by handgrip dynamometry using a hydraulic dynamometer (Saehan Corporation), which measures the strength of a grip in pounds-force. Compared with Jamar dynamometer, the Saehan hydraulic dynamometer is also a valid and trusty instrument [28].

BSCL and healthy subjects were kept in a seated position and received verbal instructions for completing the assessment. We used the mean of four grip trials as compared to either a single grip trial or the highest reading of four trials. The predicted values for grip strength were measured according to the Brazilian population previously described by Caporrino et al. [29]. Measurements of maximal respiratory pressures and peripheral muscle strength were performed by the same investigator.

Statistical analysis

The data were analyzed using *GraphPad Prism* software, version 6.0. The Shapiro–Wilk test was used to analyze normality data distribution. Continuous and normally distributed variables are expressed as mean ± standard deviation (SD). Proportions are presented as number (%) for categorical variables. Parametric comparisons between the groups were performed by unpaired T-test. The intragroup analysis was performed by repeated measures ANOVA followed by a Bonferroni post hoc test. To evaluate the correlation between MIP and peripheral muscle strength, Pearson (parametric variables) and Spearman (non-parametric variables) correlation coefficients were used. Associations between categorical variables were analyzed by the chi-square test. Statistical significance was set at $p < 0.05$.

Results

Eleven BSCL subjects were included in this study. Clinical, metabolic, and genetic data were obtained (Table 1). We found that the majority of BSCL subjects were Type 2, presenting a specific mutation in the BSCL2 gene (*325dupA*). Only one patient was Type 1 (case 1), presenting the *A712T* mutation in the AGPAT2 gene. There were no significant differences between BSCL and control subjects for gender, age, height, weight, and BMI (Table 2). Table 3 summarizes the weekly frequency of

Table 2 Physiological and metabolic data (mean ± SD) of BSCL subjects and healthy volunteers (Control)

(*n* = 11)	BSCL	Control	*p*
Age (years)	31.45 ± 8.04	30.91 ± 8.13	0.8759
Height (m)	1.65 ± 0.09	1.63 ± 0.08	0.6531
Weight (kg)	59.3 ± 13.45	64.85 ± 14.80	0.3680
BMI (kg/m^2)	21.56 ± 3.08	24.18 ± 4.41	0.1223
Diabetes Mellitus (n/%)	11 (100)	0 (0)	< 0.0001
Fasting glycemia (mg/dL)	268 ± 124	NA	–
Serum triglycerides (mg/dL)	173 ± 94.84	NA	–
Total cholesterol (mg/dL)	151.3 ± 63.65	NA	–

p values were based on independent t-tests. For categorical variables, the *p* value was calculated using the chi-square test
BMI body mass index, *NA* Not available

Table 3 Physical activity data of BSCL subjects and healthy volunteers (Control)

Classification[a]	BSCL (n/%)	Control (n/%)
Sedentary	4 (36.36)	7 (63.63)
Irregularly active B	1 (9.09)	1 (9.09)
Irregularly active A	1 (9.09)	2 (18.18)
Active	4 (36.36)	1 (9.09)
Very active	1 (9.09)	0 (0.00)
Total	11 (100)	11 (100)

[a]According to IPAQ [17–19]

physical activities according to IPAQ. We found that 63.6% ($n = 7$) of the BSCL group were classified as irregularly active B to very active, while 36.4% ($n = 3$) were classified as sedentary. On the other hand, 36.5% of the control group were classified as irregularly active B to very active, while 63.6% were classified as sedentary. These data indicate that in 2015 the BSCL group were more active than the healthy volunteers.

The BSCL group showed lower MIP and MEP pressures but no changes in handgrip strength. Although BSCL case 8 was a smoker, he presented a similar profile of these variables compared to all BSCL subjects. For this purpose, we decided to maintain case 8 in this research. Controls have shown significantly higher values for MIP and MEP in comparison to BSCL individuals in the first year. No significant difference between the groups was found for grip strength (PMS) (Table 4; Fig. 1).

Additionally, even if MIP, MEP, and peripheral muscle strength gradually increased after the first investigation, these variations were not statistically significant among the three evaluations, revealing that BSCL subjects presented maintenance of respiratory dysfunction over the years (Table 5; Fig. 2). To better understand the role of metreleptin in the respiratory and peripheral muscle strength of BSCL subjects, we divided the BSCL subjects according to the use of metreleptin (Table 6 and Fig. 2). The data revealed that the metreleptin replacement did not result in an improvement of MIP, MEP, and peripheral muscle in BSCL subjects. Moreover, we also examined the results of these tests for each BSCL patient

Table 4 MIP, MEP, and PMS measurements (mean ± SD and [95% confidence interval]) in BSCL subjects and healthy volunteers (Control)

($n = 11$)	MIP (predicted %)	MEP (predicted %)	PMS (predicted %)
BSCL subjects	70.24 ± 14.89	49.78 ± 23.81	81.77 ± 20.71
	[60.24–80.24]	[33.79–65.78]	[67.85–95.68]
Controls	129.3 ± 17.56	90.83 ± 17.83	93.76 ± 16.84
	[117.5–141.5]	[78.85–102.8]	[82.45–105.1]
p	*< 0.0001*	*0.0002*	0.1517

p values were based on independent unpaired t-tests

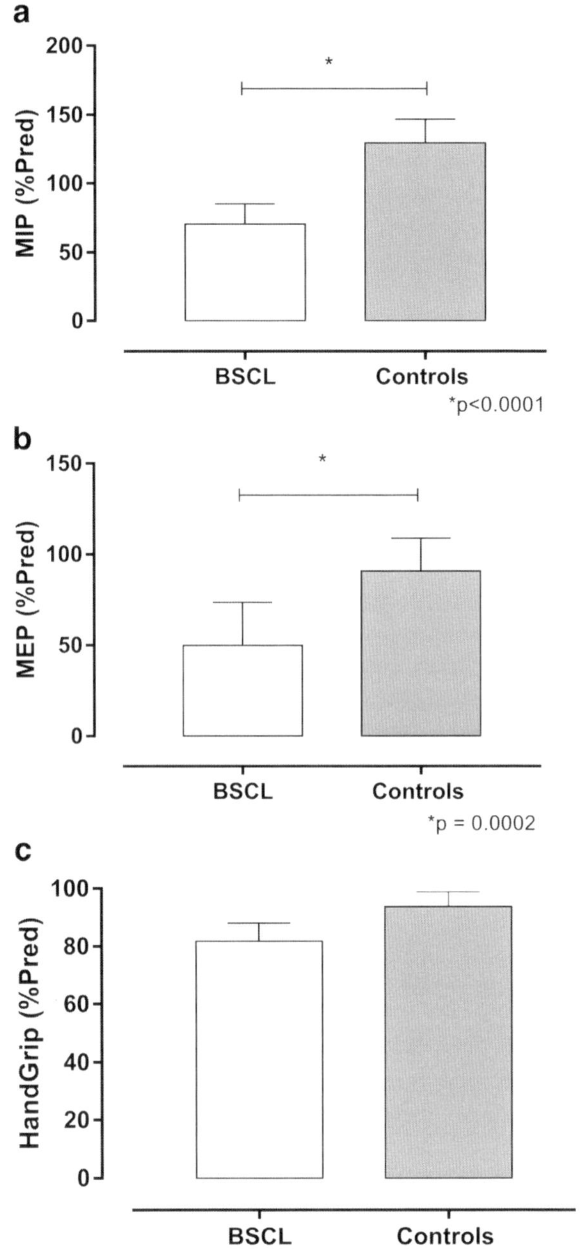

Fig. 1 Maximum Inspiratory Pressure (MIP), Maximum Expiratory Pressure (MEP) and peripheral muscle strength (PMS) values of the 11 BSCL patients and healthy subjects at the first year. **a** MIP, (**b**) MEP, and (**c**) PMS indices are expressed as % of predicted values. The results are represented as the mean ± SD. The differences were considered statistically significant when $^*p < 0.05$ using unpaired Student's t-test

separately. As shown in Fig. 3, metreleptin did not improve MIP, MEP, and peripheral muscle strength, since a similar profile was observed for subjects without (7, 8, and 10 - solid black lines) and with (1, 3, 4, and 5 - dashed blue lines) metreleptin replacement.

Afterward, we investigated the weekly frequency of physical exercise practices among the three evaluations.

Table 5 MIP, MEP, and PMS measurements (mean ± SD and [95% confidence interval]) in all BSCL subjects after three evaluations

(*n* = 7)	2015	2016	2017	*P*
MIP (predicted %)				
All BSCL subjects	66.34 ± 14.2	65.04 ± 17.14	89.5 ± 24.96	0.0580
	[53.21–79.47]	[49.18–80.9]	[66.41–112.6]	
MEP (predicted %)				
All BSCL subjects	55.24 ± 18.42	50.89 ± 15.35	49.68 ± 15.52	0.4573
	[38.20–72.28]	[36.69–65.09]	[35.33–64.03]	
PMS (predicted %)				
All BSCL subjects	85.34 ± 25	85.41 ± 26.28	85.05 ± 23.73	0.9914
	[62.22–108.5]	[61.11–109.7]	[63.1–107]	

p values were based on repeated measures ANOVA

We observed that 42.8% ($n = 3$) of BSCL subjects presented the same profile during the 2 years of investigation (Additional file 1: Table S1). Instead, 57.2% ($n = 4$) showed changes in their physical activity profile, varying from active to sedentary, and irregularly active to sedentary. Even if we consider all BSCL subjects with one of the active profiles in the same group, our data confirm that the BSCL group were more active in 2015 and 2017 (Fig. 4).

In addition, we found that grip strength and MIP were not correlated in these subjects (Additional file 2: Figure S1). We also investigated whether the respiratory and peripheral muscle strength were correlated with the metabolic variables assessed in this study. We found that the tests used to study the respiratory and peripheral strength did not present an association with age, BMI, glucose, triglycerides, and total cholesterol (Additional file 1: Table S2).

Discussion

In this study, we showed a decrease in the maximum static respiratory pressures of subjects with BSCL. This condition was not modified after 2 years as indicated by the maintenance of the low levels of MIP and MEP observed from 2015 to 2017. No changes were observed in the peripheral muscle strength of those subjects. To our knowledge, this is the first study that verified respiratory and peripheral muscle strength in this population.

Several studies showed a decrease in static respiratory pressures in patients with metabolic, renal, and cardiovascular complications [30–33], findings that were also described in BSCL patients [3–5, 16, 34]. All BSCL subjects from our research had diabetes, as shown in Table 1, which is in accordance with the previously published data from our population [3, 14].

There is evidence that the lung is a target organ in diabetes mellitus and pulmonary complications, as a respiratory muscle strength weakness was found in diabetic patients, correlating with a poor metabolic control [13]. Some mechanisms were proposed to explain the role of diabetes mellitus in pulmonary function. An association between autonomic neuropathy related to the respiratory muscles and lung impairment was previously identified [35]. Diabetic autonomic neuropathy is a complication of diabetes mellitus that has been associated with cardiovascular and respiratory dysfunctions in several studies [36–41]. Concerning BSCL, Faria et al. [5] previously showed abnormal autonomic modulation in BSCL patients of our cohort by heart rate variability (HRV) analysis, and this was independent of the presence of metabolic and hemodynamic disturbances. Atypical autonomic modulation was also recently confirmed in BSCL patients from Ceará, a Northeast state located near our patients' state [16].

Furthermore, subjects presenting type 2 diabetes mellitus with autonomic neuropathy also showed reduced muscle strength and less HR variability and the researchers found a positive correlation between MIP and HRV [12]. Together, these results suggest that BSCL subjects could present respiratory muscle weakness. The results of the present study revealed a reduction of MIP and MEP in BSCL subjects that persisted for over two years of evaluation.

In both studies, almost all BSCL patients presented the *325dupA* mutation in the BSCL2 gene that encodes Seipin. BSCL type 2 is the most severe form of this lipodystrophy, and the propensity to premature death is higher in these patients [3, 7], which could explain the low average age found for this BSCL group (31.4 ± 8.0 years). There are many Seipin-related motor neuropathies, named Seipinopathy. Lipodystrophy occurs due to Seipin loss-of-function, and the nervous system is slightly affected when compared with Seipinopathies, which occur due to Seipin gain-of-function [1, 42].

Seipin also plays an important role in regulating excitatory synaptic transmission [43]. We hypothesize that Seipin deficiency could affect the contraction of inspiratory and expiratory musculatures due to an imbalance of excitatory and inhibitory synaptic transmission. Sympathetic activation can be induced by inspiratory muscle fatigue, resulting in increased cardiac debt and arterial pressure and, consequently, leading to a reduction in arterial blood flow to the lower limbs. These findings indicate an interaction between ventilatory muscle activity and cardiovascular control mechanisms, which could potentiate previous abnormal autonomic control [12, 44, 45]. However, since these explanations were most pronounced in diabetic patients presenting autonomic neuropathies [12], new investigations are needed to address the role of Seipin in the regulation of autonomic neuropathies and its relationship with respiratory muscle strength.

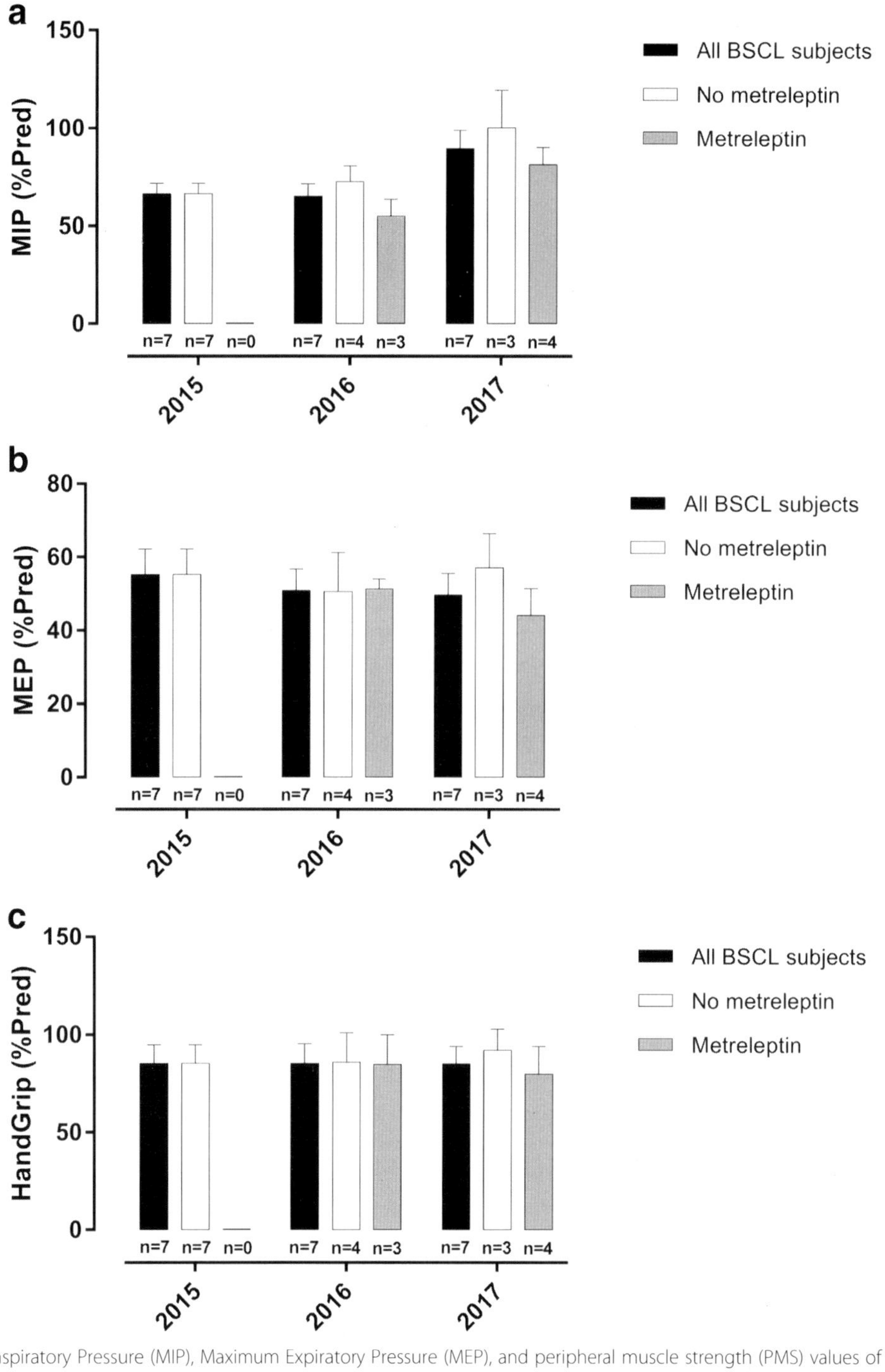

Fig. 2 Maximum Inspiratory Pressure (MIP), Maximum Expiratory Pressure (MEP), and peripheral muscle strength (PMS) values of all BSCL subjects and after stratification according to the use of metreleptin from 2015 to 2017. **a** MIP, (**b**) MEP, and (**c**) PMS indices are expressed as % of predicted values. The results are represented as the mean ± SD. For the analysis of all BSCL subjects, the differences were considered statistically significant when $*p < 0.05$ using repeated measures ANOVA. For the analysis after stratification according to the use of metreleptin, the differences were considered statistically significant when $*p < 0.05$ using repeated measures ANOVA for the group without metreleptin and using unpaired Student's t-test for the group with metreleptin

Seipin is also implicated in ER stress, and this phenomenon was widely studied in liver, adipose tissue, pancreatic islets, and mammary gland alveolar epithelial cells [46–49]. However, there is a lack of information about ER stress and Seipin's role in skeletal muscle pathophysiology. While Seipinopathy was shown to be related to ER stress, Lipodystrophy was not associated with ER stress in non-adipogenic cells. In Silver Syndrome, a type

Table 6 MIP, MEP, and peripheral muscle strength measurements (mean ± SD and [95% confidence interval]) in BSCL subjects without and with metreleptin replacement

(*n* = 7)	2015 (n/%)	2016 (n/%)	2017 (n/%)	*P*
MIP (predicted %)				
No Metreleptin	7 (100)	4 (57.2)	3 (42.8)	–
	70.24 ± 14.89	72.62 ± 16.14	100.4 ± 33.27	[b]0.0719
	[60.24–80.24]	[46.93–98.30]	[17.71–183.00]	–
Metreleptin	0 (0)	3 (42.8)	4 (57.2)	–
	–	54.93 ± 14.93	81.35 ± 17.36	[a]0.0892
	–	[17.84–92.03]	[53.73–109]	
p^a	–	0.7524	0.3644	
MEP (predicted %)				
No Metreleptin	7 (100)	4 (57.2)	3 (42.8)	–
	55.24 ± 18.42	50.56 ± 21.34	57.1 ± 16.19	[b]0.8881
	[38.2–72.28]	[16.6–84.52]	[16.87–97.33]	–
Metreleptin	0 (0)	3 (42.8)	4 (57.2)	–
	–	51.31 ± 4.67	44.11 ± 14.51	[a]0.4541
	–	[39.69–62.93]	[21.03–67.19]	–
p^a	–	0.9556	0.3142	–
PMS (predicted %)				
No Metreleptin	7 (100)	4 (57.2)	3 (42.8)	–
	85.34 ± 25	85.87 ± 30.34	92.03 ± 18.78	[b]0.9270
	[62.22–108.5]	[37.6–134.1]	[45.38–138.7]	–
Metreleptin	0 (0)	3 (42.8)	4 (57.2)	–
	–	84.8 ± 26.27	79.81 ± 28.39	[a]0.8219
	–	[19.53–150.1]	[34.63–125]	–
p^a	–	0.9632	0.5504	–

[a]*p* values were based on independent unpaired t-tests
[b]*p* values were based on repeated measures ANOVA for the group without metreleptin

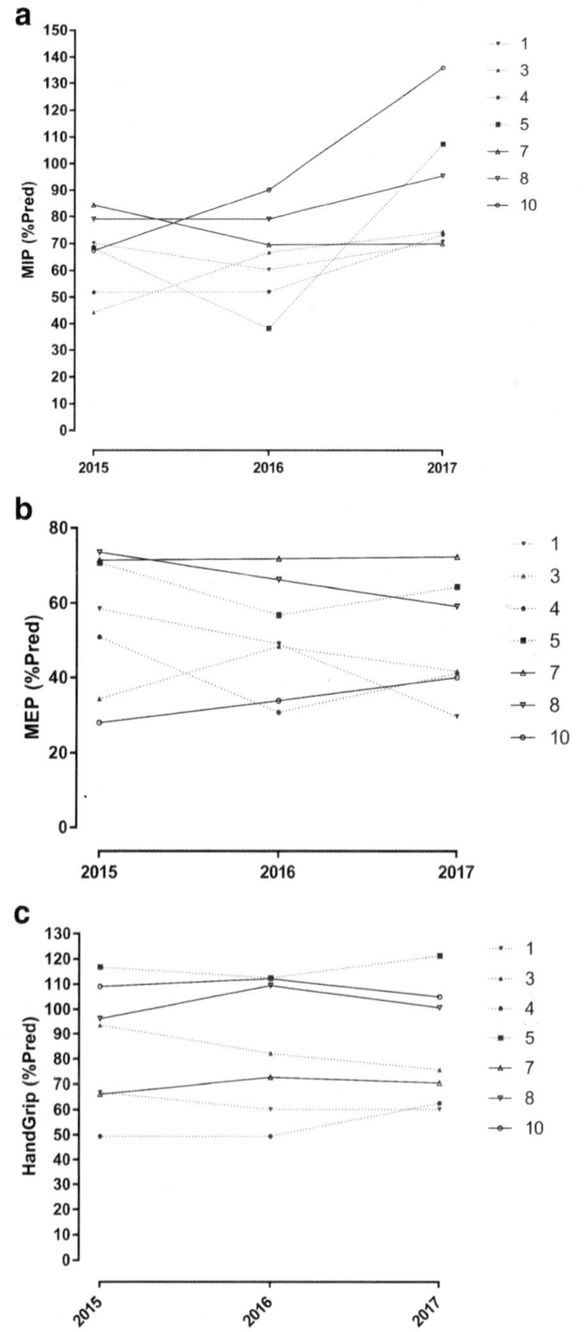

Fig. 3 Maximum Inspiratory Pressure (MIP), Maximum Expiratory Pressure (MEP), and peripheral muscle strength (PMS) values for each BSCL subject at 2015, 2016, and 2017. **a** MIP, (**b**) MEP, and (**c**) PMS indices are expressed as % of predicted values

of Seipinopathy, a weakness of upper body strength was observed, indicating that Seipin gain of function can affect the upper musculature [50]. In fact, *Bscl2* is robustly expressed in the XI cranial nerve, the main source of efferent motor fibers to the muscle groups of the shoulder and neck [50]. We suppose that there is a relationship between ER stress and Seipin in respiratory skeletal muscles that may not be per se associated with Seipinopathy, since our BSCL type 2 patients (*325dupA* mutation) did not present any signs related to neurological disturbances that were described for Seipinopathy.

The diaphragm is the most important skeletal muscle for respiratory function and, together with other respiratory muscles, acts as a respiratory pump, generating during inspiration the tidal volume necessary for the proper alveolar ventilation. Hyperglycemia can lead to loss of diaphragm muscle strength due to increased production of reactive oxygen species (ROS), which can damage contractile proteins, such as troponin T [51]. In addition, it is possible that insulin resistance, caused by intramuscular triglyceride accumulation, especially in mitochondria, generates negative adaptations in the diaphragm morphology and function, leading to the development of respiratory muscle weakness [52]. In this research all of the BSCL subjects presented hypertriglyceridemia and diabetes mellitus, indicating that these comorbidities

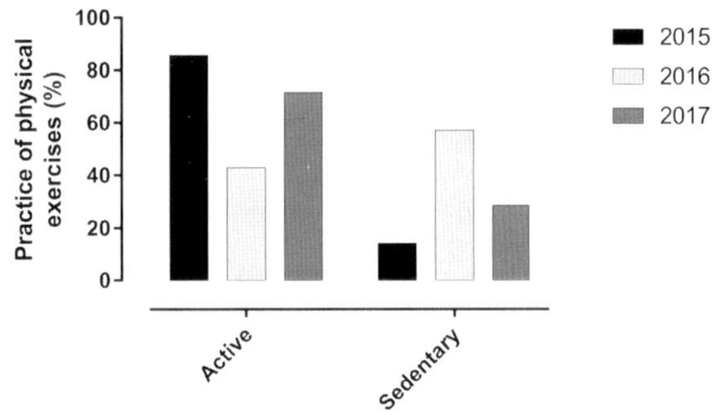

Fig. 4 Profile of physical exercise practices of BSCL subjects from 2015 to 2017 according to IPAQ classification. The results are represented as %. The differences were considered statistically significant when $*p < 0.05$ using two-way ANOVA with multiple comparisons (Bonferroni post hoc test)

may be associated with inspiratory muscle weakness found in these subjects.

Although leptin has been shown to be related to diabetic complications, no data from exploring its role in respiratory function are available. Since high levels of leptin were associated with autonomic neuropathy in diabetic patients [53–55] and these patients presented decreased muscle strength [12], we hypothesized that a relationship could exist between leptin and respiratory function. We observed a tendency to an increase in MIP and MEP after leptin replacement when all BSCL subjects were examined together (Fig. 2; Table 4). However, since only four BSCL subjects of our study started the metreleptin replacement, we were not able to conclude that administration of metreleptin can result in an improvement of respiratory muscle strength because BSCL subjects without metreleptin replacement also presented a slight increase in MIP and MEP when compared to those with metreleptin replacement (Figs. 2 and 3; Table 5).

The association between respiratory and peripheral muscle strength was previously studied in the literature. It was postulated that MIP could equally reflect the peripheral muscle strength and that the reverse is similarly true [56, 57]. In this context, we also evaluated the occurrence of peripheral muscle strength in our BSCL subjects, and the occurrence of a correlation between MIP and peripheral muscle strength was verified. In our study, we did not find peripheral muscle weakness in all BSCL subjects evaluated. These data reveal a difference between Lipodystrophy and Seipinopathy, since in the latter the weakness of upper limbs was previously described for Silver Syndrome [50].

Moreover, our peripheral muscle strength data are opposite to those obtained by Garg and co-workers [58]. The researchers observed reduced muscle strength of quadriceps femoris in 3 African BSCL patients. However, the genotyping of all patients evaluated in that study was not performed and no suppositions concerning the mutated gene and the specific BSCL mutation with the weakness of quadriceps muscle strength can be done. We also could not compare our results of MIP, MEP, and peripheral muscle strength according to the type of BSCL mutation since we had only 1 BSCL type 1 patient in our study. The one type 1 BSCL patient (case 1) presented maintenance of MIP during the 2 years of follow-up. Nonetheless, MEP and handgrip strength were reduced at follow-up, remaining below 70% of the predicted values. Weakness of lower muscle strength was also shown in patients with metabolic syndrome, especially in diabetic patients with or without polyneuropathy [59, 60].

To better elucidate the morphology of skeletal muscle from BSCL patients, Garg and co-workers also evaluated biopsy samples from quadriceps femoris and found an increase in glycolytic muscle fibers and a reduction in oxidative muscle fibers compared to healthy women. They postulated that insulin resistance found in those BSCL patients could be associated with the increase in glycolytic muscle fibers [58]. They proposed that the increased muscularity in BSCL is due to muscle hyperplasia and is not associated with increased muscle strength.

An inefficient metabolic control can contribute to a reduction in resistance to fatigue, which can be explained by the morphophysiological changes of respiratory and peripheral muscles, resulting in microvascular perturbations related to insulin resistance that compromises muscle strength and endurance [13, 58]. Nevertheless, we did not find any correlation between the respiratory and peripheral strength with the metabolic variables studied in our research. We suggest that the difference observed in our study, compared with Garg [58], can be explained by the specific characteristics of upper and lower limbs. The latter are more resistant to fatigue, mainly the quadriceps, when compared with upper limbs. In the case of BSCL patients from Garg's research [58], the increased levels of glycolytic fibers resulted in a reduction in muscle strength probably due to the commitment of the muscle performance. Currently, no data are available about the morphology of upper muscles from BSCL patients. In addition, the lower limbs may be more affected by the disuse. Domestic and personal care activities may prevent muscle weakness in the upper limbs, which are more affected in the advanced stages of metabolic comorbidities [61–64].

It has been shown that inspiratory muscle training could improve inspiratory muscle function with no consequences in functional capacity or autonomic modulation [65, 66]. Inspiratory muscle training applied for patients with metabolic syndrome has been essential to prevent and/or treat respiratory muscle weakness [65]. The lack of physical exercise is a central mechanism in the development of diabetes mellitus and can contribute to reduced muscle strength. We believe that it is essential to verify MIP and MEP in healthy diabetic subjects to compare with our data found in diabetic BSCL patients. In addition, since metabolic disturbances, including diabetes, are a marked commitment found in BSCL patients, new physical interventions are required to improve the metabolic conditions and respiratory muscle strength of these patients.

Conclusions

We found an association between BSCL and decreased respiratory muscle strength during the 2 years of evaluation, suggesting that this lipodystrophy may be related to respiratory muscle weakness, which was not recovered by metreleptin treatment. The accurate molecular and pathophysiological mechanisms to explain these results require further investigation to reveal the impact of metabolic control and the practice of physical activity on respiratory muscle strength of Berardinelli-Seip Congenital Lipodystrophy subjects.

Study limitations

The measurement of respiratory muscle strength by maximum static respiratory pressure tests may be considered a study limitation due to its volitional characteristic. Non-volitional tests, such as the magnetic and electrical stimulation of phrenic nerve, are highly specific. However, the application of non-volitional tests presents high cost and is less applicable in the clinical practice. Furthermore, it is important to increase the number of BSCL subjects with type 1 BSCL and include the younger type 2 BSCL subjects to better understand the role of 1-AGPAT2 and Seipin on respiratory and peripheral muscle strength. The increase of BSCL subjects will also allow better description of the difference between Lipodystrophy and Seipinopathy regarding the weakness of upper limbs.

Additional files

Additional file 1: Table S1. Physical activity data of BSCL subjects after three evaluations. **Table S2.** Correlations between respiratory and peripheral strength tests and metabolic parameters of BSCL subjects. (DOCX 18 kb)

Additional file 2: Figure S1. Correlation between MIP and peripheral muscle strength (PMS) values of BSCL subjects. MIP indices at 2015, 2016, and 2017 were used. r values of a Pearson correlation coefficient and *p* values are included. (TIF 345 kb)

Abbreviations

AGPAT: Acylglycerol-3-phosphate O-acyltransferase; ANOVA: Analysis of variance; *ASPOSBERN*: Association of Parents and People with Berardinelli Syndrome of *Rio Grande do Norte* (*Associação dos Pais e Pessoas com a Síndrome de Berardinelli do Estado do Rio Grande do Norte*); ATS/ERS: *American Thoracic Society* and *European Respiratory Society*; BMI: Body mass index; BSCL: Berardinelli-Seip Congenital Generalized Lipodystrophy; CI: Confidence interval; ER: Endoplasmic reticulum; FACISA: *Faculdade de Ciências da Saúde do Trairi*; HRV: Heart rate variability; MEP: Maximum Expiratory Pressure; MIP: Maximum Inspiratory Pressure; PMS: Peripheral Muscle Strength; PMW: Peripheral Muscle Weakness; RMS: Respiratory Muscle Strength; RMW: Respiratory Muscle Weakness; RN: Rio Grande do Norte; UFRN: Universidade Federal do Rio Grande do Norte

Acknowledgments

The authors would like to thank *ASPOSBERN* for kindly providing all the necessary data for analysis.

Funding

This research did not receive any specific grant from funding agencies in the public, commercial, or not-for-profit sectors.

Authors, contributions

JLDM, BCB, TABA, MSLC, TTXN and JTAMC collected and compiled data. ASCS, JTAMC, LBAM, JGL and LPG assisted in writing and formatting the text. All authors assisted with the data analysis and read and approved the final manuscript.

Competing interests

The authors declare that they have no competing interests.

Author details

[1]Faculdade de Ciências da Saúde do Trairi, Universidade Federal do Rio Grande do Norte, Santa Cruz, RN, Brazil. [2]Laboratório de Biologia Molecular e Genômica, Departamento de Biologia Celular e Genética, Centro de Biociências, Universidade Federal do Rio Grande do Norte, Natal, RN, Brazil. [3]Departamento de Medicina Clínica, Hospital Universitário Onofre Lopes (HUOL)/UFRN, Natal, RN, Brazil.

References

1. Patni N, Garg A. Congenital generalized lipodystrophies—new insights into metabolic dysfunction. Nat rev Endocrinol. Nature publishing group. 2015; 11(9):522–34.
2. Filho PPF, Val AC, Diamante R, Cunha CF, Norton RC, Lamounier JA, et al. Congenital generalized lipodystrophy. J Pediatr. 2004;80:333–6.
3. Lima JG, Nobrega LHC, de Lima NN, do Nascimento Santos MG, Baracho MFP, Jeronimo SMB. Clinical and laboratory data of a large series of patients with congenital generalized lipodystrophy. Diabetol Metab Syndr. 2016;8:23.
4. Guedes Do Rêgo A, Mesquita ET, De Faria CA, Álvares M, Do Rêgo G, De Fátima M, et al. Cardiometabolic abnormalities in patients with berardinelli-seip syndrome. Arq Bras Cardiol. 2010;94:102–10.
5. Faria CA, Moraes RS, Sobral-Filho DC, Rego AG, Baracho MFPP, Egito ESTT, et al. Autonomic modulation in patients with congenital generalized lipodystrophy (berardinelli-seip syndrome). Europace. 2009;11:763–9.
6. Garg A. Lipodystrophies. Am J Med. 2000;108:143–52.

7. Medeiros LBA, Dantas VKC, Sarmento ASC, Agnez-Lima LF, Meireles AL, Nobre TTX, et al. High prevalence of Berardinelli-Seip congenital lipodystrophy in Rio Grande do Norte state, Northeast Brazil. Diabetol Metab Syndr. 2017;9:80.
8. Gomes Lima J, Helena L, Nobrega C, Lima NN, Ferreira MC, Santos D, et al. Causes of death in patients with Berardinelli- Seip congenital generalized lipodystrophy. [cited 2018 Jun 13]; Available from: http://journals.plos.org/plosone/article/file?id=10.1371/journal.pone.0199052&type=printable.
9. Park JH, Kang S-W, Lee SC, Choi WA, Kim DH. How respiratory muscle strength correlates with cough capacity in patients with respiratory muscle weakness. Yonsei Med J [Internet]. 2010 [cited 2018 Aug 13];51:392. Available from: http://www.ncbi.nlm.nih.gov/pubmed/20376892
10. Ribeiro JP, Chiappa GR, Neder JA, Frankenstein L. Respiratory muscle function and exercise intolerance in heart failure. Curr Heart Fail Rep. 2009;6:95–101.
11. Wong E, Selig S, Hare DL. Respiratory muscle dysfunction and training in chronic heart failure. Hear Lung Circ. Australasian Society of Cardiac and Thoracic Surgeons and The Cardiac Society of Australia and New Zealand. 2011;20:289–94.
12. Kaminski DM, D'Agord Schaan B, da Silva AMV, Soares PP, Plentz RDM, Dall'Ago P. Inspiratory muscle weakness is associated with autonomic cardiovascular dysfunction in patients with type 2 diabetes mellitus. Clin Auton Res. 2011;21:29–35.
13. Fuso L, Pitocco D, Longobardi A, Zaccardi F, Contu C, Pozzuto C, et al. Reduced respiratory muscle strength and endurance in type 2 diabetes mellitus. Diabetes Metab Res Rev. 2012;28:370–5.
14. Van Maldergem L, Magré J, Khallouf TE, Gedde-Dahl T, Delépine M, Trygstad O, et al. Genotype-phenotype relationships in Berardinelli-Seip congenital lipodystrophy. J Med Genet. 2002;39:722–33.
15. Seip M, Trygstad O. Generalized lipodystrophy. Arch Dis Child. 1963;38:447–53.
16. Ponte CMM, Fernandes VO, Gurgel MHC, Vasconcelos ITGF, Karbage LB de AS, Liberato CBR, et al. Early commitment of cardiovascular autonomic modulation in Brazilian patients with congenital generalized lipodystrophy. BMC Cardiovasc Disord. 2018;18:6.
17. Hagströmer M, Oja P, Sjöström M. The International Physical Activity Questionnaire (IPAQ): a study of concurrent and construct validity. Public Health Nutr [Internet]. 2006 [cited 2018 Aug 13];9:755–762. Available from: http://www.ncbi.nlm.nih.gov/pubmed/16925881
18. Matsudo S, Araújo T, Matsudo V, Andrade D, Andrade E, Oliveira LC, et al. QUESTIONÁRIO INTERNACIONAL DE ATIVIDADE FÍSICA (IPAQ): ESTUDO DE VALIDADE E REPRODUTIBILIDADE NO BRASIL. Rev Bras Atividade Física Saúde [Internet]. 2001 [cited 2018 Aug 13];6:5–18. Available from: http://rbafs.org.br/RBAFS/article/view/931
19. Craig CL, Marshall AL, Sjöström M, Bauman AE, Booth ML, Ainsworth BE, et al. International Physical Activity Questionnaire: 12-Country Reliability and Validity. Med Sci Sport Exerc [Internet]. 2003 [cited 2018 Aug 13];35:1381–1395. Available from: http://www.ncbi.nlm.nih.gov/pubmed/12900694
20. Musso C, Major ML, Andres E, Simha V. Metreleptin treatment in three patients with generalized lipodystrophy. Clin Med Insights Case Reports. 2016; 9:123–127.
21. Labtest Diagnóstica S.A [Internet]. [cited 2018 Aug 24]. Available from: https://labtest.com.br/
22. Gibson GJ, Whitelaw W, Siafakas N, Supinski GS, Fitting JW, Bellemare F, et al. ATS/ERS statement on respiratory muscle testing. Am J Respir Crit Care Med. 2002;166:518–624.
23. Dornelas De Andrade A, Silva TNS, Vasconcelos H, Marcelino M, Rodrigues-Machado MG, Galindo Filho VC, et al. Inspiratory muscular activation during threshold® therapy in elderly healthy and patients with COPD. J Electromyogr Kinesiol. 2005;15:631–9.
24. Neder JA, Andreoni S, Lerario MC, Nery LE. Reference values for lung function tests. II. Maximal respiratory pressures and voluntary ventilation. Brazilian J Med Biol Res. 1999;32:719–27.
25. Evans JA, Whitelaw WA. The assessment of maximal respiratory mouth pressures in adults. Respir Care. 2009;54:1348–59.
26. Horizonte B, Therapist P, Federal U, Gerais DM, Parreira V, França D, et al. Maximal respiratory Pressures : actual and predicted values in healthy subjects. Rev bras fisioter. 2007;11:361–8.
27. Bravo de Souza R. Diretrizes para Testes de Função Pulmonar. J Bras Pneumol. 2002;28(Supl 3). Chapter 8: Pressões respiratórias estáticas máximas. Available from: http://www.jornaldepneumologia.com.br/detalhe_suplemento.asp?id=45.
28. Reis MM, Arantes PMM. Medida da força de preensão manual- validade e confiabilidade do dinamômetro saehan. Fisioter e Pesqui. 2011;18: 176–81.
29. Caporrino FA, Faloppa F, Santos JBGDOS, Réssio C, Soares FHDC, Segre NG, et al. Estudo populacional da força de preensão palmar com dinamômetro Jamar. Rev Bras Ortop. 1998;33:150–4.
30. Bessa EJC, Lopes AJ, Rufino R. A importância da medida da força muscular respiratória na prática da pneumologia. Pulmão RJ. 2015;24:37–41.
31. Alberto L, Junior F, Rubleski A, Garcia D, Tieppo J, Vercelino R, et al. Avaliação da Força Muscular Respiratória e da Função Pulmonar em Pacientes com Insuficiência Cardíaca. Arq Bras Cardiol. 2007;89:36–41.
32. Bonjorni LA, Jamami M, Di Lorenzo VAP, Pessoa BV. Influência da doença de Parkinson em capacidade física, função pulmonar e índice de massa magra corporal. Fisioter em Mov. 2012;25:727–36.
33. Cury JL, Brunetto AF, Aydos RD. Efeitos negativos da insuficiência renal crônica sobre a função pulmonar e a capacidade funcional Negative effects of chronic kidney failure on lung function and functional capacity. Rev Bras Fisioter. 2010;14:91–8.
34. Bande-Fernández JJ, García-Castro R, Sánchez-Alvarez JE, Rodríguez-Suárez C, Coronel-Aguilar D, Hidalgo C, et al. Síndrome de Berardinelli-Seip en diálisis peritoneal. Nefrología. Sociedad Española de Nefrología. 2015;35:493–6.
35. Klein OL, Krishnan JA, Glick S, Smith LJ. Systematic review of the association between lung function and type 2 diabetes mellitus. Diabet Med. 2010;27:977–87.
36. Ziegler D, Gries FA, Mühlen H, Rathmann W, Spüler M, Lessmann F. Prevalence and clinical correlates of cardiovascular autonomic and peripheral diabetic neuropathy in patients attending diabetes centers. The Diacan multicenter study group. Diabete Metab. 1993;19:143–51.
37. Vinik AI, Ziegler D. Diabetic cardiovascular autonomic neuropathy. Circulation. 2007;115:387–97.
38. Maser R, Mitchell B, Vinik A, Freeman R. The association between cardiovascular autonomic neuropathy and mortality in individuals with diabetes: a meta-analysis. Diabetes Care. 2003;26:1895–901.
39. Douglas NJ, Campbell IW, Ewing DJ, Clarke BF, Flenley DC. Reduced airway vagal tone in diabetic patients with autonomic neuropathy. Clin Sci. 1981; 61:581–4.
40. Heaton RW, Guy RJC, Gray BJ. Diminished bronchial reactivity to cold air in diabetic patients with autonomic neuropathy. Br Med J. 1984;289:149–51.
41. Bertherat J, Lubetzki J, Lockhart A, Regnard J. Decreased bronchial response to methacholine in IDDM patients with autonomic neuropathy. Diabetes. 1991;40:1100–6.
42. Ito D, Fujisawa T, Iida H, Suzuki N. Characterization of seipin/BSCL2, a protein associated with spastic paraplegia 17. Neurobiol Dis. 2008;31:266–77.
43. Wei S, Soh SLY, Qiu W, Yang W, Seah CJY, Guo J, et al. Seipin regulates excitatory synaptic transmission in cortical neurons. J Neurochem. 2013; 124:478–89.
44. Chiappa GR, Roseguini BT, Vieira PJC, Alves CN, Tavares A, Winkelmann ER, et al. Inspiratory muscle training improves blood flow to resting and exercising limbs in patients with chronic heart failure. J Am Coll Cardiol. 2008; 51:1663–71.
45. Croix CMS, Morgan BJ, Wetter TJ, Dempsey JA. Fatiguing inspiratory muscle work causes reflex sympathetic activation in humans. J Physiol. 2000;529: 493–504.
46. El Z, AE, Li R, Chen W, Ye X. Seipin deficiency leads to increased ER stress and apoptosis in mammary gland alveolar epithelial cells during lactation. Biol Reprod. 2017;(98)4:570–578.
47. Qiu W, Wee K, Takeda K, Lim X, Sugii S, Radda GK, et al. Suppression of Adipogenesis by pathogenic Seipin mutant is associated with inflammatory response. PLoS One. 2013;8(3):e57874.
48. Rayavarapu S, Coley W, Nagaraju K. Endoplasmic reticulum stress in skeletal muscle homeostasis and disease. Curr Rheumatol Rep. 2012;14:238–43.
49. Hölttä-Vuori M, Salo VT, Ohsaki Y, Suster ML, Ikonen E. Alleviation of seipinopathy-related ER stress by triglyceride storage. Hum Mol Genet. 2013;22:1157–66.
50. Garfield AS, Chan WS, Dennis RJ, Ito D, Heisler LK, Rochford JJ. Neuroanatomical characterisation of the expression of the lipodystrophy and motor-neuropathy gene Bscl2 in adult mouse brain. PLoS One. 2012;7(9):e45790.
51. Callahan LA, Supinski GS. Hyperglycemia-induced diaphragm weakness is mediated by oxidative stress. Crit Care [Internet]. BioMed Central; 2014 [cited 2018 Aug 8];18:R88. Available from: http://www.ncbi.nlm.nih.gov/pubmed/24886999
52. Moro C, Bajpeyi S, Smith SR. Determinants of intramyocellular triglyceride turnover: implications for insulin sensitivity. Am J Physiol Metab [Internet]. 2008 [cited 2018 Aug 8];294:E203–E213. Available from: http://www.ncbi.nlm.nih.gov/pubmed/18003718

53. Asakawa H, Tokunaga K, Kawakami F. Relationship of leptin level with metabolic disorders and hypertension in Japanese type 2 diabetes mellitus patients. J Diabetes Complicat. 2001;15:57–62.
54. Jung C-H, Kim B-Y, Mok J-O, Kang S-K, Kim C-H. Association between serum adipocytokine levels and microangiopathies in patients with type 2 diabetes mellitus. J Diabetes Investig. 2014;5:333–9.
55. Rodríguez AJ, Nunes VDS, Mastronardi CA, Neeman T, Paz-Filho GJ, Jung C-H, et al. Association between circulating adipocytokine concentrations and microvascular complications in patients with type 2 diabetes mellitus: a systematic review and meta-analysis of controlled cross-sectional studies. J Diabetes Complicat. 2016;30:357–67.
56. Bahat G, Tufan A, Ozkaya H, Tufan F, Akpinar TS, Akin S, et al. Relation between hand grip strength, respiratory muscle strength and spirometric measures in male nursing home residents. Aging Male. 2014;17:136–40.
57. Efstathiou ID, Mavrou IP, Grigoriadis KE. Correlation between maximum inspiratory pressure and hand-grip force in healthy young and middle-age individuals. Respir Care. 2016;61:925–9.
58. Garg A, Stray-Gundersen J, Parsons D, Bertocci LA. Skeletal muscle morphology and exercise response in congenital generalized lipodystrophy. Diabetes Care. 2000;23:1545–50.
59. Ijzerman TH, Schaper NC, Melai T, Meijer K, Willems PJB, Savelberg HHCM. Lower extremity muscle strength is reduced in people with type 2 diabetes, with and without polyneuropathy, and is associated with impaired mobility and reduced quality of life. Diabetes Res Clin Pract Elsevier Ireland Ltd. 2012; 95:345–51.
60. Leenders M, Verdijk LB, van der Hoeven L, Adam JJ, van Kranenburg J, Nilwik R, et al. Patients with type 2 diabetes show a greater decline in muscle mass, muscle strength, and functional capacity with aging. J Am Med Dir Assoc Elsevier Ltd. 2013;14:585–92.
61. Tatsuya Nagai MD, Koichi Okita MD, Kazuya Yonezawa MD, Yutaka Yamada MD, Akiko Hanada MD, Mitsunori Ohtsubo MD, Noriteru Morita M, Murakami T, Nishijima H, Akira Kitabatake M. Comparisons of the skeletal muscle metabolic abnormalities in the arm and leg muscles of patients with chronic heart failure. Circ J. 2004;68(6):573–9.
62. Venturelli M, Saggin P, Muti E, Naro F, Cancellara L, Toniolo L, et al. In vivo and in vitro evidence that intrinsic upper- and lower-limb skeletal muscle function is unaffected by ageing and disuse in oldest-old humans. Acta Physiol [Internet]. 2015 [cited 2018 Aug 13];215:58–71. Available from: http://www.ncbi.nlm.nih.gov/pubmed/25965867
63. Brooks NE, Myburgh KH. Skeletal muscle wasting with disuse atrophy is multi-dimensional: the response and interaction of myonuclei, satellite cells and signaling pathways. Front Physiol [Internet]. Frontiers Media SA; 2014 [cited 2018 Aug 13];5:99. Available from: http://www.ncbi.nlm.nih.gov/pubmed/24672488
64. Orlando G, Balducci S, Bazzucchi I, Pugliese G, Sacchetti M. Muscle fatigability in type 2 diabetes. Diabetes Metab Res Rev [Internet]. 2017 [cited 2018 Aug 13];33:e2821. Available from: http://www.ncbi.nlm.nih.gov/pubmed/27155086
65. Corrêa APS, Ribeiro JP, Balzan FM, Mundstock L, Ferlin EL, Moraes RS. Inspiratory muscle training in type 2 diabetes with inspiratory muscle weakness. Med Sci Sports Exerc. 2011;43:1135–41.
66. Cauza E, Hanusch-Enserer U, Strasser B, Ludvik B, Metz-Schimmerl S, Pacini G, et al. The relative benefits of endurance and strength training on the metabolic factors and muscle function of people with type 2 diabetes mellitus. Arch Phys Med Rehabil. 2005;86:1527–33.

4

What have we learned from observational studies and clinical trials of mild to moderate COPD?

Miriam Barrecheguren[1], Cruz González[2] and Marc Miravitlles[1*]

Abstract

Chronic obstructive pulmonary disease (COPD) is a major cause of morbidity and mortality worldwide. It is well established that patients with mild to moderate disease represent the majority of patients with COPD, and patients with mild COPD already have measurable physiological impairment with increased morbidity and a higher risk of mortality compared with healthy non-smoking individuals. However, this subpopulation is both underdiagnosed and undertreated. In addition, most clinical trials include cohorts of patients with worse lung function and quality of life, which are very different from the milder patients usually seen in primary care.

Clinical trials have shown that mild-moderate COPD patients present an improvement in lung function after treatment with long-acting bronchodilators (LABD). Inhaled therapy has also shown benefits in terms of symptoms, health-related quality of life (HRQL) and exacerbation prevention in this population. Early intervention might have also a positive effect to prevent functional impairment. Nevertheless, there is scarce evidence from randomised clinical trials and real-life studies about the importance of pharmacological treatment in early stages of COPD to improve long-term outcomes. New concepts such as clinically important deterioration may help to investigate the impact of interventions on the natural history of the disease.

Keywords: COPD, Diagnosis, Epidemiology, Guidelines, Mild-moderate disease, Physical activity, Quality of life, Treatment

Background

Chronic obstructive pulmonary disease (COPD) is characterised by chronic airflow limitation, which is usually progressive. This disease is a major cause of morbidity and is currently the fourth leading cause of death worldwide [1, 2]. Although it is mostly related to exposure to tobacco smoking, patients exposed to biomass and pollution are also at risk of developing COPD.

The impact of COPD on each patient depends on the degree of airflow limitation, the severity of symptoms and comorbidities. The Global Initiative for Chronic Obstructive Lung Disease (GOLD) staging system categorises COPD into 4 severity stages (based on post-bronchodilator FEV1): stage I or mild, FEV1 ≥ 80% predicted; stage II or moderate, FEV1 ≥ 50% and < 80% predicted; stage III or severe, FEV1 ≥ 30% and < 50% predicted; and stage IV or very severe, FEV1 < 30% predicted [3]. As the disease progresses, there is greater restriction in daily activity with impaired quality of life and an increase of symptoms and exacerbations.

Nonetheless, the reduction in daily activity is already present in mild disease [4]. Since COPD is progressive, it is important to identify and treat patients at early stages in order to prevent further deterioration. Patients with mild (stage I) COPD already have measurable physiological impairment with increased morbidity and a higher risk of mortality compared with healthy non-smoking controls [5]. It is well established that patients with mild to moderate disease represent the majority of patients with COPD [6]. However, this subpopulation is both underdiagnosed and undertreated [7]. In addition, most clinical trials include cohorts of patients with worse lung function and worse quality of life, which are very different from those usually seen in primary care (PC) [8].

Encouragement of smoking cessation, in conjunction with management of symptoms and treating activity limitations and exacerbations by appropriate pharmacologic

* Correspondence: mmiravitlles@vhebron.net
[1]Pneumology Department, Hospital General Universitari Vall d'Hebron, CIBER de Enfermedades Respiratorias (CIBERES), P. de la Vall d'Hebron, 119-129, 08035 Barcelona, Spain
Full list of author information is available at the end of the article

and non-pharmacologic management at the earliest possible stage can positively affect the impact and progression of the disease [9]. In recent years, newer strategies and a growing number of new pharmacologic agents to treat COPD have also been introduced and show promise in improving the management of COPD [10]. New disease lung models to predict patient-specific drug deposition are also being developed in order to individualise therapy [11].

The aim of this article is to review the current evidence on the epidemiology, natural history and management of mild to moderate COPD (defined as an FEV1 > 50% predicted), highlighting the importance of treatment in earlier stages of the disease to try to prevent progression.

Epidemiology and natural history

The World Health Organization estimates that up to 328 million people around the world have COPD with a global prevalence of 1% [12]. This prevalence increases to 8–10% for individuals above 40 years old [13]. A recent systematic review aimed at estimating the prevalence of COPD across world regions among people aged 30 years or more found an overall prevalence of 10.7% in 1990, which increased to 11.7% in 2010 (14.3% in men and 7.6% in women) [14]. However, the prevalence of COPD varied widely among world regions, being the highest in the American region (14.1%), and the lowest in South East Asia (7.8%) [14]. This variability might be explained by differences in exposures and environmental and genetic factors. Indeed, according to the BOLD study, conducted at 12 sites around the world ($n = 8775$), the overall prevalence of COPD ranged from 11.4 to 26.1%; the prevalence of GOLD I being between 1.4–15.5% and the prevalence of GOLD II between 5.1 and 12.4% [6]. The Latin American Project for the Investigation of Obstructive Lung Disease (PLATINO) examined the prevalence of COPD in adults > 40 years of age and reported crude rates of GOLD stage I between 5.2 and 12.5% and GOLD II between 1.9 and 6.4% in five Latin American countries [15]. Another systematic review estimated a pooled prevalence for GOLD I of 9.8% (95% confidence interval (CI) 5.9–15.8) and of 5.5% for GOLD II (95%CI 3.3–9.0) [13].

In Europe, a systematic review by Atsou et al. [16] found a prevalence of COPD from 2.1 to 26.1% depending on the country, the age group and the methods used, the majority being GOLD I and II.

In Spain, the IBERPOC study conducted in 1997 showed a mean prevalence of COPD of 9.1% in subjects between 40 and 69 years of age [17]. Ten years later, the EPI-SCAN trial estimated a prevalence of 10.2% in subjects between 40 and 80 years of age [18]. A sub-analysis of these studies reported an increase of patients in milder stages over time, ranging from 38.3% for mild and 39.7% for moderate in the 1997 study to 85.6% for mild and 13.0% for moderate in the 2007 study [19]. Despite the wide variability of the results found in these population-based studies, the majority of the patients diagnosed had mild or moderate COPD, independently of the classification criteria used (Table 1).

One of the main concerns in COPD is underdiagnosis, which is more marked in early stages of the disease. It has been estimated that 73–78% of patients with GOLD stages I-II COPD remain undiagnosed [18]. Llordés et al.

Table 1 Prevalence of COPD GOLD I and II in some epidemiological studies of COPD

Study	Country	Prevalence (%)	
		GOLD I	GOLD II
Halbert et al. [13]	Worldwide	All 7.6 (6.0–9.5)	
		9.8 (5.9–15.8)	5.5 (3.3–9.0)
Buist AS, et al. (BOLD) [6]	Guangzhou	5.9%	7.6%
	Salzburg	16.3%	9.3%
	Cape town	6.5%	14.2%
	Reykjavik	9.7%	6.7%
	Krakow	14.4%	10.3%
	Manila	0.9%	11.3%
Menezes AM, et al. (PLATINO) [15]	Sao Paulo	10.1%	4.6%
	Santiago	11%	4.9%
	Mexico City	5.2%	1.9%
	Montevideo	12.5%	6.4%
	Caracas	6.4%	4.9%
Miravitlles M et al. (EPISCAN) [18]	Spain	All 10.2%	
		5.7%	3.9%

carried out a study to quantify the rate of underdiagnosis and the accuracy of COPD diagnosis in PC [20]. The study included 1738 subjects over the age of 45 with a history of smoking and found a rate of underdiagnosis of 73%. Recently, the same group performed a case-finding study in smokers or former smokers older than 40 years and found a prevalence of COPD of 26.7%, with the majority of patients being in GOLD stages I and II (42.1 and 49.1%, respectively) [21]. Up to 29% of patients with underdiagnosed COPD are asymptomatic [22], which contributes to late detection. In addition, patients often under-recognize the significance of respiratory symptoms, or they may accept that their symptoms are caused by smoking and ignore them rather than consult. Another cause for underdiagnosis might also be a deficient active search for COPD by health care professionals [21]. Some of the diagnostic initiatives that have been tested to improve COPD diagnosis are early detection programs [23] and other tools such as the use of peak-flow meters or mini spirometers [24], and screening questionnaires [21, 25].

In contrast to underdiagnosis, the definition of COPD based on FEV1/FVC instead of lower limit of normality (LLN) might lead to the overdiagnosis of mild COPD in individuals older than 65 years old [26].

The natural history of COPD is usually described by the rate of decline in lung function. The rate of decline in FEV1 in GOLD stages I-II is faster than in patients with stages III-IV [27–29]. Recently, in a cohort of smokers and ex-smokers, the COPD Gene group showed that functional alteration of the small airways measured by computerized tomography was significantly associated with a decline of FEV1, particularly in mild to moderate stages of the disease, and this association was also evident even before the detection of obstruction in the spirometry [30].

Exacerbations have a negative impact on the natural history of COPD, and their presence has been associated with a faster decline of FEV1, in particular in GOLD stagesI and II [31], in which the effect of each exacerbation on rate of FEV1 decline has been estimated to be − 23 ml/year in GOLD 1 and − 10 ml/year in GOLD 2 for any exacerbation, increasing up to -87 ml/year and -20 ml/year for GOLD 1 and 2 respectively for each severe exacerbation. Frequent exacerbators also have a worse quality of life and an increased risk of death [32–34]. Thus, the prevention of exacerbations should be a target for every COPD patient, irrespective of the severity of the disease.

Symptoms, quality of life and physical activity

COPD is defined by the presence of chronic respiratory symptoms, among which exertional dyspnoea, cough and sputum production are the most frequent [35]. Although more severe patients present a higher intensity of symptoms, there is not always a clear relationship between the degree of airflow obstruction and the presence and impact of respiratory symptoms in a patient with COPD [35, 36]. The observational study ASSESS characterised the symptoms of COPD during 24 h and assessed their relationship with patient-reported outcomes [37]. The analysis showed that the frequency of symptom occurrence was high for any degree of bronchial obstruction, with a prevalence of symptoms in GOLD stages I-II of 84–88%.

The presence of respiratory symptoms in patients with early COPD may modify long-term FEV1 decline and health-related quality of life. Symptomatic subjects with GOLD I COPD have a more rapid long-term decline in lung function than asymptomatic subjects [38, 39].

Despite referring fewer symptoms, mild COPD patients present exercise limitation that leads to changes in lifestyle and deconditioning, with an increasing burden of the disease beyond the degree of airflow obstruction. Indeed, around two thirds of GOLD stage II patients may have significant lung hyperinflation [40]. This hyperinflation is manifested as exertional dyspnoea, and furthermore, dyspnoea significantly contributes to a worse quality of life due to the high impact on their daily activities [41]. Even mild patients may have severe dyspnoea; a study carried out in 5299 subjects found that 7.5 and 18.3% of subjects with GOLD stages I and II, respectively, had a Medical Research Council (MRC) score ≥ 3 [42]. Similarly, a large European observational study conducted in 1817 patients in PC showed a high prevalence of symptoms in GOLD II patients (cough 76.6%, sputum 64.1%, and dyspnoea 67.3%). Moreover, 31% had a MRC dyspnoea grade ≥ 3. [43]. In a recent analysis carried out in 49,438 COPD patients, 50.2% were GOLD stage II, and 37.1% had a MRC dyspnoea grade ≥ 3, demonstrating that significant dyspnoea can be present in early stages of the disease [44]. In addition to being the most frequent symptom, dyspnoea has proven to be a better predictor of death at 5 years than airway obstruction in patients with COPD [45].

Concerning quality of life, the study by Jones et al. [43] using the St. George's Respiratory Questionnaire [SGRQ] and the 12-Item Short Form Survey [SF-12] demonstrated that GOLD I and II patients had an impaired quality of life compared with healthy individuals. These results are similar to those obtained in the EPI-SCAN study, which observed a significant impairment of health-related quality of life in all severities of COPD, even GOLD I and II and undiagnosed COPD patients [18].

Physical activity significantly deteriorates in patients with COPD as the disease progresses [46], and the reduction in physical activity is one of the best predictors for COPD survival [47]. In addition, physical inactivity is strongly associated with the presence of comorbidities [48]. In contrast, regular physical activity reduces hospitalisation and the risk of death in COPD [49]. However, even in early stages of the disease, most patients with COPD spend less time walking (and walking more slowly) and standing, and more time sitting and lying compared with sedentary healthy elderly subjects [50].

Treatment of mild to moderate COPD

The main objectives for the treatment of COPD are the reduction of symptoms, the reduction of frequency and severity of the exacerbations and the improvement of prognosis [3, 51]. Non-pharmacological treatment, especially smoking cessation, is essential for every COPD patient and ha sproven to be the most efficient and cost-effective therapeutic strategy [3, 51]. Smoking cessation slows the loss of lung function and improves survival. Indeed, the benefits may be more evident in milder patients than in individuals with a more established disease [52]. Psychotherapy might be beneficial in addition to exercise and medication. Other non-pharmacological approaches include regular physical activity, an adequate nutrition status, management of comorbidities, and vaccination against pneumococcal and influenza viruses is also recommended for all patients. Pulmonary rehabilitation has shown to improve symptoms, exercise tolerance and health-related quality of life, and to reduce the risk of morbidity from acute exacerbations of COPD [53]. Both a meta-analysis and a systematic review concluded that patients with mild to moderate COPD also benefit from short- and long-term rehabilitation [54, 55]. Hence, considering the benefits of physical activity, patients with COPD should be encouraged to increase their level of exercise from early stages.

Real-life experience of treatment of mild-moderate COPD

Mild COPD patients are frequently followed in a PC setting, and they are usually not included in randomised controlled trials (RCT) [8], therefore, database studies could provide interesting data on the management of these subjects. An analysis of real-life prescribing patterns in primary care in the UK described the treatment of 24,957 COPD patients among which half were GOLD II [56]. Up to 17.7% did not receive any treatment for their disease, and 14% were treated only with short-acting β-agonists (SABA) despite being symptomatic. In fact, two thirds of the untreated patients referred a COPD Assessment Test (CAT) score > 10, while 22.7% had a modified MRC ≥ 2, consistent with highly symptomatic disease. Moreover, a high percentage of treated patients remained symptomatic: 36.6% of patients had a modified MRC ≥ 2, and 76.4% had a CAT score ≥ 10 with their current treatment regimen.

In a similar study that included 7881 newly diagnosed COPD patients in PC, 54.3% had GOLD stage II at the time of diagnosis. Initially, 37.9% were treated only with short-acting bronchodilators (SABD) or did not receive any inhaled treatment, while only one third of the patients were prescribed a long-acting bronchodilator (LABD), alone or in combination with inhaled corticosteroids (ICS) [57]. Raluy-Callado et al. [58] described the treatment patterns in a population of prevalent and incident COPD patients, of whom 53.5 and 61% were GOLD stage II, respectively. The authors found that almost half of the incident patients with FEV1 > 50% and infrequent exacerbations were prescribed monotherapy, being SABD the most frequent (29.3%) [58]. Similar results have been observed in other countries. In Catalonia (Spain), a recent study showed that 55.2% of the patients diagnosed in PC had GOLD stage II COPD. After the diagnosis of the disease, GOLD II patients frequently remained untreated (28.1%) or were treated only with a SABD (18.5%) [59].

The reasons for undertreatment are varied. COPD patients often do not seek medical help until the symptoms interfere with their daily life, and asymptomatic patients are also less likely to be identified and to receive treatment. In addition, some patients tend to reduce their physical activity even at early stages of the disease, which might help to minimize symptom perception. Moreover, mild COPD patients are more likely to experience unreported exacerbations [60], which may contribute to an underestimation of the impact of COPD. Another possible reason for undertreatment is a lack of awareness of guideline recommendations.

Clinical trials of pharmacological treatment of mild to moderate COPD

Clinical trials usually include patients with moderate or severe COPD; hence, the data available on the benefits of inhaled treatment in mild COPD patients are limited. This is in contrast with the distribution of severity in a real-life setting, with up to 50% of the COPD patients controlled in PC being GOLD stage II [16, 59]. However, there is some evidence of the efficacy of treatments in GOLD stage II COPD patients derived from studies on mild-moderate COPD and subgroup analysis of RCTs (Table 2).

Lung function

The effects of the treatments are measured by different outcomes: lung function, dyspnoea, quality of life and exacerbations. In terms of lung function, in a 12-week placebo-controlled study conducted in Germany, treatment with tiotropium showed a significant increase of trough FEV1 (+ 79 ml), which was even more pronounced in COPD patients with a FEV1 between 50 and

Table 2 Results in GOLD stage II COPD patients in randomised clinical trials

Study	Treatment	GOLD stage II patients (n)	Results
Decramer M, et al. UPLIFT study [66]	Tiotropium vs. placebo	2739	- Lower rate of decline of mean postbronchodilator FEV1 - improvement in the SGRQ - increase in the time to first exacerbation
Beeh KM, et al. [61]	Tiotropium vs. placebo	586	- increment in trough FEV1
Duser D, et al. Mistral study [68]	Tiotropium vs. placebo	426	- reduction in the number of exacerbations
Freeman D, et al. SPRUCE study [62]	Tiotropium	185	- improvement in trough FEV1 - reduction in the number of exacerbations
Singh D, et al. OTEMTO study [64]	Tiotropium/olodaterol vs. tiotropium or placebo	1042	- improvement in the trough FEV1 - improvement in symptoms and the SGRQ
Vincken W, et al. [88]	Tiotropium vs. ipratropium	535	- improvement in trough FEV1 - improvement in PEFR, salbutamol use, TDI, and SGRQ - reduction in the number of exacerbations
Casburi R, et al. [89]	Tiotropium vs. placebo	921	- improvement in trough FEV1 - reduction in dyspnoea - improvement in health status scores - reduction in the number of exacerbations
Jenkins C, et al. TORCH study [63]	SFC vs. placebo	2156	- reduction in the risk of death - improvements in FEV1 - reduction in the annual rate of exacerbations
Jones PW, et al. ISOLDE study [90]	Fluticasone propionate vs. placebo	391 (mild) 359 (moderate-severe)	- reduction in the number of exacerbations (less in mild disease)
Vestbo J, et al. SUMMIT study [77]	Fluticasone fuorate vs. placebo vs. vilanterol vs. combination therapy	4135 vs 4121 vs 4118	- reduction in the rate of decline in FEV1 - reduction in the rate of moderate and severe exacerbation
Vogelmeier CF, et al. CRYSTAL study [65]	Indacaterol/glycopyrronium vs. LABA/ICS vs. LABA or LAMA	811 vs. 269 811 vs. 268	- greater improvement on trough FEV1 - greater improvement in dyspnoea - greater improvement in health status - lower rescue medication use
Wedzicha JA, et al. [69]	Indacaterol/glycopyrronium vs. SFC	1680 vs. 1682	- superiority in reducing annual rate of exacerbations - longer time to the first exacerbation

FEV1 forced expiratory volume in one second, *ICS* inhaled corticosteroids, *LABA* long-acting β2-agonist, *LAMA* long-acting muscarinic antagonist, *PEFR* peak expiratory flow rate, *SFC* inhaled salmeterol plus fluticasone propionate, *SGRQ* St George's Respiratory Questionnaire, *TDI* transition dyspnoea index

70% (trough FEV1 + 113 ml) [61]. In a PC setting, GOLD I and II patients also showed a trend to improving trough FEV1 with tiotropium compared with placebo after 12 weeks [effect size 40 ml (95%CI -30, 100)] [62].

The efficacy of the inhaled salmeterol/fluticasone combination (SFC) in patients with mild COPD is limited. A post hoc analysis of the TORCH study, which included 2156 subjects with FEV1 > 50% showed an increase in FEV1 in GOLD II patients treated with 101 ml of SFC compared with placebo [63].

The combination of a long-acting antimuscarinic agent (LAMA) and a long-acting beta-2 agonist (LABA) (tiotropium/olodaterol) has also shown to improve trough FEV1 compared to placebo (149 ml versus – 10 ml, respectively) in GOLD stage II patients [64]. In the CRYSTAL study, which included 2160 patients with moderate COPD, the effect of the LABA/LAMA indacaterol/glycopyrronium was superior to LABA/ICS in trough FEV1 at week 12 (treatment difference + 71 ml) and to LABA or LAMA monotherapies (difference + 101 ml) [65].

Dyspnoea

Inhaled therapy has also shown benefits in GOLD II patients in terms of symptoms. Treatment with tiotropium/olodaterol improved dyspnoea measured by the Transition Dyspnea Index (TDI) compared to placebo (1.67*versus* 0.39) [64]. The CRYSTAL study also showed superior improvement in the total TDI score with indacaterol/glycopyrronium versus LABA/ICS (difference 1.10 units) and versus LABA or LAMA (difference 1.26 units) in GOLD stage II COPD patients [65].

Quality of life

Regarding quality of life, in the UPLIFT study, the authors observed an improvement in health status measured by the SGRQ at all time points in the tiotropium group ($p \leq 0.006$ for all time points) [66]. In the TORCH study, GOLD II COPD patients also experienced a better health status when treated with SFC in comparison with placebo (change in the SGRQ – 2.3), although the minimal clinically important difference was not reached [67]. The combination of tiotropium/olodaterol showed a greater improvement, with a change from baseline in the SGRQ score of – 4.7 compared with – 2.2 in the tiotropium arm, and – 0.7 in the placebo arm in GOLD II patients [64].

Exacerbations

The effects of treatment on exacerbation prevention in moderate COPD have been demonstrated in several studies. Tiotropium has shown to prevent exacerbations in patients with less severe COPD. In the MISTRAL study, the number of exacerbations in the subgroup of patients with a FEV1 ≥ 50% was lower for those receiving tiotropium compared to placebo (1.21 versus 1.97, respectively; $p < 0.01$) [68]. The UPLIFT study also showed that the time to the first exacerbation and the time to exacerbation resulting in hospital admission were longer in the tiotropium group than in the control group in the GOLD II subgroup (hazard ratio 0.82, 95% CI 0.75–0.90, and 0.74, 0.62–0.88, respectively) [66]. In PC, patients with FEV1 > 50% that received tiotropium in addition to their usual treatment were less likely to have ≥1 exacerbation during follow-up compared to the placebo group (6.8% versus 16.8%) [62].

Treatment with SFC has also demonstrated to reduce the annual rate of exacerbations by 31% in GOLD stage II COPD patients compared with placebo (mean of 0.57/year versus 0.82/year, respectively) [68]. The combination LABA/LAMA is also effective in reducing exacerbations. In fact, the superiority of indacaterol/glycopyrronium over monotherapies and LABA/ICS was demonstrated in several phase III clinical trials, including the FLAME study, which showed that this combination was superior to SFC in reducing the annual rate of exacerbations, although in patients with moderate COPD the difference did not reach significance, probably due to an insufficient sample size of patients with this level of severity (HR 0.93 (0.82–1.06)) [69].

These studies suggest that in general, treatment of mild to moderate COPD should be started with one or a combination of two LABD. The only exception would be asthma-COPD overlap (ACO) patients, who usually have more respiratory symptoms, but especially a better response to ICS [70].

Impact of early treatment on the natural history of COPD

Since the decline in lung function is faster in early stages of the disease, early intervention is required to prevent functional impairment [71]. However, there are only a few large-scale clinical trials on long-term interventions in patients in early stages of COPD. The Lung Health Study, carried out in 3926 smokers with mild to moderate airway obstruction for a period of 5 years showed that participants who stopped smoking experienced an improvement in FEV1 in the year after quitting (average of 47 ml or 2%), and that the subsequent rate of decline in FEV1 among sustained quitters was half the rate of that of continuing smokers (31 ml versus 62 ml, respectively), and comparable to that of never-smokers [72]. A post hoc analysis of the UPLIFT study that included only GOLD II patients observed that the rate of decline for postbronchodilator FEV1 was lower in the tiotropium group than in the control group (43 ml per year [SE 2] vs. 49 ml per year [SE 2], $p = 0.024$) [66]. Another sub-analysis from UPLIFT assessed the efficacy of treatment with tiotropium in patients without previous maintenance treatment (naïve patients) and included a majority of GOLD II (60%). The annual FEV1 decline was slower in the tiotropium group (35 ml (SD 3) in the tioptropium arm vs. 45 ml (SD 4) in the placebo arm) [73].

More recently, in a randomised placebo-controlled trial which included 841 mild to moderate COPD patients, Zhou et al. [74] observed that the annual FEV1 decline in early stage COPD was lower in patients treated with tiotropium (29 ml ±5) than in the placebo group (51 ml ± 6; difference 22 ml (95% CI 6 to 37). In the TORCH study, SFC also showed a reduction in the rate of decline in FEV1 versus placebo in the GOLD II group (difference 16 ml/year, 95% CI: 0, 32) [63]. These results were confirmed in the SUMMIT study, in which GOLD II patients also had a lower rate of decline in FEV1 in the fluticasone furoate/vilanterol arm compared to placebo (38 ml (2.4) vs. -46 ml (2.5) respectively, $p = 0.019$) [75]. These results should be considered in the context of both studies failing to reach their primary outcome of mortality (Table 3).

With regard to mortality, the TORCH study showed a 33% reduction in the risk of death in GOLD stage II COPD patients (HR 0.67; 95% CI: 0.45, 0.98) with SFC compared with placebo [63]. In UPLIFT, there was a non significant reduction in mortality with tiotropium compared to placebo (hazard ratio [HR], 0.89; 95% CI, 0.79 to 1.02, $p = 0.09$) [76]. More recently, treatment with fluticasone furoate/vilanterol showed no effect on mortality in COPD patients with FEV1 > 50% and cardiovascular risk (HR 0·88 [95% CI 0·74–1·04]; 12% relative reduction; $p = 0.137$) [77].

Table 3 Impact of early pharmacological treatment on rate of FEV1 decline

Study	Participants	Follow-up	Intervention	Outcome
Scanlon PD et al. [72]	3926 smokers	5 years	Quitting smoking	Improvement in FEV1 (47 ml or 2%)
Decreamer M, et al. [66]	2375 GOLD II	4 years	Tiotropium vs. placebo	Reduction in rate of FEV1 decline (43 ml/year vs. 49 ml/year, $p = 0.024$)
Troosters T et al. [73]	120 GOLD II	4 years	Tiotropium vs. placebo	Reduction in rate of FEV1 decline (35 ml vs. 45 ml)
Zhou Y et al. [74]	841 GOLD I and II	2 years	Tiotropium vs. placebo	Reduction in rate of FEV1 decline (29 ml vs. 51 ml)
Jenkins CR et al. [63]	2156 GOLD II	3 years	SFC vs. placebo	Reduction in rate of FEV1 decline (difference 16 ml/year, 95% CI 0,32)
Calverley PMA, et al. [75]	6981 GOLD II	15 to 44 months	SFC vs. placebo	Reduction in rate of FEV1 decline (38 ml vs −46 ml, $p = 0.019$))

FEV1 forced expiratory volume in one second, *SFC* salmeterol/fluticasone fixed dose combination

Deterioration prevention

Improvement of clinical and/or spirometric parameters are the endpoints routinely assessed to evaluate the effects of treatments in COPD in most RCTs. However, many patients do not improve and suffer progressive deterioration of their disease. Taking into account that deterioration of lung function, exacerbation frequency, and health status are important parameters to reflect the impact of treatment on COPD management [32, 78–81], the evaluation of composite endpoints may be more sensitive than individual measures to the effects of therapeutic interventions. One of the proposed composite endpoints is the so-called clinically important deterioration (CID). This endpoint allows assessing the rate of deterioration of lung function, exacerbation rate and/or health status of the patient and evaluates the effects of treatment. In addition, this composite endpoint is consistent with the current GOLD strategy, which recommends that lung function, COPD exacerbation risk, and health status are considered when assessing disease progression and severity [3].

A post hoc pooled analysis of three RCTs assessed short-term CID in maintenance-naïve patients with COPD receiving the combination of umeclidinium and vilanterol(LAMA/LABA) compared with tiotropium for 6 months [82].The results showed that early use of dual-bronchodilator therapy has superior efficacy in lung function and may reduce the risk of short-term CID compared to monotherapy in symptomatic patients with COPD [82].

Another analysis described the effect of the combination of another LAMA/LABA, indacaterol/glycopirronium versus both tiotropium or SFC on the prevention of CID using patient data from three large phase 3 RCTs [83]. The study used two different definitions for CID: definition 1 was a composite of ≥100 ml decrease in FEV1, a ≥ 4-unit increase in SGRQ, and a moderate to severe COPD exacerbation, while for definition 2, the FEV1 component was replaced by a ≥ 1-unit decrease in the TDI. This analysis confirmed the utility of the CID endpoint as a measurement of COPD worsening in patients with moderate to severe COPD and using this endpoint the analysis showed that the combination of indacaterol/glycopyrronium offers significant benefits over treatment with a LAMA or a LABA/ICS both in terms of the incidence and time to CID.

Another post hoc analysis evaluated CID using data from two randomised phase III studies that assessed the efficacy and safety of the combination of aclidinium/formoterol in patients with COPD [84]. The results demonstrated that this combination reduced the risk of a first CID, providing greater airway stability, and therefore, fewer deteriorations in lung function, dyspnoea, risk of exacerbations, and health status compared with placebo or monotherapies.

Current treatment guidelines

A recent review of COPD treatment guidelines published in Europe and Russia in the last 7 years found that although there were differences in some recommended treatments, there was a general agreement on treatment goals and the use of LABD as the cornerstone of COPD treatment [85].

The GOLD strategy establishes pharmacologic treatment algorithms by groups of different risk and intensity of symptoms. For patients in GOLD group A (low risk and low symptom burden), a bronchodilator should be offered to reduce breathlessness. For patients in GOLD group B (low risk and high symptom burden), the preferred initial therapy should be a LABD. If the symptoms persist, therapy with two bronchodilators may be considered [3].

The National Institute for Health and Care Excellence (NICE) guidelines updated in 2010 recommended that patients with FEV1 > 50% predicted with exacerbations or persistent airflow obstruction should be offered LABDs, and in the case of persistence of symptoms, patients should receive either LABA/ICS or LAMA/LABA [86].

The Spanish COPD guidelines (GesEPOC) were developed based on risk stratification and clinical phenotypes [51]. They use an easy risk classification (low or high risk) based on lung function, dyspnoea grade, and history of exacerbations. The four clinical phenotypes identified were: non-exacerbator, ACO, exacerbator with emphysema, and exacerbator with chronic bronchitis. However, they only recommend the determination of clinical phenotype in high-risk patients. Pharmacological recommendations for low-risk patients consist of LABD without any type of anti-inflammatory treatment, and the initial treatment for most high risk patients consists of LAMA/LABA [51].

The newest position statement of the Canadian Thoracic Society in COPD gives more weight to symptoms and exacerbations when it comes to increasing or decreasing therapy. In symptomatic patients with stable COPD without frequent exacerbations, treatment should be started with a LABD, and if experiencing persistent or increased dyspnoea, exercise intolerance, and/or reduced health status despite the use of monotherapy, patients should be considered for "step up" treatment with a LAMA/LABA. In patients with stable COPD experiencing exacerbations despite the use of LAMA or LABA monotherapy, "step up" treatment with inhaled LAMA/LABA should be considered. If a patient is still experiencing exacerbations despite the use of LAMA/LABA, "step up" treatment with LAMA plus LABA/ICS can be considered. Since inhaled triple or dual therapy may not prove to be superior in every patient, the notion of "step down" treatment may be a consideration in some patients. For patients with suspected ACO, a combination of LABA/ICS is recommended [87]. Figure 1 presents a treatment algorithm for mild-moderate COPD patients.

Conclusions

Although patients with mild to moderate disease represent the majority of patients with COPD, most studies and in particular RCTs are focused on severe COPD patients. Moreover, mild to moderate patients tend to be underdiagnosed and undertreated, affecting their prognosis and quality of life. Since COPD is progressive, it is important to identify and treat patients at early stages in order to prevent further deterioration, even more considering that patients with mild COPD already have measurable physiological impairment that leads to changes in lifestyle and deconditioning.

Smoking cessation, management of symptoms and treating activity limitations and exacerbations by appropriate pharmacologic and non-pharmacologic management at the earliest possible stage could positively affect the impact and progression of the disease, symptoms, exacerbations, and quality of life. These benefits may be more evident in milder patients than in COPD individuals with a more established disease. Non-pharmacological management includes regular physical activity, pulmonary rehabilitation, an adequate nutrition status, and management of comorbidities, and vaccination against pneumococcal and influenza viruses is also recommended for all patients. On the other hand, early treatment with one LABD or the combination of two bronchodilators has shown to produce a slightly greater

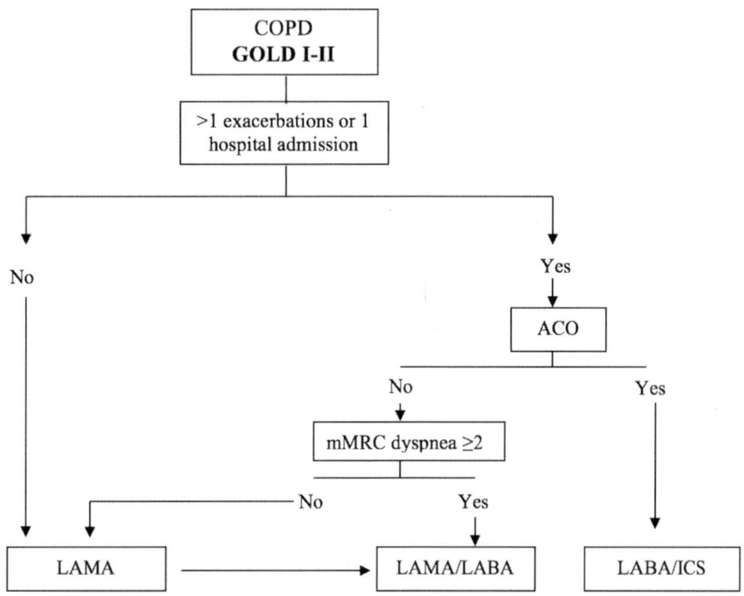

Fig. 1 Proposal of treatment algorithm for the management of GOLD 1–2 COPD patients. COPD: chronic obstructive pulmonary disease; ACO: asthma-COPD overlap; LAMA: long acting anti muscarinic; LABA: long acting b-2 agonists; ICS: inhaled corticosteroids

improvement in lung function in patients with GOLD stage II than in those with more advanced stages of COPD, and this improvement was associated with an improvement of symptoms, health-related quality of life and a reduction in the risk of exacerbations.

New studies suggest that early treatment with dual bronchodilators may prevent disease deterioration, but this interesting concept should be tested in large clinical trials specifically designed for this objective.

Abbreviations

CAT: COPD Assessment Test; CID: Clinically important deterioration; COPD: Chronic obstructive pulmonary disease; FEV1: Forced expiratory volume in the first second; GOLD: Global Initiative for Chronic Obstructive Lung Disease; ICS: Inhaled corticosteroids; LABA: Long-acting β-2 agonist; LABD: Long-acting bronchodilator; LAMA: Long-acting antimuscarinic agent; MRC: Medical Research Council; PC: Primary care; RCT: Randomised clinical trial; SABA: Short-acting β-agonists; SABD: Short-acting bronchodilators; SF-12: 12-item short form survey; SFC: Salmeterol/fluticasone combination; SGRQ: St. George's Respiratory Questionnaire; TDI: Transition dyspnoea index

Acknowledgements

Miriam Barrecheguren is the recipient of a Rio Hortega contract in the 2017 Strategic Action Health Call from the Instituto de Salud Carlos III for the years 2018-2019.

Funding

This work has been funded by an unrestricted grant from Laboratorios Esteve S.A. (Barcelona, Spain). The funding body did not participate in any stage of the preparation of the manuscript.

Authors' contributions

MM, MB and CG have contributed equally to the development of the manuscript. All authors read and approved the final manuscript.

Competing interests

Marc Miravitlles has received speaker fees from Boehringer Ingelheim, Chiesi, Cipla, Menarini, Rovi, Grifols and Novartis, and consulting fees from Boehringer Ingelheim, Chiesi, GlaxoSmithKline, Gebro Pharma, CSL Behring, Novartis and Grifols.

Cruz González has received speaker fees from Novartis, Astra, Boehringer Ingelheim, Chiesi, Menarini, and Rovi, and consulting fees from Astra, Boehringer Ingelheim, Novartis and Esteve.

Miriam Barrecheguren has received speaker fees from Grifols and Menarini, and consulting fees from GlaxoSmithKline.

Author details

[1]Pneumology Department, Hospital General Universitari Vall d'Hebron, CIBER de Enfermedades Respiratorias (CIBERES), P. de la Vall d'Hebron, 119-129, 08035 Barcelona, Spain. [2]Pneumology Department, Hospital Clínic Universitari, Valencia, Spain.

References

1. Decramer M, Janssens W, Miravitlles M. Chronic obstructive pulmonary disease. Lancet. 2012;379(9823):1341–51.
2. Buist AS, McBurnie MA, Vollmer WM, Gillespie S, Burney P, Mannino DM, et al. International variation in the prevalence of COPD (the BOLD study): a population-based prevalence study. Lancet. 2007;370(9589):741–50.
3. Vogelmeier CF, Criner GJ, Martínez FJ, Anzueto A, Barnes PJ, Bourbeau J, et al. Global strategy for the diagnosis, management, and prevention of chronic obstructive lung disease 2017 report: GOLD executive summary. Arch Bronconeumol. 2017;53:128–49.
4. Van Remoortel H, Hornikx M, Demeyer H, Langer D, Burtin C, Decramer M, et al. Daily physical activity in subjects with newly diagnosed COPD. Thorax. 2013;68(10):962–3.
5. Elbehairy AF, Ciavaglia CE, Webb KA, Guenette JA, Jensen D, Mourad SM, et al. Pulmonary gas exchange abnormalities in mild chronic obstructive pulmonary disease. Implications for dyspnea and exercise intolerance. Am J Respir Crit Care Med. 2015;191(12):1384–94.
6. Buist AS, Vollmer WM, McBurnie MA. Worldwide burden of COPD in high- and low-income countries. Part I. the burden of obstructive lung disease (BOLD) initiative. Int J Tuberc Lung Dis. 2008;12(7):703–8.
7. Bernd L, Joan BS, Michael S, Bernhard K, Lowie EV, Louisa G, et al. Determinants of underdiagnosis of COPD in national and international surveys. Chest. 2015;148(4):971–85.
8. Kruis AL, Ställberg B, Jones RC, Tsiligianni IG, Lisspers K, van der Molen T, et al. Primary care COPD patients compared with large pharmaceutically-sponsored COPD studies: an UNLOCK validation study. PLoS One. 2014;9(3): e90145.
9. Maltais F, Dennis N, Chan CK. Rationale for earlier treatment in COPD: a systematic review of published literature in mild-to-moderate COPD. COPD. 2013;10(1):79–103.
10. Narsingam S, Bozarth AL, Abdeljalil A. Updates in the management of stable chronic obstructive pulmonary disease. Postgrad Med. 2015;127(7):758–70.
11. Kannan RR, Singh N, Przekwas A. A quasi-3D compartmental multi-scale approach to detect and quantify diseased regional lung constriction using spirometry data. Int J Numer Method Biomed Eng. 2018;34:e2973.
12. Vos T, Flaxman AD, Naghavi M, Lozano R, Michaud C, Ezzati M, et al. Years lived with disability (YLDs) for 1160 sequelae of 289 diseases and injuries 1990-2010: a systematic analysis for the global burden of disease study 2010. Lancet. 2012;380:2163–96.
13. Halbert RJ, Natoli JL, Gano A, Badamqarav E, Buist AS, Mannino DM. Global burden of COPD: systematic review and meta-analysis. Eur Respir J. 2006;28: 523–32.
14. Adeloye D, Chua S, Lee C, Basquill C, Papana A, Theodoratou E, et al. Global and regional estimates of COPD prevalence: systematic review and meta-analysis. J Glob Health. 2015;5(2):020415.
15. Menezes AM, Perez-Padilla R, Jardim JR, Muiño A, López MV, Valdivia G, et al. Chronic obstructive pulmonary disease in five Latin American cities (the PLATINO study): a prevalence study. Lancet. 2005;366(9500):1875–81.
16. Atsou K, Chouaid C, Hejblum G. Variability of the chronic obstructive pulmonary disease key epidemiological data in Europe: systematic review. BMC Med. 2011;9:7.
17. Peña VS, Miravitlles M, Gabriel R, Jiménez-Ruiz CA, Villasante C, Masa JF, et al. Geographic variations in prevalence and underdiagnosis of COPD: results of the IBERPOC multicentre epidemiological study. Chest. 2000; 118(4):981–9.
18. Miravitlles M, Soriano JB, García-Río F, Munoz L, Durán-Tauleria E, Sánchez G, et al. Prevalence of COPD in Spain: impact of undiagnosed COPD on quality of life and daily life activities. Thorax. 2009;64(10):863–8.
19. Soriano JB, Ancochea J, Miravitlles M, García-Río F, Duran-Tauleria E, Muñoz L, et al. Recent trends in COPD prevalence in Spain: a repeated cross-sectional survey 1997-2007. Eur Respir J. 2010;36(4):758–65.
20. Llordés M, Jaén Á, Almagro P, Heredia JL, Morera J, Soriano JB, et al. Prevalence, risk factors and diagnostic accuracy of COPD among smokers in primary care. COPD. 2015;12(4):404–12.
21. Llordés M, Zurdo E, Jaén Á, Vázquez I, Pastrana L, Miravitlles M. Which is the best screening strategy for COPD among smokers in primary care? COPD. 2017;14(1):43–51.
22. Almagro P, Soriano J. Under diagnosis in COPD: a battle worth fighting. Lancet Respir Med. 2017;5(5):367–8.
23. Ulrik CS, Lokke A, Dahl R, Dollerup J, Hansen G, Cording PH, Andersen KK. Early detection of COPD in general practice. Int J COPD. 2011;6:123–7.
24. Thorat YT, Salvo SS, Kodgule RR. Peak flow meter with a questionnaire and mini-spirometer to help detect asthma and COPD in real-life clinical practice: a cross-sectional study. NPJ Prim Care Respir Med. 2017;27:32.

25. Price DB, Tinkelman DG, Halbert RJ, Nordyke RJ, Isonaka S, Nonikov D, et al. Symptom-based questionnaire for identifying COPD in smokers. Respir Int Rev Thorac Dis. 2006;73(3):285–95.
26. Karrasch S, Bruske I, Smith MP, Thorand B, Huth C, Ladwig KH, et al. What is the impact of different spirometric criteria on the prevalence of spirometrically defined COPD and its comorbidities? Results from the population-based KORA study. Int J Chron Obstruct Pulmon Dis. 2016;11:1881–94.
27. Lung Health Study Research Group, Wise R, Connett J, Weinmann G, Scanlon P, Skeans M. Effect of inhaled triamcinolone on the decline in pulmonary function in chronic obstructive pulmonary disease. N Engl J Med. 2000;343(26):1902–9.
28. Tantucci C, Modina D. Lung function decline in COPD. Int J Chron Obstruct Pulmon Dis. 2012;7:95–9.
29. Kim J, Yoon HI, Oh YM, Lim SY, Lee JH, Kim TH, et al. Lung function decline rates according to GOLD group in patients with chronic obstructive pulmonary disease. Int J Chron Obstruct Pulmon Dis. 2015;10:1819–27.
30. Bhatt SP, Soler X, Wang X, Murray S, Anzueto AR, Beaty TH, et al. Association between functional small airway disease and FEV1 decline in chronic obstructive pulmonary disease. Am J Respir Crit Care Med. 2016;194(2):178–84.
31. Dransfield MT, Kunisaki KM, Strand MJ, Anzueto A, Bhatt SP, Bowler RP, et al. Acute exacerbations and lung function loss in smokers with and without chronic obstructive pulmonary disease. Am J Respir Crit Care Med. 2017; 195(3):324–30.
32. Donaldson GC, Seemungal TA, Bhowmik A, Wedzicha JA. Relationship between exacerbation frequency and lung function decline in chronic obstructive pulmonary disease. Thorax. 2002;57(10):847–52.
33. Miravitlles M, Ferrer M, Pont A, Zalacain R, Álvarez-Sala JL, Masa F, et al. Effect of exacerbations on quality of life in patients with chronic obstructive pulmonary disease: a 2 year follow up study. Thorax. 2004;59(5):387–95.
34. Soler-Cataluña JJ, Martínez-García MA, Roman Sánchez P, Salcedo E, Navarro M, Ochando R. Severe acute exacerbations and mortality in patients with chronic obstructive pulmonary disease. Thorax. 2005;60(11):925–31.
35. Miravitlles M, Ribera A. Understanding the impact of symptoms on the burden of COPD. Respir Res. 2017;18:67.
36. Miravitlles M, Menezes A, Lopez Varela MV, Casas A, Ugalde L, Ramírez-Venegas A, et al. Prevalence and impact of respiratory symptoms in a population of patients with COPD in Latin America: the LASSYC observational study. Respir Med. 2018;134:62–9.
37. Miravitlles M, Worth H, Soler Cataluña JJ, Price D, De Benedetto F, Roche N, et al. Observational study to characterise 24-hour COPD symptoms and their relationship with patient-reported outcomes: results from the ASSESS study. Respir Res. 2014;15:122.
38. Bridevaux PO, Gerbase MW, Probst-Hensch NM, Schindler C, Gaspoz JM, Rochat T. Long-term decline in lung function, utilisation of care and quality of life in modified GOLD stage 1 COPD. Thorax. 2008;63(9):768–74.
39. Rennard SI, Drummond MB. Early chronic obstructive pulmonary disease: definition, assessment, and prevention. Lancet. 2015;385(9979):1778–88.
40. Chen C, Jian W, Gao Y, Xie Y, Song Y, Zheng J. Early COPD patients with lung hyperinflation associated with poorer lung function but better bronchodilator responsiveness. Int J Chron Obstruct Pulmon Dis. 2016;11: 2519–26.
41. Anzueto A, Miravitlles M. Pathophysiology of dyspnea in COPD. Postgrad Med. 2017;129(3):366–74.
42. Fabricius P, Lokke A, Marott JL, Vestbo J, Lange P. Prevalence of COPD in Copenhagen. Respir Med. 2011;105(3):410–7.
43. Jones PW, Brusselle G, Dal Negro RW, Ferrer M, Kardos P, Levy ML, et al. Health-related quality of life in patients by COPD severity within primary care in Europe. Respir Med. 2011;105(1):57–66.
44. Mullerova H, Lu C, Li H, Tabberer M. Prevalence and burden of breathlessness in patients with chronic obstructive pulmonary disease managed in primary care. PLoS One. 2014;9(1):e85540.
45. Nishimura K, Izumi T, Tsukino M, Oga T. Dyspnea is a better predictor of 5-year survival than airway obstruction in patients with COPD. Chest. 2002; 121(5):1434–40.
46. Ramón MA, Esquinas C, Barrecheguren M, Pleguezuelos E, Molina J, Quintano JA, et al. Self-reported daily walking time in COPD: relationship with relevant clinical and functional characteristics. Int J Chron Obstruct Pulmon Dis. 2017;12:1173–81.
47. Waschki B, Kirsten A, Holz O, Muller KC, Meyer T, Watz H, et al. Physical activity is the strongest predictor of all-cause mortality in patients with COPD: a prospective cohort study. Chest. 2011;140(2):331–42.
48. Van Remoortel H, Hornikx M, Langer D, Burtin C, Everaerts S, Verhamme P, et al. Risk factors and comorbidities in the preclinical stages of chronic obstructive pulmonary disease. Am J Respir Crit Care Med. 2014;189(1):30–8.
49. García-Aymerich J, Lange P, Benet M, Schnohr P, Anto JM. Regular physical activity reduces hospital admission and mortality in chronic obstructive pulmonary disease: a population based cohort study. Thorax. 2006;61(9):772–8.
50. Pitta F, Troosters T, Spruit MA, Probst VS, Decramer M, Gosselink R. Characteristics of physical activities in daily life in chronic obstructive pulmonary disease. Am J Respir Crit Care Med. 2005;171(9):972–7.
51. Miravitlles M, Soler-Cataluña JJ, Calle M, Molina J, Almagro P, Quintano JA, et al. Spanish guidelines for Management of Chronic Obstructive Pulmonary Disease (GesEPOC) 2017. Pharmacological treatment of stable phase. Arch Bronconeumol. 2017;53(6):324–35.
52. Price D, Freeman D, Cleland J, Kaplan A, Cerasoli F. Earlier diagnosis and earlier treatment of COPD in primary care. Prim Care Respir J. 2011;20(1):15–22.
53. Puhan MA, Gimeno-Santos E, Scharplatz M, Troosters T, Walters EH, Steurer J. Pulmonary rehabilitation following exacerbations of chronic obstructive pulmonary disease. Cochrane Database Syst Rev. 2011;10:CD005305.
54. Corhay JL, Dang DN, Van Cauwenberge H, Louis R. Pulmonary rehabilitation and COPD: providing patients a good environment for optimizing therapy. Int J Chron Obstruct Pulmon Dis. 2014;9:27–39.
55. Jacome CIO, Marques ASPD. Pulmonary rehabilitation for mild chronic obstructive pulmonary disease: a systematic review. Respir Care. 2014 Apr; 59:588–94.
56. Price D, West D, Brusselle G, Gruffydd-Jones K, Jones R, Miravitlles M, et al. Management of COPD in the UK primary-care setting: an analysis of real-life prescribing patterns. Int J Chron Obstruct Pulmon Dis. 2014;9:889–904.
57. Wurst KE, Shukla A, Muellerova H, Davis KJ. Respiratory pharmacotherapy use in patients newly diagnosed with chronic obstructive pulmonary disease in a primary care setting in the UK: a retrospective cohort study. COPD. 2014;11(5):521–30.
58. Raluy-Callado M, Lambrelli D, MacLachlan S, Khalid JM. Epidemiology, severity, and treatment of chronic obstructive pulmonary disease in the United Kingdom by GOLD 2013. Int J Chron Obstruct Pulmon Dis. 2015;10: 925–37.
59. Barrecheguren M, Monteagudo M, Ferrer J, Borrell E, Llor C, Esquinas C, et al. Treatment patterns in COPD patients newly diagnosed in primary care. A population-based study. Respir Med. 2016;111:47–53.
60. Langsetmo L, Platt RW, Ernst P, Bourbeau J. Underreporting exacerbation of chronic obstructive pulmonary disease in a longitudinal cohort. Am J Respir Crit Care Med. 2008;177:396–401.
61. Beeh KM, Beier J, Buhl R, Stark-Lorenzen P, Gerken F, Metzdorf N, et al. Efficacy of tiotropium bromide (Spiriva) in patients with chronic-obstructive pulmonary disease (COPD) of different severities. Pneumologie. 2006;60(6):341–6.
62. Freeman D, Lee A, Price D. Efficacy and safety of tiotropium in COPD patients in primary care--the SPiRiva usual CarE (SPRUCE) study. Respir Res. 2007;8:45.
63. Jenkins CR, Jones PW, Calverley PM, Celli B, Anderson JA, Ferguson GT, et al. Efficacy of salmeterol/fluticasone propionate by GOLD stage of chronic obstructive pulmonary disease: analysis from the randomised, placebo-controlled TORCH study. Respir Res. 2009;10:59.
64. Singh D, Gaga M, Schmidt O, Bjermer L, Gronke L, Voss F, et al. Effects of tiotropium + olodaterol versus tiotropium or placebo by COPD disease severity and previous treatment history in the OTEMTO(R) studies. Respir Res. 2016;17(1):73.
65. Vogelmeier CF, Gaga M, Aalamian-Mattheis M, Greulich T, Marin JM, Castellani W, et al. Efficacy and safety of direct switch to indacaterol/ glycopyrronium in patients with moderate COPD: the CRYSTAL open-label randomised trial. Respir Res 2017;18(1):140.
66. Decramer M, Celli B, Kesten S, Lystig T, Mehra S, Tashkin DP, et al. Effect of tiotropium on outcomes in patients with moderate chronic obstructive pulmonary disease (UPLIFT): a prespecified subgroup analysis of a randomised controlled trial. Lancet. 2009;374(9696):1171–8.
67. Jones PW, Anderson JA, Calverley PMA, Celli BR, Ferguson GT, Jenkins C, et al. Health status in the TORCH study of COPD: treatment efficacy and other determinants of change. Respir Res. 2011;12(1):71.
68. Dusser D, Bravo ML, Iacono P. The effect of tiotropium on exacerbations and airflow in patients with COPD. Eur Respir J. 2006;27(3):547–55.
69. Wedzicha JA, Banerji D, Chapman KR, Vestbo J, Roche N, Ayers RT, et al. Indacaterol-Glycopyrronium versus salmeterol-fluticasone for COPD. N Engl J Med. 2016;374(23):2222–34.

70. Barrecheguren M, Esquinas C, Miravitlles M. The asthma-chronic obstructive pulmonary disease overlap syndrome (ACOS): opportunities and challenges. Curr Opin Pulm Med. 2015 Jan;21(1):74–9.
71. Decramer M, Miravitlles M, Price D, Román-Rodríguez M, Llor C, Welte T, et al. New horizons in early stage COPD – improving knowledge, detection and treatment. Respir Med. 2011;105:1576–87.
72. Scanlon PD, Connett JE, Waller LA, Altose MD, Bailey WC, Buist AS, et al. Smoking cessation and lung function in mild-to-moderate chronic obstructive pulmonary disease. The lung health study. Am J Respir Crit Care Med. 2000;161(2 Pt 1):381–90.
73. Troosters T, Celli B, Lystig T, Kesten S, Mehra S, Tashkin DP, et al. Tiotropium as a first maintenance drug in COPD: secondary analysis of the UPLIFT trial. Eur Respir J. 2010;36(1):65–73.
74. Zhou Y, Zhong NS, Li X, Chen S, Zheng J, Zhao D, et al. Tiotropium in early-stage chronic obstructive pulmonary disease. N Engl J Med. 2017;377(10):923–35.
75. Calverley PMA, Anderson JA, Brook RD, Crim C, Gallot N, Kilbride S, et al. SUMMIT (study to understand mortality and morbidity) investigators. Fluticasone Furoate, Vilanterol, and Lung Function Decline in Patients with Moderate Chronic Obstructive Pulmonary Disease and Heightened Cardiovascular Risk. Am J Respir Crit Care Med. 2018;197(1):47–55.
76. Tashkin DP, Celli B, Senn S, Burkhart D, Kesten S, Menjoge S, Decramer M. A 4-year trial of tiotropium in chronic obstructive pulmonary disease. N Engl J Med. 2008;359:1543–54.
77. Vestbo J, Anderson JA, Brook RD, Calverley PM, Celli BR, Crim C, et al. Fluticasone furoate and vilanterol and survival in chronic obstructive pulmonary disease with heightened cardiovascular risk (SUMMIT): a double-blind randomised controlled trial. Lancet. 2016;387(10030):1817–26.
78. Celli BR, Thomas NE, Anderson JA, Ferguson GT, Jenkins CR, Jones PW, et al. Effect of pharmacotherapy on rate of decline of lung function in chronic obstructive pulmonary disease: results from the TORCH study. Am J Respir Crit Care Med. 2008;178(4):332–8.
79. Spencer S, Calverley PM, Sherwood Burge P, Jones PW. Isolde study group - inhaled steroids in obstructive lung disease. Health status deterioration in patients with chronic obstructive pulmonary disease. Am J Respir Crit Care Med. 2001;163(1):122–8.
80. Wilke S, Jones PW, Mullerova H, Vestbo J, Tal-Singer R, Franssen FM, et al. One-year change in health status and subsequent outcomes in COPD. Thorax. 2015;70(5):420–5.
81. Anzueto A. Impact of exacerbations on COPD. Eur Respir Rev. 2010;19(116): 113–8.
82. Maleki-Yazdi MR, Singh D, Anzueto A, Tombs L, Fahy WA, Naya I. Assessing short-term deterioration in maintenance-naive patients with copd receiving umeclidinium/vilanterol and tiotropium: a pooled analysis of three randomized trials. Adv Ther. 2017;33(12):2188–99.
83. Anzueto AR, Vogelmeier CF, Kostikas K, Mezzi K, Fucile S, Bader G, et al. The effect of indacaterol/glycopyrronium versus tiotropium or salmeterol/fluticasone on the prevention of clinically important deterioration in COPD. Int J Chron Obstruct Pulmon Dis. 2017;12:1325–37.
84. Singh D, D'Urzo AD, Chuecos F, Muñoz A, García GE. Reduction in clinically important deterioration in chronic obstructive pulmonary disease with aclidinium/formoterol. Respir Res. 2017;18(1):106.
85. Miravitlles M, Vogelmeier C, Roche N, Halpin D, Cardoso J, Chuchalin AG, et al. A review of national guidelines for management of COPD in Europe. Eur Respir J. 2016;47(2):625–37.
86. O'Reilly J, Jones MM, Parnham J, Lovibond K, Rudolf M, Guideline Development Group. Management of stable chronic obstructive pulmonary disease in primary and secondary care: summary of updated NICE guidance. BMJ. 2010;340:c3134.
87. Bourbeau J, Bhutani M, Hernandez P, Marciniuk DD, Aaron SD, Balter M, et al. CTS position statement: pharmacotherapy in patients with COPD—an update. Can J Resp Crit Care Sleep Med. 2017;1(4):222–41.
88. Vincken W, van Noord JA, Greefhorst AP, Bantje TA, Kesten S, Korducki L, et al. Improved health outcomes in patients with COPD during 1 yr's treatment with tiotropium. EurRespir J. 2002;19(2):209–16.
89. Casaburi R, Mahler DA, Jones PW, Wanner A, San PG, ZuWallack RL, et al. A long-term evaluation of once-daily inhaled tiotropium in chronic obstructive pulmonary disease. Eur Respir J. 2002;19(2):217–24.
90. Jones PW, Willits LR, Burge PS, Calverley PM. Inhaled steroids in obstructive lung disease in Europe study investigators. Disease severity and the effect of fluticasone propionate on chronic obstructive pulmonary disease exacerbations. Eur Respir J. 2003;21(1):68–73.

5

Elevated serum soluble programmed cell death ligand 1 concentration as a potential marker for poor prognosis in small cell lung cancer patients with chemotherapy

Jianjun Jin*, Jiming Si, Yuanhua Liu, Huanqin Wang, Ran Ni and Jing Wang

Abstract

Background: Potential relationship between serum soluble programmed cell death ligand 1 and prognosis of small cell lung cancer is not well explored. The aim of the study was to reveal the prognostic significance of serum soluble programmed cell death ligand 1 in patients with small cell lung cancer.

Methods: A total of 250 small cell lung cancer patients and 250 controls were included. Research information was obtained from their medical records. Blood samples were collected on admission. Serum concentration of programmed cell death ligand 1 was measured using Enzyme-Linked Immunosorbent Assay. The patients underwent cisplatin-etoposide chemotherapy with a maximum of six cycles. Subsequently, they were followed-up for 12 months, and therapeutic response and cancer death were recorded.

Results: Serum concentration of programmed cell death ligand 1 was higher in the patients than in the controls on admission ($P < 0.001$). After chemotherapy, 112 patients had no response to this therapy. In the 12-month follow up period, 118 patients died due to this cancer. Multivariate Cox regression model revealed that the higher serum concentration of programmed cell death ligand 1 on admission was associated with the higher risk of no response to chemotherapy or cancer caused death (HR: 1.40, 95% CI: 1.05 ~ 1.87; HR: 1.43, 95% CI: 1.08 ~ 1.87).

Conclusion: Elevated serum concentration of soluble programmed cell death ligand 1 might be an independent risk factor for non-response to chemotherapy and cancer caused death in small cell lung cancer patients.

Keywords: Chemotherapy, Prognosis, Programmed cell death ligand 1, Response, Small cell lung carcinoma

Background

Lung cancer is the most common cause of cancer death in men and the second common cause in women around the world [1, 2]. There are two major histological lung cancers: non-small cell lung cancer (NSCLC) and small cell lung cancer (SCLC). SCLC accounts for about 15% of the cases [2]. Patients with SCLC primarily received systemic chemotherapy [3]. Cisplatin, etoposide, carboplatin, gemcitabine, paclitaxel, vinorelbine, topotecan, irinotecan and their combinations are commonly used in these patients [4, 5].

Programmed death 1 receptor (PD-1) and its ligand programmed death ligand 1 (PD-L1) are ectopically up-regulated in tumor tissue [6]. They attenuate the activation of T-cells and inhibit the anti-tumor immune response [7]. Due to these characteristics, PD-1 and PD-L1 are regarded as a novel target for immunotherapy, and their inhibitors have been adopted in NSCLC patients [8–10].

Several studies suggested that tissue expressions of PD-1 and PD-L1 were associated with survival in patients with SCLC or NSCLC [11, 12]. Furthermore, Okuma et al. in their study suggested that high serum level of soluble PD-L1 was prognostic for reduced survival in advanced lung cancer, but this study only included seven SCLC patients [13]. Therefore, prognostic significance of soluble PD-L1 in SCLC patients has not been well investigated.

* Correspondence: jinjianjun2423@163.com
Department of Respiratory and Critical Medicine, the First Affiliated Hospital of Zhengzhou University, No. 1, Jianshe East Road, Zhengzhou 450052, Henan Province, China

A potential relationship between PD-L1 expression and chemotherapeutic response in NSCLC patients has been reported. Zhang et al. suggested that high expression of PD-L1 after cisplatin-based neo-adjuvant chemotherapy could be an indication of therapeutic resistance and poor prognosis in patients with NSCLC [14]. On the contrary, Ishii et al. reported that PD-L1 expression was associated with high immunoscore, and the highest immunoscore tended to have a favorable disease-free survival in NSCLC [15]. However, studies focusing on this relationship in SCLC patients are lacking.

This study aimed to evaluate the prognostic significance of soluble PD-L1 in SCLC, and explore the relationship between soluble PD-L1 and chemotherapeutic response in this disease.

Methods

The study was approved by the ethics committee of the First Affiliated Hospital of Zhengzhou University.

Subjects

A total of 250 patients with SCLC were continuously included from Department of Respiratory and Critical Medicine, the First Affiliated Hospital of Zhengzhou University between January 2010 and December 2016. Adequate histological samples with abundant tumor cells from these patients were available, and all these patients were diagnosed by pathology. Patients who did not have enough histological samples were excluded from this study. And, 250 health volunteers were randomly selected from medical examination center, the First Affiliated Hospital of Zhengzhou University in the same period, and served as controls. The patients did not receive any type of anti-tumor therapy before. The subjects did not have acute myocardial infarction, unstable angina, acute cerebral infarction/hemorrhage, severe infection, autoimmune disease or other kind of cancer. The patients and controls agreed to take part in this study, and signed the written informed consents.

Data collection

Demographic and clinical information were obtained from their medical records. Tumor tissue expressions of epidermal growth factor receptor (EGFR) and kirsten rat sarcoma viral oncogene (KRAS) were obtained from their pathological records.

Enzyme-linked immunosorbent assay

Blood samples were collected from the patients and controls on admission, and were immediately centrifuged at 1000 rpm for 12 min. Serum samples were stored at −70 °C for following determination.

Serum concentration of PD-L1 was measured using a Human/Cynomolgus Monkey PD-L1/B7-H1 Quantikine Enzyme-Linked Immunosorbent Assay (ELISA) Kit (R&D Systems, Minneapolis, MN, USA) according to the manufacturer's instruction. Sensitivity was 4.52 pg/ml, and assay range was 25.0–1600 pg/ml. Each sample was measured twice, and the mean was reported.

Immunohistochemistry

Of the 250 SCLC patients, 98 provided available tumor tissue samples, which were stored at −196 °C (liquid nitrogen) for further measurement.

Mature and reliable immunohistochemical staining technique was adopted to detect the PD-L1 expression in tumor tissue, and its steps were briefly introduced. First, the tissue samples were fixed in formalin (10%), embedded in paraffin and cut into 4 μm slice. Second, the slices were dewaxed in xylene, rehydrated using graded ethanol and rinsed in phosphate buffer saline. Third, antigen retrieval was performed in citrate buffer (0.01 mol/l, pH 6.0). Fourth, the slices were heated using microwave and then cooled at room temperature for 30 min. Fifth, the slices were infiltrated in hydrogen peroxide (3%) at room temperature for 20 min and incubated in goat serum at 37 °C for 40 min. Sixth, the slices were incubated with primary anti- PD-L1 monoclonal antibodies (Catalog Number: 66248–1-Ig; Proteintech, Wuhan, Hubei, China; 1:500 Dilution) at 4 °C overnight. Seventh, after washing in phosphate buffer saline, the slices were incubated with goat anti-mouse IgG (H + L), biotin conjugate secondary antibodies (Catalog Number: SA00004–1; Proteintech, Wuhan, Hubei, China; 1:500 Dilution) at 37 °C for 30 min. Eighth, the slices were exposed to 3, 3′-diaminobenzidine and counterstained in hematoxylin. Percentage of the positive staining SCLC cells was reported. If more than 5% of the SCLC cells in one tissue slice exhibited positive staining, it was considered as positive result [16].

Definition

Tumor staging was determined by the veterans administration lung cancer group (VALG) staging system [17]. Limited disease (LD) was defined as an area that was tolerably treated by one radiotherapy area, but excluded cancers with pleural or pericardial effusions. All other SCLCs were regarded as extensive disease (ED). Performance status was measured according to the eastern cooperative oncology group (ECOG) score [18].

Smoker was defined as a subject who had at least one cigarette per week for six months or more in his or her life. Other subjects were defined as non-smokers.

Therapy

The patients underwent chemotherapy with a maximum of six cycles. Their chemotherapy regimen was cisplatin and etoposide. Therapeutic response was defined according to the Response Evaluation Criteria in Solid Tumors (RECIST) [19]. There were four categories: complete response (CR), partial response (PR), stable disease (SD) and progressive disease (PD). In this study, CR and PR were grouped as response, and SD and PD were combined as non-response.

Follow up

All the patients were followed-up for 12 months by telephone. The process was conducted by a well-trained investigator. Major endpoint was SCLC-caused death.

Statistical analysis

Continuous variable was expressed as mean ± standard deviation (SD), and categorical variable was showed as frequency and constituent ratio. Difference of continuous variables was analyzed using independent sample t test, and difference of categorical variables was detected using chi-square test. A two-sided $P < 0.05$ was regarded to be statistically significant. A cutoff value for serum concentration of PD-L1 was calculated by receiver operating characteristic curve analysis. Relationship between serum concentration of PD-L1 and prognosis of SCLC patients was analyzed using multivariate Cox regression analysis. Hazard ratio (HR) and 95% confidence interval (CI) were reported. If a 95%CI included value one, it was considered statistically significant. All statistical analyses were conducted using SPSS 19.0 (SPSS Inc., Chicago, IL, USA).

Table 1 Baseline characteristics of the patients and controls

	SCLC [a]	Control	*P* value
Total (*n*)	250	250	–
Age (*n*)	64.5 ± 5.8	65.0 ± 5.8	0.381
Gender (*n*)			
Female	53	67	0.143
Male	197	183	
Smoking history (*n*)			
Non-smoker	107	135	0.012
Smoker	143	115	
Performance status			
0–1	218	–	–
2	32	–	–
Tumor grade (*n*)			
High-middle	193	–	–
Low	57	–	–
Tumor stage (*n*)			
LD[a]	143	–	–
ED[a]	107	–	–
EGFR (*n*)[a]			
Negative	202	–	–
Positive	48	–	–
KRAS (*n*)[a]			
Negative	234	–	–
Positive	16	–	–
Serum PD-L1 (ng/ml)[a]	7.0 ± 3.0	1.2 ± 0.6	<0.001

[a]*SCLC* Small cell lung cancer, *LD* Limited disease, *ED* Extensive disease, *EGFR* Epidermal growth factor receptor, *KRAS* Kirsten rat sarcoma viral oncogene, *PD-L1* Programmed death ligand 1

Results

As shown in Table 1, there were 250 SCLC patients and 250 health controls in the study. There was no difference in age and gender between these two groups ($P = 0.381$, $P = 0.143$). Smokers were more common in the SCLC patients than in the health controls ($P = 0.012$). Serum concentration of PD-L1 was higher in the SCLC patients than in the controls ($P < 0.001$).

As shown in Table 2, a total of 138 patients had a response and 112 patients had no response to chemotherapy. Age, gender, smoking history, performance status, tumor grade and tumor stage were equivalent between the patients with a response and the patients without a response to chemotherapy ($P = 0.472$, $P = 0.817$, $P = 0.127$, $P = 0.076$, $P = 0.169$, $P = 0.312$). Serum concentration of PD-L1, tissue expressions of EGFR and KRAS were higher in the patients without a response than in the patients with a response to chemotherapy ($P = 0.008$, $P = 0.016$, $P = 0.046$).

As shown in Tables 3, 118 patients died due to SCLC in the follow up period, and the remaining 132 patients were still living at the end of the follow up. There was no difference in age, gender, smoking history, performance status, tissue expressions of EGFR and KRAS between the dead patients and the living patients ($P = 0.573$, $P = 0.532$, $P = 0.370$, $P = 0.063$, $P = 0.086$, $P = 0.074$). More dead patients had low-grade or ED-stage tumors ($P = 0.014$, $P = 0.007$). More dead patients had no response to chemotherapy ($P < 0.001$). Serum concentration of PD-L1 was higher in the dead patients than in the living patients ($P = 0.003$).

A cutoff point for serum concentration of soluble PD-L1 was 7.0 ng/ml in predicting the risk of chemotherapeutic non-response (Sensitivity = 68.7%, Specificity = 69.8%, Area under the curve = 0.707, $P < 0.001$) (Fig. 1a). A cutoff point for serum concentration of soluble PD-L1 was 7.1 ng/ml in predicting the risk of cancer death (Sensitivity = 73.9%, Specificity = 71.3%, Area under the curve = 0.726, $P < 0.001$) (Fig. 1b).

Tissue expression of PD-L1 was higher in the patients without a response than in the patients with a response to chemotherapy (6.8% ± 3.6%, 4.9% ± 3.6%, $P = 0.012$) (Fig. 2a). Tissue expression of PD-L1 was higher in the dead patients than in the living patients (6.8% ± 3.4%, 4.6% ± 3.7%, $P = 0.003$) (Fig. 2b). In Fig. 2c, there is a linear relationship between serum level of soluble PD-L1 and tissue expression of PD-L1 ($r = 0.214$, $P = 0.034$).

Table 2 Baseline characteristics of the non-response and response patients

	Non-response	Response	*P* value
Total (*n*)	112	138	–
Age (*n*)	64.2 ± 6.2	64.7 ± 5.5	0.472
Gender (*n*)			
Female	23	30	0.817
Male	89	108	
Smoking history (*n*)			
Non-smoker	42	65	0.127
Smoker	70	73	
Performance status			
0–1	93	125	0.076
2	19	13	
Tumor grade (*n*)			
High-middle	91	102	0.169
Low	21	36	
Tumor stage (*n*)			
LD[a]	68	75	0.312
ED[a]	44	63	
EGFR (*n*)[a]			
Negative	83	119	0.016
Positive	29	19	
KRAS (*n*)[a]			
Negative	101	133	0.046
Positive	11	5	
Serum PD-L1 (ng/ml)[a]	7.6 ± 2.5	6.6 ± 3.2	0.008

[a]*LD* Limited disease, *ED* Extensive disease, *EGFR* Epidermal growth factor receptor, *KRAS* Kirsten rat sarcoma viral oncogene, *PD-L1* Programmed death ligand 1

Figure 2d and e showed positively and negatively immunohistochemical staining of PD-L1 in SCLC patients, respectively.

According to the cutoff values of the serum PD-L1 level, the patients were divided into several subgroups for following analysis. As shown in Tables 4 and 5, the higher serum concentration of soluble PD-L1 was associated with the higher risk of no response to chemotherapy or SCLC caused death (HR: 1.40, 95% CI: 1.05 ~ 1.87; HR: 1.43, 95% CI: 1.08 ~ 1.87). The positive expression of PD-L1 in tissue was also associated with the higher risk of no response to chemotherapy or SCLC caused death (HR: 1.76, 95% CI: 1.13 ~ 2.78; HR: 1.86, 95% CI: 1.24 ~ 2.76). In addition, the higher expressions of EGFR and KRAS were related to the higher risk of no response to chemotherapy (HR: 1.45, 95% CI: 1.09 ~ 1.93; HR: 1.57, 95% CI: 1.09 ~ 2.27). Low-grade and ED-stage tumors were associated with the higher risk of cancer death (HR: 1.41, 95% CI: 1.08 ~ 1.85; HR: 1.42, 95% CI: 1.09 ~ 1.84).

Table 3 Baseline characteristics of the cancer-dead and survival patients

	Cancer death	Survival	P value
Total (*n*)	118	132	–
Age (*n*)	64.2 ± 5.5	64.7 ± 6.1	0.573
Gender (*n*)			
Female	23	30	0.532
Male	95	102	
Smoking history (*n*)			
Non-smoker	47	60	0.370
Smoker	71	72	
Performance status			
0–1	98	120	0.063
2	20	12	
Tumor grade (*n*)			
High-middle	83	110	0.014
Low	35	22	
Tumor stage (*n*)			
LD[a]	57	86	0.007
ED[a]	61	46	
EGFR (n)[a]			
Negative	90	112	0.086
Positive	28	20	
KRAS (*n*)[a]			
Negative	107	127	0.074
Positive	11	5	
Chemotherapeutic response (*n*)			
Response	12	126	<0.001
Non-response	106	6	
Serum PD-L1 (ng/ml)[a]	7.6 ± 3.1	6.5 ± 2.7	0.003

[a]*LD* Limited disease, *ED* Extensive disease, *EGFR* Epidermal growth factor receptor, *KRAS* Kirsten rat sarcoma viral oncogene, *PD-L1* Programmed death ligand 1

Discussion

To our knowledge, this is the first published article focusing on the relationship between serum concentration of soluble PD-L1 and prognosis of SCLC patients after chemotherapy. There were 250 patients with confirmed SCLC and 250 health controls in the study. We discovered that serum concentration of soluble PD-L1 significantly elevated in the SCLC patients, which was consistent with a previous study involving several types of advanced lung cancers [13].

A previous study suggested that soluble PD-L1 originated from PD-L1 on the surface of tumor cells by a disengagement mechanism, and serum concentration of soluble PD-L1 should be related to the tumor burden [20]. In the study, we confirmed the relationship between the serum level of soluble PD-L1 and the expression of PD-L1

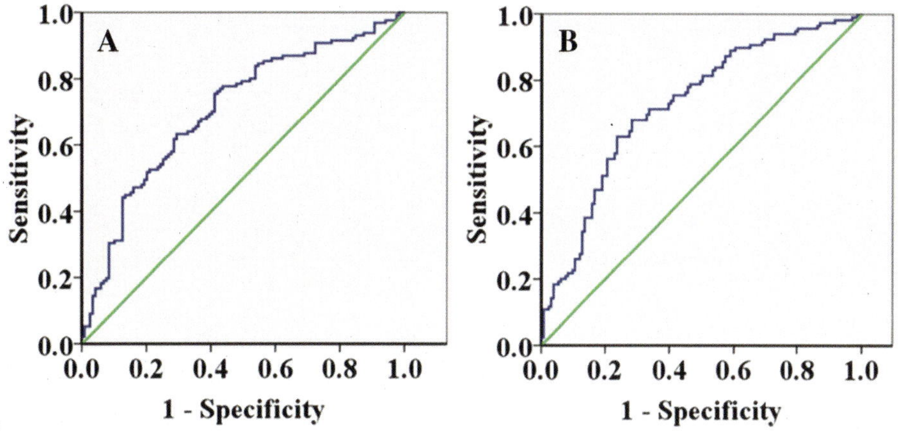

Fig. 1 Receiver operating characteristic curve analysis of serum soluble programmed cell death ligand 1 in the patients according to the prognosis. **a**. A cutoff point for serum concentration of soluble programmed cell death ligand 1 was 7.0 ng/ml in predicting the risk of chemotherapeutic non-response (Sensitivity = 68.7%, Specificity = 69.8%, Area under the curve = 0.707, $P < 0.001$). **b**: A cutoff point for serum concentration of soluble programmed cell death ligand 1 was 7.1 ng/ml in predicting the risk of cancer death (Sensitivity = 73.9%, Specificity = 71.3%, Area under the curve = 0.726, $P < 0.001$)

in tissue. However, this did not mean that the soluble PD-L1 was also associated with the tumor burden, because the expression level of PD-L1 per unit tumor volume was diverse.

Serum PD-L1 was not a specific tumor marker, but an inflammatory and immunoregulatory marker in human [21]. Soluble PD-1 and its receptor PD-1 could be produced by peripheral immunological cells, and represented an unanticipated contributing factor to immune homeostasis [22]. Greisen et al. reported that increased concentration of soluble PD-1 was associated with disease activity and radiographic progression in rheumatoid

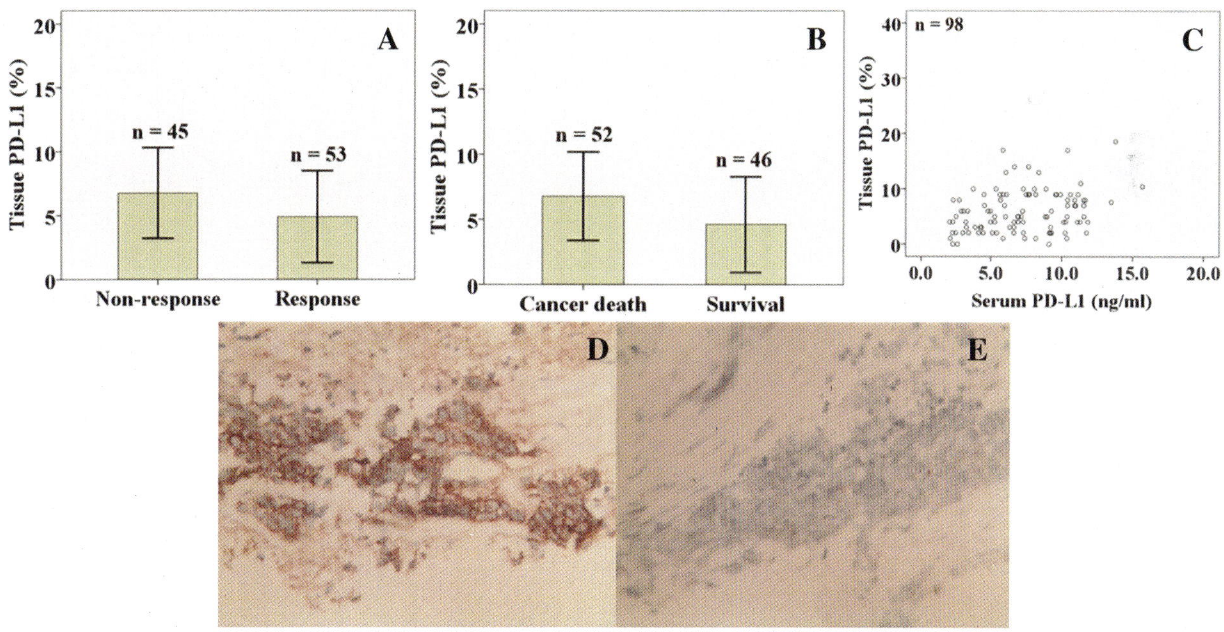

Fig. 2 Tissue expression of soluble programmed cell death ligand 1 in patients with small cell lung cancer patients. **a**: Tissue expression of programmed cell death ligand 1 was higher in the patients without a response to chemotherapy than in the patients with a response to chemotherapy (6.8% ± 3.6%, 4.9% ± 3.6%, $P = 0.012$). **b**: Tissue expression of programmed cell death ligand 1 was higher in the dead patients than in the living patients (6.8% ± 3.4%, 4.6% ± 3.7%, $P = 0.003$). **c**: There is a linear relationship between serum level of soluble programmed cell death ligand 1 and tissue expression of soluble programmed cell death ligand 1 ($r = 0.214$, $P = 0.034$). **d**: Positively immunohistochemical staining of programmed death ligand 1 in patients with small cell lung cancer patients (400×). **e**: Negatively immunohistochemical staining of programmed death ligand 1 in patients with small cell lung cancer patients (400×)

Table 4 Relationship between several markers and chemotherapeutic response

	Non-response (*n*)	Total (*n*)	Multivariate HR[a] (95% CI)[a,b]	Multivariate HR (95% CI)[c]
Total	112	250	–	–
Tumor grade				
High-middle	91	193	Reference	Reference
Low	21	57	0.78 (0.54 ~ 1.13)	0.76 (0.53 ~ 1.11)
Tumor stage				
LD[a]	68	143	Reference	Reference
ED[a]	44	107	0.86 (0.65 ~ 1.15)	0.84 (0.64 ~ 1.13)
EGFR[a]				
Negative	83	202	Reference	Reference
Positive	29	48	1.47 (1.11 ~ 1.95)	1.45 (1.09 ~ 1.93)
KRAS[a]				
Negative	101	234	Reference	Reference
Positive	11	16	1.59 (1.11 ~ 2.29)	1.57 (1.09 ~ 2.27)
Serum PD-L1[a]				
<7.0 ng/ml	45	122	Reference	Reference
≥ 7.0 ng/ml	67	128	1.42 (1.07 ~ 1.89)	1.40 (1.05 ~ 1.87)
Tissue PD-L1				
Negative	17	50	Reference	Reference
Positive	28	48	1.75 (1.12 ~ 2.77)	1.76 (1.13 ~ 2.78)

[a]LD: Limited disease; ED: Extensive disease; EGFR: Epidermal growth factor receptor; KRAS: Kirsten rat sarcoma viral oncogene; PD-L1: Programmed death ligand 1; HR: Hazard ratio; CI: Confidence interval
[b]The model was adjusted by age and gender
[c]The model was adjusted by age, gender, smoking history, performance status, tumor grade, tumor stage, tissue expressions of epidermal growth factor receptor and kirsten rat sarcoma viral oncogene

arthritis [23]. Wu et al. and Shi et al. suggested that soluble PD-1 also contributed to the aberrant activation of T cells and the development of diseases in aplastic anemia and diabetic atherosclerotic complications, respectively [24, 25]. So, an inflammatory lesion in tumor as well as an extra-tumor inflammatory lesion could elevate the concentration of soluble PD-L1. In SCLC patients without other inflammation and immune related diseases, serum concentration of soluble PD-L1 indicated the extents of anti-tumor T cell response and immune suppression induced by PD-1 and PD-L1.

In the study, we reported a 40% increased risk of non-response to chemotherapy in the patients with relatively higher concentration of soluble PD-L1, which was consistent with one previous study by Zhang et al. [14] and was contrary to another study by Ishii et al. [15]. Both these studies included NSCLC patients and measured the tissue expression of PD-L1, but not the serum concentration of PD-L1.

Some studies had revealed the effect of PD-L1 on chemoresistance in other type of cancer. Black et al. suggested that the activation of PD-1/PD-L1 immune checkpoint conferred breast cancer cell chemoresistance associated with increased metastasis [26]. Ishibashi et al. found that the interaction between PD-1 and PD-L1 not only inhibited tumor-specific cytotoxic T lymphocytes, but also induced drug resistance in myeloma cells [27]. Tamura et al. reported that the bone marrow microenvironment up-regulated PD-1 expression on myeloma cells, which linked to aggressive myeloma-cell characteristics and insensitivity to anti-myeloma chemotherapy [28].

Tumor infiltrating lymphocyte (TIL) was regarded to be a protective factor for cancer, and it improved survival in NSCLC patients [29]. Zhang et al. suggested that the higher TIL expression rate was usually found in chemosensitive samples in NSCLC [14]. Potential association between PD-L1 and TILs was also confirmed in lung cancer patients [30]. Furthermore, miR-197/CKS1B/STAT3-mediated network regarded the tumor expression of PD-L1 as a biomarker of this cascade, and the biological interaction between PD-L1 and chemoresistance occurred through this microRNA regulatory cascade [31]. Therefore, the effect of PD-L1 on chemoresistance might be involved in the inhibition of TILs and the dysregulation of miR-197/CKS1B/STAT3-mediated cascade. These findings partly explained the effect of PD-L1 on chemotherapeutic response.

Table 5 Relationship between several markers and cancer caused death

	Cancer death (*n*)	Total (*n*)	Multivariate HR[a] (95% CI)[a, b]	Multivariate HR (95% CI) [c]
Tumor grade				
High-middle	83	193	Reference	Reference
Low	35	57	1.43 (1.10 ~ 1.86)	1.41 (1.08 ~ 1.85)
Tumor stage				
LD[a]	57	143	Reference	Reference
ED[a]	61	107	1.43 (1.10 ~ 1.85)	1.42 (1.09 ~ 1.84)
EGFR[a]				
Negative	90	202	Reference	Reference
Positive	28	48	1.31 (0.99 ~ 1.74)	1.30 (0.98 ~ 1.73)
KRAS[a]				
Negative	108	234	Reference	Reference
Positive	10	16	1.35 (0.90 ~ 2.03)	1.33 (0.88 ~ 2.01)
Serum PD-L1[a]				
<7.1 ng/ml	48	124	Reference	Reference
≥ 7.1 ng/ml	70	126	1.44 (1.09 ~ 1.88)	1.43 (1.08 ~ 1.87)
Tissue PD-L1				
Negative	19	50	Reference	Reference
Positive	33	48	1.85 (1.24 ~ 2.75)	1.86 (1.24 ~ 2.76)

[a]*LD* Limited disease, *ED* Extensive disease, *EGFR* Epidermal growth factor receptor, *KRAS* Kirsten rat sarcoma viral oncogene, *PD-L1* Programmed death ligand 1, *HR* Hazard ratio, *CI* Confidence interval
[b]The model was adjusted by age and gender
[c]The model was adjusted by age, gender, smoking history, performance status, tumor grade, tumor stage, tissue expressions of epidermal growth factor receptor and kirsten rat sarcoma viral oncogene

Furthermore, our study revealed a relationship between soluble PD-L1 and prognosis of SCLC patients, and the patients with higher concentration of soluble PD-L1 showed a 40% increased risk of cancer caused death in the 12-month follow up period. This result was consistent with a previous study exploring the prognostic significance of soluble PD-L1 in advanced lung cancer [13]. In the study, most of the dead patients had no response to chemotherapy. Therefore, prognostic significance of soluble PD-L1 might be related to the effect of this ligand on chemotherapeutic response.

Prognostic significance of soluble PD-L1 in other type of cancer had also been explored. Zheng et al. suggested that circulating PD-L1 expression was significantly correlated with differentiation and lymph node metastasis in total advanced gastric cancer patients [32]. Ha et al. reported that advanced biliary tract cancer patients with high soluble PD-L1 showed worse overall survival than patients with low soluble PD-L1, and high soluble PD-L1 was an independent poor prognostic factor in multivariate analysis [33]. Wang et al. revealed that overall response rate to treatment in multiple myeloma patients was higher in low soluble PD-L1 patients than in high soluble PD-L1 patients, and higher soluble PD-L1 level was an independent prognostic factor for shorter 3-year progression free survival [34]. Finkelmeier et al. discovered that soluble PD-L1 level positively correlated with the stage of cirrhosis and with stage of HCC, and patients with high serum PD-L1 concentration had an increased mortality risk, while very low PD-L1 level seemed to come along with better prognosis [35]. Rossille et al. suggested that diffuse large B-cell lymphoma patients with elevated soluble PD-L1 experienced a poorer prognosis with a 3-year overall survival of 76% versus 89% [36]. A meta-analysis from Zhu et al. indicated that high PD-L1 expression was likely to be a negative factor for patients with sarcomas and that it predicted worse survival outcomes [37].

PD-1 and PD-L1 had become a target for anti-tumor therapy. According to this understanding, a novel targeted drug nivolumab had been produced, which was an IgG4 monoclonal antibody against PD-1. It exerted its biological function through inhibiting the PD-1/PD-L1 signal pathway and allowing the immune system to scavenge the tumor cells [38]. Around the world, nivolumab had been used in the treatment of metastatic melanoma, squamous non-small cell lung cancer and renal cell carcinoma [39–41]. Potential therapeutical effect of the drug on SCLC had also been explored. A multicentre, open-label, phase 1/2 trial at 23 hospitals in six countries

(CheckMate 032) reported that nivolumab monotherapy and nivolumab plus ipilimumab had an anti-tumor activity with durable responses and manageable safety profiles in previously treated patients with SCLC [42]. Furthermore, Hellmann et al. in their study reported that the efficacy of nivolumab monotherapy and nivolumab plus ipilimumab was enhanced in SCLC patients with high tumor mutational burden [43]. This promising finding required further confirmation in phase 3 randomized controlled trials in SCLC.

Conclusion

In conclusion, elevated serum concentration of soluble PD-L1 might be an independent risk factor for non-response to chemotherapy and cancer caused death in SCLC patients. Further studies should be conducted to explore the mechanisms involved.

Abbreviations

CI: Confidence interval; CR: Complete response; ECOG: Eastern cooperative oncology group; ED: Extensive disease; EGFR: Epidermal growth factor receptor; ELISA: Enzyme Linked Immunosorbent Assay; HR: Hazard ratio; KRAS: Kirsten rat sarcoma viral oncogene; LD: Limited disease; NSCLC: Non-small cell lung cancer; PD: Progressive disease; PD-1: Programmed death 1 receptor; PD-L1: Programmed death ligand 1; PR: Partial response; RECIST: Response Evaluation Criteria in Solid Tumors; SCLC: Small cell lung cancer; SD: Stable disease; SD: Standard deviation; TIL: Tumor infiltrating lymphocyte; VALG: Veterans administration lung cancer group

Authors' contributions

JJ and SJ contributed to the study concept and design. JJ, SJ, LY, WH, NR and WJ were involved in the acquisition of data. JJ, SJ, LY, WH, NR and WJ conducted the analysis and interpretation of data. JJ, SJ, LY, WH, NR and WJ worked on the preparation of the manuscript. All authors read and approved the final manuscript.

Competing interests

The authors declared that they had no competing interests.

References

1. Didkowska J, Wojciechowska U, Mańczuk M, Łobaszewski J. Lung cancer epidemiology: contemporary and future challenges worldwide. Ann Transl Med. 2016;4:150.
2. Temraz S, Charafeddine M, Mukherji D, Shamseddine A. Trends in lung cancer incidence in Lebanon by gender and histological type over the period 2005-2008. J Epidemiol Glob Health. 2017;7:161–7.
3. Hann CL, Rudin CM. Management of small-cell lung cancer: incremental changes but hope for the future. Oncology (Williston Park). 2008;22:1486–92.
4. Murray N, Turrisi AT 3rd. A review of first-line treatment for small-cell lung cancer. J Thorac Oncol. 2006;1:270–8.
5. Azim HA Jr, Ganti AK. Treatment options for relapsed small-cell lung cancer. Anti-Cancer Drugs. 2007;18:255–61.
6. Herbst RS, Soria JC, Kowanetz M, Fine GD, Hamid O, Gordon MS, Sosman JA, McDermott DF, Powderly JD, Gettinger SN, Kohrt HE, Horn L, Lawrence DP, Rost S, Leabman M, Xiao Y, Mokatrin A, Koeppen H, Hegde PS, Mellman I, Chen DS, Hodi FS. Predictive correlates of response to the anti-PD-L1 antibody MPDL3280A in cancer patients. Nature. 2014;515:563–7.
7. Gatalica Z, Snyder C, Maney T, Ghazalpour A, Holterman DA, Xiao N, Overberg P, Rose I, Basu GD, Vranic S, Lynch HT, Von Hoff DD, Hamid O. Programmed cell death 1 (PD-1) and its ligand (PD-L1) in common cancers and their correlation with molecular cancer type. Cancer Epidemiol Biomark Prev. 2014;23:2965–70.
8. Topalian SL, Hodi FS, Brahmer JR, Gettinger SN, Smith DC, McDermott DF, Powderly JD, Carvajal RD, Sosman JA, Atkins MB, Leming PD, Spigel DR, Antonia SJ, Horn L, Drake CG, Pardoll DM, Chen L, Sharfman WH, Anders RA, Taube JM, McMiller TL, Xu H, Korman AJ, Jure-Kunkel M, Agrawal S, McDonald D, Kollia GD, Gupta A, Wigginton JM, Sznol M. Safety, activity, and immune correlates of anti-PD-1 antibody in cancer. N Engl J Med. 2012;366:2443–54.
9. Fehrenbacher L, Spira A, Ballinger M, Kowanetz M, Vansteenkiste J, Mazieres J, Park K, Smith D, Artal-Cortes A, Lewanski C, Braiteh F, Waterkamp D, He P, Zou W, Chen DS, Yi J, Sandler A, Rittmeyer A, POPLAR Study Group. Atezolizumab versus docetaxel for patients with previously treated non-small-cell lung cancer (POPLAR): a multicentre, open-label, phase 2 randomised controlled trial. Lancet. 2016;387:1837–46.
10. Rittmeyer A, Barlesi F, Waterkamp D, Park K, Ciardiello F, von Pawel J, Gadgeel SM, Hida T, Kowalski DM, Dols MC, Cortinovis DL, Leach J, Polikoff J, Barrios C, Kabbinavar F, Frontera OA, De Marinis F, Turna H, Lee JS, Ballinger M, Kowanetz M, He P, Chen DS, Sandler A, Gandara DR; OAK Study Group. Atezolizumab versus docetaxel in patients with previously treated non-small-cell lung cancer (OAK): a phase 3, open-label, multicentre randomised controlled trial. Lancet 2017;389:255–265.
11. Cui S, Su X, Dong L Qian J, Ye L, Zhang T, Fu H, Han H, Huang J, Yao Y, Gu Y, Jiang L. Programmed cell death ligand 1 protein levels predicted survival of non-small cell lung cancer. J Cancer. 2017;8:4075–82.
12. Ishii H, Azuma K, Kawahara A, Yamada K, Imamura Y, Tokito T, Kinoshita T, Kage M, Hoshino T. Significance of programmed cell death-ligand 1 expression and its association with survival in patients with small cell lung cancer. J Thorac Oncol. 2015;10:426–30.
13. Okuma Y, Hosomi Y, Nakahara Y, Watanabe K, Sagawa Y, Homma S. High plasma levels of soluble programmed cell death ligand 1 are prognostic for reduced survival in advanced lung cancer. Lung Cancer. 2017;104:1–6.
14. Zhang P, Ma Y, Lv C, Huang M, Li M, Dong B, Liu X, An G, Zhang W, Zhang J, Zhang L, Zhang S, Yang Y. Upregulation of programmed cell death ligand 1 promotes resistance response in non-small-cell lung cancer patients treated with neo-adjuvant chemotherapy. Cancer Sci. 2016;107:1563–71.
15. Ishii H, Azuma K, Kawahara A, Matsuo N, Tokito T, Kinoshita T, Yamada K, Sasada T, Akiba J, Hoshino T. Programmed cell death-ligand 1 expression and immunoscore in stage II and III non-small cell lung cancer patients receiving adjuvant chemotherapy. Oncotarget. 2017;8:61618–25.
16. Jotatsu T, Oda K, Yatera K. PD-L1 immunohistochemistry in patients with non-small cell lung cancer. J Thorac Dis. 2018;10:2127–9.
17. van Meerbeeck JP, Fennell DA, De Ruysscher DK. Small-cell lung cancer. Lancet. 2011;378:1741–55.
18. Oken MM, Creech RH, Tormey DC, Horton J, Davis TE, McFadden ET, Carbone PP. Toxicity and response criteria of the eastern cooperative oncology group. Am J Clin Oncol. 1982;5:649–55.
19. Therasse P, Arbuck SG, Eisenhauer EA, Wanders J, Kaplan RS, Rubinstein L, Verweij J, Van Glabbeke M, van Oosterom AT, Christian MC, Gwyther SG. New guidelines to evaluate the response to treatment in solid tumors. European Organization for Research and Treatment of Cancer, National Cancer Institute of the United States, National Cancer Institute of Canada. J Natl Cancer Inst. 2000;92:205–16.
20. Chen Y, Wang Q, Shi B, Xu P, Hu Z, Bai L, Zhang X. Development of a sandwich ELISA for evaluating soluble PD-L1 (CD274) in human sera of different ages as well as supernatants of PD-L1+ cell lines. Cytokine. 2011;56:231–8.
21. Sharpe AH, Wherry EJ, Ahmed R, Freeman GJ. The function of programmed cell death 1 and its ligands in regulating autoimmunity and infection. Nat Immunol. 2007;8:239–45.
22. Frigola X, Inman BA, Krco CJ, Liu X, Harrington SM, Bulur PA, Dietz AB, Dong H, Kwon ED. Soluble B7-H1: differences in production between dendritic cells and T cells. Immunol Lett. 2012;142:78–82.
23. Greisen SR, Rasmussen TK, Stengaard-Pedersen K, Hetland ML, Hørslev-Petersen K, Hvid M, Deleuran B. Increased soluble programmed death-1 (sPD-1) is associated with disease activity and radiographic progression in early rheumatoid arthritis. Scand J Rheumatol. 2014;43:101–8.

24. Wu H, Miao M, Zhang G, Hu Y, Ming Z, Zhang X. Soluble PD-1 is associated with aberrant regulation of T cells activation in aplastic anemia. Immunol Investig. 2009;38:408–21.
25. Shi B, Du X, Wang Q, Chen Y, Zhang X. Increased PD-1 on CD4(+)CD28(−) T cell and soluble PD-1 ligand-1 in patients with T2DM: association with atherosclerotic macrovascular diseases. Metabolism. 2013;62:778–85.
26. Black M, Barsoum IB, Truesdell P, Cotechini T, Macdonald-Goodfellow SK, Petroff M, Siemens DR, Koti M, Craig AW, Graham CH. Activation of the PD-1/PD-L1 immune checkpoint confers tumor cell chemoresistance associated with increased metastasis. Oncotarget. 2016;7:10557–67.
27. Ishibashi M, Tamura H, Sunakawa M, Kondo-Onodera A, Okuyama N, Hamada Y, Moriya K, Choi I, Tamada K, Inokuchi K. Myeloma drug resistance induced by binding of myeloma B7-H1 (PD-L1) to PD-1. Cancer Immunol Res. 2016;4:779–88.
28. Tamura H, Ishibashi M, Yamashita T, Tanosaki S, Okuyama N, Kondo A, Hyodo H, Shinya E, Takahashi H, Dong H, Tamada K, Chen L, Dan K, Ogata K. Marrow stromal cells induce B7-H1 expression on myeloma cells, generating aggressive characteristics in multiple myeloma. Leukemia. 2013; 27:464–72.
29. Horne ZD, Jack R, Gray ZT, Siegfried JM, Wilson DO, Yousem SA, Nason KS, Landreneau RJ, Luketich JD, Schuchert MJ. Increased levels of tumor-infiltrating lymphocytes are associated with improved recurrence-free survival in stage 1A non-small-cell lung cancer. J Surg Res. 2011;171:1–5.
30. Chen YB, Mu CY, Huang JA. Clinical significance of programmed death-1 ligand-1 expression in patients with non-small cell lung cancer: a 5-year-follow-up study. Tumori. 2012;98:751–5.
31. Fujita Y, Yagishita S, Hagiwara K, Yoshioka Y, Kosaka N, Takeshita F, Fujiwara T, Tsuta K, Nokihara H, Tamura T, Asamura H, Kawaishi M, Kuwano K, Ochiya T. The clinical relevance of the miR-197/CKS1B/STAT3-mediated PD-L1 network in chemoresistant non-small-cell lung cancer. Mol Ther. 2015;23: 717–27.
32. Zheng Z, Bu Z, Liu X, Zhang L, Li Z, Wu A, Wu X, Cheng X, Xing X, Du H, Wang X, Hu Y, Ji J. Level of circulating PD-L1 expression in patients with advanced gastric cancer and its clinical implications. Chin J Cancer Res. 2014;26:104–11.
33. Ha H, Nam AR, Bang JH, Park JE, Kim TY, Lee KH, Han SW, Im SA, Kim TY, Bang YJ, Oh DY. Soluble programmed death-ligand 1 (sPDL1) and neutrophil-to-lymphocyte ratio (NLR) predicts survival in advanced biliary tract cancer patients treated with palliative chemotherapy. Oncotarget. 2016;7:76604–12.
34. Wang L, Wang H, Chen H, Wang WD, Chen XQ, Geng QR, Xia ZJ, Lu Y. Serum levels of soluble programmed death ligand 1 predict treatment response and progression free survival in multiple myeloma. Oncotarget. 2015;6:41228–36.
35. Finkelmeier F, Canli Ö, Tal A, Pleli T, Trojan J, Schmidt M, Kronenberger B, Zeuzem S, Piiper A, Greten FR, Waidmann O. High levels of the soluble programmed death-ligand (sPD-L1) identify hepatocellular carcinoma patients with a poor prognosis. Eur J Cancer. 2016;59:152–9.
36. Rossille D, Gressier M, Damotte D, Maucort-Boulch D, Pangault C, Semana G, Le Gouill S, Haioun C, Tarte K, Lamy T, Milpied N, Fest T, Groupe Ouest-Est des Leucémies et Autres maladies du sang; Groupe Ouest-Est des Leucémies et Autres maladies du sang. High level of soluble programmed cell death ligand 1 in blood impacts overall survival in aggressive diffuse large B-cell lymphoma: results from a French multicenter clinical trial. Leukemia. 2014;28:2367–75.
37. Zhu Z, Jin Z, Zhang M, Tang Y, Yang G, Yuan X, Yao J, Sun D. Prognostic value of programmed death-ligand 1 in sarcoma: a meta-analysis. Oncotarget. 2017;8:59570–80.
38. Gunturi A, McDermott DF. Nivolumab for the treatment of cancer. Expert Opin Investig Drugs. 2015;24:253–60.
39. Nomura M, Otsuka A, Kondo T, Nagai H, Nonomura Y, Kaku Y, Matsumoto S, Muto M. Efficacy and safety of retreatment with nivolumab in metastatic melanoma patients previously treated with nivolumab. Cancer Chemother Pharmacol. 2017;80:999–1004.
40. Grossi F, Crinò L, Logroscino A, Canova S, Delmonte A, Melotti B, Proto C, Gelibter A, Cappuzzo F, Turci D, Gamucci T, Antonelli P, Marchetti P, Santoro A, Giusti S, Di Costanzo F, Giustini L, Del Conte A, Livi L, Giannarelli D, de Marinis F. Use of nivolumab in elderly patients with advanced squamous non-small-cell lung cancer: results from the Italian cohort of an expanded access programme. Eur J Cancer. 2018;100:126–34.
41. Gunjur A. Nivolumab plus ipilimumab in advanced renal-cell carcinoma. Lancet Oncol. 2018;19:e232.
42. Antonia SJ, López-Martin JA, Bendell J, Ott PA, Taylor M, Eder JP, Jäger D, Pietanza MC, Le DT, de Braud F, Morse MA, Ascierto PA, Horn L, Amin A, Pillai RN, Evans J, Chau I, Bono P, Atmaca A, Sharma P, Harbison CT, Lin CS, Christensen O, Calvo E. Nivolumab alone and nivolumab plus ipilimumab in recurrent small-cell lung cancer (CheckMate 032): a multicentre, open-label, phase 1/2 trial. Lancet Oncol. 2016;17:883–95.
43. Hellmann MD, Callahan MK, Awad MM, Calvo E, Ascierto PA, Atmaca A, Rizvi NA, Hirsch FR, Selvaggi G, Szustakowski JD, Sasson A, Golhar R, Vitazka P, Chang H, Geese WJ, Antonia SJ. Tumor mutational burden and efficacy of Nivolumab monotherapy and in combination with Ipilimumab in small-cell lung Cancer. Cancer Cell. 2018;33:853–61.

6

Short and long-term effects of pulmonary rehabilitation in interstitial lung diseases

Silvia Perez-Bogerd[1,2], Wim Wuyts[2], Veronica Barbier[2], Heleen Demeyer[3], Alain Van Muylem[1], Wim Janssens[2,3,4] and Thierry Troosters[2,3*]

Abstract

Background: Few data are available on the long-term effect of pulmonary rehabilitation (PR) and on long PR programs in interstitial lung diseases (ILD).
We aimed to evaluate the effects of PR on exercise capacity (6-Minute Walking Distance, 6MWD; Peak Work Rate, W_{max}), quality of life (St George's Respiratory Questionnaire, SGRQ), quadriceps force (QF) and objectively measured physical activity in ILD after the 6-month PR-program and after 1 year.

Methods: 60 patients (64 ± 11 years; 62% males; 23% with IPF) were randomly assigned to receive a 6 month-PR program or usual medical care.

Results: Exercise capacity, quality of life and muscle force increased significantly after the program as compared to control (mean,95%CI[ll to ul]; 6MWD + 72,[36 to 108] m; W_{max} 19, [8 to 29]%pred; SGRQ − 12,[− 19 to − 6] points; QF 10, [1 to 18] %pred). The gain was sustained after 1 year (6MWD 73,[28 to 118] m; Wmax 23, [10 to 35]%pred; SGRQ − 11,[− 18 to − 4] points; QF 9.5, [1 to 18] %pred). Physical activity did not change.

Conclusions: PR improves exercise tolerance, health status and muscle force in ILD. The benefits are maintained at 1-year follow-up. The intervention did not change physical activity.

Background

Interstitial lung diseases (ILD) are a group of disorders characterized by progressive dyspnoea, exercise limitation and poor quality of life [1, 2]. Treatment typically involves corticosteroids or cytotoxic drugs and, in some cases, anti-fibrotic agents [3]. While these therapies tackle the respiratory problems to some degree, strategies that further reduce complaints, improve health status and delay extra-pulmonary disease progression are therefore needed.

It has been shown that quadriceps weakness [4] and physical inactivity [5] are present in idiopathic pulmonary fibrosis (IPF) and poor exercise capacity, physical inactivity and, recently, a low fat-free mass index have been related to mortality [5–7]. Therefore, enhancing exercise tolerance, physical activity and muscle function in IPF must be treatment goals that were not shown to be altered by pharmacotherapy [3]. These factors have been proven to be tackled by pulmonary rehabilitation (PR) in other chronic lung diseases, such as COPD [8].

Rare randomised controlled trials exist about the effectiveness of PR in ILD [9–13]. A Cochrane review [14] accumulated 168 patients for the most studied outcome measure (6-min walking distance, 6MWD) and reported clinically significant benefits on this outcome after short programs (8–12 weeks). A recent large Australian trial reported somewhat smaller effects [9]. None of these studies propose long programs and only one small trial showed limited long-term effects (beyond 6 months) [15].

* Correspondence: thierry.troosters@kuleuven.be;
Thierry.troosters@kuleuven.be
[2]University Hospitals Leuven, Department of Respiratory Diseases, B-3000 Leuven, Belgium
[3]KU Leuven, Department of Rehabilitation Sciences, B-3000 Leuven, Belgium
Full list of author information is available at the end of the article

The aim of this study was to evaluate the feasibility and effectiveness of a longer (6-month) multidisciplinary PR program on exercise tolerance, muscle strength, quality of life and physical activity in a randomized controlled trial. In addition, long-term benefits of the program were investigated.

Methods

Study subjects

Patients with chronic ILD referred to the ILD clinic in the University Hospital of Leuven were considered for enrolment. According to eligibility criteria, potential candidates were informed about the protocol and written informed consent was obtained, between March 2009 and September 2011. The study was approved by the local ethics committee (B32220095560) of this hospital.

Inclusion criteria were a diagnosis of ILD according to internationally established criteria with a formal workup and multidisciplinary discussion [1, 2], dyspnoea on exertion and having a stable medical therapy with no infection/exacerbation in the previous 4 weeks.

Exclusion criteria were comorbidities (unstable angina, recent myocardial infarction or cerebrovascular accident, active cancer, severe orthopedic disorders) or systemic manifestations (active myopathy, arthralgia, synovitis) that do not allow training and a life expectancy below 3 months.

Study design

Patients were randomly assigned to the rehabilitation or control group using sealed envelopes prepared and shuffled before the start of the study by an independent person unrelated to the study protocol. The envelope was opened by the allocator sequentially, only after the participant's name was written on it.

Patients assigned to the rehabilitation group were invited to attend a 6-month outpatient rehabilitation program with a total of 60 sessions, 3 times per week for the first 3 months and thereafter twice weekly. The program was performed in accordance with the guidelines [16] and is detailed in the Additional file 1 (online data supplement). Patients assigned to the control group were treated with maximal medical care and with an identical medical follow-up, similarly to the active intervention arm.

Assessments

All measurements were made at enrolment and at 3, 6 and 12 months after the start of the study.

The primary outcome of the study, functional exercise capacity, was measured as the distance walked during the best of two 6-minute walking tests (6MWD) [17] and also expressed as percentage of the predicted values [18]. Use of oxygen was standardized to a minimal flow rate of 2 l-per-minute and subsequent follow-up tests were conducted in the same conditions as at baseline. The difference in 6MWD between treatment and control group at 6 months was considered as the primary endpoint.

The secondary outcomes were forced vital capacity (FVC); slow vital capacity (SVC); diffusing capacity for carbon monoxide (DL_{CO}); arterial partial pressure of oxygen (PaO_2); maximal work rate (W_{max}); 6MWD; quadriceps (QF) and hand grip (HF) muscle force; quality of life evaluated by the the St George's respiratory (SGRQ) and the chronic respiratory disease questionnaires (CRQ) and dyspnoea (MRC 1 to 5). More details on the assessments are provided in the Additional file 1 (online data supplement).

Patients were provided with an activity monitor SenseWear Armband (Bodymedia, Pittsburgh, USA), in order to assess objectively their physical activity. They were instructed to wear the monitor for at least 7 consecutive days, from waking up until going to bed. Days with less than 8 h of wearing time during waking (defined as 7 AM-8 PM) were excluded. Only week days were used to minimize the variability. A valid measurement was defined as having at least 2 valid weekdays. The influence of the duration of the daylight time was included as a covariate [19].

Mean step count and mean time in at least moderate intense physical activity (MPA) were chosen as the physical activity outcomes. MPA was defined as any activity with an energy expenditure above 3 METs [20]. The SenseWear has been validated in COPD patients [21], a respiratory population with a comparable inactive lifestyle.

Physical activity at 1 year was not included in the analysis due to the large number of missing data at this time point, caused by incompliance of patients and technical problems. For this reason the data were not judged as being representative of the entire sample and therefore not included in the analyses.

All adverse events during the rehabilitation program were registered.

Statistics

All variables were expressed as means ± standard deviation (SD) or 95% confidence interval (95% CI). A minimal 6MWD benefit of 38 ± 43 m might be expected after 3 months [10]. To anticipate a similar difference of 40 ± 45 m, a sample size of 20 patients in each arm is needed to show a statistically significant difference at the 0.05 p-level with 80% power. Anticipating on 40% of dropouts, a total number of 60 patients were randomized. Statistical analysis was performed using mixed models including the outcomes as measured in the 4 visits (baseline, after 3, 6 and 12 months). 'Visit' was included as a class variable. *P* values below 0.05 were considered as significant in all analyses (R version 3.2.1) [22]. Group, time and group*time interactions were retrieved. This interaction term assesses the pure effect of rehabilitation since it is the difference, at each time-point, between changes from baseline in the rehabilitation group and in the control group. Duration of daylight was including as a (time varying) covariate when investigating the physical activity outcomes [19]. The number needed to treat (NNT) to achieve an increase in functional exercise capacity was defined as a clinically significant improvement (> 30 m) in the 6MWD.

Results

Study recruitment and population characteristics

Figure 1 shows the Consort flow diagram. From 271 patients referred to the ILD clinic, 209 were eligible for inclusion; 60 (22%; 37 M/23F) were randomized.

Sixty-seven percent of patients completed the rehabilitation program and 60% of the randomized patients were followed up at 1 year.

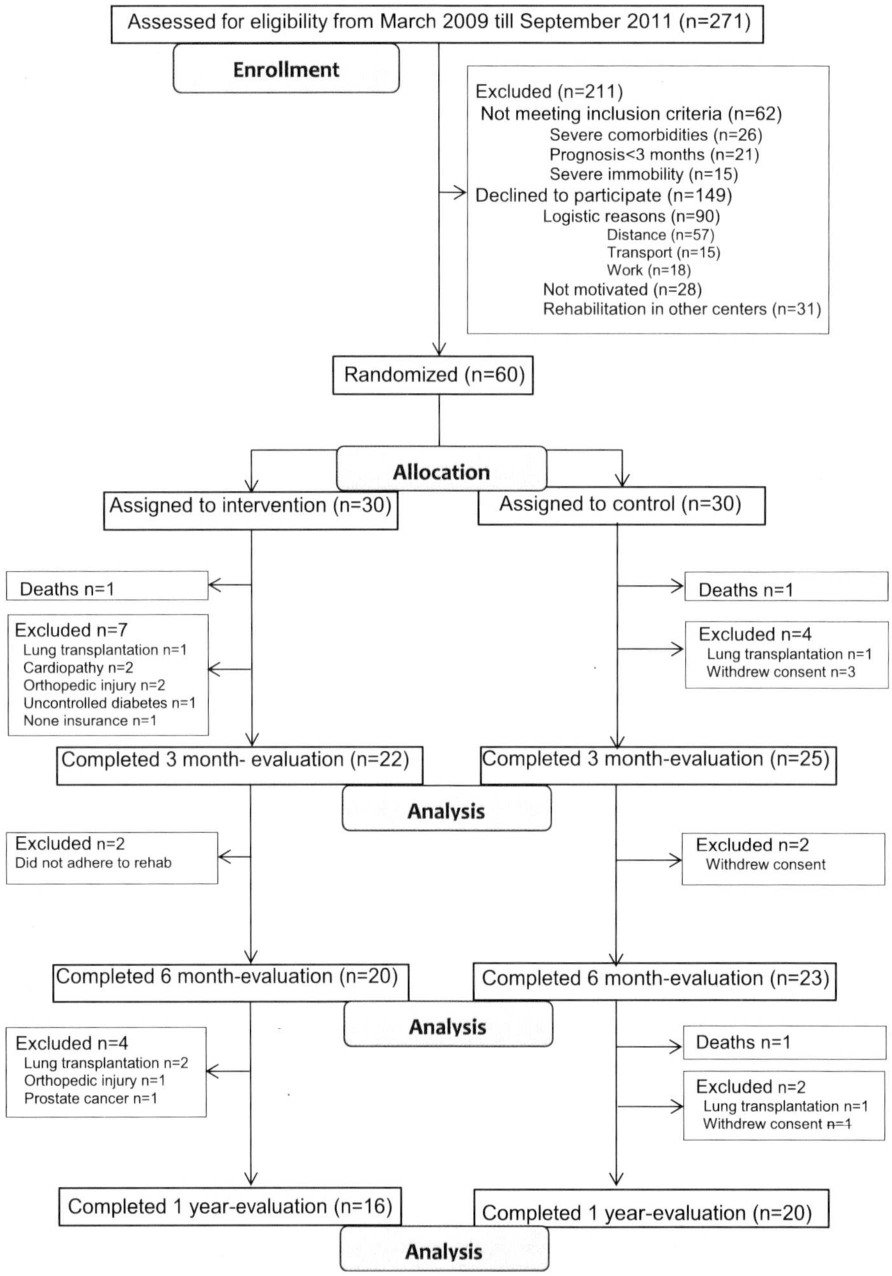

Fig. 1 Consort Flow Diagram

Table 1 shows the baseline characteristics of the participants. At baseline, 6MWD (expressed as percentage of the predicted value) was slightly lower ($p = 0.045$) and hypersensitivity pneumonitis was more represented in the rehabilitation group. The groups were matched for other parameters (Table 1, Additional file 1: Table S1). Patients who dropped out did not differ from those who completed the study in the rehabilitation group; in the control group, drop-outs appeared to be younger and to have worse diffusing capacity (Additional file 1: Table S2).

Table 1 Baseline characteristics

	Control $n = 30$	*Rehabilitation* $n = 30$	*p- Value*
Age (years)	64 (8)	64 (13)	0.81
Gender (men)	15 (50%)	22 (73%)	0.06
BMI (Kg/m^2)	26 (5)	28 (4)	0.21
Diagnosis			
IIP	10 (33%)	11 (37%)	0.79
• IPF	7 (23%)	7 (23%)	1.0
• NSIP	3 (10%)	3 (10%)	1.0
• DIP	0	1 (3%)	0.50
KNOWN CAUSES	12 (40%)	16 (53%)	0.30
• Chronic HP	4 (13%)	12 (40%)	**0.02**
• Asbestosis	0	1 (3%)	0.50
• Drug induced ILD	1 (3%)	1 (3%)	1.0
• CTD-ILD	7 (23%)	2 (7%)	0.14
UNCLASSIFIABLE ILD	8 (27%)	3 (10%)	0.09
Steroids	14 (47%)	15 (50%)	0.80
SVC (L)	2.6 (1.1)	2.9 (0.7)	0.35
SVC (%pred)	77 (22)	76 (20)	0.86
DL_{CO} ($mmol.min^{-1}.kPa^{-1}$)	3,4 (1,1)	4 (1,6)	0.11
DL_{CO} (%pred)	41 (13)	45 (16)	0.30
PaO_2 (mmHg)	77 (14)	76 (11)	0.71
6MWD (m)	491 (95)	462 (123)	0.32
6MWD (%pred)	79 (14)	71 (16)	**0.045**
W_{max} (%pred)	71 (26)	61 (20)	0.10
QF (%pred)	81 (36)	78 (23)	0.70
HF (%pred)	85 (27)	89 (23)	0.61
SGRQ total (points)	40 (18)	42 (14)	0.68
Physical Activity (PA)			
• Steps per day	7182 (3523)	5745 (3312)	0.12
• MPA	57 (21–158)	36 (10–130)	0.14

Data expressed as mean (SD) or numbers and MPA as geometric mean (geometric interval): geometric mean is antilog(m) and geometric interval is (antilog(m-SD) – antilog(m + SD)), m and SD being the mean and the standard deviation of the log-transformed MPA, respectively. *BMI* body mass index, *IIP* idiopathic interstitial pneumonia, *IPF* idiopathic pulmonary fibrosis, *NSIP* nonspecific interstitial pneumonia, *DIP* desquamative interstitial pneumonia, *HP* hypersensitivity pneumonitis, *CTD-ILD* connective tissue disease-related ILD, *SVC* slow vital capacity, *DLco* diffusion capacity for carbon monoxide, PaO_2 partial pressure of oxygen at breathing room air, *6MWD* six-minute walking distance, W_{max} maximal workload, *QF* quadriceps force, *SGRQ* St George's respiratory questionnaire, *MPA* moderate intense physical activity (dailt time spent in activities with an intensity of at least 3 METs)a. *p*-values in bold indicate a statistically significant difference between intervention and control group

Effects

At 6 months, the 6MWD of the intervention group was mean, 95% CI [ll to ul] +72, [36 to 108]m better as compared to the usual care group (Table 2, Fig. 2). The benefit was largely maintained between groups at 1-year follow-up (73, [28 to 118] m). Taking a conservative intention to treat approach where none of the dropouts in either group is counted as a responder, 11 patients (37% of the initially selected 30 patients) had a clinically significant improvement in their 6MWD at the 1-year time point, whereas only 5 (17%) of the controls had such an improvement. This results in a NNT of 5.

Similarly, the intervention yielded significant increases in maximal exercise capacity (W_{max}), health status (in all the domains) and quadriceps force at the end of PR (Table 2, Fig. 2, Additional file 1: Tables S3-S4), as compared to usual care. Most of these benefits were maintained at 1 year. A significant improvement was already shown after 3 months of PR for exercise tolerance, muscle force, total scores of health status, SGRQ activity domain and CRQ dyspnoea, emotion and mastery (Table 2, Additional file 1: Tables S3-S4).

The rehabilitation program did not change MRC dyspnoea and physical activity significantly as compared to the control group at any time point (Table 3, Fig. 2, Additional file 1: Table S4).

PR did not influence lung function and arterial blood gases with the exception of forced vital capacity which was slightly better in the rehabilitation group as compared to usual care (Table 2, Additional file 1: Table S5).

Missing data

The mixed model assumes that a patient with a missing data follows the general trend of the group. We challenged this option by considering a more penalizing hypothesis: in the intervention group, missing data were assumed to follow the general trend of the control group whereas, in the control group, missing data were assumed to be equal to the baseline values. With this hypothesis, the PR-effect on 6MWD, W_{max}, QF and CRQ remained significant at any time-point (Additional file 1: Table S6).

Feasibility and adverse events

The patients participated in a mean of 50 ± 13 sessions. Aerobic training intensity for cycling started at 65 ± 8% of the initial W_{max}. Walking was initiated at 72 ± 8% of the baseline mean 6MWD speed. These intensities were

Table 2 Effects of PR and at 1-year on exercise capacity, muscle force and health status

	Control	Rehabilitation	Rehabilitation effect mean (95% CI ll,ul)	p- Value
6MWD (m)				
Baseline	491 (57)	462 (57)		0.36
3 months	474 (57)	504 (57)	59 (33, 85)	**< 0.001**
6 months	468 (57)	511 (57)	72 (36, 108)	**< 0.001**
1 year	456 (57)	501 (57)	73 (28, 118)	**0.002**
W_{max} (%pred)				
Baseline	71 (18)	61 (18)		0.15
3 months	68 (18)	68 (18)	10 (2, 19)	**0.01**
6 months	62 (18)	71 (18)	19 (8, 29)	**< 0.001**
1 year	61 (18)	74 (18)	23 (10, 35)	**< 0.001**
SVC (%pred)				
Baseline	77 (21)	76 (21)		0.86
3 months	77 (21)	78 (21)	2 (−2, 6)	0.23
6 months	75 (21)	77 (21)	3 (−1, 7)	0.20
1 year	76 (21)	79 (21)	4 (−0.2, 9)	0.06
DL_{CO} (%pred)				
Baseline	42 (13)	45 (13)		0.31
3 months	39 (13)	44 (13)	1.2 (− 2.4, 4.8)	0.52
6 months	39 (13)	43(13)	0.9 (−3.6, 5.3)	0.70
1 year	38 (13)	45 (13)	3.2 (−1.8, 8.2)	0.21
QF (%pred)				
Baseline	81 (27)	78 (27)		0.69
3 months	81 (27)	88 (27)	10 (2, 18)	**0.01**
6 months	83 (27)	90 (27)	10 (1, 18)	**0.02**
1 year	88 (27)	94 (27)	9.5 (1, 18)	**0.04**
HF (%pred)				
Baseline	73 (17)	76(17)		0.56
3 months	76 (17)	91 (17)	12.5 (5, 20)	**0.002**
6 months	75 (17)	90 (17)	12 (4, 20)	**0.004**
1 year	79 (17)	88 (17)	6 (−3, 15)	0.20
SGRQ total				
Baseline	40 (14)	42 (14)		0.68
3 months	44 (14)	39 (14)	−7 (−13, −2)	**0.005**
6 months	46 (14)	35 (14)	−12 (−19, −6)	**< 0.001**
1 year	45 (14)	35 (14)	−11 (− 18, −4)	**0.002**

Data are expressed as mean (SD) from the mixed model. The rehabilitation effect at each time point is the difference (and its 95% confidence interval) between changes from baseline in the rehabilitation group and in the control group. *6MWD* six-minute walking distance, W_{max} maximal workload, *SVC* slow vital capacity, *DLco* diffusion capacity for carbon monoxide, *QF* quadriceps force, *HF* handgrip force, *SGRQ* St George's respiratory questionnaire. The rehabilitation effect at each time point is the interaction term between time points and group effects. The *p*-Value on the baseline line assesses differences in baseline values, the other ones assess the effect of rehabilitation at each time point. *p*-values in bold indicate a statistically significance

progressed to 95 ± 17% and 106 ± 15%, respectively. The resistance training load also increased significantly over time (Fig. 3).

No adverse events related to the exercise training were recorded during the PR program.

Discussion

This is the first trial showing long-term benefits (at 1-year follow-up) after a 6-month outpatient PR program in ILD and the first study investigating the PR-effect on objectively measured physical activity (PA). As hypothesized, exercise capacity, health status and muscle force improved significantly after PR; these benefits were maintained after 1 year in those patients that completed the program. PR did not change the physical activity level.

The improvements in exercise capacity (6MWD) and quality of life (total scores; symptoms and impact of SGRQ; and dyspnea, emotion and mastery of CRQ) are relevant, as they exceeded the minimal clinically important difference (MCID) after PR and at 1-year follow-up (Table 2 and Additional file 1: Table S4) [23–26]. In IPF, the MCID of the 6MWD (22–45 m) [23, 26] and the SGRQ (5–8 points) [27] have been established [24], but, to our knowledge, the MCID of the CRQ has not been validated yet in ILD, only in COPD (0,5 points per item) [25]. Clinically relevant strategies, such as pulmonary rehabilitation, are very important for ILD patients whose quality of life is seriously deteriorated.

Short-term benefits

To our knowledge, there are only 5 randomized controlled trials [9–13] and a meta-analysis [14] demonstrating improvements in exercise performance and symptoms after exercise training in ILD. Only one non-randomised study showed a benefit on muscle force after PR [28]. Overall, the magnitude of the effect in our trial was more pronounced than in previous shorter studies [10, 11, 13, 28–33].

Unfortunately, the large benefits after PR in ILD were not translated in objective gains in PA. This is in line with research in COPD [34]: some trials showed an increase in PA after PR and others failed to do so. In the negative studies, the lack of improvement was also observed despite gains in physiological function and health status. This is the first trial measuring the PR-effect on PA in ILD objectively. Previously, 2 studies [6, 35] have evaluated IPF patients with PA questionnaires and have suggested small benefits. However, questionnaires may not provide a reliable estimation of true PA behaviour. In our study, no specific interventions were introduced to coach patients towards more PA. Future studies could consider for instance the

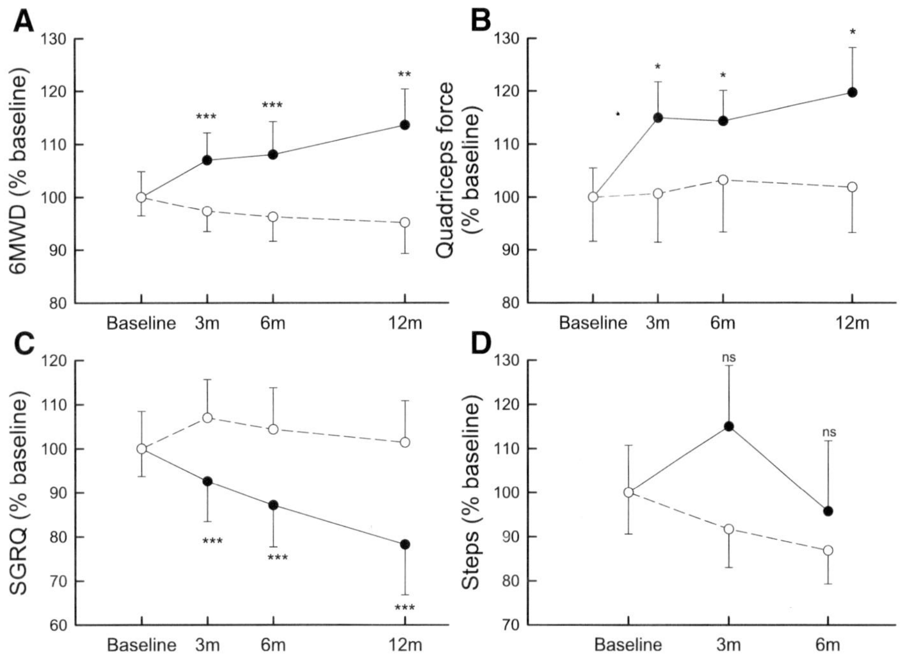

Fig. 2 Effects of PR and at 1-year on exercise capacity, muscle force, health status, physical activity. 6-min walking distance (6MWD) (Panel **a**), quadriceps force (Panel **b**), St-Georges respiratory questionnaire (SGRQ) (Panel **c**) and steps per day (Steps) (Panel **d**) expressed as percentage (%) of the baseline value as a function of time. Closed circles (solid lines) and open circles (dashed lines) are the mean values and SEM at each time points of rehabilitation and control groups, respectively. Rehabilitation and control groups were compared for rehabilitation effects at each time points: *** $p < 0.001$; ** $p < 0.01$; * $p \leq 0.05$; ns $p > 0.05$

Table 3 Effects of PR on physical activity

	Control	*Rehabilitation*	*Rehabilitation effect mean (95% CI ll,ul)*	*p-Value*
Steps				
Baseline	7013 (2598)	5671 (2598)		0.10
3 months	6593 (2598)	5721 (2598)	470 (− 920, 1860)	0.50
6 months	6118 (2598)	5540 (2598)	764 (− 746, 2274)	0.32
MPA				
Baseline	54 (38, 78)	36 (25, 52)		0.46
3 months	44 (31, 64)	37 (26, 54)	1.3 (0.7, 2.2)	0.42
6 months	41 (29, 60)	33 (23, 48)	1.2 (0.6, 2.3)	0.57

Steps expressed as mean (SD) and MPA as geometric mean (geometric interval): geometric mean is antilog(m) and geometric interval is (antilog(m-SD), antilog(m + SD)), m and SD being the mean and the SD of the log-transformed MPA, respectively. *MPA* moderate intense physical activity (daily time spent in activities with an intensity of at least 3 METs). The rehabilitation effect at each time point is the difference (and its 95% confidence interval) between changes from baseline in the rehabilitation group and in the control group. As computation was made on log-transformed MPA, rehabilitation effect is expressed as a ratio (1.3 means + 30% in favor of rehabilitation). The *p*-Value on the baseline line assesses differences in baseline values, the other ones assess the effect of rehabilitation at each time point

provision of feedback on PA using step-counters providing promising results in COPD [36].

Feasibility

The high number of attended sessions and the high exercise intensity reached during the training sessions indicate that PR is feasible to be implemented in ILD in a similar way as in COPD [8]. In the present study, ILD patients trained alongside patients with COPD and other chronic respiratory conditions. However, it remains a point of attention that many patients refuse the offer for rehabilitation and 33% dropped out during the program although the reasons were not related to the provided intervention.

All ILD patients used oxygen supplements per protocol in order to avoid desaturation [37] and all the exercise tests were performed with oxygen in order to better show the improvements related to the training [38].

Long-term benefits

The novel finding of this trial is the maintenance of the benefits in exercise capacity, health status and muscle force at 1 year in a subgroup of patients. So far, 5 studies [10, 13, 15, 28, 39] have evaluated long-term effects. Only 1 randomized trial [15] did find a discrete gain in quality of life at 1 year and one non-randomized study [39]

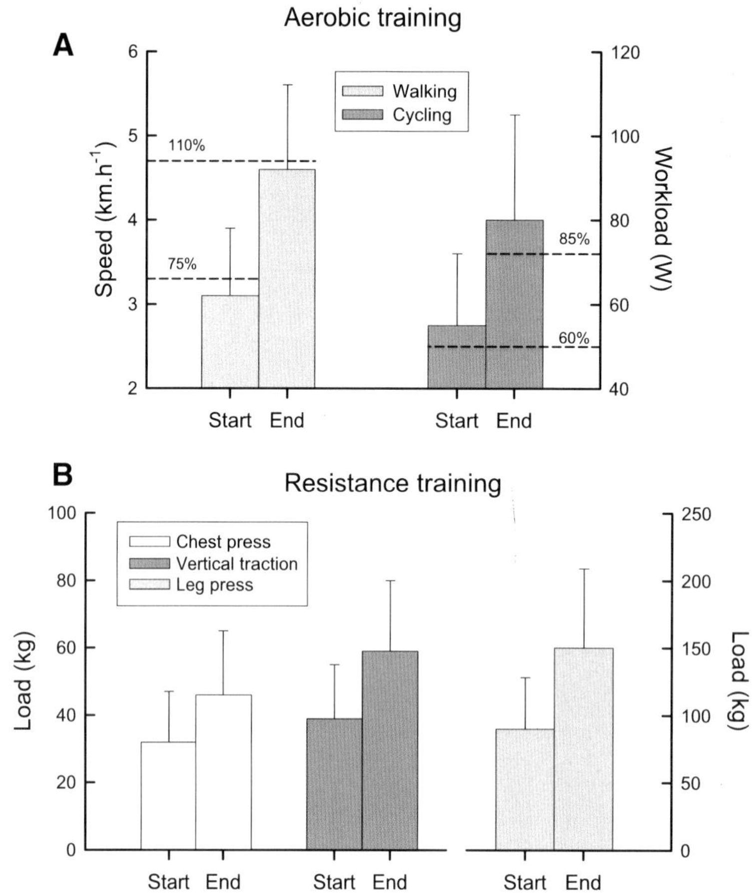

Fig. 3 Feasability of the training. Training intensity at the Start and the End of the 6 month PR program, expressed as mean (SD). Aerobic training: patients started the Cycling at 60% of the initial maximal workload on the cycle ergometer and the Walking at 75% of their maximal walking speed during the initial 6-min walking test. Based on subjective Borg scale scores, the intensity was progressively increased up to 85% of the maximal workload and up to 110% of the maximal walking speed (Dashed lines, Panel **a**). Resistance training: patients started the program on a multi-gym device in 3 series of 8 repetitions at 70% of the initial 1-Repetition Maximum (1RM) load for each muscle group (chest press, vertical traction, leg press) and this load was progressively incremented (Panel **b**)

showed an improvement on 6MWD and health status at 6 months.

The larger and long-term benefits in our study could potentially be explained by the differences in the rehabilitation program, the differences in disease aetiology and disease severity.

First, our regimen proposed a longer training than reported previously [9–13, 28–30, 32, 33, 35, 39]. In COPD, longer programs showed to have more effects than shorter programs [8, 40]. In addition, in line with recommendations for PR [16], a multidisciplinary approach consisting of occupational therapy, psychosocial and nutritional support was offered in our program.

Second, the lower proportion of IPF patients (23% in our trial compared to 100% [11–13] or around 50% of the patients [9, 10] in the other 5 randomised trials) could explain the more pronounced treatment effects. Indeed, the magnitude of improvement following PR in IPF was less than other ILD [10, 41, 42] or COPD [28]. However, a mixed population reflects more the clinical reality of most of ILD units.

Third, greater PR-benefits were described in patients with less functional impairment [9, 10, 28]. Our patients had better baseline 6MWD and muscle force [10, 11, 13, 28–33], whereas, the impairment in health status was comparable [43]. In fact, one trial with a similar baseline 6MWD did find similar PR-gains [12]. However, this remains controversial since other studies found greater improvements in the most disabled patients [29, 39].

Finally, it is important to note that, among the immunosuppressive medications proposed in the majority of non-IPF [2] and the recent recommended antifibrotic agents in IPF [3], none of them did increase exercise capacity, only pirfenidone has demonstrated to reduce the decline in 6MWD [44–47]; and nintedanib [48, 49] showed a discrete, not clinically significant, improvement in quality of life in 1 of the 2 phase three trials [49]. The fact that PR showed a large and maintained benefit on health status and exercise tolerance and without any clinically meaningful side effects is of utmost importance to ILD patients.

Natural evolution of the disease

In contrast to previous trials, our study did not show a lung function decline over time in the whole group [9, 10]. This finding might be due to our larger amount of non-IPF patients.

Curiously, our study showed an improvement over time of muscle force in the entire group. Steroid therapy contributes to muscle dysfunction in ILD [50], a treatment often proposed to non-IPF patients [1, 2, 51]. In our study, 47% were under prednisolone at baseline or during the preceding 6 months (Table 2) and only 28% at 1 year. We suggest that muscle dysfunction of our ILD patients might be partly explained by the steroid therapy and the improvement over time by the gradual steroid tapering.

Limitations

First, an a priori expected limitation of the study was the dropout rate (33%) over the course of the 6-month PR program. This number was slightly higher than observed in ILD following some shorter programs [10–13, 30, 33, 39], but similar as the Australian trial [9] and long programs in COPD [8, 40]. However, since the patients who dropped out from the rehabilitation group were very similar to those who completed the PR program, this has likely had minimal impact on the main results of the study. In addition, it is important to see that long-term benefits were obtained in a significant fraction of patients in the rehabilitation group resulting in a very acceptable NNT of 5 for the outcome 6MWD. Finally, a treatment of missing data penalizing the PR-effect did not affect the significance at any time-point.

Second, assessors were not blinded for 6MWD (main outcome) which may have led to an overestimation of the benefit, however this probably will not have affected the results of quality of life.

Third, only 20% from the eligible candidates were randomized in the present study (Fig. 1). This may compromise the external validity of the study. Whereas it shows the general difficulty of performing randomised controlled trials in rare diseases like ILD and patients may have considerable travel distances to attend our centre of reference. This has likely not impacted on the observed differences between groups.

Conclusion

We conclude that a 6-month outpatient pulmonary rehabilitation program resulted in improvements in functional and maximal exercise capacity, health status and muscle force but not in physical activity in patients with ILD. The benefits were maintained at 1-year follow-up.

Abbreviations

1RM: One-Repetition maximum; 6MWD: Six-minute walking distance; CRQ: Chronic respiratory disease questionnaire; CTD-ILD: Connective tissue disease-related ILD; DIP: Desquamative interstitial pneumonia; DL_{CO}: Diffusion capacity for carbon monoxide; HF: Handgrip force; HP: Hypersensitivity pneumonitis; IIP: Idiopathic interstitial pneumonia; ILD: Interstitial lung diseases; IPF: Idiopathic pulmonary fibrosis; MPA: Moderate to intense physical activity; NNT: Number needed to treat; NSIP: Nonspecific interstitial pneumonia; PA: Physical activity; PaO_2: Partial pressure of oxygen at breathing room air; PR: Pulmonary rehabilitation; QF: Quadriceps force; SGRQ: St-George's respiratory questionnaire; VC: Slow vital capacity; W_{max}: Maximal workload

Acknowledgements

The authors would like to thank the physiotherapists, Ilse Muylaert and Iris Coosemans, and the other staff of the Respiratory Rehabilitation Department for their assistance with the clinical tests and the supervision of the rehabilitation sessions. We would also like to thank the staff of the Pulmonary Function Department for their assistance with the lung function and exercise tests. We are also grateful to the researchers, Daniel Langer, Chris Burtin, Hans Van Remoortel and Miek Hornikx, for the help in collection and analysis of the physical activity data.

Funding

HD is a post-doctoral research fellow of the Flemish Research Foundation (FWO #G.0871.13). WJ is a senior clinical investigator of the FWO. TT is supported by the FWO #G.0871.13.

Prior abstract publication/presentation

As an oral presentation at the ERS Congress in Amsterdam (September 2011). Silvia Pérez Bogerd, Wim Wuyts, Veronica Barbier, Daniel Langer, Chris Burtin, Hans Van Remoortel, Marc Decramer, Thierry Troosters, Wim Janssens. Preliminary results of pulmonary rehabilitation in interstitial lung diseases: a randomised controlled trial. *Eur Respir J.* 2011; 38 (Suppl 55): P1451.

Authors' contributions

Conception, design and protocol development: SPB VB WW WJ TT. Conception, design and protocol development: SPB VB WW WJ TT. Data collection: SPB VB HD. Analysis and interpretation of the data: SPB HD AVM WJ TT. Writing of the manuscript: SPB. Critical review of the manuscript: WW HD AVM WJ TT. All authors approved the manuscript to be published.

Competing interests

SPB, VB, HD and TT have nothing to disclose. WW reports grants from Roche and Boehringer Ingelheim, outside the submitted work. WJ reports grants from Chiesi, Astra Zeneca, Boehringer Ingelheim, GSK, Novartis, outside the submitted work.

Author details

[1]Erasme University Hospital, Chest Department, Université Libre Bruxelles, B-1060 Brussels, Belgium. [2]University Hospitals Leuven, Department of Respiratory Diseases, B-3000 Leuven, Belgium. [3]KU Leuven, Department of Rehabilitation Sciences, B-3000 Leuven, Belgium. [4]KU Leuven, Department of Chronic Diseases, Metabolism and Ageing, B-3000 Leuven, Belgium.

References

1. Raghu G, Collard HR, Egan JJ, Martinez FJ, Behr J, Brown KK, Colby TV, Cordier JF, Flaherty KR, Lasky JA, et al. An official ATS/ERS/JRS/ALAT statement: idiopathic pulmonary fibrosis: evidence-based guidelines for diagnosis and management. Am J Respir Crit Care Med. 2011;183:788–824.
2. Travis WD, Costabel U, Hansell DM, King TE Jr, Lynch DA, Nicholson AG, Ryerson CJ, Ryu JH, Selman M, Wells AU, et al. An official American Thoracic Society/European Respiratory Society statement: update of the international multidisciplinary classification of the idiopathic interstitial pneumonias. Am J Respir Crit Care Med. 2013;188:733–48.
3. Raghu G, Rochwerg B, Zhang Y, Garcia CA, Azuma A, Behr J, Brozek JL, Collard HR, Cunningham W, Homma S, et al. An official ATS/ERS/JRS/ALAT clinical practice guideline: treatment of idiopathic pulmonary fibrosis. An update of the 2011 clinical practice guideline. Am J Respir Crit Care Med. 2015;192:e3–19.
4. Nishiyama O, Taniguchi H, Kondoh Y, Kimura T, Ogawa T, Watanabe F, Arizono S. Quadriceps weakness is related to exercise capacity in idiopathic pulmonary fibrosis. Chest. 2005;127:2028–33.
5. Wallaert B, Monge E, Le Rouzic O, Wemeau-Stervinou L, Salleron J, Grosbois JM. Physical activity in daily life of patients with fibrotic idiopathic interstitial pneumonia. Chest. 2013;144:1652–8.
6. Vainshelboim B, Kramer MR, Izhakian S, Lima RM, Oliveira J. Physical activity and exertional desaturation are associated with mortality in idiopathic pulmonary fibrosis. J Clin Med. 2016;5:73.
7. Nishiyama O, Yamazaki R, Sano H, Iwanaga T, Higashimoto Y, Kume H, Tohda Y. Fat-free mass index predicts survival in patients with idiopathic pulmonary fibrosis. Respirology. 2017;22:480–5.
8. McCarthy B, Casey D, Devane D, Murphy K, Murphy E, Lacasse Y. Pulmonary rehabilitation for chronic obstructive pulmonary disease. Cochrane Database Syst Rev. 2015;2.
9. Dowman LM, McDonald CF, Hill CJ, Lee AL, Barker K, Boote C, Glaspole I, Goh NSL, Southcott AM, Burge AT, et al. The evidence of benefits of exercise training in interstitial lung disease: a randomised controlled trial. Thorax. 2017;72:610–9.
10. Holland AE, Hill CJ, Conron M, Munro P, McDonald CF. Short term improvement in exercise capacity and symptoms following exercise training in interstitial lung disease. Thorax. 2008;63:549–54.
11. Nishiyama O, Kondoh Y, Kimura T, Kato K, Kataoka K, Ogawa T, Watanabe F, Arizono S, Nishimura K, Taniguchi H. Effects of pulmonary rehabilitation in patients with idiopathic pulmonary fibrosis. Respirology. 2008;13:394–9.
12. Vainshelboim B, Oliveira J, Yehoshua L, Weiss I, Fox BD, Fruchter O, Kramer MR. Exercise training-based pulmonary rehabilitation program is clinically beneficial for idiopathic pulmonary fibrosis. Respiration. 2014;88:378–88.
13. Jackson RM, Gomez-Marin OW, Ramos CF, Sol CM, Cohen MI, Gaunaurd IA, Cahalin LP, Cardenas DD. Exercise limitation in IPF patients: a randomized trial of pulmonary rehabilitation. Lung. 2014;192:367–76.
14. Dowman L, Hill CJ, Holland AE. Pulmonary rehabilitation for interstitial lung disease. Cochrane Database Syst Rev. 2014;10.
15. Vainshelboim B, Oliveira J, Fox BD, Soreck Y, Fruchter O, Kramer MR. Long-term effects of a 12-week exercise training program on clinical outcomes in idiopathic pulmonary fibrosis. Lung. 2015;193:345–54.
16. Spruit MA, Singh SJ, Garvey C, ZuWallack R, Nici L, Rochester C, Hill K, Holland AE, Lareau SC, Man WD, et al. An official American Thoracic Society/European Respiratory Society statement: key concepts and advances in pulmonary rehabilitation. Am J Respir Crit Care Med. 2013;188:e13–64.
17. Brooks D, Solway S, Gibbons WJ. ATS statement on six-minute walk test. Am J Respir Crit Care Med. 2003;167:1287.
18. Troosters T, Gosselink R, Decramer M. Six minute walking distance in healthy elderly subjects. Eur Respir J. 1999;14:270–4.
19. Demeyer H, Burtin C, Van Remoortel H, Hornikx M, Langer D, Decramer M, Gosselink R, Janssens W, Troosters T. Standardizing the analysis of physical activity in patients with COPD following a pulmonary rehabilitation program. Chest. 2014;146:318–27.
20. Haskell WL, Lee IM, Pate RR, Powell KE, Blair SN, Franklin BA, Macera CA, Heath GW, Thompson PD, Bauman A. Physical activity and public health: updated recommendation for adults from the American College of Sports Medicine and the American Heart Association. Med Sci Sports Exerc. 2007;39:1423–34.
21. Van Remoortel H, Raste Y, Louvaris Z, Giavedoni S, Burtin C, Langer D, Wilson F, Rabinovich R, Vogiatzis I, Hopkinson NS, et al. Validity of six activity monitors in chronic obstructive pulmonary disease: a comparison with indirect calorimetry. PLoS One. 2012;7:e39198.
22. Vainshelboim B, Fox BD, Kramer MR, Izhakian S, Gershman E, Oliveira J. Short-term improvement in physical activity and body composition after supervised exercise training program in idiopathic pulmonary fibrosis. Arch Phys Med Rehabil. 2016;97:788–97.
23. Swigris JJ, Wamboldt FS, Behr J, du Bois RM, King TE, Raghu G, Brown KK. The 6 minute walk in idiopathic pulmonary fibrosis: longitudinal changes and minimum important difference. Thorax. 2010;65:173–7.
24. Swigris JJ, Brown KK, Behr J, du Bois RM, King TE, Raghu G, Wamboldt FS. The SF-36 and SGRQ: validity and first look at minimum important differences in IPF. Respir Med. 2010;104:296–304.
25. Jaeschke R, Singer J, Guyatt GH. Measurement of health status Ascertaining the minimal clinically important difference. Control Clin Trials. 1989;10:407–15.
26. du Bois RM, Weycker D, Albera C, Bradford WZ, Costabel U, Kartashov A, Lancaster L, Noble PW, Sahn SA, Szwarcberg J, et al. Six-minute-walk test in idiopathic pulmonary fibrosis: test validation and minimal clinically important difference. Am J Respir Crit Care Med. 2011;183:1231–7.
27. Jones PW, Quirk FH, Baveystock CM. The St George's respiratory questionnaire. Respir Med. 1991;85:25–31 Suppl B discussion 33–27.
28. Kozu R, Senjyu H, Jenkins SC, Mukae H, Sakamoto N, Kohno S. Differences in response to pulmonary rehabilitation in idiopathic pulmonary fibrosis and chronic obstructive pulmonary disease. Respiration. 2011;81:196–205.
29. Ferreira A, Garvey C, Connors GL, Hilling L, Rigler J, Farrell S, Cayou C, Shariat C, Collard HR. Pulmonary rehabilitation in interstitial lung disease: benefits and predictors of response. Chest. 2009;135:442–7.
30. Rammaert B, Leroy S, Cavestri B, Wallaert B, Grosbois JM. Home-based pulmonary rehabilitation in idiopathic pulmonary fibrosis. Rev Mal Respir. 2011;28:e52–7.
31. Salhi B, Troosters T, Behaegel M, Joos G, Derom E. Effects of pulmonary rehabilitation in patients with restrictive lung diseases. Chest. 2010;137:273–9.
32. Jastrzebski D, Gumola A, Gawlik R, Kozielski J. Dyspnea and quality of life in patients with pulmonary fibrosis after six weeks of respiratory rehabilitation. J Physiol Pharmacol. 2006;57(4):139–48.
33. Huppmann P, Sczepanski B, Boensch M, Winterkamp S, Schonheit-Kenn U, Neurohr C, Behr J, Kenn K. Effects of inpatient pulmonary rehabilitation in patients with interstitial lung disease. Eur Respir J. 2013;42:444–53.
34. Watz H, Pitta F, Rochester CL, Garcia-Aymerich J, ZuWallack R, Troosters T, Vaes AW, Puhan MA, Jehn M, Polkey MI, et al. An official European Respiratory Society statement on physical activity in COPD. Eur Respir J. 2014;44:1521–37.
35. Gaunaurd IA, Gomez-Marin OW, Ramos CF, Sol CM, Cohen MI, Cahalin LP, Cardenas DD, Jackson RM. Physical activity and quality of life improvements of patients with idiopathic pulmonary fibrosis completing a pulmonary rehabilitation program. Respir Care. 2014;59:1872–9.
36. Demeyer H, Louvaris Z, Frei A, Rabinovich RA, de Jong C, Gimeno-Santos E, Loeckx M, Buttery SC, Rubio N, Van der Molen T, et al. Physical activity is increased by a 12-week semiautomated telecoaching programme in patients with COPD: a multicentre randomised controlled trial. Thorax. 2017;72:415–23.
37. Bye PT, Anderson SD, Woolcock AJ, Young IH, Alison JA. Bicycle endurance performance of patients with interstitial lung disease breathing air and oxygen. Am Rev Respir Dis. 1982;126:1005–12.
38. Holland AE. Exercise limitation in interstitial lung disease - mechanisms, significance and therapeutic options. Chron Respir Dis. 2010;7:101–11.
39. Ryerson CJ, Cayou C, Topp F, Hilling L, Camp PG, Wilcox PG, Khalil N, Collard HR, Garvey C. Pulmonary rehabilitation improves long-term outcomes in interstitial lung disease: a prospective cohort study. Respir Med. 2014;108:203–10.
40. Troosters T, Casaburi R, Gosselink R, Decramer M. Pulmonary rehabilitation in chronic obstructive pulmonary disease. Am J Respir Crit Care Med. 2005;172:19–38.
41. Holland A, Hill C. Physical training for interstitial lung disease. Cochrane Database Syst Rev. 2008;4.
42. Holland AE, Hill CJ, Glaspole I, Goh N, McDonald CF. Predictors of benefit following pulmonary rehabilitation for interstitial lung disease. Respir Med. 2012;106:429–35.
43. De Vries J, Seebregts A, Drent M. Assessing health status and quality of life in idiopathic pulmonary fibrosis: which measure should be used? Respir Med. 2000;94:273–8.
44. Azuma A, Nukiwa T, Tsuboi E, Suga M, Abe S, Nakata K, Taguchi Y, Nagai S, Itoh H, Ohi M, et al. Double-blind, placebo-controlled trial of pirfenidone in patients with idiopathic pulmonary fibrosis. Am J Respir Crit Care Med. 2005;171:1040–7.

45. Taniguchi H, Ebina M, Kondoh Y, Ogura T, Azuma A, Suga M, Taguchi Y, Takahashi H, Nakata K, Sato A, et al. Pirfenidone in idiopathic pulmonary fibrosis. Eur Respir J. 2010;35:821–9.
46. Noble PW, Albera C, Bradford WZ, Costabel U, Glassberg MK, Kardatzke D, King TE Jr, Lancaster L, Sahn SA, Szwarcberg J, et al. Pirfenidone in patients with idiopathic pulmonary fibrosis (CAPACITY): two randomised trials. Lancet. 2011;377:1760–9.
47. King TE Jr, Bradford WZ, Castro-Bernardini S, Fagan EA, Glaspole I, Glassberg MK, Gorina E, Hopkins PM, Kardatzke D, Lancaster L, et al. A phase 3 trial of pirfenidone in patients with idiopathic pulmonary fibrosis. N Engl J Med. 2014;370:2083–92.
48. Richeldi L, Costabel U, Selman M, Kim DS, Hansell DM, Nicholson AG, Brown KK, Flaherty KR, Noble PW, Raghu G, et al. Efficacy of a tyrosine kinase inhibitor in idiopathic pulmonary fibrosis. N Engl J Med. 2011;365:1079–87.
49. Richeldi L, du Bois RM, Raghu G, Azuma A, Brown KK, Costabel U, Cottin V, Flaherty KR, Hansell DM, Inoue Y, et al. Efficacy and safety of nintedanib in idiopathic pulmonary fibrosis. N Engl J Med. 2014;370:2071–82.
50. Hanada M, Sakamoto N, Ishimatsu Y, Kakugawa T, Obase Y, Kozu R, Senjyu H, Izumikawa K, Mukae H, Kohno S. Effect of long-term treatment with corticosteroids on skeletal muscle strength, functional exercise capacity and health status in patients with interstitial lung disease. Respirology. 2016;21:1088–93.
51. American Thoracic S, European Respiratory S. American Thoracic Society/European Respiratory Society international multidisciplinary consensus classification of the idiopathic interstitial pneumonias. This joint statement of the American Thoracic Society (ATS), and the European Respiratory Society (ERS) was adopted by the ATS board of directors, June 2001 and by the ERS executive committee, June 2001. Am J Respir Crit Care Med. 2002;165:277–304.

7

Serum phosphate and phosphate-regulatory hormones in COPD patients

Alexandra Stroda[1], Vincent Brandenburg[3,4], Ayham Daher[1], Christian Cornelissen[1], Claudia Goettsch[2], András Keszei[3] and Michael Dreher[1,4*]

Abstract

Background: Fibroblast growth factor 23 (FGF23) regulates phosphate metabolism by increasing renal phosphate excretion and decreasing 1.25-dihydroxyvitamin D synthesis. Reports about hypophosphatemia in patients with chronic obstructive pulmonary disease (COPD) suggest altered phosphate metabolism. Therefore, we hypothesized that disturbances in phosphate-regulatory hormones such as FGF23 and parathyroid hormone (PTH) are present in COPD patients.

Methods: We investigated 40 COPD patients (63.5 ± 9.9 years, 27 male), each matched with two age- and sex-matched controls without any primary lung disease. COPD patients underwent lung function testing in advance. All patients had a glomerular filtration rate (GFR) > 60 mL/min/1.73m^2. We measured concentrations of intact FGF23 (iFGF23) and c-terminal FGF23 (c-term FGF23), phosphate, parathyroid hormone (PTH) and C-reactive protein (CRP) levels in COPD patients and controls.

Results: Phosphate (1.0 ± 02 vs. 1.1 ± 0.2 mmol/L; $p = 0.027$), PTH (54.2 ± 29.4 vs. 68.7 ± 31.8 pg/mL; $p = 0.002$) and iFGF23 (46.3 ± 29.0 vs. 57.5 ± 33.5 pg/mL; $p = 0.026$) levels were significantly lower in COPD patients compared with controls. There was a significant negative correlation between c-term FGF23 and total lung capacity ($r = -0.4$; $p = 0.01$), and between c-term FGF23 and CRP in COPD patients ($r = 0.48$; $p = 0.002$). iFGF23 and c-term FGF23 were positively correlated with phosphate and PTH in the control group.

Conclusion: We confirmed lower average serum phosphate levels in COPD patients compared with controls. However, our data do not suggest a causative role for FGF23 or PTH in COPD because levels of both phosphate-lowering hormones appear to be adaptively decreased as well. Therefore, further investigations are needed to identify the pathogenesis of low phosphate levels in patients with COPD and the relationship between phosphate-regulatory hormones and disease progression.

Keywords: Chronic obstructive pulmonary disease, Fibroblast growth factor 23, Phosphate, Parathyroid hormone

Background

Chronic obstructive pulmonary disease (COPD) is a serious condition that is increasing in incidence and is and is one of the leading causes of death worldwide [1]. COPD affects 5–15% of adults in Western countries [2] and it is predicted to cause 4.1% of all deaths in these countries by 2030 [1].

Several lines of evidence indicate that phosphate-fibroblast growth factor-23 (FGF23) signaling pathways deserve attention in patients with COPD, in whom a tendency for hypophosphatemia has been described [3, 4]. FGF23 is a major regulator of phosphate metabolism leading to increased renal phosphate excretion and diminished synthesis of 1,25-dihydroxyvitamin D [5–7]. Genetic deficiency of FGF23 results in a lethal phenotype in mice, including premature aging and severe pulmonary emphysema [8]. It equals the lethal phenotype of the klotho-knockout mouse, which can be ameliorated by phosphate restriction, showing that phosphate drives a large extent the phenotypic changes characterizing the aging process [9].

* Correspondence: mdreher@ukaachen.de
[1]Department of Pneumology and Intensive Care Medicine, University Hospital Aachen, Aachen, Germany
[4]Department of Cardiology and Nephrology, Rhein-Maas Klinikum Würselen, Aachen, Germany
Full list of author information is available at the end of the article

Genetic ablation of FGF23 associates in vivo with a phenotype of premature aging but accumulating data points to circulating levels of FGF23 in serum being a potentially independent risk factor for increased cardiovascular risk and is associated with elevated cardiovascular and all-cause mortality in various patient cohorts, especially those with chronic kidney and cardiac diseases [10–12].

Preliminary data from earlier studies indicate that COPD is linked with low phosphate levels in both muscles and the circulation [3, 4]. In addition, hypophosphatemia predicted poor outcome in hospitalized COPD patients [13]. Only one study so far, conducted in Saudi Arabia, has addressed a potentially causative relation between FGF23 and COPD. However, this study has several limitations, including the exclusion and inclusion criteria, use of concomitant medications, and glomerular filtration rate (GFR) as confounding factor [14]. Thus, existing data are limited and cannot establish a clear cause-and-effect relationship.

We hypothesize that phosphate metabolism and its major regulator FGF23 play a role in COPD. Here, we investigated a well-characterized cohort of COPD patients with respect to phosphate metabolism status, including FGF23 and parathyroid hormone (PTH), and compared these results with age- and sex-matched controls without COPD. The aim was to determine whether COPD patients have relevant changes in serum phosphate levels and phosphate-regulatory hormones or factors.

Methods

This cross-sectional case-control study was conducted at the University Hospital RWTH Aachen, Aachen, Germany. The study protocol was approved by the local ethics committee (190/50,07-22-2015). Blood samples were taken from November 2015 until June 2017. All patients signed informed consent prior to the study. The implemented methods are in accordance with the latest revision of the Declaration of Helsinki.

Participants

COPD patients underwent a lung function test, and were then assigned two sex- and aged- matched controls who did not have COPD or any other primary lung disease. Exclusion criteria for COPD patients were a GFR < 60 mL/min/1.73 m^2 and any other primary pulmonary diseases except for COPD. Exclusion criteria for control patients were a GFR < 60 mL/min/1.73 m^2 or any primary pulmonary disease. Gender, age, height, weight and body mass index (BMI) were recorded for all participants.

Lung function testing

All but one of the COPD patients had previously undergone whole-body plethysmography (the remaining patient had spirometry). All COPD patients were classified according to the Global Initiative for Chronic Obstructive Lung Disease (GOLD) guidelines [15].

Measurements and laboratory values

iFGF23 and c-term FGF23 concentrations in plasma were measured using a two-site enzyme-linked immunosorbent assay (ELISA) kit (Immutopics, Inc., 96 Test Kit, Cat. # 60–6600 for iFGF23 and Immutopics, Inc., 96 Test Kit, Cat. # 60–6100 for c-term FGF23) according to the manufacture protocol [16]. To detect the amino-terminal and carboxyl-terminal portions of iFGF23, two antibodies were used: a murine monoclonal antibody, which was biotinylated for capture and an affinity purified goat polyclonal antibody conjugated with the enzyme horseradish peroxidase (HRP) for detection. As instructed, 50 µL of standard, control and sample were pipetted into the streptavidin-coated microtiter well followed by 50 µL of biotinylated antibody. After incubation and washing five times, 100 µL of HRP-conjugated human FGF23 antibody was pipetted into the wells. The well was then incubated and washed another five times. 100 µL of ELISA HRP substrate was added followed by incubation. Absorbance was read before (OD_{595nm}) and after (OD_{450nm}) adding 50 µL of Stop Solution. The detection is limit 1.5 pg/mL. The intra- and interassay coefficients of variation were 2.0–4.1% and 3.5–9.1%, respectively.

C-term FGF23 was assayed in a similar way. However, in this assay the biotinylated capture antibody was also an affinity-purified goat antibody. The used antibodies only detected epitopes within the c-term portion of FGF23 and bound to the intact molecule and the large carboxyl terminal fragments of human FGF23. As per the instructions, 100 µL of standard, control and sample were pipetted into streptavidin-coated wells. Afterwards, 50 µL of Working Antibody Solution, containing both antibodies, was added. After incubation, the wells were washed five times and 150 µL of ELISA HRP Substrate was added. The remaining steps were as described above. The detection is limit 1.5 RU/mL. The intra- and interassay coefficients of variation were 1.4–2.4% and 2.4–4.7%, respectively.

All samples were assayed in duplicate. Serum concentrations of C-reactive protein (CRP), phosphate, plasma PTH, GFR, creatinine, urea and hemoglobin (Hb) were quantified using standardized laboratory procedures implemented by the laboratory diagnostic center (LDZ) of the university hospital Aachen.

Statistical analysis

Statistical analysis was performed using the SPSS 25.0 statistical package (IBM Corp. Released 2017. IBM SPSS Statistics for Windows, Version 25.0. Armonk, NY: IBM Corp.) and R (R Core Team (2016). R: A language and environment for statistical computing. R Foundation for Statistical Computing, Vienna, Austria.).

Baseline characteristics, laboratory values and lung function parameters are presented as mean ± standard deviation (SD) with *p*-values calculated using a Student's t-test for normally distributed data. All skewed continuous parameters are also presented as median (quartile [Q] 1 – Q3) with p-values determined using a Mann-Whitney U-test for non-normally distributed data. *p*-values of < 0.05 were considered statistically significant.

IFGF23 and c-term FGF23 level data were statistically analyzed using a logarithmic transformation of iFGF23 and c-term FGF23 concentrations. We designed a linear mixed model with fixed effects for case-control status and random effects of matched groups and subjects. The logarithmic transformations of iFGF23 and c-term FGF23 were maintained during correlation analysis using Pearson's correlation coefficient. We investigated correlations between FGF23 and lung function parameters in the COPD group by determining Pearson's correlation coefficient due to approximate linear regression seen in the scatterplots. Correlations between FGF23 and phosphate, PTH and CRP were determined using Spearman's correlation coefficient, because we could not determine linear correlation between these parameters using the scatterplot.

Results

Baseline characteristics, laboratory values, lung function

A total of 119 participants were enrolled in the study (40 patients with COPD and 79 controls) (Table 1). Fifty-one of the control subjects had no COPD based on the GOLD classification or whole-body plethysmography; COPD was not mentioned in medical records for the 28 control group subjects who did not have a lung function test during hospitalization. One control subject was excluded from the analysis because of a previous blood transfusion. Patients with COPD were in GOLD stage I (n = 3, 7.5%), II (n = 13, 32.5%), III (n = 10, 25%) or IV (n = 14, 35%).

There were no significant differences in sex, height, weight and BMI between COPD patients and controls (Table 1). Although GFR differed significantly between the two groups (Table 1), all patients could be clinically classified as chronic kidney disease stage I-II (CKD I-II)

Table 1 Baseline characteristics, laboratory values and lung function parameters for patients and controls

	COPD patients (n = 40)	Controls (n = 79)	*p*-value
Male sex, n (%)	27 (67.5)	54 (68.4)	
Age, years	63.5 ± 9.9	63.7 ± 9.8	0.908
Height, m	1.7 ± 0.1	1.7 ± 0.1	0.598
Weight, kg	83.2 ± 19.2	84.9 ± 16.5	0.624
Body mass index, kg/m^2	27.3 ± 5.9	28.3 ± 5.1	0.387
GFR, mL/min/1.73m^2	88.9 ± 11.3	82.7 ± 12.9	0.026
Creatinine, mg/dL	0.8 ± 0.2	0.9 ± 0.2	0.022
Urea, mg/dL[a]	30.1 ± 8.8	35.5 ± 14.2	0.013
Hemoglobin, g/dL	13.6 ± 1.5	13.0 ± 1.8	0.058
Lung function[b]			
FEV_1, L	1.4 ± 0.8	2.6 ± 0,8	< 0.0001
FEV_1, % predicted	47.5 ± 22.5	87.3 ± 17.6	< 0.0001
FEV_1/FVC ratio, %	49.8 ± 14.2	80.6 ± 6.6	< 0.0001
TLC, L	7.7 ± 1.7	6.1 ± 1.5	< 0.0001
TLC, % predicted	118.7 ± 17.5	95.4 ± 18.1	< 0.0001
RV, L	4.9 ± 1.7	2.8 ± 0.9	< 0.0001
RV, % predicted	208.1 ± 62.5	123.0 ± 39.5	< 0.0001
VC, L	2.8 ± 1.0	3.3 ± 0.9	0.021
VC, % predicted	71.6 ± 21.4	84.3 ± 16.4	0.003
R total	0.76 ± 0.46 (0.65; 0.46–0.91)	0.31 ± 0.13 (0.3; 0.25–0.34)	< 0.0001
R total, % predicted	252.9 ± 155.2 (216.6; 153.2–302.9)	104.1 ± 43.1 (98.2; 84.4–114.9)	< 0.0001

[a]Urea data available for 39 COPD patients; [b]Overall, lung function was assessed in 51 patients from the control group; data for TLC, RV, VC and R were available for 39 patients with COPD

Values are number of patients (%) or mean ± SD, with median; Q1-Q3 values shown for skewed continuous parameters

FEV_1, forced expiratory volume in 1 s; *Q* quartile; *R* resistance; *RV* residual volume; *VC* vital capacity.

[17]. Lung function was significantly impaired in COPD patients versus controls (Table 1). Coronary heart disease (CHD) was present in 17 patients with COPD and 57 controls.

iFGF23 and c-term FGF23 concentrations

Table 2 shows concentrations of iFGF23, c-term FGF23, CRP, PTH and phosphate in patients with COPD and the control group. Application of the model suggested that iFGF23 concentration was 27% higher in controls than in COPD patients. The effect estimate on transformed scale for case-control status was 0.24 with a 95% confidence interval (CI) of 0.03–0.45; $p = 0.026$. When the model was adjusted for GFR, the between-group difference remained significant (estimate 0.23; 95% CI 0.01–0.45; $p = 0.04$).

The model representing the results for c-term FGF23 was developed in a similar manner to the one for iFGF23. One specimen showed values > 1478.5 RU/mL and the ELISA kit could not give more exact data. Working with estimators, we could retain a result representing all measured concentrations. The case-control comparison did not show a significant difference of c-term FGF23 in controls compared with COPD patients. The effect estimate (on transformed scale) for case-control status was 0.09 with a 95% CI of – 0.17, 0.36; $p = 0.494$.

Correlation between iFGF23 and c-term FGF23 and lung function parameters in COPD

Scatterplots suggest approximately linear correlations between iFGF23 and FEV_1/FVC ratio, FEV_1 and TLC. There was no significant correlation between logarithmic transformed iFGF23 and FEV_1, FEV_1/FVC ratio and TLC. Pearson's correlation coefficient with logarithmic transformed iFGF23 in patients with COPD were as follows: FEV_1, $r = -0.24$, $p = 0.13$; FEV_1/FVC ratio, $r = -0.09$, $p = 0.59$; TLC, $r = -0.22$, $p = 0.18$. There was an approximately linear correlation between logarithmic transformed c-term FGF23 and TLC ($r = -0.4$, $p = 0.01$) (Fig. 1). The other correlations with logarithmic transformed c-term FGF-23 in cases were: FEV_1, $r = -0.25$, $p = 0.13$; FEV_1/FVC ratio, $r = -0.10$, $p = 0.58$.

CRP, phosphate and PTH levels in COPD patients and controls

Hypophosphatemia (phosphate < 0.8 mmol/L) was detected in 12.5% of COPD patients and 5% of controls ($p = 0.25$). There was no significant difference in CRP levels between COPD patients and controls, but levels of PTH and phosphate were significantly lower in COPD patients versus controls (Tab. 2).

Correlation of CRP, phosphate and PTH with FGF23 in COPD patients and controls

Because there was no distinct linear relationship for PTH and phosphate with iFGF23 and c-term FGF23, Spearman's correlation coefficients were calculated (Table 3). This was also the case for the correlation between CRP and either iFGF23 or c-term FGF23. In the control group, there was a significant positive correlation for phosphate and PTH with iFGF23 and c-term FGF23. In patients with COPD, there was a significant positive correlation between c-term FGF23 and CRP.

Discussion

To the best of our knowledge, this study is the most detailed investigation of disturbed phosphate metabolism in COPD patients to date. We have confirmed that serum phosphate levels are lower in COPD patients, which is consistent with previous studies showing that COPD patients have low phosphate levels in both muscles and the circulation [3, 4]. Our data expand previous findings by providing a sophisticated analysis of important phosphate-regulatory hormones in COPD patients [18], showing that the level of iFGF23 and PTH are reduced in COPD

Table 2 Laboratory findings and concentrations of serum phosphate and phosphate-regulatory hormones

	COPD patients($n = 40$)	Controls($n = 79$)	p-value
CRP, mg/L	14.3 ± 22.8 (5.9; 1.3–10.6)	14.4 ± 17.4 (7.5; 2.4–20.8)	0.226[a]
Phosphate, mmol/L	1.0 ± 0.2	1.1 ± 0.2	0.027[b]
PTH, pg/mL	54.2 ± 29.4 (44; 36.4–62.1)	68.7 ± 31.8 (61.1; 46.9–83.3)	0.002[a]
iFGF23, pg/mL	46.3 ± 29.0 (38.9; 29.0–55.9)	57.5 ± 33.5 (51.9; 34.3–71.7)	0.026[c]
c-term FGF23, RU/mL	121.6 ± 191.6 (65.2; 54.2–88.2)	120.6 ± 98.8 (93.2; 55.8–143.8)	0.5[c]

[a] Mann-Whitney-U. [b]T-test. [c]Difference calculated using the model described in the methods section

Values are number of patients (%) or mean ± SD, with median; Q1–Q3 values shown for skewed continuous parameters.

CRP C-reactive protein; *c-term FGF23* c-terminal fibroblast growth factor-23; *GFR* glomerular filtration rate; *iFGF23* intact fibroblast growth factor-23; *PTH* parathyroid hormone.

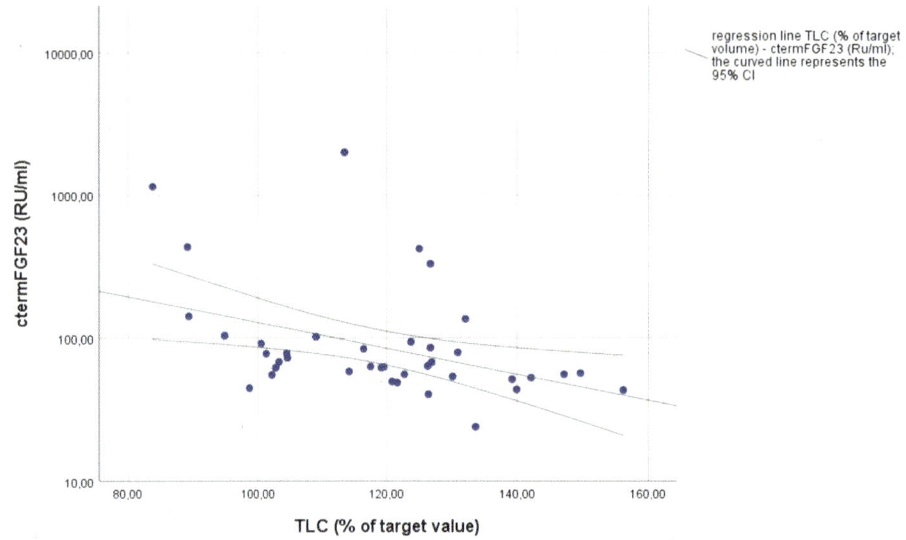

Fig. 1 Relationship between total lung capacity (TLC) and c-term FGF23 in chronic obstructive pulmonary disease patients

patients compared with controls. This suggests the possibility that the alteration in serum phosphate is the primary modification, which is followed by reductions in phosphate-lowering hormones. What is causing low phosphate levels and the tendency to develop hypophosphatemia in COPD patients cannot be determined from our data. Changes in the two major phosphate regulatory hormones PTH and iFGF23 appear to be adaptive to primary phosphate alterations assuming a physiological feedback loop between phosphate and its regulators.

In contrast to our findings, a previous cross-sectional study conducted in Saudi Arabia partly reported higher FGF23 and PTH levels in COPD patients versus controls [14]. Several aspects differ between the two studies and potentially explain the different results, including the distribution of GOLD stages within the COPD group, ethnicity, and different exclusion and inclusion criteria. The Saudi Arabian study excluded patients taking medications that could affect bone metabolism, but did not focus explicitly on GFR as confounding factor. Moreover, they did not distinguish between c-term FGF23 and iFGF23, and it is not clear which of these has been measured [14]. The disparate findings of these two studies investigating the role of FGF23 in COPD patients highlights the need for further investigations in this field to clearly elucidate the role of FGF23 in COPD patients.

Table 3 Correlation coefficients for intact and c-terminal fibroblast growth factor-23 (FGF23) with phosphate and parathyroid hormone (PTH) levels

FGF23	Variable	Group	Correlation coefficient	*p*-value
intact	Phosphate	Case	0.3	0.057
intact	Phosphate	Control	0.31	0.006
intact	PTH	Case	0.29	0.067
intact	PTH	Control	0.25	0.02
c-term	Phosphate	Case	0.23	0.15
c-term	Phosphate	Control	0.29	0.01
c-term	PTH	Case	0.3	0.064
c-term	PTH	Control	0.27	0.016
intact	CRP	Case	0.16	0.31
intact	CRP	Control	−0.16	0.157
c-term	CRP	Case	0.48	0.002
c-term	CRP	Control	0.05	0.683

Regarding correlation of both iFGF23 and c-term FGF23 with lung function parameters in humans, we showed a significant moderate negative correlation between the metabolic product c-term FGF23 and TLC. We are the first to show that patients with an abnormal distension of the lung have lower levels of the degradation product c-term FGF23. In our opinion, further investigations are needed to determine whether this is a cause-effect relationship and to identify whether there is a direct effect of FGF23 in the lung tissue.

Earlier studies showed a significant association between inflammation, including CRP, and FGF23 levels [19, 20]. In our study there was no significantly difference in CRP levels between COPD patients and controls, suggesting a similar level of systemic inflammation in the two groups. Therefore, inflammation is unlikely to be a confounder of FGF23 levels in our study.

FGF23 is known to be higher in patients with CKD, especially in severe stages [21]. Therefore, we excluded patients with a GFR < 60 mL/min/1.73 m^2. This means that our results were not influenced by a low GFR. The only exclusion criteria for the control group was a lack of primary lung diseases, meaning that we included a diverse and representative sample of hospitalized individuals.

The study has several limitations that should be highlighted. Firstly, not all control patients underwent lung function assessment to exclude COPD. Therefore, some control patients may have had undetected COPD. However, lung function testing was performed in the majority of control patients and none had COPD mentioned in previous medical reports. Another limitation was the small sample size in our study. Studies with a larger sample size may be able to detect a statistically significant relationship between iFGF23 and the severity of COPD based on FEV_1 and TLC. Furthermore, many patients in the control group had CHD, which could have influenced our results because FGF23 is a known risk factor for cardiovascular disease [11]. A confounding factor regarding phosphate levels might be varying medication among the patients potentially contributing to hypophosphatemia. Especially ß2-agonists, corticosteroids, xanthine derivates and hydrochlorothiazide (HCT) are known to influence phosphate homeostasis [22]. Among the controls three persons were medicated with ß2-agonists, three with corticosteroids, none with xanthine derivates and 15 with HCT. Regarding the COPD-patients 29 were medicated with ß2-agonists, 12 with corticosteroids, one with xanthine derivates and eight with HCT. Finally, a potential limitation of our trial is, that we cannot comment on tissue levels of FGF23 and its receptors. Moreover, we have not assessed circulating klotho levels in our studies. The density and distribution of klotho influences FGF23 metabolism and also the FGF23 signalling cascade. However, currently available klotho assays lack specifity and have only limited diagnostic power regarding biological activity of the klotho-FGF23-system [23].

In conclusion, iFGF23 level and concentrations of PTH and phosphate were lower in our cohort of COPD patients compared with non-COPD controls. These data suggest that PTH and FGF23 react to, rather than induce, changes in phosphate homeostasis, which we therefore consider to be the primary defect. Causes of this low serum phosphate remain unknown and we acknowledge that we cannot provide data about phosphate distribution within deeper compartments (e.g. muscles) or intracellularly. Therefore, further investigations are needed including investigations about renal phosphate handling and the role of klotho in this setting.

Abbreviations

BMI: Body mass index; CHD: Coronary heart disease; CI: Confidence interval; CKD: Chronic kidney disease; COPD: Chronic obstructive pulmonary disease; CRP: C-reactive protein; c-term FGF23: C-terminal fibroblast growth factor 23; ELISA: Enzyme-linked immunosorbent assay; FEV_1: Forced expiratory volume in 1 s; FGF23: Fibroblast growth factor 23; GFR: Glomerular filtration rate; GOLD: Global Initiative for Chronic Obstructive Lung Disease; Hb: Hemoglobin; HCT: Hydrochlorthiazide; HRP: Horseradish peroxidase; iFGF23: Intact fibroblast growth factor 23; PTH: Parathyroid hormone; Q: Quartile; RV: Residual volume; SD: Standard deviation; TLC: Total lung capacity; VC: Vital capacity

Acknowledgements

English language editing assistance was provided by Nicola Ryan, independent medical writer.

Funding

The study was not funded.

Author's contributions

M.D. and V.B. designed the study, contributed to the interpretation of the results and reviewed the manuscript. A.S. was responsible for sample handling and database management, contributed to data analysis and interpretation and wrote the manuscript. C.G. organized and supervised the FGF23 measurements and reviewed the manuscript. A.K. conducted the statistical analyses. All co-authors contributed to the interpretation of the results and reviewed and edited the manuscript. All authors have read and approved the final version of the manuscript as submitted.

Competing interests

The authors declare no conflict of interest regarding the manuscript.

Author details

[1]Department of Pneumology and Intensive Care Medicine, University Hospital Aachen, Aachen, Germany. [2]Department of Cardiology, Angiology and Intensive Care Medicine, University Hospital Aachen, Würselen, Germany. [3]Department of Cardiology, Angiology and Intensive Care Medicine, University Hospital Aachen, Aachen, Germany. [4]Department of Cardiology and Nephrology, Rhein-Maas Klinikum Würselen, Aachen, Germany.

References

1. Mathers CD, Loncar D. Projections of global mortality and burden of disease from 2002 to 2030. PLoS Med. 2006;3:e442.
2. Anto JM, Vermeire P, Vestbo J, Sunyer J. Epidemiology of chronic obstructive pulmonary disease. Eur Respir J. 2001;17:982–94.
3. Fiaccadori E, Coffrini E, Ronda N, Vezzani A, Cacciani G, Fracchia C, Rampulla C, Borghetti A. Hypophosphatemia in course of chronic obstructive pulmonary disease. Chest. 1990;97:857–68.
4. Fiaccadori F, Coffrini E, Fracchia C, Rampulla C, Montagna T, Borghetti A. Hypophosphatemia and phosphorus depletion in respiratory and peripheral muscles of patients with respiratory failure due to COPD. Chest. 1994;105:1392–8.
5. Gattineni J, Bates C, Twombley K, Dwarakanath V, Robinson ML, Goetz R, Mohammadi M, Baum M. FGF23 decreases renal NaPi-2a and NaPi-2c expression and induces hypophosphatemia in vivo predominantly via FGF receptor 1. Am J Physiol Renal Physiol. 2009;297:F282–91.

6. Saito H, Kusano K, Kinosaki M, Ito H, Hirata M, Segawa H, Miyamoto K, Fukushima N. Human fibroblast growth factor-23 mutants suppress Na+ –dependent phosphate co-transport activity and 1alpha,25-dihydroxyvitamin D3 production. J Biol Chem. 2003;278:2206–11.
7. Shimada T, Hasegawa H, Yamazaki Y, Muto T, Hino R, Takeuchi Y, Fujita T, Nakahara K, Fukumoto S, Yamashita T. FGF-23 is a potent regulator of vitamin D metabolism and phosphate homeostasis. J Bone Miner Res. 2004; 19:429–35.
8. Razzaque MS, Sitara D, Taguchi T, St-Arnaud R, Lanske B. Premature aging-like phenotype in fibroblast growth factor 23 null mice is a vitamin D-mediated process. FASEB J. 2006;20:720–2.
9. Ohnishi M, Razzaque MS. Dietary and genetic evidence for phosphate toxicity accelerating mammalian aging. FASEB J. 2010;24:3562–71.
10. Parker BD, Schurgers LJ, Brandenburg VM, Christenson RH, Vermeer C, Ketteler M, Shlipak MG, Whooley MA, Ix JH. The associations of fibroblast growth factor 23 and uncarboxylated matrix Gla protein with mortality in coronary artery disease: the heart and soul study. Ann Intern Med. 2010;152:640–8.
11. Brandenburg VM, Kleber ME, Vervloet MG, Tomaschitz A, Pilz S, Stojakovic T, Delgado G, Grammer TB, Marx N, Marz W, Scharnagl H. Fibroblast growth factor 23 (FGF23) and mortality: the Ludwigshafen risk and cardiovascular health study. Atherosclerosis. 2014;237:53–9.
12. Isakova T, Xie H, Yang W, Xie D, Anderson AH, Scialla J, Wahl P, Gutierrez OM, Steigerwalt S, He J, et al. Fibroblast growth factor 23 and risks of mortality and end-stage renal disease in patients with chronic kidney disease. JAMA. 2011;305:2432–9.
13. Farah R, Khamisy-Farah R, Arraf Z, Jacobson L, Makhoul N. Hypophosphatemia as a prognostic value in acute exacerbation of COPD. Clin Respir J. 2013;7:407–15.
14. Elsammak M, Attia A, Suleman M. Fibroblast growth Factor-23 and hypophosphatemia in chronic obstructive pulmonary disease patients. J Med Biochem. 2012;31.
15. Vestbo J, Hurd SS, Agusti AG, Jones PW, Vogelmeier C, Anzueto A, Barnes PJ, Fabbri LM, Martinez FJ, Nishimura M, et al. Global strategy for the diagnosis, management, and prevention of chronic obstructive pulmonary disease: GOLD executive summary. Am J Respir Crit Care Med. 2013;187:347–65.
16. El-Maouche D, Dumitrescu CE, Andreopoulou P, Gafni RI, Brillante BA, Bhattacharyya N, Fedarko NS, Collins MT. Stability and degradation of fibroblast growth factor 23 (FGF23): the effect of time and temperature and assay type. Osteoporos Int. 2016;27:2345–53.
17. Kidney Disease: Improving Global Outcomes (KDIGO) CKD Work Group: KDIGO. Clinical practice guideline for the evaluation and Management of Chronic Kidney Disease. Kidney Int Suppl. 2012;2013(3):1–150.
18. Bergwitz C, Juppner H. Regulation of phosphate homeostasis by PTH, vitamin D, and FGF23. Annu Rev Med. 2010;61:91–104.
19. Hanks LJ, Casazza K, Judd SE, Jenny NS, Gutierrez OM. Associations of fibroblast growth factor-23 with markers of inflammation, insulin resistance and obesity in adults. PLoS One. 2015;10:e0122885.
20. Munoz Mendoza J, Isakova T, Ricardo AC, Xie H, Navaneethan SD, Anderson AH, Bazzano LA, Xie D, Kretzler M, Nessel L, et al. Fibroblast growth factor 23 and inflammation in CKD. Clin J Am Soc Nephrol. 2012;7:1155–62.
21. Chudek J, Kocelak P, Owczarek A, Bozentowicz-Wikarek M, Mossakowska M, Olszanecka-Glinianowicz M, Wiecek A. Fibroblast growth factor 23 (FGF23) and early chronic kidney disease in the elderly. Nephrol Dial Transplant. 2014;29:1757–63.
22. Liamis G, Milionis HJ, Elisaf M. Medication-induced hypophosphatemia: a review. QJM. 2010;103:449–59.
23. Olauson H, Larsson TE. FGF23 and klotho in chronic kidney disease. Curr Opin Nephrol Hypertens. 2013;22:397–404.

8

The impact of HIV on the prevalence of asthma in Uganda: a general population survey

Bruce J. Kirenga[1*], Levicatus Mugenyi[2], Corina de Jong[3,4], J. Lucian Davis[5], Winceslaus Katagira[6], Thys van der Molen[3,4], Moses R. Kamya[7] and Marike Boezen[8]

Abstract

Background: HIV and asthma are highly prevalent diseases in Africa but few studies have assessed the impact of HIV on asthma prevalence in high HIV burden settings. The objective of this analysis was to compare the prevalence of asthma among persons living with HIV (PLHIV) and those without HIV participating in the Uganda National Asthma Survey (UNAS).

Methods: UNAS was a population-based survey of persons aged ≥12 years. Asthma was diagnosed based on either self-reported current wheeze concurrently or within the prior 12 months; physician diagnosis; or use of asthma medication. HIV was defined based on confidential self-report. We used Poisson regression with robust standard errors to estimate asthma prevalence and the prevalence ratio (PR) for HIV and asthma.

Results: Of 3416 participants, 2067 (60.5%) knew their HIV status and 103 (5.0%) were PLHIV. Asthma prevalence was 15.5% among PLHIV and 9.1% among those without HIV, PR 1.72, (95%CI 1.07–2.75, $p = 0.025$). HIV modified the association of asthma with the following factors, PLHIV vs. not PLHIV: tobacco smoking (12% vs. 8%, $p = < 0.001$), biomass use (11% vs. 7%, $p = < 0.001$), allergy (17% vs. 11%, $p = < 0.001$), family history of asthma (17% vs. 11%, $p = < 0.001$), and prior TB treatment (15% vs. 10%, $p = < 0.001$).

Conclusion: In Uganda the prevalence of asthma is higher in PLHIV than in those without HIV, and HIV interacts synergistically with other known asthma risk factors. Additional studies should explore the mechanisms underlying these associations. Clinicians should consider asthma as a possible diagnosis in PLHIV presenting with respiratory symptoms.

Keywords: Asthma, HIV, Prevalence, Uganda

Background

Human Immunodeficiency Virus (HIV) and asthma are both highly prevalent diseases globally [1, 2]. An estimated 334 million people have asthma and 36.7 million people have HIV [1, 2]. Both diseases disproportionately affect Africa and other low and middle income countries (LMICs) [2, 3]. The weighted mean prevalence of asthma in Africa is 7.0% in the rural areas (2.5–11.5) and 9.6% (3.9–15.2) in urban areas. The prevalence of asthma and HIV in Uganda is 10% and 6.2% respectively [4, 5].

Epidemiological studies have found increased prevalence of asthma among HIV infected persons [6–13]. However, the number of studies is small and most are either clinical or hospital based and most of them have been conducted in high income low HIV burden settings. Examples of available studies include a study that included 248 HIV infected and 236 HIV uninfected males. This study found that the prevalence of wheezing was 54.4%, vs. 21.2%, $p < 0.001$ [9]. In another study among 223 HIV patients in the USA, the prevalence of doctor diagnosed asthma was 20.6 compared to 8.2% in the general population [13]. In a study comparing 14,005

* Correspondence: bruckirenga@yahoo.co.uk
[1]Makerere University Lung Institute & Division of Pulmonary Medicine, Department of Medicine, Makerere University College of Health Sciences, Kampala, Uganda
Full list of author information is available at the end of the article

HIV infected with age matched HIV uninfected controls in Canada, the prevalence ratio for asthma was 1.31 (95% CI 1.20–1.43) [12].

Several mechanisms through which HIV increases the prevalence of asthma have been proposed [14–16]. Notable among these is the HIV associated persistent immune activation and inflammation [17]. It is also postulated that HIV proteins such as the nef protein or activation of memory CD4 T cells directly increase the risk of asthma [18]. Studies indicate that the higher the viral loads, the worse the lung function in HIV infected populations [14, 17]. HIV infected persons have been found to have higher levels of Immunoglobulin E (IgE) and this increases with increasing immunosuppression [15]. IgE is a well-known mediator of allergy and asthma. HIV could also drive asthma through its association with predominance of T-helper 2 (Th2) pathway. Priming of the Th2 pathway is known to increase the risk of asthma and other allergic diseases [19, 20]. In a cohort of 223 HIV infected persons, doctor diagnosed asthma appeared to be more common in participants with high sputum interleukin 4 (IL-4) (27% with asthma if high IL-4 vs.10.5% with asthma if low IL-4, $p = 0.02$) [13]. Antiretroviral therapy (ART) medications used to treat HIV have also be implicated in increasing the risk of asthma among HIV infected persons [21].

An interaction between HIV and asthma is important in high HIV burden settings because with the availability of highly active antiretroviral therapy and efficient health systems to deliver them, many HIV infected people are living longer into age groups where non-communicable diseases (NCDs) are common. In addition, prevention of HIV may lead to reduction in the burden of asthma. Data on the burden of asthma in HIV may also lead to assessment of asthma in HIV and routine HIV testing among persons with asthma. Drug-drug interactions in the management of patients with asthma-HIV comorbidity is also a key consideration.

In this study we analyzed data from the Uganda national asthma survey (UNAS) to determine if the prevalence of asthma was higher among persons with self-reported HIV infection. We also aimed to determine if HIV interacts with other known asthma risk factors namely tobacco smoking, biomass use, TB, family history of asthma and allergy.

Methods

Design and study participants

UNAS was a cross sectional general population-based survey conducted in Uganda in 2016. Participants were selected in clusters (villages) selected by probability proportionate to size by the Uganda Bureau of Statistics using the Uganda National population and housing census of 2014. Households (HHs) within clusters were selected by simple random sampling from a HH list generated by village leaders. All persons aged ≥12 years who were members of selected HH and provided written informed consent (and assent in case of minors) were surveyed. Exclusion criteria were: residing in congregate settings (schools, prisons, homes) and temporary residents (less than 2 weeks in household of selected villages).

Asthma diagnosis

Sampled participants were interviewed by trained research assistants using a standardized questionnaire developed by adapting questions from internationally recognized questionnaires, including the World Health Organization (WHO) health survey [1, 22], the international study of asthma and allergies in children (ISAAC) [22] and the European community respiratory health survey (ECRHS) surveys [23]. Asthma was defined as self-report of physician diagnosis, prescribed use of breathing medications for asthma or report of a wheeze in the last 12 months.

HIV diagnosis

HIV status in this survey was established by self-report. All participants were asked about their HIV status in private interviews. Responses were either HIV positive, HIV negative or unknown HIV status. HIV positive participants were classified as persons living with HIV (PLHIV).

Statistical analysis

Participants with unknown HIV status were excluded from this analysis. Participants' demographic and social characteristics and known asthma risk factors (tobacco smoking, allergy, family history of asthma, biomass use, and history of TB treatment) were summarized as proportions and compared between PLHIV and those who were not using Chi-square and Fisher's exact test statistics as appropriate.

We used Poisson regression with robust standard errors to estimate asthma prevalence and prevalence ratios (PR) between PLHIV and those who were not [24]. The Poisson model, an alternative for the log-binomial, was used due to convergence problems with the latter approach. The prevalence of asthma and the corresponding PRs among patients with key asthma risk factors namely tobacco smoking, biomass smoke exposure, family history of asthma, tuberculosis (TB) and allergy were also calculated. The PR ratio of asthma between PLHIV and those who were not living with HIV was then finally adjusted for these risk factors. Exposure to biomass smoke was defined as cooking in the living space (same room where participants slept), tobacco smoking was by self-report of being a smoker while allergy was considered to be present if a participant reported suffering in the past 12 months from any of the following: suffering in the past 12 months from any of watery itchy eyes, recurrent skin rash, or having sneezing, nasal congestion or rhinorrhea in the absence of an upper respiratory tract infection). To assess for the interaction between HIV and known asthma risk factors (tobacco smoking, biomass use, history of TB treatment, allergy, family history), we calculated age-dependent asthma prevalence comparing PLHIV and those who were not while keeping all other factors at zero and then by each factor. A graphical aid was used to visualize the age-dependent asthma prevalence by these factors.

Results

Characteristics of study participants

Of 3416 UNAS participants, 2067 (60.5%) knew their HIV status and 103 reported to be living with HIV (5.0% of the group that knew their HIV status). The characteristics of these participants by HIV status are shown in Table 1. The proportions of participants with respiratory symptoms of cough, sputum production and wheezing did not differ by HIV status. However, the proportions with the symptom breathlessness differed significantly by HIV status, positive vs. negative (17.5% vs. 9.0%, $p = 0.004$). Tobacco smoking was higher among PLHIV (12.6% vs. 7.9%, $p = 0.086$) as well as having history of TB treatment (9.7% vs.1.5%, $p < 0.001$).

Table 1 Participant characteristics Please see my feedback in the previous file

	PLHIV (*N* = 103)	Not PLHIV (*N* = 1964)	*P*-value
Characteristic			
Male gender, *n*(%)	31 (30.1)	763 (38.8)	0.076
Age groups *n*(%)			< 0.001
< 15	1 (1.0)	91 (4.6)	
15–24	10 (9.7)	474 (24.1)	
25–34	27 (26.2)	510 (25.9)	
35–44	33 (32.0)	388 (19.7)	
45–54	27 (26.2)	304 (15.5)	
55–64	4 (3.9)	131 (6.7)	
65+	1 (1.0)	68 (3.5)	
Respiratory Symptoms *n*(%)			
Cough	23 (22.3)	404 (20.6)	0.665
Sputum	7 (6.8)	140 (7.1)	0.900
Wheezing	11 (10.7)	131 (6.7)	0.116
Shortness of breath	18 (17.5)	177 (9.0)	0.004
Risk factors and co-morbid conditions *n* (%)			
History of smoking	13 (12.6)	155 (7.9)	0.086
Exposure to bio-mass	24 (23.3)	385 (19.6)	0.357
Ever been treated for TB	10 (9.7)	30 (1.5)	< 0.001
Allergy	42 (40.8)	721 (36.7)	0.400
Family history of asthma	15 (14.6)	220 (11.2)	0.295

PLHIV people living with HIV, *TB* tuberculosis

Prevalence of asthma by HIV status

The prevalence of asthma among PLHIV was 15.5% while that among those without HIV was 9.1%, PR 1.72 (95% CI: 1.07–2.75, $p = 0.025$). After adjusting for gender, age, tobacco smoking, biomass exposure, TB treatment, family history of asthma and allergy, the PR ratio decreased to 1.54 (95% CI: 0.94–2.51, $p = 0.085$), Table 2. A high prevalence of asthma among PLHIV was maintained at all ages irrespective of absence or presence of other risk factors of tobacco smoking, biomass use, allergy, family history of asthma and previous TB treatment (Fig. 1). Considering only participants younger than 35 years the prevalence of asthma was still higher among PLHIV, PR 3.06 (Fig. 2). The prevalence of asthma among participants with known HIV status and unknown HIV status did not differ significantly (9.4% vs.9.0%, $p = 0.689$), Table 3. HIV modified the association between asthma and other asthma risk factors, positive vs. negative: tobacco smoking (12% vs.8%, $p = < 0.001$) biomass use (11% vs. 7%, $p = < 0.001$), allergy (17% vs. 11%, $p = < 0.001$), family history asthma (17% vs. 11%, $p = < 0.001$) and TB treatment (15% vs. 10%, $p = < 0.001$), Fig. 3.

Prevalence of asthma by other factors

Other factors associated with increased prevalence of asthma in this study were biomass use adjusted PR 1.56 (95% CI: 1.18–2.07, $p = 0.002$), tobacco smoking 1.79 (95% CI: 1.23–2.60, $p = 0.002$), history of TB treatment 2.20 (95% CI: 1.26–3.84, $p = 0.005$), family history of asthma 2.41 (95% CI: 1.81–3.23, $p = < 0.001$), and allergy 2.45 (95% CI: 1.85–3.26, $p = < 0.001$), Table 2.

Discussion

This study has established that the prevalence of asthma among PLHIV is higher than among those without HIV and that HIV modifies the associations of asthma with tobacco smoking, biomass use, TB, allergy and family history of asthma. The study also shows that the only respiratory symptom more prevalent in PLHIV than without PLHIV is breathlessness. In terms of asthma risk factors the study found that PLHIV have high rates of tobacco smoking and history of TB treatment.

A higher prevalence of asthma among PLHIV has been reported in previous studies in clinic-based studies in high income with low HIV prevalence [6–12]. In 248 HIV infected and 236 HIV uninfected males, the prevalence of wheezing was 54.4%, vs. 21.2%, $p < 0.001$

Table 2 Asthma prevalence by HIV and potential confounding factors

	n (%)	Prevalence of asthma %	Crude PR (95% CI)	*p*	Adjusted PR[b] (95% CI)	*p*-value
Characteristic						
HIV status						
Infected	103 (5.0)	15.5	1.72 (1.07–2.75)	0.025	1.54 (0.94–2.51)	0.085
Uninfected	1966 (95.0)	9.1	Reference		Reference	
Gender						
Female	1275 (61.6)	9.9	1.15 (0.87–1.53)	0.319	1.24 (0.92–1.68)	0.159
Male	794 (38.4)	8.6	Reference		Reference	
Smoking						
Yes	168 (8.1)	16.7	1.91 (1.32–2.76)	0.001	1.79 (1.23–2.60)	0.002
No	1901 (91.9)	8.7	Reference		Reference	
Biomass use						
Yes	409 (19.8)	14.2	1.74 (1.31–2.32)	< 0.001	1.56 (1.18–2.07)	0.002
No	1659 (80.2)	8.1	Reference		Reference	
TB treatment						
Yes	40 (1.9)	22.5	2.46 (1.36–4.45)	0.003	2.20 (1.26–3.84)	0.005
No	2026 (98.1)	9.1	Reference		Reference	
Family history of asthma						
Yes	235 (11.4)	23.8	3.16 (2.39–4.18)	< 0.001	2.41 (1.81–3.23)	< 0.001
No	1832 (88.6)	7.5	Reference		Reference	
Allergy						
Yes	763 (36.9)	16.0	2.90 (2.20–3.83)	< 0.001	2.45 (1.85–3.26)	< 0.001
No	1306 (63.1)	5.5	Reference		Reference	
TB/HIV (HIV infected and history of TB treatment)						
Yes	10 (0.5)	10.0	1.07 (0.17–6.89)	0.946	0.20 (0.02–1.66)	0.135
No	2059 (99.5)	9.4	Reference		Reference	
Age in years[a]			2.09 (1.52–2.88)	< 0.001	1.83 (1.30–2.58)	0.001

[a]log transformed due to skewness, [b]Adjusted for age, gender, smoking, biomass smoke exposure, allergy, history of TB and family history of asthma, *CI* confidence interval, *TB* tuberculosis, *PR* prevalence ratio

[9] while in a study comparing 14,005 HIV infected patients with age matched HIV uninfected controls in Canada, the PR for asthma was 1.31 (95% CI 1.20–1.43) [12]. In another study among 223 HIV patients in the USA, the prevalence of doctor diagnosed asthma was 20.6 compared to 8.2% in the general population [13]. Although after adjusting for other risk factors of asthma such as smoking, biomass smoke, TB, allergy the PR ratio for asthma in PLHIV reduced to 1.54 with a trend *p*-value of 0.085. The results are however line with the findings from the studies above which increases the possibility that HIV is associated with asthma even in the present study.

We investigated the effect HIV had on the risk of asthma from other asthma risk factors. We found that PLHIV had higher rates of smoking as previously reported [25, 26]. The prevalence of asthma among tobacco smoking PLHIV was 12.6% compared to 7.9% of smokers who were not living with HIV. The finding of high smoking rates among PLHIV in this study has been reported in previous studies [25, 26]. This finding therefore calls for heightened efforts to reduce smoking among PLHIV."

We compared respiratory symptoms between HIV infected and HIV uninfected participants and found that there were no differences except for breathlessness. George et al. found that HIV infected persons had high rates of most respiratory symptoms [21]. We cannot explain why we failed to observe these differences in respiratory symptoms apart from breathlessness. The excess breathlessness in the HIV infected participants might be due to interstitial and diffusion derangements that are so prevalent among HIV infected persons [27–29]. Gingo et al. in a cross-sectional analysis

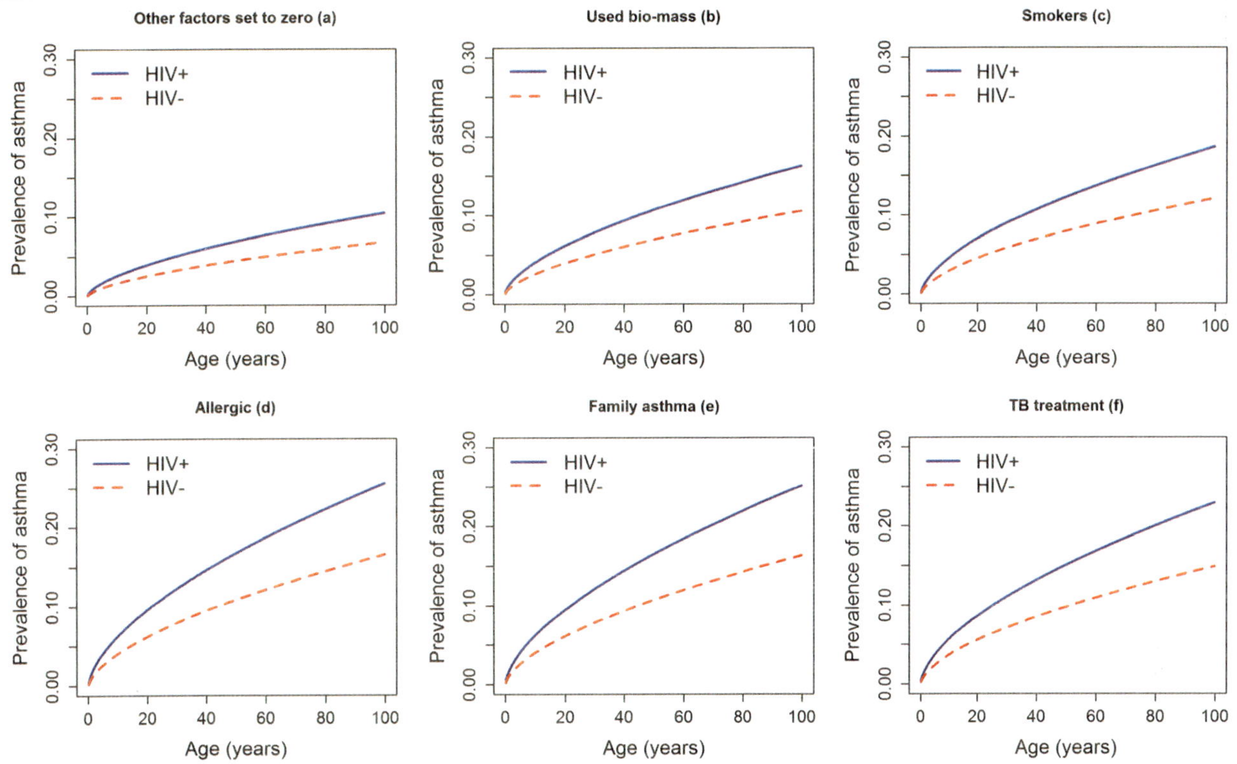

Fig. 1 Prevalence of asthma by age stratified by HIV status and other asthma risk factors: **a** Prevalence of asthma by age and HIV status keeping all other factors at zero. **b** Prevalence of asthma by age and HIV status among participants exposed to biomass smoke (**c**) Prevalence of asthma by age and HIV status among smokers. **d** Prevalence of asthma by age and HIV status among participants with history of allergy. **e** Prevalence of asthma by age and HIV status among participants with family history of asthma **f**) Prevalence of asthma by age and HIV status among participants with history of TB treatment

of 158 HIV-infected individuals without acute respiratory symptoms or infection found that 55 (34.8%) participants had a significantly reduced DL_{CO} (< 60% predicted) [29].

This study had limitations. Most notably the use of self-report to determine HIV infection. Self-report as a means of determining HIV status has been reported to have low sensitivity but high specificity [30, 31]. Among older adults (≥40 years) in South Africa, Rohr et al. report a sensitivity of HIV self-report of 51.2% (95% CI: 48.2–54.3) and specificity was 99.0% (95% CI: 98.7–99.4) [30, 31]. The low sensitivity of self-report may also be present in our study, the self-reported prevalence of HIV in our survey is 3.1%,

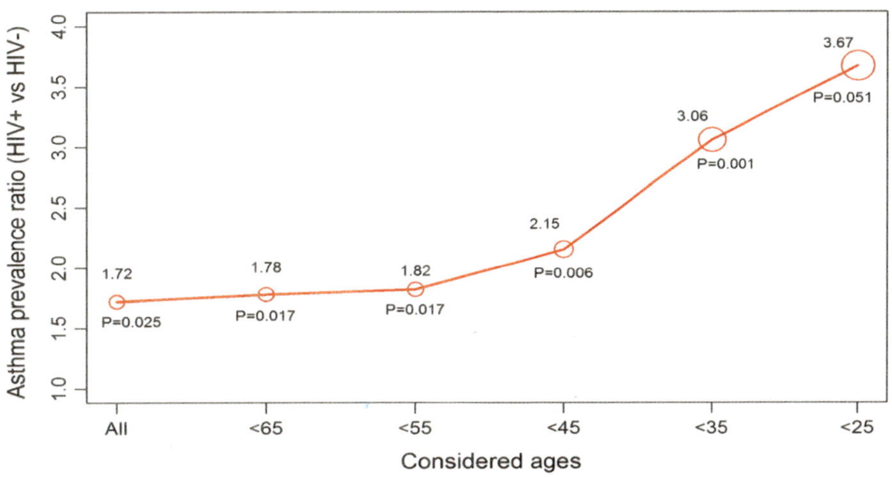

Fig. 2 Asthma prevalence ratios (HIV+ vs HIV-) considering different ages of participants

Table 3 Participants characteristics by HIV status (known vs. unknown status)

	HIV status known (*N* = 2069)	HIV status unknown (*N* = 1347)	*P*-value
Characteristic			
Male gender	794 (38.4)	533 (39.6)	0.484
Age groups			< 0.001
< 15	92 (4.5)	280 (20.8)	
15–24	484 (23.4)	400 (29.7)	
25–34	537 (26.0)	144 (10.7)	
35–44	421 (20.4)	156 (11.6)	
45–54	331 (16.0)	144 (10.7)	
55–64	135 (6.5)	90 (6.7)	
65+	69 (3.3)	133 (9.9)	
Respiratory Symptoms			
Cough	427 (20.7)	284 (21.1)	0.751
Sputum	147 (7.1)	110 (8.2)	0.250
Wheezing	142 (6.9)	84 (6.2)	0.471
Shortness of breath	195 (9.4)	114 (8.5)	0.337
Risk factors and co-morbid conditions			
History of smoking	168 (8.1)	74 (5.5)	0.004
Exposure to bio-mass	409 (19.8)	289 (21.5)	0.235
Ever been treated for TB	40 (1.9)	10 (0.7)	0.005
Allergy	763 (36.9)	433 (32.2)	0.005
Family history of asthma	235 (11.4)	142 (10.6)	0.455
Asthma			
Positive	194 (9.4)	121 (9.0)	0.698

TB tuberculosis

which is much lower than the national prevalence of 6.2% [4]. We believe that differential classification of HIV by asthma status is unlikely, but if present would likely tend to underestimate the prevalence ratio if patients without HIV are less likely to report HIV status. We performed further analysis on our data comparing demographic characteristics and asthma prevalence between participants with known HIV status and those with unknown HIV status, Table 3. As can be seen in this table the prevalence of asthma among these two groups did not significantly differ.

Another limitation of our study is that asthma was diagnosed based on history or current wheeze, prior physician diagnosis and being currently on asthma medications. However the methods used in this study are the standard methods that are used in most asthma surveys including the ISAAC), ECRHS)and the WHO health survey [1, 22, 23]. We recognise that wheezing could be due to other diseases such as chronic obstructive pulmonary disease (COPD). Therefore, it is possible that some of the participants classified as asthma could have had COPD which is also known to be associated with HIV. We performed sensitivity analysis considering only participants who are younger than 35 years, the age below which the diagnosis of COPD is unlikely and found that the prevalence of asthma in age group was still higher among the HIV infected participants (Fig. 1 left panel) implying that the association between asthma and HIV in this study might be a true one. There are however other conditions that can cause wheezing such as bronchiectasis, heart failure and mechanical airway obstruction [32, 33] that we could not exclude although these conditions are deemed to be rare.

Despite the limitations, our findings have several scientific, healthcare and programmatic implications. Firstly, HIV care programs need to build capacity for diagnosis of asthma and its management. At the same time there may be need to test for HIV among asthma patients in high HIV burden settings and to know their ART status and the medications they are taking. Asthma and HIV co-morbidity can be associated with complexities that can arise while managing the two diseases notably drug-drug interactions and increased rates of adverse events as can occur with

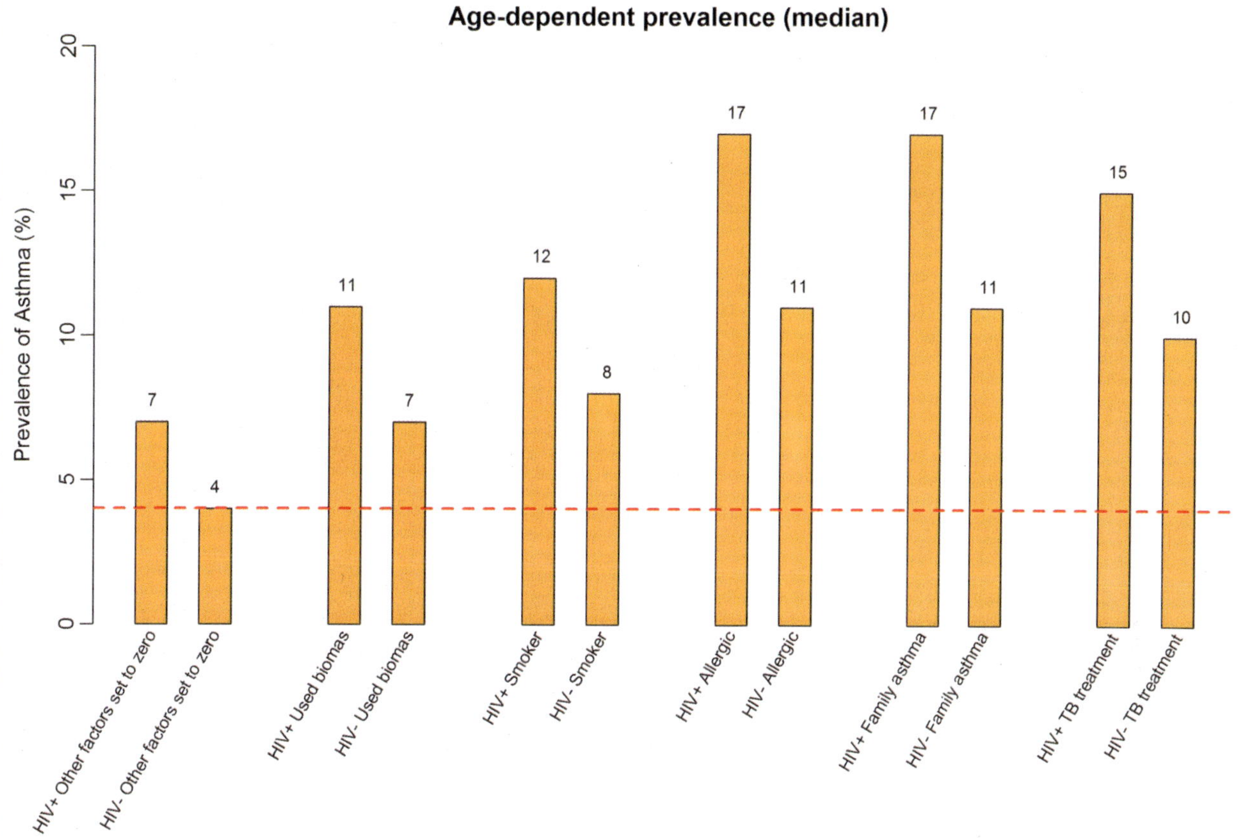

Fig. 3 Asthma prevalence considering different known asthma risk factors (all *p*-values < 0.001)

corticosteroids used in the management of asthma. Corticosteroids use in HIV infected persons has been associated with adverse outcomes such as the development of cancers like Kaposi's sarcoma and TB [34–36]. Another key drug-drug interaction to consider is that between protease inhibitors and corticosteroids, which is mediated through the effects of PIs on the cytochrome CYP450 3A4 drug metabolism pathway [37, 38]. This interaction can lead to complications such as Cushing's syndrome, hypertension and poor CD4 cell count recovery [38]. We found that HIV modified the risk of asthma from other risk factors. This calls for vigorous prevention of these risk factors among PLHIV. PLHIV in this study had higher rates of tobacco smoking. This calls for heightened efforts to reduce smoking among PLHIV since they may be more likely to develop tobacco associated lung diseases. In terms of science, our findings call for more research on the impact of HIV on asthma in high HIV burden settings and the mechanistic pathways of the HIV asthma interaction especially in settings with high rates of factors like TB and biomass smoke exposure. The impact of HIV on asthma prognosis also needs to be studied.

Conclusion

In conclusion, the prevalence of asthma among PLHIV in this survey is higher than among those without HIV. HIV also modifies the risk of asthma from other asthma risk factors such as tobacco smoking, TB, exposure to biomass, allergy and family history of asthma. PLHIV should be assessed for asthma and asthma patients should undergo HIV testing.

Abbreviations

ART: Antiretroviral therapy; CD4: Cluster of differentiation 4; CI: Confidence interval; COPD: Chronic obstructive pulmonary disease; CY: Cytochrome; ECRHS: European community respiratory health survey; HIV: Human immune deficiency virus; HHs: Households; IgE: Immunoglobulin E; IL-4: Interleukin-4; ISAAC: International study of asthma and allergies in children; LMICs: Low and middle-income countries; NCDs: Non-communicable diseases; PLHIV: People living with HIV; PR: Prevalence ratio; TB: Tuberculosis; UNAS: Uganda National asthma survey; USA: Unites States of America; WHO: World Health Organization

Acknowledgements

The authors thank all study participants and research assistants as well as research managers who were involved in this study. Special thanks go to the data management team headed by Mr. Rogers Sekibira that ensured all data were entered, cleaned and available for analysis in a timely manner.

Funding

This work was funded by the National Institutes of Health (NIH) (Award No. R24 TW008861) and NCS, UMCG, The Netherlands.

Authors' contributions

BJK, TVDM, MRK and CDJ conceived and designed the original survey, supervised data collection and interpreted the data. BJK and LJD conceived the idea of the current analysis of the survey data. BJK and LM analyzed the data. BJK, and WK participated in and supervised data collection. All authors reviewed and contributed to the manuscript writing. All authors read and approved the final manuscript.

Competing interests

The authors declare that they have no competing interests.

Author details

[1]Makerere University Lung Institute & Division of Pulmonary Medicine, Department of Medicine, Makerere University College of Health Sciences, Kampala, Uganda. [2]Makerere University Lung Institute, Makerere University College of Health Sciences, Kampala, Uganda. [3]GRIAC-Primary Care, Department of General Practice and Elderly Care, University of Groningen, University Medical Center Groningen (UMCG), Groningen, The Netherlands. [4]Groningen Research Institute for Asthma COPD (GRIAC), University of Groningen, University Medical Center Groningen (UMCG), Groningen, The Netherlands. [5]Department of Epidemiology of Microbial Diseases, Yale School of Public Health, and Pulmonary, Critical Care, and Sleep Medicine Section, Yale School of Medicine, New Haven, CT, USA. [6]Makerere University Lung Institute, Makerere University College of Health Sciences, Kampala, Uganda. [7]Department of Medicine, Makerere University College of Health Sciences, Kampala, Uganda. [8]Department of Epidemiology, University of Groningen, Groningen, The Netherlands.

References

1. To T, Stanojevic S, Moores G, Gershon AS, Bateman ED, Cruz AA, et al. Global asthma prevalence in adults: findings from the cross-sectional world health survey. BMC Public Health. 2012;12(1):204.
2. Marais BJ. Childhood tuberculosis: epidemiology and natural history of disease. The Indian Journal of Pediatrics. 2011;78(3):321–7.
3. Adeloye D, Chan KY, Rudan I, Campbell H. An estimate of asthma prevalence in Africa: a systematic analysis. Croatian medical journal. 2013; 54(6):519–31.
4. Ayles H, Muyoyeta M, Du Toit E, Schaap A, Floyd S, Simwinga M, et al. Effect of household and community interventions on the burden of tuberculosis in southern Africa: the ZAMSTAR community-randomised trial. Lancet. 2013; 382(9899):1183–94.
5. Morgan BW, Siddharthan T, Grigsby MR, Pollard SL, Kalyesubula R, Wise RA, et al. Asthma and allergic disorders in Uganda: a population-based study across urban and rural settings. In Practice: The Journal of Allergy and Clinical Immunology; 2018.
6. Puri A, Gingo M, Morris A. Asthma in HIV-infected population: a review of respiratory symptoms, pulmonary function abnormalities and pathophysiology. Epidemiol. 2014;4:164. https://doi.org/10.4172/2161-1165.1000164·
7. Wallace JM, Stone GS, Browdy BL, Tashkin DP, Hopewell PC, Rosen MJ, et al. Nonspecific airway hyperresponsiveness in HIV disease. Chest 1997;111(1): 121–127.
8. O'Donnell CR, Bader MB, Zibrak JD, Jensen WA, Rose RM. Abnormal airway function in individuals with the acquired immunodeficiency syndrome. Chest. 1988;94(5):945–8.
9. Poirier CD, Inhaber N, Lalonde RG, Ernst P. Prevalence of bronchial hyperresponsiveness among HIV-infected men. Am J Respir Crit Care Med. 2001;164(4):542–5.
10. Crothers K, Huang L, Goulet JL, Goetz MB, Brown ST, Rodriguez-Barradas MC, et al. HIV infection and risk for incident pulmonary diseases in the combination antiretroviral therapy era. Am J Respir Crit Care Med. 2011; 183(3):388–95.
11. Lin RY, Lazarus TS. Asthma and related atopic disorders in outpatients attending an urban HIV clinic. Ann Allergy Asthma Immunol. 1995;74(6):510–5.
12. Kendall CE, Wong J, Taljaard M, Glazier RH, Hogg W, Younger J, et al. A cross-sectional, population-based study measuring comorbidity among people living with HIV in Ontario. BMC Public Health. 2014;14(1):161.
13. Gingo MR, Wenzel SE, Steele C, Kessinger CJ, Lucht L, Lawther T, et al. Asthma diagnosis and airway bronchodilator response in HIV-infected patients. Journal of allergy and clinical immunology. 2012;129(3):708–14. e8.
14. Drummond MB, Kirk GD, Astemborski J, Marshall MM, Mehta SH, McDyer JF, et al. Association between obstructive lung disease and markers of HIV infection in a high-risk cohort. Thorax. 2011:thoraxjnl-2011-200702.
15. Wright DN, Nelson RP Jr, Ledford DK, Fernandez-Caldas E, Trudeau WL, Lockey RF. Serum IgE and human immunodeficiency virus (HIV) infection. J Allergy Clin Immunol. 1990;85(2):445–52.
16. Thuesen B, Husemoen L, Hersoug LG, Pisinger C, Linneberg A. Insulin resistance as a predictor of incident asthma-like symptoms in adults. Clin Exp Allergy. 2009;39(5):700–7.
17. Drummond MB, Merlo CA, Astemborski J, Marshall MM, Kisalu A, Mcdyer JF, et al. The effect of HIV infection on longitudinal lung function decline among injection drug users: a prospective cohort. AIDS (London, England). 2013;27(8):1303.
18. Gingo MR, Morris A. Pathogenesis of HIV and the lung. Current HIV/AIDS Reports. 2013;10(1):42–50.
19. Kidd P. Th1/Th2 balance: the hypothesis, its limitations, and implications for health and disease. Altern Med Rev. 2003;8(3):223–46.
20. Deo SS, Mistry KJ, Kakade AM, Niphadkar PV. Role played by Th2 type cytokines in IgE mediated allergy and asthma. Lung India. 2010;27(2):66.
21. George MP, Kannass M, Huang L, Sciurba FC, Morris A. Respiratory symptoms and airway obstruction in HIV-infected subjects in the HAART era. PLoS One. 2009;4(7):e6328.
22. Asher M, Anderson H, Stewart A, Crane J, Ait-Khaled N, Anabwani G, et al. Worldwide variations in the prevalence of asthma symptoms: the international study of asthma and allergies in childhood (ISAAC). Eur Respir J. 1998;12(2):315–35.
23. Fitzpatrick C, Floyd K. A systematic review of the cost and cost effectiveness of treatment for multidrug-resistant tuberculosis. PharmacoEconomics. 2012; 30(1):63–80.
24. Coutinho L, Scazufca M, Menezes PR. Methods for estimating prevalence ratios in cross-sectional studies. Revista de saude publica. 2008;42(6):992–8.
25. Mdege ND, Shah S, Ayo-Yusuf OA, Hakim J, Siddiqi K. Tobacco use among people living with HIV: analysis of data from demographic and health surveys from 28 low-income and middle-income countries. Lancet Glob Health. 2017;5(6):e578–e92.
26. Mdodo R, Frazier EL, Dube SR, Mattson CL, Sutton MY, Brooks JT, et al. Cigarette smoking prevalence among adults with HIV compared with the general adult population in the United States: cross-sectional surveys. Ann Intern Med. 2015;162(5):335–44.
27. Doffman SR, Miller RF. Interstitial lung disease in HIV. Clin Chest Med. 2013; 34(2):293–306.
28. Semenzato G, Agostini C. HIV-related interstitial lung disease. Curr Opin Pulm Med. 1995;1(5):383–91.
29. Gingo MR, He J, Wittman C, Fuhrman C, Leader JK, Kessinger C, et al. Contributors to diffusion impairment in HIV-infected persons. Eur Respir J. 2014;43(1):195–203.
30. Rohr JK, Xavier Gómez-Olivé F, Rosenberg M, Manne-Goehler J, Geldsetzer P, Wagner RG, et al. Performance of self-reported HIV status in determining true HIV status among older adults in rural South Africa: a validation study. Journal of the International AIDS Society. 2017;20(1).
31. Validity of data on self-reported hiv status and implications for measurement of arv coverage in malawi. [cited 2018 June 7]; Available from: https://dhsprogram.com/pubs/pdf/WP81/WP81.pdf.
32. Clerf L. Differential diagnosis of wheezing respiration. J Am Geriatr Soc. 1953;1(9):623–6.
33. Lillington GA, Lin H-w. Differential diagnosis of asthma in adults asthma, occult asthma, and Pseudoasthma. Bronchial Asthma: Springer; 1994. p. 171–87.
34. Lee C-H, Kim K, Hyun MK, Jang EJ, Lee NR, Yim J-J. Use of inhaled corticosteroids and the risk of tuberculosis. Thorax. 2013;68(12):1105–13.
35. Brassard P, Suissa S, Kezouh A, Ernst P. Inhaled corticosteroids and risk of tuberculosis in patients with respiratory diseases. Am J Respir Crit Care Med. 2011;183(5):675–8.
36. Gill PS, Loureiro C, Bernstein-Singer M, Rarick MU, Sattler F, Levine AM. Clinical effect of glucocorticoids on Kaposi sarcoma related to the acquired immunodeficiency syndrome (AIDS). Ann Intern Med. 1989;110(11):937–40.
37. Foisy M, Yakiwchuk E, Chiu I, Singh A. Adrenal suppression and Cushing's syndrome secondary to an interaction between ritonavir and fluticasone: a review of the literature. HIV medicine. 2008;9(6):389–96.

9

PrtA immunization fails to protect against pulmonary and invasive infection by *Streptococcus pneumoniae*

Chen-Fang Hsu[1,2,3,4†], Chen-Hao Hsiao[5,6†], Shun-Fu Tseng[7], Jian-Ru Chen[7], Yu-Jou Liao[7], Sy-Jou Chen[8,9], Chin-Sheng Lin[10], Huey-Kang Sytwu[7,11] and Yi-Ping Chuang[7*]

Abstract

Background: *Streptococcus pneumoniae* is a respiratory pathogen causing severe lung infection that may lead to complications such as bacteremia. Current polysaccharide vaccines have limited serotype coverage and therefore cannot provide maximal and long-term protection. Global efforts are being made to develop a conserved protein vaccine candidate. PrtA, a pneumococcal surface protein, was identified by screening a pneumococcal genomic expression library using convalescent patient serum. The *prtA* gene is prevalent and conserved among *S. pneumoniae* strains. Its protective efficacy, however, has not been described. Mucosal immunization could sensitize both local and systemic immunity, which would be an ideal scenario for preventing *S. pneumoniae* infection.

Methods: We immunized BALB/c mice intranasally with a combination of a PrtA fragment (amino acids 144–1041) and Th17 potentiated adjuvant, curdlan. We then measured the T-cell and antibody responses. The protective efficacy conferred to the immunized mice was further evaluated using a murine model of acute pneumococcal pneumonia and pneumococcal bacteremia.

Results: There was a profound antigen-specific IL-17A and IFN-γ response in PrtA-immunized mice compared with that of adjuvant control group. Even though PrtA-specific IgG and IgA titer in sera was elevated in immunized mice, only a moderate IgA response was observed in the bronchoalveolar lavage fluid. The PrtA-immunized antisera facilitated the activated murine macrophage, RAW264.7, to opsonophagocytose *S. pneumoniae* D39 strain; however, PrtA-specific immunoglobulins bound to pneumococcal surfaces with a limited potency. Finally, PrtA-induced immune reactions failed to protect mice against *S. pneumoniae*-induced acute pneumonia and bacterial propagation through the blood.

Conclusions: Immunization with recombinant PrtA combined with curdlan produced antigen-specific antibodies and elicited IL-17A response. However, it failed to protect the mice against *S. pneumoniae*-induced infection.

Keywords: *Streptococcus pneumoniae*, IL-17A, PrtA, Curdlan

Background

Streptococcus pneumoniae is a gram-positive encapsulated coccus that generally colonizes the upper respiratory tract in humans without symptoms [1]. However, it may cause community-acquired pneumonia and invasive infections owing to mucosal translocation, such as bacterial meningitis, bacteremia, and otitis media [2, 3]. Therefore, *S. pneumoniae* remains the most common acute pneumonia-causing pathogen in infants and the elderly worldwide [4, 5]. Not only is it a common cause of primary bacterial pneumonia, *S. pneumoniae* also frequently causes secondary bacterial pneumonia following influenza virus infection, thus becoming the main cause of high mortality in adults [6, 7].

Considering *S. pneumoniae*'s impact on morbidity and mortality, healthcare providers promote vaccination to prevent pneumococcal infection. PPSV23 and conjugate

* Correspondence: ypchuang@mail.ndmctsgh.edu.tw
†Chen-Fang Hsu and Chen-Hao Hsiao contributed equally to this work.
[7]Department and Graduate Institute of Microbiology and Immunology, National Defense Medical Center, Taipei, Taiwan
Full list of author information is available at the end of the article

vaccines PCV10 and PCV13 are currently available for use as vaccines [8, 9]. The unconjugated polysaccharide PPSV23 vaccine provides higher coverage of serotypes against pneumococci than the other vaccines, but it cannot be administered to infants owing to their underdeveloped immune system. The conjugated vaccine has reduced the occurrence of invasive pneumococcal diseases since PCV7 was introduced in 2000 [10, 11]; however, cases of pneumococcal infections increased because of non-vaccine serotypes [12, 13]. In fact, invasive diseases attributable to serotypes that are included in the current polysaccharide vaccines may still threaten the protective effect [14]. Notably, capsular polysaccharide vaccines are less effective against acute otitis media and non-bacteremic pneumococcal pneumonia in adult populations [15, 16], possibly due to capsule shedding in response to the epithelium during mucosal infection [17]. Therefore, efforts are being made to develop vaccines containing highly conserved, immunogenic protein antigens, which are selected by immunoscreening with the patients' sera [18] or by reverse vaccinology [19], among other approaches.

PrtA, a cell wall-associated protein, was screened from convalescent patient serum after *S. pneumoniae* infection [20] and was identified as a serine protease. The amino terminal of PrtA, containing catalytic domains, was highly conserved among 78 clinical pneumococcal isolates displaying 22 different serotypes, including the D39 strain [21]. The deletion of the *prtA* in *S. pneumoniae* D39 reduced mortality at 36 h after intraperitoneal infection [21] and alleviated lung inflammation at 48 h after intranasal infection [22]. Furthermore, *prtA* expression in *S. pneumoniae* could be induced during epithelial cell contact, pneumococcal bacteremia, and meningitis in infected mice [23]. Although the immunogenicity, conservation, and virulence of PrtA have been reported, the efficacy of PrtA as a vaccine against pneumococcal infection has not been studied.

The Th17 response is considered effective against *S. pneumoniae* infection. The intratracheal administration of recombinant IL-17A can stimulate the local release of MIP-2 and IL-1β, leading to the recruitment of polymorphonuclear leukocytes to the lungs [24]. Th17 response also triggers the mucosal epithelium to generate anti-microbial peptides, which facilitate the elimination of mucosal pathogens [25]. Mice lacking the IL-17A receptor, but not IFN-γ or IL-4 receptors, demonstrated decreased protection against *S. pneumoniae* [26]. Thus, screening for Th17-based antigens is a feasible approach to select vaccine candidates that could reduce *S. pneumoniae* colonization [27]. Adjuvants provide an alternative approach to support ideal vaccine candidates and develop appropriate cellular immunity.

Curdlan is a linear and nonionic β-1,3-glucan isolated from the bacterium *Alcaligenes faecalis*. Due to its non-toxicity [28, 29] and heat-based gel-forming capabilities [30], curdlan has been approved as a food additive by the U.S. Food and Drug Administration. Curdlan is an agonist of Dectin-1, activating dendritic cells to induce Th17 differentiation [31], along with being a strong inducer of Th17 response [32]. Therefore, curdlan has been successfully adopted as a vaccine adjuvant against *Pseudomonas aeruginosa* pulmonary infection [33], and lethal Candida infection [34], among other infections [35]. In the present study, we investigated the efficacy of PrtA immunization combined with curdlan to prevent *S. pneumoniae* infection. We used BALB/c mice to deliver the vaccine via the nasal route to trigger both local mucosal and systemic immune responses, we also checked the vaccines' capability to reduce the severity of pneumonia as well as the incidence of invasion.

Methods

Bacterial strains and media

Escherichia coli strains DH5α and BL21 (DE3) were used for plasmid cloning and protein expression, respectively. The strains harboring plasmids were grown in Luria–Bertani medium supplemented with kanamycin (50 μg/ml). *S. pneumoniae* D39 (NCTC7466) was purchased from the National Collection of Type Cultures (London, UK), and *S. pneumoniae* TIGR4 (ATCC BAA-334) was obtained from American Type Culture Collection (Manassas, VA, USA). *S. pneumoniae* strains were cultured at 37 °C in 5% CO_2 in Todd–Hewitt broth supplemented with 0.5% yeast extract (THY) until mid-log phase for the bacterial challenge, and on sheep-blood agar plates for bacterial load examination after infection.

Construction of expression vector

The gene encoding a PrtA fragment (amino acids 144–1041) was cloned into plasmid pET29a using the primer pair F1-AATCGAGCTCCTATCCAATC and R1-TGAG CCTCGAGAGGATTTCC to construct pET-PrtA105-His. The underlined primer sequences were modified to obtain appropriate restriction sites. To generate recombinant PrtA with dual tags, another primer pair, F2-AGGGTACCG TATTCATGTCC and R2-GCAGATCGTCAGTCAGTCA C, was used to clone DNA encoding glutathione S transferase (GST) from pGEX-4 T-1, which was inserted into pET-PrtA105-His to construct pET-GST-PrtA105-His.

Purification of recombinant proteins

E. coli BL21 (DE3) was transformed with an expression vector. Protein expression was induced in the exponential phase [optical density (OD) at 600 nm = 1] using 1 mM isopropyl β-D-1-thiogalactopyranoside (IPTG). At 3 h after induction, the bacteria were harvested and resuspended in lysis buffer [20 mM Tris (pH 8.0), 5 mM imidazole, 500 mM NaCl, 10% glycerol, 1% Triton X-100, 1 mM phenylmethylsulfonyl fluoride, 1× protease inhibitor cocktail (Roche)], followed by sonication on ice. The recombinant protein PrtA105-His (PrtA1) was purified using Ni-NTA resin (GE Healthcare) according to the manufacturer's instructions. The other recombinant protein, GST-PrtA105-His (PrtA2), was further purified with glutathione-Sepharose® 4B (Millipore). Lipopolysaccharide (LPS) contamination was reduced by using 0.1% Triton X-114 in the washing step [36]. The residual LPS was less than 1 EU/μg protein, as determined by a ToxinSensor™ Gel Clot Endotoxin Assay Kit (GenScript).

Mice

BALB/c mice used in the immunization and challenge experiments were purchased from the National Laboratory Animal Center, NARLabs, Taiwan.

Mice immunization

Male mice (3–4 weeks old) were treated intranasally with 8 μg recombinant PrtA1 combined with 0.2 mg curdlan (Sigma) in 20 μl phosphate-buffered saline (PBS) once a week for 3 weeks under anesthesia (intramuscular injection of 40 μl PBS containing Zoletil 50 and 1% Rompun®). One week after the last immunization, mice were restrained to collect saliva before sacrificing them to collect nasal washes, sera, bronchoalveolar lavage fluid (BALF), and spleens.

For PPSV23 vaccination, Pneumovax®23 (Merck & Co., Inc.) vaccines were 10^{-1} diluted in saline, and 100 μl was injected intraperitoneally into five-week-old mice. Booster immunizations were administered after 2 weeks.

Identification of CD4⁺ T cell subsets

$CD4^+$ T cell subsets (Th1 [IFN-γ-producing $CD4^+$ T cells], Th2 [IL-4-producing $CD4^+$ T cells], and Th17 [IL-17A-producing $CD4^+$ T cells]) were identified by intracellular cytokine staining. To estimate the total effector T cell ratio, splenocytes (2×10^6 cell/ml) were seeded in 24-well plates and stimulated with phorbol 12-myristate13-acetate (PMA) (20 ng/ml) and ionomycin (1 μM) for 6 h while incubating with 4 μM monensin. The antibodies used were FITC-anti-IFN-γ (XMG1.2), PE-anti-IL-4 (11B11), APC-anti-CD4 (RM4–5) (eBioscience), and PE-anti-IL-17A (TC11-18H10) (BD Biosciences). Intracellular staining was performed after treatment with permeabilization buffer (eBioscience) containing 0.1% saponin according to the instructions provided by eBioscience, and the effector T cell ratio was analyzed by flow cytometry using a FACSCalibur™ (BD Biosciences).

PrtA-specific cytokine responses

Splenocytes were prepared and seeded at 4×10^5/well using ten wells of a 96-well plate. Recombinant PrtA2 was added at 10 μg/ml and incubated for 48 h. Then, the supernatants were pooled and stored at − 80 °C until use. The cytokine levels were measured using a DuoSet® ELISA (enzyme-linked immunosorbent assay) Development System (R&D Systems).

PrtA-specific antibody titers

PrtA-specific isotype antibody titers were measured in the sera, saliva, nasal washes, and BALF, as described previously [37, 38]. In brief, a 96-well plate was coated with 100 ng/50 μl PrtA2 in PBS and incubated overnight at 4 °C. After blocking with a 50 μl blocking buffer [0.5% bovine serum albumin (BSA), 0.05% Tween-20, and 1 mM EDTA in PBS], 50 μl of twofold serially diluted samples were added and incubated at room temperature for 2 h. Following three washes, horseradish peroxidase-labeled goat anti-mouse IgG or rat anti-mouse IgA (Southern Biotech) was added, and the plate was incubated at room temperature for 2 h. The color was developed using tetramethylbenzidine (Science Products, Inc.). The endpoint titer was expressed as the reciprocal $\log_2$ of the last dilution that gave an OD of 0.1 or 0.2 at 450 nm for IgG and IgA, respectively.

To analyze the titers of PrtA-specific IgG subclasses, modified mouse Ig isotyping ELISA was used. Slightly, diluted rat anti-mouse Ig isotype antibodies (1×10^{-3}; IgG1, IgG2a, IgG2b, and IgG3) (Affymetrix, eBioscience) were used to detect the levels of PrtA-bound IgG subclasses in 96-well plates as described earlier. HRP-labeled donkey anti-rat Ig antibodies (Jackson ImmunoResearch) were pre-adsorbed with 2% nonimmune mouse sera to minimize the cross-reaction.

Detection of PrtA on pneumococcal surfaces using vaccinated mouse sera

A. Flow cytometry assay

Bacteria cultured from stock for less than 13 h were diluted 1:50 in THY broth and cultured until the mid-log phase. Next, 1 ml bacterial broth was centrifuged and resuspended in filtered PBS containing 1% BSA. PrtA was detected using vaccinated mouse sera (1:20 dilution) by incubating at 37 °C for 20 min. The mouse sera collected from adjuvant-treated littermates were used as controls. The pneumococcal surface-bound Ig was detected using FITC-anti-mouse IgG antibody (eBioscience) and was analyzed by flow cytometry using a FACSCalibur™. Anti-cell wall polysaccharide (CWPS) antisera (SSI Diagnostica) were diluted 1:100 to interact with D39 cells as another control. Surface-bound Ig was identified using FITC-anti-rabbit IgG antibody (BD).

B. Immunofluorescence assay

S. pneumoniae D39 cells were labeled with 0.5 mg/mL FITC, as described previously [39, 40], and were resuspended in PBS. The whole-cell immunofluorescence assay was performed according to the method published by Jose et al. [41] with slightly modification. The cells dried on the round coverslips were first fixed with 4% paraformaldehyde for 20 min and then washed by PBS for three times. After blocking with 3% BSA in PBS, FITC-labeled D39 cells were incubated with 1/150 diluted antisera at room temperature for 1 h. The pneumococcal surface-bound Ig was identified using DyLight™ 649-conjugated anti-mouse IgG antibody (1:150) (BioLegend) or Cy5-anti-rabbit IgG antibody (Abcam) (1:150), and then was visualized using immunofluorescence microscopy with DeltaVision™ Elite.

Opsonophagocytosis assay

The opsonophagocytosis assay was performed according to the method published by Martinez et al. [42], by using murine RAW264.7 macrophages. An aliquot of 20 µl of bacterial suspension containing 8×10^6 CFU FITC-labeled D39 cells was mixed in a 96-well round bottom plate with 1:1 serially diluted antiserum from the vaccinated mice. The plate was incubated at 37 °C for 30 min with shaking at 200 rpm. Opsonized bacterial cells were then co-cultivated with RAW264.7 macrophages in 24-well plates, that were activated with 100 nM PMA for 3 days. The opsonophagocytosis was conducted at 37 °C for 30 min with shaking at 200 rpm. The bacterial cells were then washed twice with cold PBS, and RAW264.7 macrophages were detached with 2% EDTA in PBS. Extracellular FITC was quenched with 20 µg/ml trypan blue followed by flow cytometry analysis by using FACSCalibur™.

Bacterial challenge of immunized mice

Bacteria cultured overnight were diluted 1:50 in THY broth and cultured until the mid-log phase. Following washing with PBS, and the OD at 580 nm was adjusted to 3.0 before aliquots were stored at − 80 °C. The bacterial counts were estimated after plating. Mice with complete vaccinations were challenged with *S. pneumoniae* D39 on day 14 after the last boost. The mice were injected with 2.5×10^4 CFU of *S. pneumoniae* D39 in 100 µl PBS via the retro-orbital venous sinus or anesthetized and infected with $1–3 \times 10^7$ CFU of D39 in 40 µl PBS intranasally. Bacterial counts in the blood were monitored at 1–3 days after infection. Blood was collected by submandibular bleeding using a lancet. At 1–3 days after infection, the mice were sacrificed to remove the lungs, which were homogenized to examine bacterial load during acute infection. The humane endpoint was applied to the survival experiment to reduce distress to the animals. We monitored the health of the mice every 12 h for 6 days after the bacterial challenge. If the mice were found to experience labored breathing, lethargy, or inability to ambulate, then they were killed instead of letting them suffer and progress to the experimental endpoint.

Statistics

Significant differences between groups were analyzed using Student's *t*-test or Mann-Whitney test. The value indicated in the figures represents mean and standard deviation (SD). The survival rate was investigated using the Kaplan–Meier estimation, and the significance was evaluated by the log-rank test.

Results

Expression and purification of the conserved amino terminal of PrtA

The PrtA fragment containing the catalytic triad was cloned into the pET29a expression vector, and its expression was induced under an optimal IPTG concentration and temperature. The expressed PrtA1 recombinant protein was in-frame with the histidine (His) tag and purified using Ni-NTA resin. Additionally, a PrtA fragment in-frame with both the GST and His tags (PrtA2) was purified using Ni-NTA resin and glutathione-Sepharose 4B. The molecular weight of PrtA1 and PrtA2 were approximately 105 and 130 kDa, respectively (Fig. 1). PrtA2 had a higher purity than PrtA1. However, PrtA2 yield dramatically decreased after complete purification. Thus, PrtA1 was used for vaccination and PrtA2 was used to analyze the antigen-specific immune response in vitro.

PrtA1 vaccination elicited an antigen-specific cellular immune response

IL-17A is crucial in the pulmonary defense of a host, therefore, the PrtA1 immunogen was combined with curdlan to induce a strong IL-17A response when administered intranasally [43]. Since pulmonary pneumococcal infection still threatens neonates and infants in a clinical setting, immunization was induced in infant mice (3–4 weeks old) to evaluate the efficacy of vaccination. After exposure to the immunogen on three occasions, the immune response was determined 1 week after the last immunization.

After three rounds of immunization, vaccine-sensitized splenocytes were treated with PMA and ionomycin to determine whether immunization with PrtA1 combined with curdlan (PrtA1/curdlan) could activate effector T cells. PrtA1/curdlan did not increase the proportion of Th1 nor Th2 cells within the total number of CD4 T cells. However, PrtA1/curdlan induced an increase in the number of Th17 cells by over twofold compared with the adjuvant control group (Fig. 2a). Antigen-recall assay showed that the spleens belonging to the mice in the PrtA1/curdlan group exhibited higher levels of antigen-specific Th17 cells

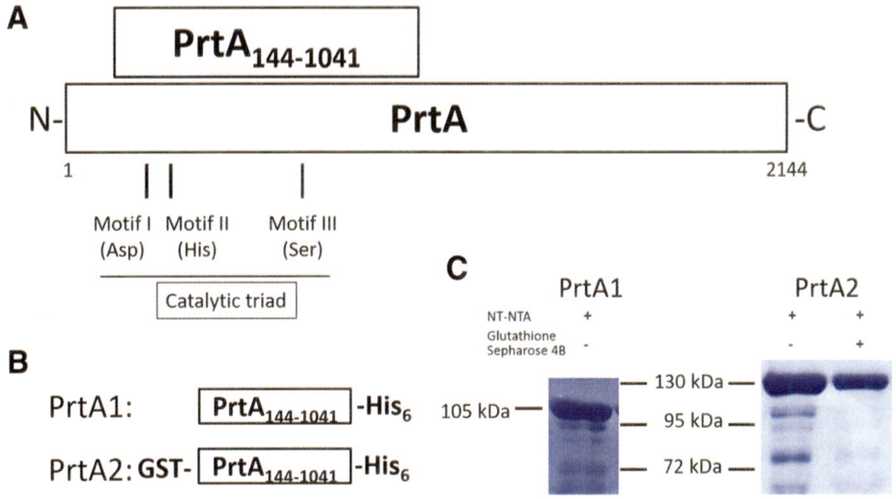

Fig. 1 Purification of the amino terminal of PrtA. **a** The PrtA fragment (amino acids 144–1041) containing the catalytic triad was cloned and expressed. **b** Illustration of the PrtA fragment used for expression and purification. **c** PrtA1 and PrtA2 purified using Ni-NTA resin alone or with glutathione-Sepharose 4B were resolved by SDS-polyacrylamide gel electrophoresis and visualized by Coomassie Brilliant Blue staining

than those of the mice in the adjuvant control group (Fig. 2b). After recombinant PrtA protein stimulation in vitro for 48 h, the splenocytes belonging to the PrtA1/curdlan immunization group showed a higher potential to produce antigen-specific IL-17A than those belonging to the adjuvant control group (Fig. 2c). Although in vitro stimulation of PrtA did not recall a high percentage of IFN-γ-positive $CD4^+$ effector T cells (Fig. 2b), it triggered PrtA1/curdlan-immunized splenocytes to produce high levels of antigen-specific IFN-γ (Fig. 2c). In contrast, PrtA1/curdlan immunization did not induce antigen-specific Th2 cells (Fig. 2b). For the reason that the levels of PrtA-specific IL-4/IL-13 production by splenocytes were lower than the assay's limit of detection, we

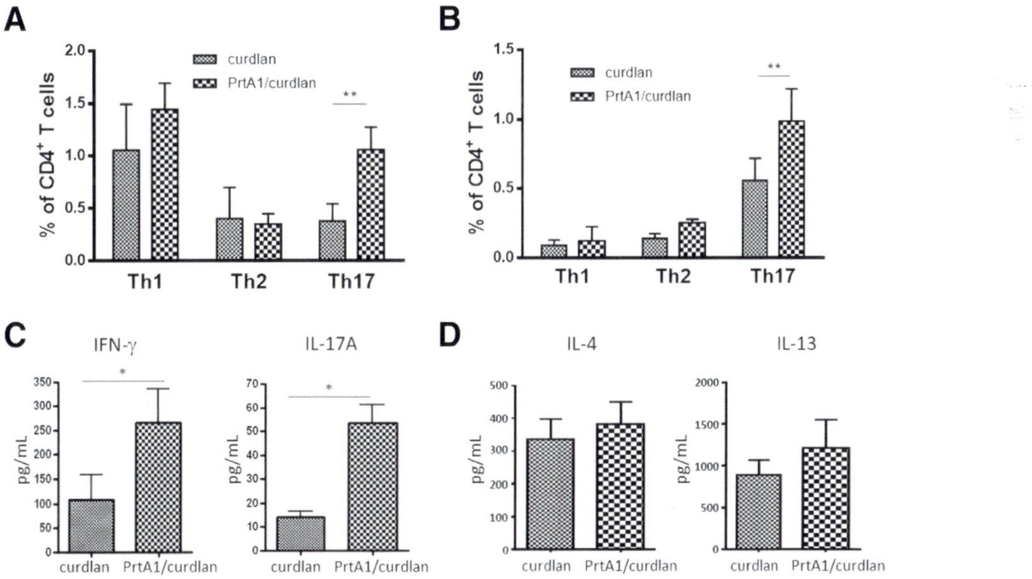

Fig. 2 PrtA immunization induced effector T cell responses. At 3 weeks after immunization, mouse splenocytes were stimulated with (**a**) PMA and ionomycin for 6 h or (**b**) PrtA for 48 h before T cell subsets were examined by flow cytometry. The Th1 (IFN-γ^+CD4^+), Th2 (IL-4^+CD4^+), and Th17 (IL-$17A^+CD4^+$) ratios relative to the total $CD4^+$ T cells were compared between the PrtA1/curdlan groups and the curdlan control group ($n \geq 4$). $^{**}p < 0.01$, Student's *t*-test. **c** IL-17A and IFN-γ production levels after PrtA stimulation in vitro were compared between the immunization groups and the adjuvant control group ($n = 4$). $^{*}p < 0.05$, Mann–Whitney test. **d** IL-4 and IL-13 production levels were detected after anti-CD3 (0.1 μg/mL) and anti-CD28 (0.2 μg/mL) antibody activation for 24 h ($n = 5$)

measured IL-4/IL-13 levels after the splenocytes were treated with anti-CD3/CD28 antibodies for 24 h. The levels of both IL-4 and IL-13 produced by the splenocytes of mice belonging to the PrtA1/curdlan-immunized and adjuvant control groups were similar (Fig. 2d). Splenocytes from the mice immunized with PrtA1 alone produced undetectable levels of PrtA-responsive cytokines (data not presented). This indicates that curdlan induced PrtA to produce antigen-specific IL-17A and IFN-γ, but not Th2 response.

PrtA induced an antigen-specific humoral response

To assess the antibody response after PrtA immunization, sera and mucosal secretions (BALF, nasal washes, and saliva) were collected from the mice to measure PrtA-specific IgG and IgA responses. The anti-PrtA IgG titer in the sera and BALF was significantly higher after immunization with PrtA1/curdlan than that of the adjuvant control group and PrtA1-only group (Fig. 3a). This indicated that curdlan supplementation improved the PrtA-specific IgG titers in the sera and BALF. The PrtA-specific IgA titer also increased markedly in the sera when it was combined with curdlan. Mucosal secretions, saliva, and nasal washes showed higher PrtA-specific IgA titers for the immunized mice than the control mice; however, the IgA titer did not increase in BALF (Fig. 3a). The titers of the IgG subclasses after immunization were also measured and showed that PrtA-specific IgG1, IgG2a, IgG2b, and IgG3 titers of PrtA1/curdlan-immunized mice increased significantly (Fig. 3b).

To check whether the PrtA-specific antibody could bind to the surface of *S. pneumoniae* cells, *S. pneumoniae* strains D39 and TIGR4 were incubated with the sera from immunized mice and IgG binding was evaluated using an anti-mouse IgG-FITC antibody. The sera from PrtA1/curdlan-immunized mice showed that the PrtA-specific antibody bound to the surface of D39 cells [serotype 2] and not TIGR4 cells [serotype 4]; the sera from adjuvant control group failed to elicit antibodies specific to the bacterial cells (Fig. 3c). However, the anti-PrtA antisera did not interact with the entire pneumococcal population. We used an anti-cell wall polysaccharide antibody (anti-CWPS antisera, SSI Diagnostica) to rule out the possibility that the bacterial capsule impeded with the binding of the bacterial cells to the antigen-specific antibody. It showed that the anti-CWPS antisera could access the target cells independent of the capsular serotype with more than 90% of conjugation on the whole population (Fig. 3c). These results indicated that although PrtA immunization elicited antigen-specific antibodies, PrtA-immunized antisera selectively bound to the surface of the pneumococcal cells with limited potency.

PrtA-specific antisera facilitated opsonophagocytosis of *S. pneumoniae*

We further checked the efficacy of PrtA1/curdlan-immunized antisera in assisting the opsonophagocytosis of FITC-labeled D39 cells. The capability of immunized antisera-opsonized bacterial cells was first accessed with immunofluorescence assay. It showed that PrtA-specific antisera potentiated opsonization of the D39 cells, while adjuvant control antisera bound to the D39 cell surface with little efficacy (Fig. 4a). The PPSV23-immunized antisera were used as positive control and PBS-treated control antisera functioned as parallel negative control. Compared with PPSV23, antisera from PrtA-immunized mice revealed considerably weaker activity when bound to pneumococcal surfaces, suggesting that surface-bound Ig levels were lower in PrtA-antisera than in PPSV23-antisera. Although PrtA-immunized antisera could conjugate to D39 cell surface, the distribution of surface-bound Ig signal was not well correlated with that of FITC-labeled D39 cells (Additional file 1). In contrast, signals from capsule targeting Ig in PPSV23 antisera were well distributed and superimposed on where FITC signals (D39 cells) presented (Additional file 1). It suggested portion of bacterial cells eluding PrtA-specific Ig recognition, which was in accordance with the result of our flow cytometry assay (Fig. 3c).

We then co-cultivated the activated RAW264.7 macrophages and the opsonized bacterial cells with shaking to reduce non-specific interaction. It revealed that PrtA-immunized antisera facilitated the phagocytosis of D39 cells by the macrophages (Fig. 4b) owing to its higher capability of opsonizing pneumococci compared with adjuvant control antisera. We found that the bacterial cells opsonized by PrtA-antisera could be ingested by the phagocytes as potently as by PPSV23-antisera regardless of the quantity of Ig on the surface of the bacterial cells (Fig. 4a, b). This suggests phagocytes could clear opsonized bacterial cells with similar potency irrespective of the degree of Ig conjugation on the bacterial cell surface. The data indicates that intranasal immunization with PrtA1/curdlan triggered systemic humoral immune responses and facilitated opsonophagocytosis of *S. pneumoniae* cells.

PrtA combined with curdlan immunization failed to protect against pneumococcal pneumonia and systemic invasion

PrtA1/curdlan immunization induced high IgA titers in sera as well as nasal washes and also induced a higher level of PrtA-specific IL-17A production. Therefore, we tested the efficacy of PrtA immunization against pneumococcal pneumonia. BALB/c mice with complete immunizations were challenged with $1{-}3 \times 10^7$ CFU of *S. pneumoniae* D39 in 40 μl PBS via nasal administration. After 1–3 days of infection, bacterial colonization was

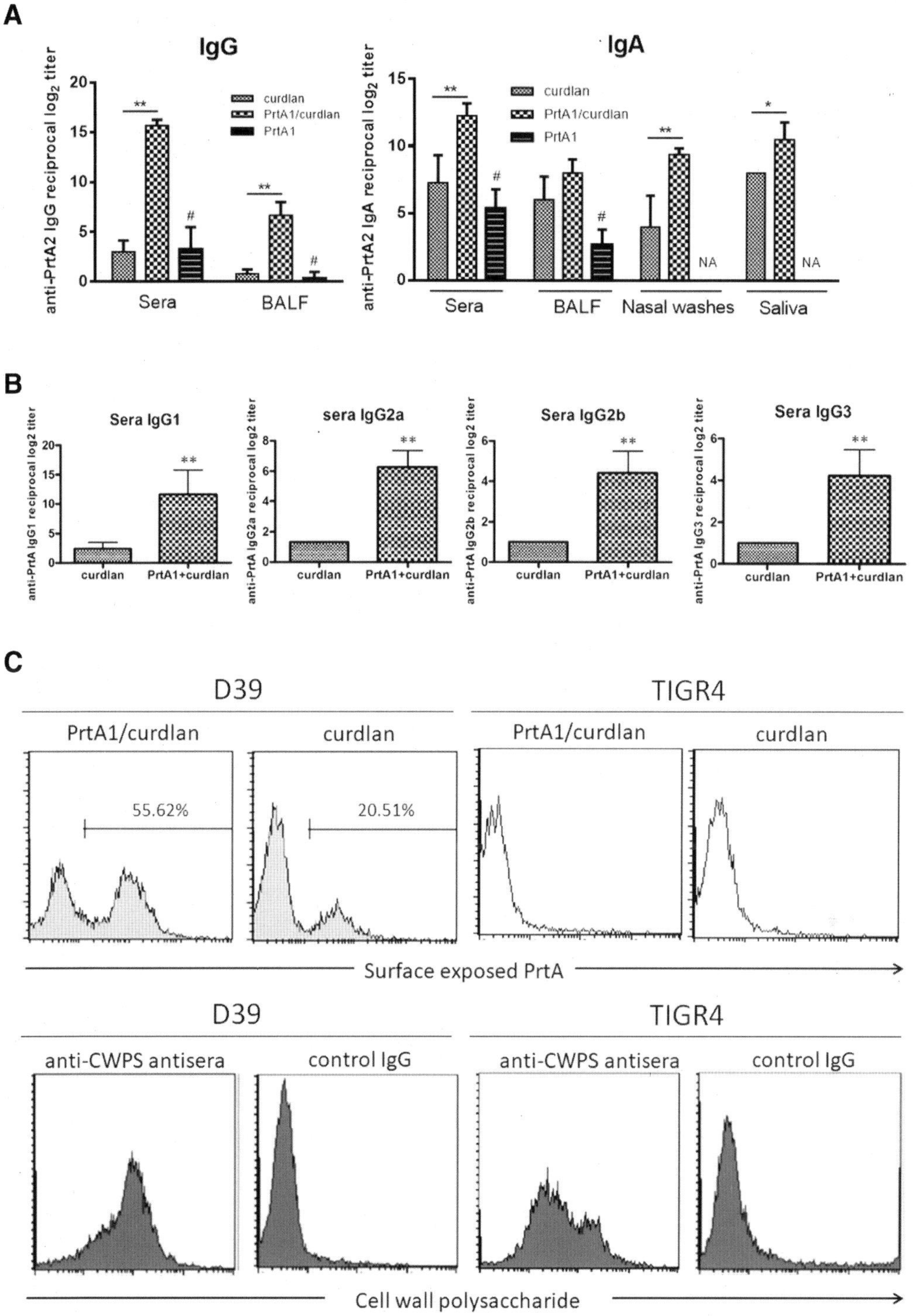

Fig. 3 PrtA immunization increased the antigen-specific immunoglobulin titer and responses. **a** Sera, nasal washes, saliva, and the BALF were collected from the PrtA1/curdlan-immunized group and the adjuvant control group after three vaccinations ($n \geq 4$). Sera and BALF were also collected from mice immunized with PrtA1 protein alone ($n = 3$). The antigen-specific Ig titer was measured using PrtA-specific ELISA. IgG and IgA were distinguished by an isotype-specific secondary antibody. The reciprocal $\log_2$ of the last dilution yielded an OD of 0.2 at 450 nm for sera IgG and 0.1 for the others. *$p < 0.05$; **$p < 0.01$; # $p < 0.01$ compared with PrtA1/curdlan, Student's *t*-test. NA, not analyzed. **b** PrtA-specific IgG subclasses were determined by modified mouse Ig isotyping ELISA ($n \geq 4$). **$p < 0.01$, Student's *t*-test. **c** Sera from immunized mice, but not adjuvant control mice, induced pneumococcal-bound Ig in D39, but not in TIGR4. The sera were pooled from at least four mice in either immunized or adjuvant control group. Rabbit anti-CWPS antisera were used as a control. Bacterial cell-bound IgG was detected using FITC-anti-mouse IgG or FITC-anti-rabbit IgG antibodies and analyzed by flow cytometry

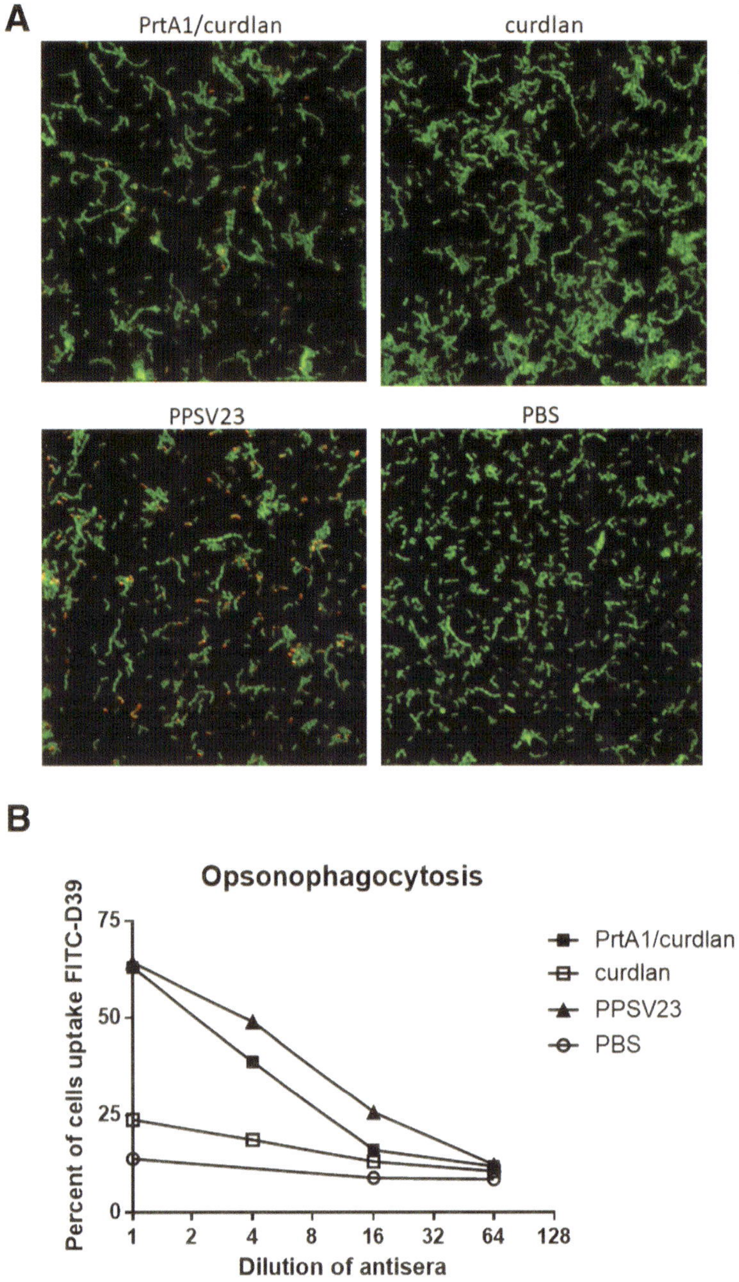

Fig. 4 PrtA immunization facilitated opsonophagocytosis. **a** FITC-labeled *S. pneumoniae* D39 cells were incubated with pooled antisera ($n = 4$) from PrtA1/curdlan- or curdlan-immunized groups. The opsonized bacterial cells were identified using Dylight™ 649-anti-mouse IgG antibody and were visualized using immunofluorescence microscopy (DeltaVision Elite) under 40× oil objective. The images were processed by deconvolution. **b** FITC-labeled D39 cells were mixed with serially diluted antisera and were incubated with PMA-activated murine macrophage RAW264.7. The proportion of RAW264.7 cells to internalized bacterial cells was examined using flow cytometry after extracellular fluorescence quenching with trypan blue. The sera were pooled from four mice in each group, and the results were a representative of two independent experiments

examined by plating out the lung homogenates. Although PrtA immunization elicited a high IgG titer in the BALF, it did not promote D39 clearance in the lungs during acute infection (Fig. 5a). The bacterial load in the blood was further examined, and there was no significant difference in the D39 count between the immunization group and adjuvant control group (Fig. 5b). PrtA1/curdlan seemed to reduce the bacterial load in the infected lungs of the mice on day 3 and tended to alleviate the mucosal invasion; however, day 3 data might reveal a biased trend since some mice in both groups (four in curdlan group; three in PrtA1/curdlan group) died due to severe pneumonia or

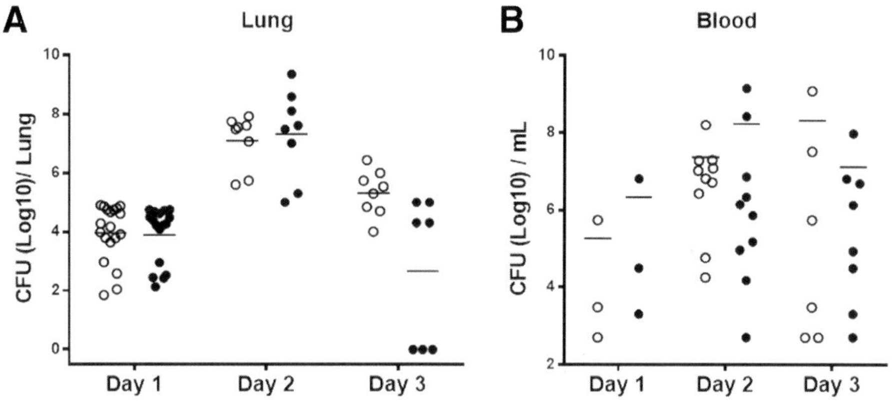

Fig. 5 PrtA immunization failed to protect mice against acute pneumococcal pneumonia. *S. pneumoniae* D39 was intranasally administered to immunized group and the adjuvant control group. **a** Bacterial load in the lungs and (**b**) subsequent bloodstream invasion were examined 1, 2, and 3 days post infection. The open circle represents the curdlan-treated mice, and the filled circle represents the PrtA1/curdlan-immunized mice. The data were pooled from one or two experiments. At least three mice per experiment were used

bacteremia at midnight, which were excluded in the experimental results. These data suggest that PrtA1/curdlan did not effectively protect the mice against *S. pneumoniae*-induced acute pneumonia and the resulting systemic invasion.

PrtA immunization failed to suppress blood propagation of *S. pneumoniae* cells

Although PrtA1/curdlan immunization increased the PrtA-specific IgA titer in most mucosal secretions as shown earlier, the rising antibody titer in paired samples seemed to be insufficient in controlling bacterial burden in the respiratory tract. Because PrtA/curdlan immunization markedly increased antigen-specific IgG and IgA titers in the sera, we checked the protective efficacy against blood propagation of *S. pneumoniae.* D39 cells were injected intravenously into immunized and nonimmunized mice, and the bacterial load after infection as well as the approximative survival rate was ascertained to evaluate the vaccine efficacy. The bacterial burden in the blood of curdlan control mice increased from day 1 to day 2, whereas it was restrained in PrtA1/curdlan immunized mice (Fig. 6a), suggesting that the PrtA-specific Ig potentiated bacterial clearance during the early infection phase. However, PrtA immunization did not increase the survival rate of mice compared with adjuvant control group or untreated mice (Fig. 6b). Clinical PPSV23 vaccine was administered as the positive control, which protected the mice from lethality. PPSV23 prevented bacterial propagation via the blood from day 1 of infection, which was examined by the plating count (data not presented). Our results indicate that although PrtA1/curdlan immunization reduced bacterial load in the blood during the early phase of infection, it failed to alleviate the severity of pneumococcal bacteremia.

Discussion

Overall results indicate that on one hand PrtA/curdlan immunization activated antigen-specific antibody and IL-17A response in the mice, but on the other, it failed to protect against pneumococcal pneumonia and invasive infection. PrtA mediates human apolactoferrin cleavage to yield an N-terminal lactoferricin-like peptide that is more efficient than apolactoferrin as a bactericide against *S. pneumoniae* [44]. It suggested that human innate immunity provided defense against pneumococci with assistance from PrtA and considered PrtA inadequate as a vaccine candidate. It is unknown if mouse apolactoferrin is the PrtA substrate, but a *prtA* mutation reduced the virulence of *S. pneumoniae* in a murine pneumonia model [21, 22, 45], thereby suggesting that it plays a pathogenic role.

PrtA was selected using convalescent-phase serum [20] and was considered an immunogen. Zysk et al. could not confirm the immunoreactivity of PrtA based on 45 serum samples from patients with invasive pneumococcal diseases [46]. However, they used part of the *prtA* gene (nucleotides 330–1041) to express recombinant PrtA as an antigen and that it was highly hydrophobic indicated by TopPred 2 [47]; thus it might not have been an ideal T or B cell receptor ligand in all patients. Another study also observed no significant difference in the anti-PrtA IgG titer in sera from acute and convalescent patients with pneumococcal bacteremia [48]. They further indicated that anti-PrtA IgG titers were higher among healthy children with pneumococcal carriage [49], thereby suggesting that higher antibody titers are insufficient against pneumococcal colonization. In the present study, immunization with recombinant PrtA generated anti-PrtA IgG that bound to the surface of D39 pneumococci but failed to mediate protection against pneumococcal pneumonia and blood stream invasion. It is well known that prior exposure to whole *S.*

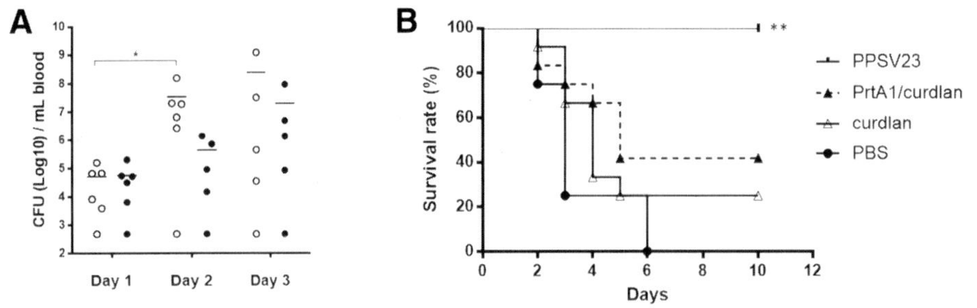

Fig. 6 PrtA immunization failed to protect mice against blood propagation of *S. pneumoniae*. *S. pneumoniae* D39 cells were intravenously administered to the immunized group or adjuvant control group ($n = 6$ in each group). **a** The bacterial load in the blood was monitored on days 1, 2, and 3 post-infection. $n = 6$; *$p < 0.05$; Mann–Whitney test. **b** The survival rate was monitored after pneumococcus infection. Mice administered with PPSV23 were used as the positive control. **$p < 0.01$; Log-rank test

pneumoniae provides immunity against pneumococcal colonization, which depends on $CD4^+$ T cells and IL-17A, a neutrophil-activating cytokine [26, 50]. This suggests that the IL-17A response aids vaccine efficacy. Curdlan is an agonist of dectin-1, which activates Syk-CARD9 signaling in dendritic cells to induce Th17 differentiation [32]. As mentioned earlier, we saw that PrtA-specific IL-17A response was induced in the mice with curdlan as an adjuvant, but it did not protect against pneumococcal pneumonia. Curdlan has been previously shown to facilitate a conserved protein vaccine, PopB, in preventing *P. aeruginosa*-induced pneumonia [33]. With the potency of Th17 stimulation, it is noteworthy to mention that PopB/curdlan could induce a 30-fold higher antigen-specific IL-17A response than PrtA/curdlan, as seen in the antigen-recall T cell activation assay. The distinct IL-17A responses induced by the vaccines used in this study, combined with curdlan, might be attributable to the innate properties of the immunogens along with the potency of being conjugated with curdlan. Curdlan retains antigen in the polymer microspheres via protein-polysaccharide interaction and is extensively used as an adjuvant. High retention of immunogens with curdlan-based support would be expected to provide ideal adjuvant activity. A high molecular weight tetanus anatoxin (150 kDa) has been previously shown to provide about 16-fold lower retention on curdlan than a low molecular weight lysozyme (14.6 kDa) [51]. PrtA is 105 kDa in size which is self-evidently higher than the 40 kDa PopB, that the inefficiency of the IL-17A response induced by PrtA was probably attributable to the low retention on curdlan.

Although PopB/curdlan confers higher protection against pulmonary infection, 40% lethality is still observed within 5 days [33], which might be correlated with an antibody response that is ineffective suppressing bacterial propagation. *S. pneumoniae* D39 is a highly invasive, encapsulated strain with the ability to mediate antiphagocytosis [52]. Clinical PPSV23 vaccine offered 100% protection to mice infected with D39 due to optimal antibody binding, which results in complement deposition or opsonophagocytosis leading to effective pneumococcal clearance. Examination of the protective efficacy of PrtA immunization by determination of the bacterial load in the blood after intravenous infection revealed that the PrtA1/curdlan immunized group, but not the adjuvant control group, restrained bacteria proliferation during the first 2 days (Fig. 6a). However, it failed to protect against lethal bacteremia (Fig. 6b). We determined the potency of PrtA-antisera bound to pneumococcal surfaces and found only a portion of the pneumococcal population was conjugated (Fig. 3c, Additional file 1), which might be the point of vulnerability leading to immune escape and disease progression.

PrtA1/curdlan did not induce marked antigen-specific Th2 response, which was possibly attributable to Th1 skewing by curdlan modulation. Because Th1/2 imbalance could limit the antibody responses, we verified the efficacy of an alternative immunization with PrtA combined with traditional complete Freund's adjuvant-incomplete Freund's adjuvant (CFA-IFA), which was assumed to efficiently enhance global immune responses. When combined with CFA-IFA, PrtA immunization induced a considerably higher antigen-specific Th1 and Th2 response than did PrtA1/curdlan; Th17 induction was comparable with PrtA1/curdlan (Fig. 2, Additional file 2). Although CFA-IFA facilitated Th2 activation, PrtA-specific antibody titers did not improve in the sera or mucosal secretions compared with PrtA1/curdlan (Fig. 3, Additional file 3). Unlike the limited interaction of PrtA1/curdlan antisera with TIGR4 cells (Fig. 3c), the antisera from PrtA/CFA-IFA-immunized mice could successfully recognize D39 as well as TIGR4 cells (Additional file 3), possibly because of the T-cell receptor repertoire induced by CFA-IFA [53]. However, the potency of antigen-specific antibody conjugation on the pneumococcal cell surface was still limited

(Additional file 3). Moreover, it failed to improve bacterial clearance from the blood and could not stop the progression of bacteremia (Additional file 4).

The number of effective immunoglobulins from both PrtA-immunized antisera (PrtA/curdlan and PrtA/CFA-IFA) bound to pneumococcal cell surfaces was lower than that from PPSV23-immunized antisera (Additional file 1). This suggested that fewer epitopes on the pneumococcal cell surface were recognized by the PrtA-antisera than by PPSV23 antisera. Moreover, higher number of pneumococci were not conjugated by Ig in PrtA-antisera than in PPSV23 antisera, highlighting the imperfect reactivity of PrtA-antisera against the pneumococci due to population heterogeneity [54, 55]. The inefficiency of PrtA/curdlan antisera was not different from that of PPSV23 antisera in the opsonophagocytosis assay (Fig. 4b). It seemed that the ratio of bacterial cells opsonized by either PrtA- or PPSV23 antisera versus phagocytes in the assay could be large enough to ignore the proportion of bacterial cells eluding Ig recognition. These escaped pneumococci might have continued to replicate; thereby, breaching the infectivity threshold. This is in accordance with the outcome of the systemic invasion murine model, which restrained bacteria load in day 2 but could not stop the bacterial propagation and disease severity to the end of experiment. The mechanism underlying the variable expression of PrtA on the pneumococcal surface remains unclear, and if elucidated, might partly explain the failure of PrtA immunization against *S. pneumoniae* invasion.

Although the PrtA/curdlan vaccine did not suppress pneumococcal invasion, we found that it tended to reduce the bacterial load in the lung after 3 days of infection, in addition to seemingly restricting the bacterial propagation during the early phase of blood invasion, despite the limited potency of the antibody response. We have previously found that BABL/c mice might not be suitable for evaluating vaccine efficacy because they are more resistant to *S. pneumoniae* infection than other mouse strains [56]. Furthermore, a high dose of infection, which is needed to potentiate pneumococcal disease, could exceed the threshold of protection conferred by the PrtA/curdlan vaccine. This limitation might also partly explain the failure of the PrtA vaccine.

Global efforts are being made to develop efficient protein vaccine candidates against *S. pneumoniae.* An effective mucosal Th2 response and IgA titer, in addition to antigen-specific Th17 are essential to prevent pneumococcal colonization of the lungs. A high titer of antigen-specific IgG and sufficient potency to bind to the surface of all bacteria in population, are critical to prevent pneumococcal invasion. Thus, the variable expression of selected pneumococcal vaccine candidates needs to be considered in the field.

Conclusions

Combining a PrtA fragment (amino acids 144–1041) with curdlan induced antigen-specific Th17 and antibody response in BALB/c mice after immunization. However, the PrtA/curdlan vaccine did not effectively protect the mice against acute pneumonia, along with failing to suppress pneumococcal propagation in the blood. The failure of the vaccine might be attributable to the limited potency of PrtA-specific antibodies bound to the pneumococcal cell surface.

Additional files

Additional file 1: PrtA-induced antibody conjugated with pneumococci with limited potency. FITC-labeled *S. pneumoniae* D39 cells were incubated with antisera as indicated. The opsonized bacterial cells were identified using Dylight™ 649-conjugated secondary antibody and were visualized by immunofluorescence microscopy (DeltaVision Elite) under 40× oil objective. The inserts show higher magnification (with 60× oil objective) of Ig-conjugated bacteria. The images were processed by deconvolution. The antisera were pooled from at least four mice in either immunized or adjuvant control group. (TIF 19843 kb)

Additional file 2: PrtA1/CFA-IFA immunization induced effector T cell responses. PrtA1 combined with 100 μL of CFA or IFA (PrtA/CFA-IFA) was injected subcutaneously in the neck of the mice with the same antigen dosage and administration schedule as the curdlan adjuvant (see details in Materials and Methods). PrtA1, CFA, and IFA were mixed sufficiently to create an emulsion before immunization with the CFA mixture for the first week and the IFA mixture for the following two weeks. One week after completion of the immunization, the spleens were isolated from immunized mice. (A) The splenocytes were stimulated with PMA and ionomycin for 6 h before T cell subset examination by flow cytometry. Th1 (IFN-γ^+CD4$^+$), Th2 (IL-4$^+$CD4$^+$), and Th17 (IL-17A$^+$CD4$^+$) numbers relative to the total CD4$^+$ T cells were compared between the immunized groups and the adjuvant control group ($n \geq 4$). (B) After recombinant PrtA protein stimulation in vitro for 48 h, the supernatant was collected for cytokine analysis. *$p < 0.05$; **$p < 0.01$; Student's *t*-test. (TIF 11486 kb)

Additional file 3: PrtA1/CFA-IFA immunization increased the antigen-specific immunoglobulin titer and responses. (A) Sera, BALF, and nasal washes were collected from the immunized mice and the adjuvant control group (n ≥ 4) one week after three vaccinations. The antigen-specific Ig titer was measured using PrtA-specific ELISA. IgG and IgA were distinguished using an isotype-specific secondary antibody. The reciprocal $\log_2$ of the last dilution yielded an OD of 0.2 at 450 nm for sera IgG and 0.1 for the others. **$p < 0.01$; Student's *t*-test. (B) Pneumococcal-bound IgG in antisera from vaccinated mice and adjuvant control mice were evaluated using two pneumococcal strains, D39 and TIGR4. Bacterial-bound IgG was detected using an FITC-anti-mouse IgG antibody and flow cytometry. The ratio was representative of the percentage of total pneumococci being conjugated by antigen-specific IgG. (C) FITC-labeled *S. pneumoniae* D39 cells were incubated with antisera from PrtA1/CFA-IFA-immunized or adjuvant control groups. The opsonized bacterial cells were identified using Dylight™ 649-anti-mouse IgG antibody and were visualized by immunofluorescence microscopy (DeltaVision Elite) under 40× oil objective. The images were processed by deconvolution. The antisera used in (B) and (C) were pooled from at least four mice in either immunized or adjuvant control groups. (TIF 9038 kb)

Additional file 4: PrtA1/CFA-IFA immunization failed to protect mice against pneumococcal bacteremia. *S. pneumoniae* D39 cells were intravenously administered to immunized group or adjuvant control group ($n \geq 6$). (A) The bacterial loads in the blood from PrtA1/CFA-IFA- or CFA-IFA- immunized mice were monitored on days 1, 2, and 3 post infection. *$p < 0.05$; Mann–Whitney test. (B) The survival rate was monitored after pneumococcal infection. The humane endpoint was replaced with experimental endpoint. (TIF 13629 kb)

Abbreviations

BALF: Bronchoalveolar lavage fluid; CFA: Complete Freund's adjuvants; ELISA: Enzyme-linked immunosorbent assay; IFA: Incomplete Freund's adjuvants; IFN: Interferon; IL: Interleukin; Th: T helper

Acknowledgements

The authors acknowledge the technical services (supports) provided by Instrument Center of National Defense Medical Center and would like to thank Enago (http://www.enago.com/) for the English language review.

Funding

This study was supported by the grants from Chi Mei Medical Center (CMNDMC10108), the Ministry of Science and Technology (NSC 102–2320-B-016 -013-MY2 to Y.-P.C.), the National Defense Medical Research (MAB102–91 and MAB106–109), and the Cheng-Hsin General Hospital (CH-NDMC-105-8, CH-NDMC-107-12).

Authors' contributions

CFH, CHH, HS, and YC designed and conceived the project; ST, JC, and YL performed the experiments and collected the data. CFH, CHH and YC analyzed and interpreted the data; SC and CL support the administration. YC wrote the manuscript. All authors have read and approved the manuscript.

Competing interests

The authors declare that they have no competing interests.

Author details

[1]Department of Pediatrics, Chi Mei Medical Center, Tainan, Taiwan. [2]Taipei Medical University, Taipei, Taiwan. [3]Kaohsiung Medical University, Kaohsiung, Taiwan. [4]Chung Shan Medical University, Taichung, Taiwan. [5]Cheng Hsin General Hospital, Taipei, Taiwan. [6]Genome and Systems Biology Degree Program, National Taiwan University and Academia Sinica, Taipei, Taiwan. [7]Department and Graduate Institute of Microbiology and Immunology, National Defense Medical Center, Taipei, Taiwan. [8]Department of Emergency Medicine, Tri-Service General Hospital, National Defense Medical Center, Taipei, Taiwan. [9]Graduate Institute of Injury Prevention and Control, College of Public Health and Nutrition, Taipei Medical University, Taipei, Taiwan. [10]Division of Cardiology, Department of Medicine, Tri-Service General Hospital, National Defense Medical Center, Taipei, Taiwan. [11]National Institute of Infectious Diseases and Vaccinology, National Health Research Institutes, Miaoli, Taiwan.

References

1. McCullers JA. Insights into the interaction between influenza virus and pneumococcus. Clin Microbiol Rev. 2006;19(3):571–82.
2. Lynch JPI, Zhanel GG. Streptococcus pneumoniae: epidemiology and risk factors, evolution of antimicrobial resistance, and impact of vaccines. Curr Opin Pulm Med. 2010;16(3):217–25.
3. Thigpen MC, et al. Bacterial meningitis in the United States, 1998-2007. N Engl J Med. 2011;364(21):2016–25.
4. Whitney CG. Changing epidemiology of pneumococcal disease in the era of conjugate vaccines. Curr Epidemiol Rep. 2016;3(2):125–35.
5. Prevention. CfDCa: Active Bacterial Core Surveillance (ABCs) Report Emerging Infections Program Network: Streptococcus pneumoniae, 2010 (ORIG). http://www.cdc.gov/abcs/reports-findings/survreports/spneu10-orig.pdf. Accessed 21 Mar 2013.
6. Morens DM, et al. Predominant role of bacterial pneumonia as a cause of death in pandemic influenza: implications for pandemic influenza preparedness. J Infect Dis. 2008;198(7):962–70.
7. Weinberger DM, et al. Impact of the 2009 influenza pandemic on pneumococcal pneumonia hospitalizations in the United States. J Infect Dis. 2012;205(3):458–65.
8. Daniels CC, et al. A review of pneumococcal vaccines: current polysaccharide vaccine recommendations and future protein antigens. J Pediatr Pharmacol Ther. 2016;21(1):27–35.
9. Hammitt LL, et al. Population effect of 10-valent pneumococcal conjugate vaccine on nasopharyngeal carriage of Streptococcus pneumoniae and non-typeable Haemophilus influenzae in Kilifi, Kenya: findings from cross-sectional carriage studies. Lancet Glob Health. 2014;2(7):e397–405.
10. Pilishvili T, et al. Sustained reductions in invasive pneumococcal disease in the era of conjugate vaccine. J Infect Dis. 2010;201(1):32–41.
11. Rosen JB, et al. Geographic variation in invasive pneumococcal disease following pneumococcal conjugate vaccine introduction in the United States. Clin Infect Dis. 2011;53(2):137–43.
12. Kwambana-Adams B, et al. Rapid replacement by non-vaccine pneumococcal serotypes may mitigate the impact of the pneumococcal conjugate vaccine on nasopharyngeal bacterial ecology. Sci Rep. 2017;7(1):8127.
13. Hicks LA, et al. Incidence of pneumococcal disease due to non-pneumococcal conjugate vaccine (PCV7) serotypes in the United States during the era of widespread PCV7 vaccination, 1998-2004. J Infect Dis. 2007;196(9):1346–54.
14. Sutcu M, et al. Empyema due to Streptococcus pneumoniae serotype 9V in a child immunized with 13-valent conjugated pneumococcal vaccine. Balkan Med J. 2017;34(1):74–7.
15. Pichichero ME, et al. Next generation protein based Streptococcus pneumoniae vaccines. Hum Vaccin Immunother. 2016;12(1):194–205.
16. Jose RJ, Brown JS. Adult pneumococcal vaccination: advances, impact, and unmet needs. Curr Opin Pulm Med. 2017;23(3):225–30.
17. Kietzman CC, et al. Dynamic capsule restructuring by the main pneumococcal autolysin LytA in response to the epithelium. Nat Commun. 2016;7:10859.
18. Giefing C, et al. Discovery of a novel class of highly conserved vaccine antigens using genomic scale antigenic fingerprinting of pneumococcus with human antibodies. J Exp Med. 2008;205(1):117–31.
19. Serruto D, et al. Genome-based approaches to develop vaccines against bacterial pathogens. Vaccine. 2009;27(25–26):3245–50.
20. Zysk G, et al. Detection of 23 immunogenic pneumococcal proteins using convalescent-phase serum. Infect Immun. 2000;68(6):3740–3.
21. Bethe G, et al. The cell wall-associated serine protease PrtA: a highly conserved virulence factor of Streptococcus pneumoniae. FEMS Microbiol Lett. 2001;205(1):99–104.
22. de Stoppelaar SF, et al. Streptococcus pneumoniae serine protease HtrA, but not SFP or PrtA, is a major virulence factor in pneumonia. PLoS One. 2013;8(11):e80062.
23. Orihuela CJ, et al. Microarray analysis of pneumococcal gene expression during invasive disease. Infect Immun. 2004;72(10):5582–96.
24. Laan M, et al. Neutrophil recruitment by human IL-17 via C-X-C chemokine release in the airways. J Immunol. 1999;162(4):2347–52.
25. Kumar P, et al. Th17 cell based vaccines in mucosal immunity. Curr Opin Immunol. 2013;25(3):373–80.
26. Lu YJ, et al. Interleukin-17A mediates acquired immunity to pneumococcal colonization. PLoS Pathog. 2008;4(9):e1000159.
27. Moffitt KL, et al. T(H)17-based vaccine design for prevention of Streptococcus pneumoniae colonization. Cell Host Microbe. 2011;9(2):158–65.
28. Spicer EJ, et al. A toxicological assessment of curdlan. Food Chem Toxicol. 1999;37(4):455–79.
29. Gordon M, et al. Curdlan sulfate (CRDS) in a 21-day intravenous tolerance study in human immunodeficiency virus (HIV) and cytomegalovirus (CMV) infected patients: indication of anti-CMV activity with low toxicity. J Med. 1997;28(1–2):108–28.
30. Harada T, et al. Curdlan: a bacterial gel-forming beta-1,3-glucan. Arch Biochem Biophys. 1968;124(1):292–8.
31. Higashi T, et al. Curdlan induces DC-mediated Th17 polarization via Jagged1 activation in human dendritic cells. Allergol Int. 2010;59(2):161–6.

32. LeibundGut-Landmann S, et al. Syk- and CARD9-dependent coupling of innate immunity to the induction of T helper cells that produce interleukin 17. Nat Immunol. 2007;8(6):630–8.
33. Wu W, et al. Th17-stimulating protein vaccines confer protection against Pseudomonas aeruginosa pneumonia. Am J Respir Crit Care Med. 2012; 186(5):420–7.
34. Bar E, et al. A novel Th cell epitope of Candida albicans mediates protection from fungal infection. J Immunol. 2012;188(11):5636–43.
35. Thompson IJ, et al. Potential of the beta-glucans to enhance innate resistance to biological agents. Expert Rev Anti-Infect Ther. 2010;8(3):339–52.
36. Reichelt P, et al. Single step protocol to purify recombinant proteins with low endotoxin contents. Protein Expr Purif. 2006;46(2):483–8.
37. Lee SE, et al. A bacterial flagellin, Vibrio vulnificus FlaB, has a strong mucosal adjuvant activity to induce protective immunity. Infect Immun. 2006;74(1): 694–702.
38. Fukuyama Y, et al. Secretory-IgA antibodies play an important role in the immunity to Streptococcus pneumoniae. J Immunol. 2010;185(3):1755–62.
39. DeVelasco EA, et al. Adjuvant Quil a improves protection in mice and enhances opsonic capacity of antisera induced by pneumococcal polysaccharide conjugate vaccines. Vaccine. 1994;12(15):1419–22.
40. Jansen WT, et al. Use of highly encapsulated Streptococcus pneumoniae strains in a flow-cytometric assay for assessment of the phagocytic capacity of serotype-specific antibodies. Clin Diagn Lab Immunol. 1998;5(5):703–10.
41. Jose J, et al. Bacterial surface display library screening by target enzyme labeling: identification of new human cathepsin G inhibitors. Anal Biochem. 2005;346(2):258–67.
42. Martinez JE, et al. A flow cytometric opsonophagocytic assay for measurement of functional antibodies elicited after vaccination with the 23-valent pneumococcal polysaccharide vaccine. Clin Diagn Lab Immunol. 1999;6(4):581–6.
43. Zygmunt BM, et al. Intranasal immunization promotes th17 immune responses. J Immunol. 2009;183(11):6933–8.
44. Mirza S, et al. Serine protease PrtA from Streptococcus pneumoniae plays a role in the killing of S. pneumoniae by apolactoferrin. Infect Immun. 2011; 79(6):2440–50.
45. Hava DL, Camilli A. Large-scale identification of serotype 4 Streptococcus pneumoniae virulence factors. Mol Microbiol. 2002;45(5):1389–406.
46. Zysk G, et al. Immune response to capsular polysaccharide and surface proteins of Streptococcus pneumoniae in patients with invasive pneumococcal disease. J Infect Dis. 2003;187(2):330–3.
47. von Heijne G. Membrane protein structure prediction. Hydrophobicity analysis and the positive-inside rule J Mol Biol. 1992;225(2):487–94.
48. Hagerman A, et al. Failure to elicit seroresponses to pneumococcal surface proteins (pneumococcal histidine triad D, pneumococcal choline-binding protein a, and serine proteinase precursor a) in children with pneumococcal bacteraemia. Clin Microbiol Infect. 2012;18(8):756–62.
49. Hagerman A, et al. Influence of age, social patterns and nasopharyngeal carriage on antibodies to three conserved pneumococcal surface proteins (PhtD, PcpA and PrtA) in healthy young children. Eur J Clin Microbiol Infect Dis. 2013;32(1):43–9.
50. Malley R, et al. CD4+ T cells mediate antibody-independent acquired immunity to pneumococcal colonization. Proc Natl Acad Sci U S A. 2005; 102(13):4848–53.
51. Mocanu G, et al. Curdlan microspheres. Synthesis, characterization and interaction with proteins (enzymes, vaccines). Int J Biol Macromol. 2009; 44(3):215–21.
52. Noske N, et al. Pneumococcal interaction with human dendritic cells: phagocytosis, survival, and induced adaptive immune response are manipulated by PavA. J Immunol. 2009;183(3):1952–63.
53. Malherbe L, et al. Vaccine adjuvants Alter TCR-based selection thresholds. Immunity. 2008;28(5):698–709.
54. Manso AS, et al. A random six-phase switch regulates pneumococcal virulence via global epigenetic changes. Nat Commun. 2014;5(5055).
55. Li J, et al. Epigenetic switch driven by DNA inversions dictates phase variation in Streptococcus pneumoniae. PLoS Pathog. 2016;12(7):e1005762.
56. Kadioglu A, Andrew PW. Susceptibility and resistance to pneumococcal disease in mice. Brief Funct Genomic Proteomic. 2005;4(3):241–7.

10

Efficacy and effectiveness of Ceftaroline Fosamil in patients with pneumonia

Giovanni Sotgiu[1], Stefano Aliberti[2,3*], Andrea Gramegna[2,3], Marco Mantero[2,3], Marta Di Pasquale[2,3], Federica Trogu[1], Laura Saderi[1] and Francesco Blasi[2,3]

Abstract

Background: Pneumonia is a relevant clinical and public health issue worldwide frequently associated with infections caused by Multi-Drug Resistant (MDR) pathogens. Ceftaroline fosamil is a promising new antibiotics with broad-spectrum bacterial activity. The aim of this systematic review and meta-analysis is to assess the efficacy and the effectiveness of ceftaroline fosamil in community-acquired (CAP), hospital-acquired (HAP), healthcare-associated (HCAP) and ventilator-associated (VAP) pneumonia.

Methods: A systematic review and meta-analysis was carried out retrieving both experimental and observational studies.

Results: A total of 2364 records was found and 14 manuscripts were finally considered eligible. The pooled efficacy/effectiveness was 81.2% (I^2: 1.2%) in all types of pneumonia. The pooled relative risk of clinical cure was 1.1 (I^2: 0.0%). The success rate was higher than 70% for infections caused by *S. pneumoniae* and *S. aureus*, including MDR pathogens.

Conclusions: Ceftaroline fosamil showed a high efficacy/effectiveness in patients with any type of pneumonia with a good safety profile.

Keywords: CAP, HAP, VAP, HCAP, MRSA, Stewardship, Safety

Background

Pneumonia is one of the major threats and leading cause of death due to infectious diseases worldwide, in both adults and children [1]. Mortality for community-acquired pneumonia (CAP) ranges from < 5% among outpatients up to 30% in those admitted in an intensive care unit [2]. Hospital-acquired pneumonia is the second most common nosocomial infection and the first in terms of mortality [3]. One of the major drivers of the high impact of pneumonia on patients' morbidity and mortality is represented by infections with multi-drug resistant (MDR) bacteria and, among them, methicillin resistant *Staphylococcus aureus* (MRSA) plays a relevant rule in both CAP and HAP [4].

Over the past two decades, antimicrobial resistance has become a tangible reality not only for patients with hospital-acquired (HAP), ventilator-associated (VAP) or healthcare-associated (HCAP) pneumonia but also for those coming from the community [5]. It has been recognized as a clinical and public health threat, which should be immediately addressed in order to avoid a dramatic back to a pre-antibiotic era. The clinical mismanagement of the antibiotics and the misuse in agriculture and in veterinary medicine are favoring the rapid increase of the rate of antibiotic resistant bacterial strains worldwide. The research and development activities of the pharmaceutical companies in the bacterial field have significantly decreased since the 1980s' for several reasons, including an increased prevalence of chronic diseases, the complex design of the clinical trials requested

* Correspondence: stefano.aliberti@unimi.it
[2]Department of Pathophysiology and Transplantation, University of Milan, Milan, Italy
[3]Internal Medicine Department, Respiratory Unit and Cystic Fibrosis Adult Center, Fondazione IRCCS Ca' Granda Ospedale Maggiore Policlinico, Milan, Italy
Full list of author information is available at the end of the article

by regulatory agencies, and the increasing antibiotic resistance rates.

One of the most promising antibiotics recently marketed is ceftaroline fosamil, a fifth-generation cephalosporin which proved a both in vitro and in vivo broad-spectrum activity against gram-positive (including methicillin susceptible and resistant *S. aureus* -MSSA and MRSA) and –negative bacteria. Ceftaroline fosamil showed clinical and bacteriological efficacy against bacterial pathogens responsible of CAP and skin infections [6]. Furthermore, during the pre-marketing studies, it showed a good safety and tolerability profile [7].

The aim of the present study was to perform a systematic review and meta-analysis to evaluate the efficacy and the effectiveness of ceftaroline fosamil in patients with any kind of pneumonia described in experimental and observational studies, respectively.

Methods

Search strategy

9pt?>Experimental and observational studies aimed to evaluate the efficacy/effectiveness of ceftaroline fosamil in adult hospitalized patients and outpatients with a diagnosis of pneumonia, including CAP, HAP, VAP, and HCAP, were selected. The search was conducted in three electronic databases: PubMed, Scopus, and Cochrane Central Register of Controlled Trials, without any time restrictions. Only publications written in English language were selected. Several key-words, combined using different strings according to the electronic database protocols, were used: "Ceftaroline", "Ceftaroline Fosamil", and "Respiratory Infections". To increase the search sensitivity, the list of references of the selected articles, as well as published systematic or narrative reviews, were manually and carefully assessed to include manuscripts not cited in the search record lists. Abstracts of the main pulmonology, infectious diseases, or microbiology conferences were not searched based on the poor information they could provide on the selection criteria and on the main clinical and bacteriological findings. Furthermore, non-peer-reviewed articles of the grey literature were not considered based on their poor clinical and methodological reliability.

Article selection

Only articles clearly describing the primary objective of this systematic review, i.e. efficacy/effectiveness of Ceftaroline fosamil in patients with pneumonia (CAP, HAP, VAP, and HCAP) were selected. At least one of the following efficacy/effectiveness-related outcomes were considered: 1) number of responders/number of subjects in group at day 4 after initiating therapy; 2) cure rate at the end of therapy (EOT); 3) cure rate at the test of cure (8–15 days after the end of therapy, TOC); 4) 14-day clinical success/cure (±1 day) from the diagnosis of pneumonia. The assessment of the outcomes and, then, the suitability of the article was carried out during the evaluation of the abstract or the full-text article if the information was not stated in the abstract. Studies were included if adult (≥18 years of age) patients, recruited in the ceftaroline fosamil or in the control arm, were at least 20.

The following exclusion criteria were adopted for the searched records: 1) papers written in languages other than English; 2) narrative or systematic reviews and meta-analyses; 3) abstracts presented in national and international conferences; 4) editorials, research letters, commentaries, correspondences; 5) case-reports or –series; 6) manuscripts focused only on efficacy/effectiveness of ceftaroline fosamil in infections other than respiratory.

Safety and tolerability profile of ceftaroline fosamil included only the collection of the adverse events.

Records were independently assessed by two researchers (LS and FT). They carefully evaluated titles and contents of the abstracts. In case of potential interesting articles, they retrieved and assessed the full-text. Inconsistencies during the first and second phase were solved by a third and senior reviewer (GS), who supervised the entire selection and review process.

Data extraction

Qualitative and quantitative data were extracted by the same reviewers (LS and FT) who selected the articles. Collection of the variables was decided during the preparation of the study protocol, as well as the implementation of an ad-hoc standardized form in an Excel format (Microsoft Office). Disparity during data collection was solved by a third reviewer (GS) by consensus. However, the final inter-rater agreement was approximately 100%. A random cross-check was carried out for ~ 20% of the selected citations.

The following variables were collected: response rate at day 4, response rate EOT, response rate TOC, 14-day clinical cure, publication year, epidemiological study design, country/ies where the study was carried out, study period, sample size (total, ceftaroline and control arm), age, gender, ethnic origin, severity of pneumonia, including the Pneumonia Severity Index (PSI) [2], lobar infiltration, pleural effusion, parenchymal or airway disease, previous episodes of pneumonia or bacteremia, previous exposure to antibiotics, asthma, etiology (i.e., *S. pneumoniae*, MSSA and MRSA), and adverse events. According to the Italian law on epidemiological studies based on anonymous and aggregated data, no ethical clearance was requested to the ethical committees of Milan and Sassari, Italy.

Study quality assessment

The systematic review and meta-analysis was carried out following the Preferred Reporting Items for Systematic

Reviews and Meta-Analyses (PRISMA) [8]. No significant inconsistencies and disparities were detected in the selection and data extraction phases. The agreement between LS and FT was higher than 97% and incongruences were solved by the intervention of GS.

Statistical analysis

A descriptive analysis of qualitative and quantitative variables was performed using proportions and central tendency/variability indicators (i.e., mean and standard deviation, SD), respectively. A meta-analysis was conducted for the efficacy/effectiveness-related outcomes. Forest plots were adopted to show the characteristics (i.e., between-study variability and sample size) of the single outcomes in comparison with the pooled estimates. Point and interval (95% confidence intervals, CI) estimates were used for studies' and pooled outcomes. The inconsistency (I^2) indicator was computed to show the variability across studies and was statistically tested with the chi-squared test for heterogeneity. Fixed or random-effects models were implemented according to the assumption that the true effect is or is not the same in all studies, respectively. Stratified analyses were conducted following the type of pneumonia (i.e., CAP, HAP, VAP, HCAP) or the etiology (i.e., *S. pneumoniae*, MSSA and MRSA). A two-tailed *p*-value less than 0.05 was considered statistically significant. The statistical software STATA version 14 (STATACorp LP, College Station, TX 77845, USA) was used to perform all statistical computations.

Results

Selection of the studies

The search of the three electronic databases found 2364 records (Fig. 1). After the removal of duplicates, 999 citations were screened and only 14 were considered suitable for a qualitative and quantitative analysis.

Characteristics of the selected studies

Six [9–14] (42.9%) studies were clinical trials, published in the time period 2010–2015, and 7 [15–21] (50.0%) were observational retrospective studies (6, 85.7%, cohort studies and 1, 14.3%, case-control study), published between 2014 and 2016 (Table 1). Only one [22] (7.1%) study was a retrospective analysis of previous clinical trials. In the majority of the cases (13/14, 92.9%), studies were carried out from 2007 to 2014 in USA; only the clinical trial of Zhong et al. [14] was conducted in five Asian countries. The efficacy/effectiveness of the

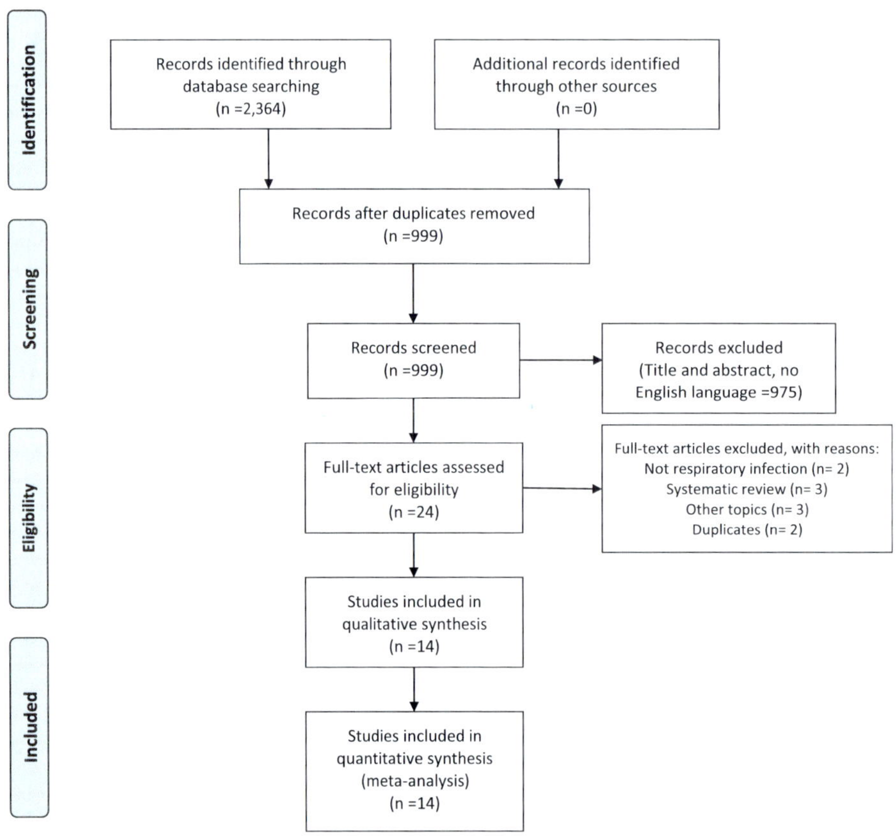

Fig. 1 Flow-chart of the systematic review

Table 1 Summary of the selected studies

First Author	Title	Publication year	Type of study	Country	Study period
Jandourek et al. [9]	Efficacy of ceftaroline fosamil for bacteremia associated with community-acquired bacterial pneumonia	2014	Clinical Trial	USA	Jul 2007-Dec 2008
File et al. [10]	FOCUS 1: a randomized, double-blinded, multicentre, Phase III trial of the efficacy and safety of ceftaroline fosamil versus ceftriaxone in community-acquired pneumonia	2011	Clinical Trial	USA	Jan 2008-Dec 2008
Low et al. [11]	FOCUS 2: a randomized, double-blinded, multicentre, Phase III trial of the efficacy and safety of ceftaroline fosamil versus ceftriaxone in community-acquired pneumonia	2011	Clinical Trial	USA	Jul 2007-Aug 2008
Shorr et al. [12]	Assessment of ceftaroline fosamil in the treatment of community-acquired bacterial pneumonia due to Streptococcus pneumoniae: insights from two randomized trials	2013	Clinical Trial	USA	Jul 2007-Dec 2008
File et al. [13]	Integrated analysis of FOCUS 1 and FOCUS 2: randomized, doubled-blinded, multicenter phase 3 trials of the efficacy and safety of ceftaroline fosamil versus. Ceftriaxone in patients with community-acquired pneumonia	2010	Clinical Trial	USA	Jul 2007-Dec 2008
Zhong et al. [14]	Ceftaroline fosamil versus ceftriaxone for the treatment of Asian patients with community-acquired pneumonia: a randomised, controlled, double-blind, phase 3, non-inferiority with nested superiority trial	2015	Clinical Trial	China, India, South Korea, Taiwan, Vietnam	Dec 2011-Apr 2013
Arshad et al. [15]	Ceftaroline fosamil for treatment of Methicillin-Resistant *Staphylococcus aureus* hospital-acquired pneumonia and health care-associated pneumonia. A 5-year matched case-control evaluation of epidemiology and outcomes	2016	Case-control study	USA	Jan 2009-May 2013
Eckburg et al. [22]	Day 4 Clinical response of ceftaroline fosamil versus ceftriaxone for community-acquired bacterial pneumonia	2012	Retrospective integrated analysis of FOCUS trials	USA	Jul 2007-Dec 2008
Guervil et al. [16]	Ceftaroline fosamil as first-line versus second-line treatment for acute bacterial skin and skin structure infections (ABSSSI) or community-acquired bacterial pneumonia (CABP)	2015	Retrospective Cohort study	USA	Aug 2011-Feb 2013
Udeani et al... [17]	Ceftaroline fosamil for the treatment of community-acquired bacterial pneumonia in elderly patients	2014	Retrospective Cohort study	USA	Aug 2011-Ap 2013
Ramani et al..... [18]	Contemporary use of ceftaroline fosamil for the treatment of community-acquired bacterial pneumonia: CAPTURE study experienc	2014	Retrospective Cohort study	USA	Aug 2011-Feb 2013
Vasquez et al... [19]	Ceftaroline Fosamil for the Treatment of Staphylococcus aureus Bacteremia Secondary to Acute Bacterial Skin and Skin Structure Infections or Community-Acquired Bacterial Pneumonia	2015	Retrospective Cohort study	USA	Aug 2011-Feb 2013

Table 1 Summary of the selected studies *(Continued)*

First Author	Title	Publication year	Type of study	Country	Study period
Casapao et al... [20]	Large retrospective study evaluation of the effectiveness and safety of Ceftaroline fosamil therapy	2014	Retrospective observational study	USA	Jan 2011-Jun 2013
Kaye et al. [21]	Ceftaroline fosamil for the treatment of hospital acquired pneumonia and ventilator associated pneumonia	2015	Retrospective Cohort study	USA	Sep 2013-Mar 2014

ceftaroline fosamil arm was compared with that of a control group in 8 (57.1%) studies [9–15, 22]; in the remaining 6 studies [16–21] no comparators were chosen. The dosage of ceftaroline fosamil was the same across all 14 studies [9–22] (i.e., 600 mg every 12 h). The ceftriaxone was the most frequently (7/8, 87.5%) prescribed antibiotic in controlled studies (Additional file 1: Table S1).

Characteristics of the enrolled cohort compared with a control group

The sample size of the studies with a control arm ranged from 45 to 1153 patients; in particular, the ceftaroline fosamil arm ranged from 23 to 580 patients, whereas the control arm sized from 22 to 573 (Table 2). The mean (SD) age of the ceftaroline and the control group was ~ 60 (15) years, ranging from 58.8 (16.1) to 66.1 (14.7) years and from 58.8 (16.4) to 65.8 (13.9) years, respectively. The proportion of males was higher than 60%, both in the ceftaroline and in the control arm, in all studies, with the only exception of that of Arshad et al. [15], where the percentage of males was ~ 50% in both treatment groups. Three (37.5%) studies [9, 12, 22] did not describe the ethnic origin of the cohort; 3 studies [10, 11, 15] showed a highest (> 80%) prevalence of white patients in both arms, whereas the studies of Zhong et al. [14] and Arshad et al. [15] had a high proportion of Asian and black patients, respectively.

The PSI was heterogeneous (Table 3); the majority of the patients were diagnosed as risk class III or IV. Only the study of Arshad et al. [15] did not provide a pneumonia severity classification. Half of the patients in the ceftaroline fosamil and control arm were diagnosed as PSI risk class III. However, the study of Jandourek et al. [9] recruited two third of the patients diagnosed as PSI risk class IV. A description of a multi-lobar infiltration, as well as of a pleural effusion, was performed by two (25.0%) studies [9, 12]. At least one chronic parenchymal or airway disease (including COPD, bronchiectasis, and interstitial fibrosis) affected a proportion of patients ranging from 20.0 to 33.2% per single arm. Asthma was described only by four (50.0%) studies [10, 11, 13, 14] and was found in less than 10% of the patients. Previous episodes of pneumonia were recorded in one fifth of the treatment group; however, this information was provided only by three (37.5%) studies [10, 11, 13]. Four (50.0%) studies [10–12, 22] found that 1/3–1/2 of the cohort was previously treated with antibiotics. The prevalence

Table 2 Demographics by treatment groups

Study	Sample size, n	Sample size, n		Mean (SD) age, y		Male, n (%)		Ethnic origin[a], n (%)	
		Ceftaroline group	Control group	Ceftaroline group	Control group	Ceftaroline group	Control group	Ceftaroline group	Control group
Jandourek et al...., *2014* [9]	45	23	22	60.6 (16.1)	63.2 (16.2)	15 (65.2)	17 (77.3)	–	–
File et al.., *2011* [10]	591	291	300	61.0 (16.6)	61.2 (16.4)	187 (64.3)	191 (63.7)	260 (89.3)	268 (83.3)
Low et al, *2011* [11]	562	289	273	60.6 (16.1)	62.0 (14.7)	175 (60.6)	175 (64.1)	278 (96.2)	264 (96.7)
Shorr et al..., *2013* [12]	139	69	70	63 (17)	62 (15)	43 (62.3)	47 (67.1)	–	–
File et al., *2010* [13]	1153	580	573	60.8 (16.4)	61.6 (15.6)	362 (62.4)	366 (63.9)	538 (92.8)	532 (92.8)
Zhong et al, *2015* [14]	763	381	382	66.1 (14.7)	65.8 (13.9)	265 (69.6)	272 (71.2)	381 (100.0) A	382 (100.0) A
Arshad et al...., *2016* [15]	149	40	109	58.8 (16.1)	58.8 (16.4)	20 (50.0)	54 (49.5)	16 (40.0) B	46 (42.2) B
Eckburg et al.., *2012* [22]	309	154	155	59.9 (17.7)	60.5 (16.0)	99 (64.3)	97 (62.6)	–	–

[a]Proportion of white patients, unless otherwise specified as black (B), or Asian (A)

Table 3 Clinical baseline characteristics by treatment groups

Study	Ceftaroline group	Control group	Ceftaroline group	Control group	Ceftaroline group	Control group	Ceftaroline group	Control group	Ceftaroline group	Control group
	PSI risk class III, n (%)		PSI risk class IV, n (%)		Severe CAP[a], n (%)		Multilobar infiltrate, n (%)		Pleural effusion, n (%)	
Jandourek et al.., *2014* [9]	5 (21.7)	5 (22.7)	18 (78.3)	15 (68.2)	–	–	5 (21.7)	5 (22.7)	5 (21.7)	5 (22.7)
File et al........, *2011* [10]	190 (65.3)	182 (60.7)	101 (34.7)	118 (39.3)	82 (28.2)	89 (29.7)	–	–	–	–
Low et al...., *2011* [11]	170 (58.8)	171 (62.6)	119 (41.2)	102 (37.4)	99 (34.3)	80 (29.3)	–	–	–	–
Shorr et al.........., *2013* [12]	34 (49.3)	37 (52.9)	35 (50.7)	33 (47.1)	22 (31.9)	32 (45.7)	18 (26.1)	21 (30.0)	15 (21.7)	13 (18.6)
File et al, *2010* [13]	360 (62.1)	353 (61.6)	220 (37.9)	220 (38.4)	–	–	–	–	–	–
Zhong et al.., *2015* [14]	255 (67.0)	265(69.4)	126 (33.1)	117 (30.6)	–	–	–	–	–	–
Arshad et al, *2016* [15]	–	–	–	–	–	–	–	–	–	–
Eckburg et al, *2012* [22]	84 (54.5)	82 (52.9)	61 (39.6)	61 (39.4)	–	–	–	–	–	–
	Structural lung disease[b], n (%)		Prior pneumonia, n (%)		Asthma, n (%)		Prior antimicrobial therapy, n (%)		Bacteremia, n (%)	
Jandourek et al, *2014* [9]	–	–	–	–	–	–	–	–	23 (100.0)	22 (100.0)
File et al, *2011* [10]	64 (22.0)	60 (20.0)	61 (21.0)	51 (17.0)	25 (8.6)	25 (8.3)	137 (47.1)	143 (47.7)	8 (2.7)	9 (3.0)
Low et al, *2011* [11]	96 (33.2)	87 (31.9)	62 (21.5)	41 (15.0)	24 (8.3)	13 (4.8)	100 (34.6)	117 (42.9)	15 (5.2)	11 (4.0)
Shorr et al, *2013* [12]	–	–	–	–	–	–	26 (37.7)	32 (45.7)	19 (27.5)	13 (18.6)
File et al, *2010* [13]	160 (27.6)	147 (25.7)	123 (21.2)	92 (16.1)	49 (8.4)	38 (6.6)	–	–	23 (4.0)	20 (3.5)
Zhong et al, *2015* [14]	120 (31.5)[c]	121 (31.7)[c]	–	–	21 (5.5)	22 (5.8)	80 (21.0)	85 (22.3)	3 (0.8)	5 (1.3)
Arshad et al, *2016* [15]	8 (20.0)	31 (28.4)	–	–	–	–	4 (11.8)	24 (23.3)	–	–
Eckburg et al, *2012* [22]	43 (27.9)	41 (26.5)	–	–	–	–	57 (37.0)	68 (43.9)	23 (14.9)	21 (13.5)
	Diabetes mellitus, n (%)									
Jandourek et al, *2014*	–	–								
File et al, *2011*	–	–								
Low et al, *2011*	–	–								
Shorr et al, *2013*	–	–								
File et al, *2010*	–	–								
Zhong et al, *2015*	62 (16.3)	62 (16.3)								
Arshad et al., *2016*	10 (25.0)	20 (18.4)								
Eckburg et al..., *2012*	–	–								

[a]Modified ATS severe CAP criteria include the presence of three or more of the following at baseline: respiratory rate ≥ 30 breaths/min; O2,90% or PaO2,60 mmHg; multilobar infiltrates; confusion/disorientation; blood urea nitrogen level ≥ 20 mg/dL; leucopenia (WBC count,4000 cells/mm3); thrombocytopenia (platelet count,100,000 cells/mm3); hypothermia (core temperature,368C); systolic blood pressure,90 mmHg; or diastolic blood pressure ≤ 60 mmHg. (*Niederman MS, Mandell LA, Anzuetto A et al........... Guidelines for the management of adults with community-acquired pneumonia: diagnosis, assessment of severity, antimicrobial therapy, and prevention. Am J Respir Crit Care Med 2001; 163: 1730–54*)
[b]Defined as any chronic parenchymal or airway disease [e.g. chronic obstructive pulmonary disease (emphysema, chronic bronchitis), bronchiectasis, or interstitial fibrosis]
[c]only COPD and chronic bronchitis

of bacteremia was very low (< 10%) per single arm in 4 (50.0%) studies [10, 11, 13, 14]. Only the study of Jandourek et al. [9] found a bacteremia prevalence of 100%.

Characteristics of the enrolled cohort without a control group

Six [16–21] out fourteen (42.9%) studies evaluated the efficacy/effectiveness of ceftaroline fosamil without a control arm. The sample size was heterogeneous, from 21 to 528 patients (Table 4). The mean (SD) age was high, ranging from 60 (18) to 64.3 (1.7) years. The proportion of males ranged from 48.3 to 57.5%.

Table 4 Demographic characteristics of subjects treated with only ceftaroline

Study	Sample size, n	Mean (SD) age, y	Male, n (%)
Guervil et al..., *2015* [16]	396	64.3 (1.7)	198 (50.0)
Udeani et al.., *2014* [17]	528	63.6 (20.2)	255 (48.3)
Ramani et al, *2014* [18]	398	63.5 (17.8)	199 (50.0)
Vasquez et al., *2015* [19]	21	60 (18)	11 (52.4)
Casapao et al..., *2014* [20]	92	–	–
Kaye et al, *2015* [21]	40	61.3 (16.8)	23 (57.5)

Table 5 Clinical characteristics of subjects treated with only ceftaroline

Study	Structural lung disease[a], n (%)	Congestive heart failure, n (%)	Prior pneumonia, n (%)	GERD, n (%)	Smoking, n (%)	Prior antimicrobial therapy, n (%)
Guervil et al, *2015* [16]	161 (40.7)	79 (20.0)	98 (24.8)	91 (23.0)	114 (28.8)	396 (100.0)
Udeani et al....., *2014* [17]	228 (43.2)	113 (21.4)	134 (25.4)	127 (24.1)	159 (30.1)	–
Ramani et al.., *2014* [18]	162 (40.7)	80 (20.1)	98 (24.6)	92 (23.1)	114 (28.6)	328 (82.4)
Vasquez et al..., *2015* [19]	–	–	–	–	–	18 (85.7)
Casapao et al......, *2014* [20]	–	–	–	–	–	–
Kaye et al., *2015* [21]	19 (47.5)	8 (0.20)	10 (25.0)	10 (25.0)	21 (52.5)	–

[a]Defined as any chronic parenchymal or airway disease [e.g. chronic obstructive pulmonary disease (emphysema, chronic bronchitis), bronchiectasis, or interstitial fibrosis]

The prevalence of patients with chronic parenchymal or airway diseases was significantly higher if compared with that found in the cohort of patients recruited in controlled studies (40.7–47.5%) (Table 5). Furthermore, in three out four studies (75%) [16–18] one fifth of those treated with ceftaroline fosamil suffered of congestive heart failure. However, the percentage of previous episodes of pneumonia was similar (range: 24.6–25.4%). Three (50.0%) studies [16, 18, 19] described previous antimicrobial exposure, which was higher than 82%.

Efficacy and effectiveness of ceftaroline fosamil

The overall efficacy/effectiveness of ceftaroline fosamil in all types of pneumonia (i.e., CAP, VAP, HCAP, HAP) cases was 81.2% (95% CI: 79.9–82.6; I^2: 1.2%) (Fig. 2). The pooled treatment success rate was equal to 81.3% (95% CI: 80.0–82.7; I^2: 7.7%) in patients with CAP, recruited in 12 (85.7%) studies (Fig. 3); a similar pooled clinical success (83.0%, 95% CI: 65.0–95.0; I^2: -) was found for patients with VAP, HCAP, and HAP, enrolled in 2 (14.3%) studies (Fig. 4).

In the 8 (57.1%) controlled studies [9–15, 22] the pooled relative risk of clinical cure was 1.1 (95% CI: 1.1–1.2; I^2: 0.0%) (Fig. 5).

The stratified analysis according to the microbiological diagnosis showed a high clinical and microbiological success: it was 82.6% (95% CI: 78.6–86.4; I^2: 0.0%) in patients with a lung infection caused by *S. pneumoniae,* 93.0% (95% CI: 77.0–100.0; I^2: 0.0%) in those with a MDR *S. pneumoniae* infection (Figs. 6 and 7). The cases of pneumonia caused by MSSA and MRSA showed a pooled success rate of 72.3% (95% CI: 64.5–79.4; I^2: 0.0%) and 71.7% (95% CI: 59.7–82.3; I^2: 67.9%), respectively (Figs. 8 and 9).

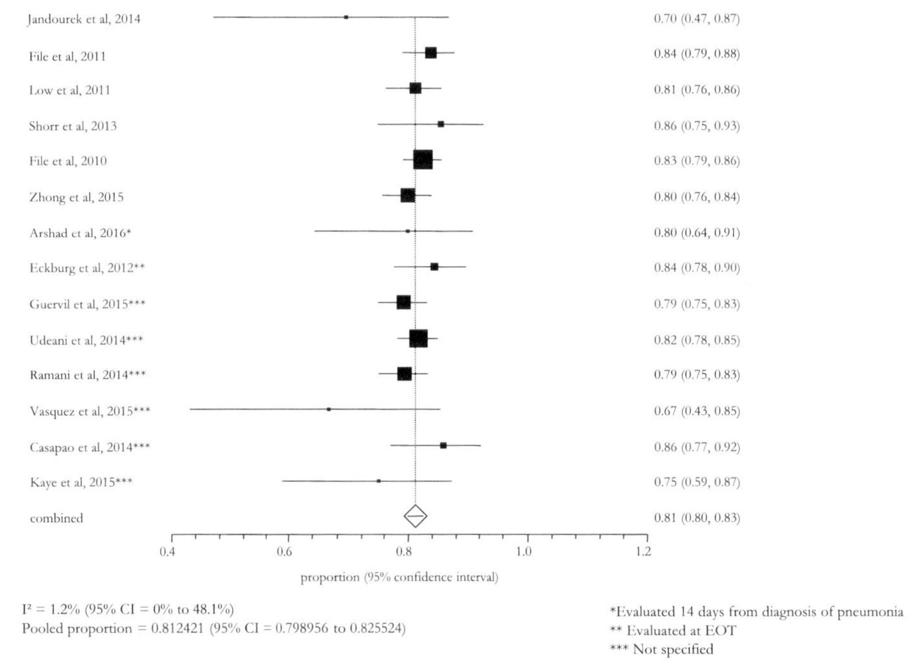

Fig. 2 Efficacy of ceftaroline in the overall pneumonia (including CAP, VAP, HCAP, HAP)

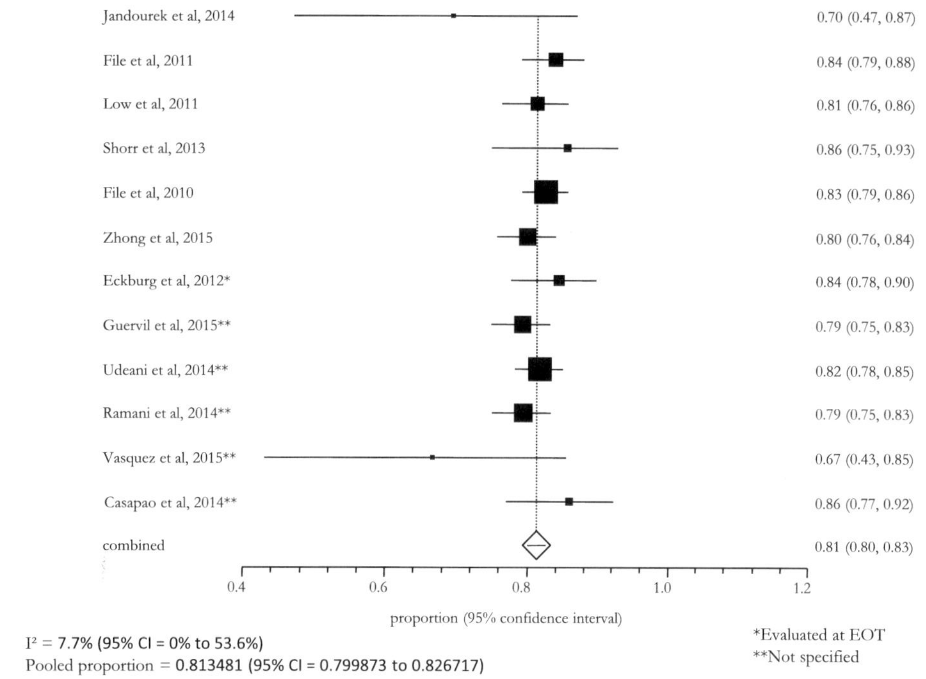

Fig. 3 Clinical success in CAP subjects treated with ceftaroline

Safety and tolerability of ceftaroline fosamil

Only 4 (28.6%) studies [10, 11, 13, 14] described the safety profile of the ceftaroline fosamil and control group: the percentage of adverse events ranged from 39.9 to 53.7% in the ceftaroline fosamil arm, whereas it ranged from 42.7 to 47.2% in the control arm (Table 6). The most frequently reported adverse events were: diarrhea, headache, insomnia, nausea, phlebitis, hypertension, and hypokalemia; however, their point prevalence was less than 5% in the ceftaroline fosamil group. Mortality rate in ceftaroline-treated arm is summarized in the Table 7.

Discussion

This systematic review and meta-analysis confirms the positive results on ceftaroline fosamil described in single observational and experimental studies. It pools observational findings from a real-world scenario as well as experimental results from the clinical trial world. The final message highlights the high efficacy

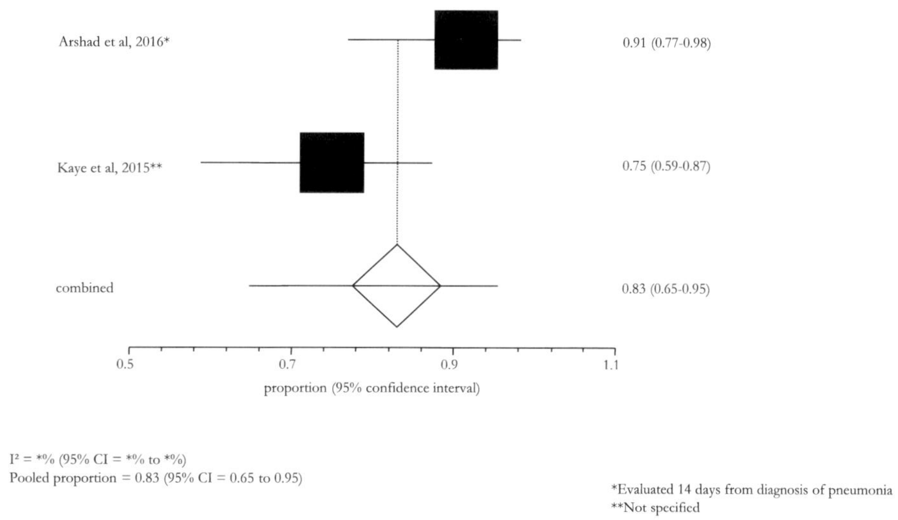

Fig. 4 Clinical success in HAP/VAP/HCAP subjects treated with ceftaroline

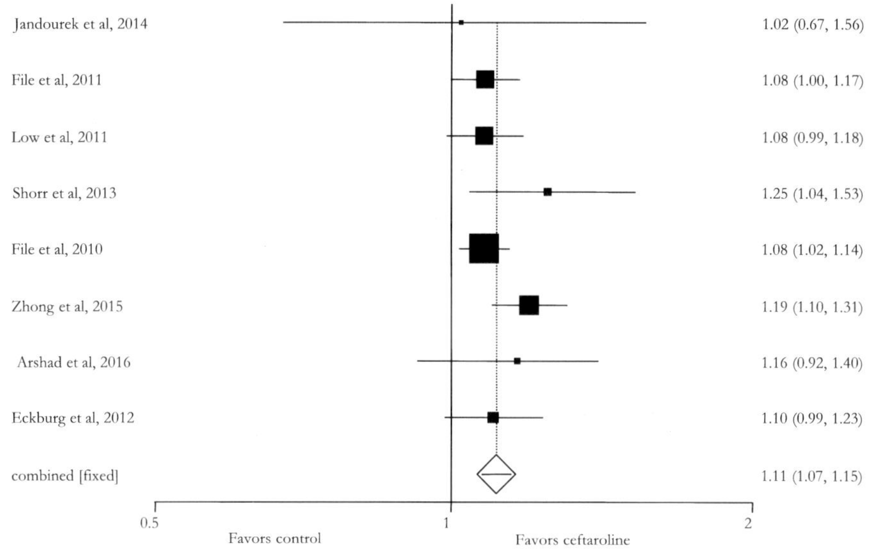

Fixed effects (Mantel-Haenszel, Rothman-Boice)
Pooled relative risk = 1.11 (95% CI = 1.07 to 1.15)
I^2 (inconsistency) = 0% (95% CI = 0% to 56.3%)

	Ceftaroline		Control			
Study	Total	Events	Total	Events	Relative risk (95% CI)	Weights, %
Jandourek et al, 2014	23	16	22	15	1.02 (0.67-1.56)	1.12
File et al, 2011	291	244	300	233	1.08 (1.00-1.17)	16.87
Low et al, 2011	289	235	273	206	1.08 (0.99-1.18)	15.60
Shorr et al, 2013	69	59	70	48	1.25 (1.04-1.53)	3.50
File et al, 2010	580	479	573	439	1.08 (1.02-1.14)	32.46
Zhong et al, 2015	381	305	382	256	1.19 (1.10-1.31)	18.79
Arshad et al, 2016	40	32	109	75	1.16 (0.92-1.40)	2.96
Eckburg et al, 2012	154	130	155	119	1.1 (0.99-1.23)	8.72

Fig. 5 Effect of ceftaroline on clinical cure

and effectiveness of ceftaroline fosamil in patients with different types of pneumonia, including CAP, HAP, VAP and HCAP, as well as its good safety and tolerability profile.

All the selected studies found a high pooled clinical success rate (> 80%) across all types of pneumonia, demonstrating poor variability between studies and between pneumonia types. However, the majority of the selected studies focused the attention on CAP and only two studies on pneumonias other than CAP [15, 21].

One of the most important findings is the high microbiological cure against drug-susceptible and –resistant *S. pneumoniae* strains. In the last two decades, it has been described the emergence and spread of MDR isolates, as well as the decreased vaccination coverage and the replacement of vaccine-related with other non-vaccine-related serotypes. The possibility of increasing the current antibiotic *armamentarium* with new effective and safe drugs can improve the prognosis of some patients.

More attention needs to be deserved to the MSSA and MRSA. The current therapeutic options (e.g., glycopeptides or linezolid) could be inappropriate or not available in some geographical settings. The high frequency of MRSA both in the hospital and in the community should be carefully monitored and adequate therapeutic options are necessary. Ceftaroline fosamil has demonstrated a high clinical cure rate (> 70%) in forms of pneumonia caused by MSSA and MRSA strains.

The broad-spectrum activity of ceftaroline fosamil against gram-positive and –negative bacteria could represent an added value in case of complicated polymicrobial infections, as well as in case of empirical therapy when the collection of respiratory specimens is negative or not feasible.

Several limitations of the present study can be detected: only experimental studies with positive and significant results on ceftaroline fosamil could have been published, representing a publication bias. Nevertheless,

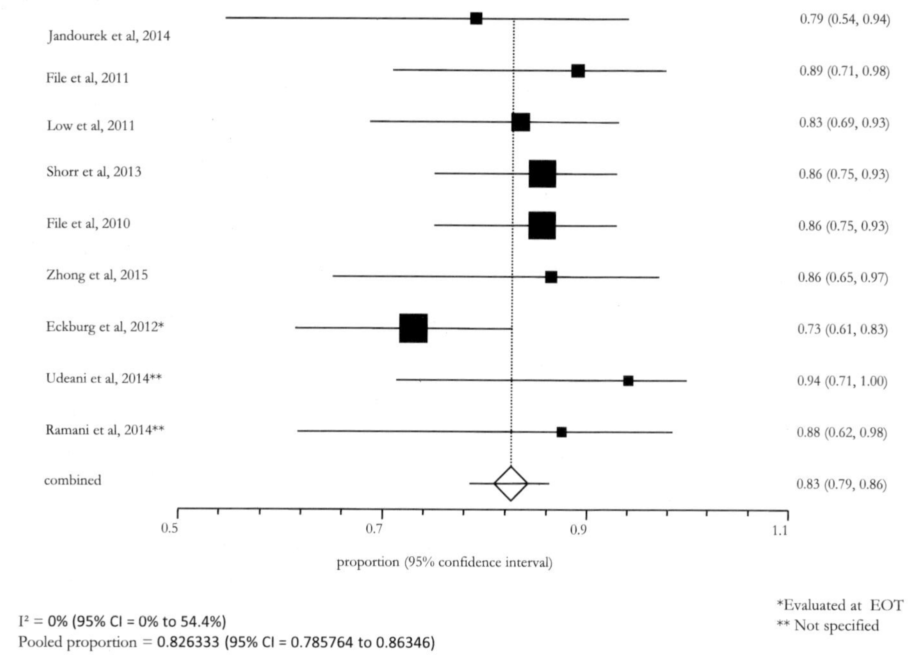

Fig. 6 Clinical and microbiological response rates in subjects with *Streptococcus pneumoniae* treated with ceftaroline

the confirmation of the experimental findings with observational and real-life results supports the reliability of the clinical and microbiological findings. The selection of non-controlled studies could reduce the statistical power of some findings and represent a methodological limitation; however, the necessity of recruiting real-life studies and the homogeneity of the results on the efficacy across the studies provide robustness to the inferential analysis. The geographical representation is partially jeopardized, with a highest prevalence of studies carried out in the USA. This could reduce the generalizability of the findings to some geographical areas (e.g., Africa, Europe), which could show differences in terms of microbial ecology (antibiotic resistance rates and different microbial burden) and of patients' characteristics. Yet, the scientific evidence provided by high-,

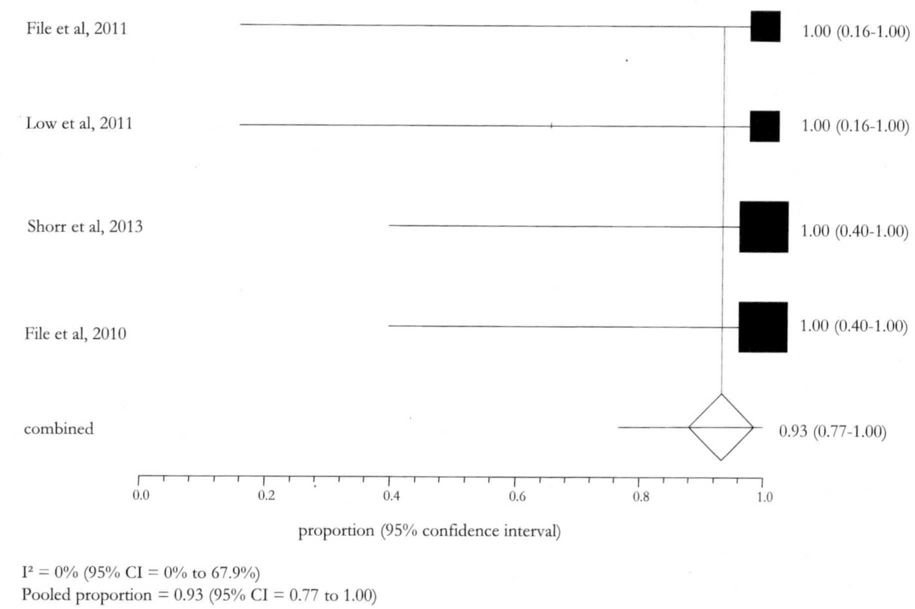

Fig. 7 Clinical cure rates in subjects with *MDR Streptococcus pneumoniae* treated with ceftaroline at TOC visit

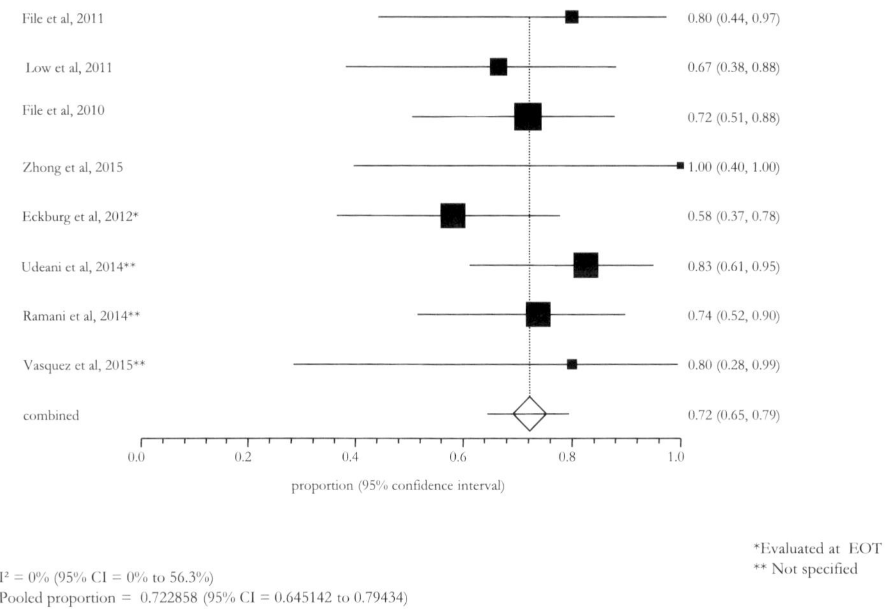

Fig. 8 Clinical and microbiological response rates in subjects with *MSSA* treated with ceftaroline

middle-, and low-income (Asian countries) settings could reduce this selection bias, as demonstrated by Aliberti et al. [4].

It was proved a clear confirmation of the efficacy and effectiveness of ceftaroline fosamil in patients with CAP but only a few studies (i.e., two) assessed its role in other pneumonia entities (e.g., HCAP), which can be caused by MDR bacteria in difficult-to-treat patients with severe clinical conditions and comorbidities. One of the main shortcomings of the published studies is the limited focus on the antibiotic safety. An individual patient data meta-analysis, with the involvement of all the authors of the published studies, could better analyze this critical point.

No studies have evaluated pharmacological interactions in randomized clinical trials with other antibiotics

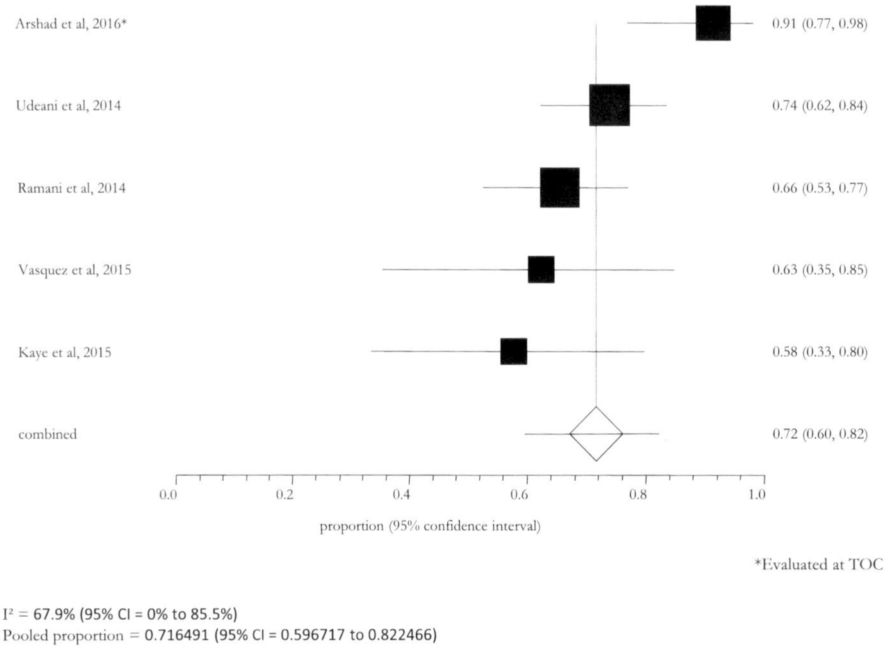

Fig. 9 Clinical and microbiological response rates in subjects with *MRSA* treated with ceftaroline

Table 6 Adverse events (safety population)

Study	Ceftaroline group	Control group	Ceftaroline group	Control group	Ceftaroline group	Control group	Ceftaroline group	Control group
	Any adverse events, n (%)		Diarrhea, n (%)		Headache, n (%)		Insomnia, n (%)	
File et al..........., *2011* [10]	119/298 (39.9)	136/308 (44.2)	14/298 (4.7)	7/308 (2.3)	10/298 (3.4)	4/308 (1.3)	9/298 (3.0)	6/308 (1.9)
Low et al., *2011* [11]	196/315 (53.7)	145/307 (47.2)	12/315 (3.8)	9/307 (2.9)	11/315 (3.5)	5/307 (1.6)	10/315 (3.2)	8/307 (2.6)
File et al, *2010* [13]	288/613 (47.0)	281/615 (45.7)	26/613 (4.2)	16/615 (2.6)	21 /613 (3.4)	9/615 (1.5)	19/613 (3.1)	14/615 (2.3)
Zhong et al..., *2015* [14]	172/381 (45.1)	163/383 (42.7)	24/381 (6.3)	13/383 (3.4)	6/381 (1.6)	9/383 (2.4)	–	–
	Nausea, n (%)		Phlebitis, n (%)		Hypertension, n (%)		Hypokalaemia, n (%)	
File et al, *2011* [10]	8/298 (2.7)	8/308 (2.6)	7/298 (2.3)	5/308 (1.6)	6/298 (2.0)	8/308 (2.6)	4/298 (1.3)	10/308 (3.2)
Low et al, *2011* [11]	6/315 (1.9)	6/307 (2.0)	10/315 (3.2)	8/307 (2.6)	8/315 (2.5)	8/307 (2.6)	10/315 (3.2)	5/307 (1.6)
File et al, *2010* [13]	14/613 (2.3)	14/615 (2.3)	17/613 (2.8)	13/615 (2.1)	14/613 (2.3)	16/615 (2.6)	14/613 (2.3)	15/615 (2.4)
Zhong et al, *2015* [14]	8/381 (2.1)	3/383 (0.8)	–	–	–	–	5/381 (1.3)	4/383 (1.1)

or drugs prescribed for chronic diseases. Furthermore, evidence should be provided for some at-risk patient categories, such as children, pregnant and breast-feeding women, elderly people. This systematic review selected clinical studies where a high proportion of patients with comorbidities was enrolled. However, more significant findings are needed, along with specific studies on the efficacy against other less incident bacterial pathogens.

In conclusion, this study provides a systematic collection and critical analysis of the present scientific evidence on ceftaroline fosamil. A few years after its distribution in the market, it has been shown its high efficacy and effectiveness, as well as its safety and tolerability. However, its effectiveness can be preserved in the near future if prescribed appropriately following antimicrobial stewardship policies and proved in vitro drug susceptibility in individual cases.

Table 7 Mortality rate in the ceftaroline and control groups

Study	Mortality rate, n (%)	
	Ceftaroline group	Control group
Jandourek et al, *2014*	–	–
File et al, *2011*	6/298 (2.0)	6/308 (1.9)
Low et al, *2011*	9/315 (2.9)	6/307 (2.0)
Shorr et al, *2013*	–	1/70 (1.4)
File et al, *2010*	15/613 (2.4)	12/615 (2.0)
Zhong et al, *2015*	3/381 (0.8)	4/383 (1.0)
Arshad et al, *2016 28-day mortality*	4/40 (10.0)[a]	16/109 (14.7)[a]
Eckburg et al, *2012*	–	–
Ramani et al, *2014*	8/398 (2.0)[b]	–
Casapao et al, *2014*	13/92 (14.1)[b]	–
Vasquez et al, *2015*	1/21 (4.8)	–
Guervil et al, *2015*	8/396 (2.0)[b]	–
Kaye et al, *2015*	5/40 (12.5)	–
Udeani et al, *2014*	15/528 (2.8)	–

[a]28-day mortality
[b] Hospital mortality

Authors' contributions

Conception and design: GS, SA. Performed research and paper revision: FT, LS. Analysis and Interpretation: GS, SA. Drafting the manuscript: GS, FT, LS. All authors participated in writing and revising the article prior to submission. All authors read and approved the final manuscript.

Competing interests

The authors declare that they have no competing interests.

Author details

[1]Clinical Epidemiology and Medical Statistics Unit, Department of Clinical and Experimental Medicine, University of Sassari, Sassari, Italy. [2]Department of Pathophysiology and Transplantation, University of Milan, Milan, Italy. [3]Internal Medicine Department, Respiratory Unit and Cystic Fibrosis Adult Center, Fondazione IRCCS Ca' Granda Ospedale Maggiore Policlinico, Milan, Italy.

References

1. Walker CL, Rudan I, Liu L, Nair H, Theodoratou E, Bhutta ZA, O'Brien KL, Campbell H, Black RE. Global burden of childhood pneumonia and diarrhoea. Lancet. 2013;381(9875):1405–16.
2. Fine MJ, Auble TE, Yealy DM, Hanusa BH, Weissfeld LA, Singer DE, Coley CM, Marrie TJ, Kapoor WN. A prediction rule to identify low-risk patients with community-acquired pneumonia. N Engl J Med. 1997;336(4):243–50.
3. Torres A, Ferrer M, Badia JR. Treatment guidelines and outcomes of hospital-acquired and ventilator-associated pneumonia. Clin Infect Dis. 2010; 51(Suppl 1):S48–53.
4. Aliberti S, Reyes LF, Faverio P, Sotgiu G, Dore S, Rodriguez AH, Soni NJ, Restrepo MI. GLIMP investigators. Global initiative for meticillin-resistant Staphylococcus aureus pneumonia (GLIMP): an international, observational cohort study. Lancet Infect Dis. 2016;16(12):1364–76.
5. Aliberti S, Cilloniz C, Chalmers JD, Zanaboni AM, Cosentini R, Tarsia P, Pesci A, Blasi F, Torres A. Multidrug-resistant pathogens in hospitalised patients coming from the community with pneumonia: a European perspective. Thorax. 2013;68(11):997–9.
6. El Hajj MS, Turgeon RD, Wilby KJ. Ceftaroline fosamil for community-acquired pneumonia and skin and skin structure infections: a systematic review. Int J Clin Pharm. 2017;39(1):26–32.
7. File TM Jr, Wilcox MH, Stein GE. Summary of ceftaroline fosamil clinical trial studies and clinical safety. Clin Infect Dis. 2012;55(Suppl 3):S173–80.

8. Moher D, Liberati A, Tetzlaff J, Altman DG. The PRISMA Group. Preferred Reporting Items for Systematic Reviews and Meta-Analyses: The PRISMA Statement. PLoS Med. 2009;6(6):e1000097.
9. Jandourek A, Smith A, Llorens L, Thye DA, Eckburg PB, Friedland HD. Efficacy of ceftaroline fosamil for bacteremia associated with community-acquired bacterial pneumonia. Hosp Pract. 2014;42(1):75–8.
10. File TM Jr, Low DE, Eckburg PB, Talbot GH, Friedland HD, Lee J, Llorens L, Critchley IA, Thye DA. FOCUS 1 investigators. FOCUS 1: a randomized, double-blinded, multicentre, Phase III trial of the efficacy and safety of ceftaroline fosamil versus ceftriaxone in community-acquired pneumonia. J Antimicrob Chemother. 2011;66(Suppl 3):iii19–32.
11. Low DE, File TM Jr, Eckburg PB, Talbot GH, David Friedland H, Lee J, Llorens L, Critchley IA, Thye DA. FOCUS 2 investigators. FOCUS 2: a randomized, double-blinded, multicentre, Phase III trial of the efficacy and safety of ceftaroline fosamil versus ceftriaxone in community-acquired pneumonia. J Antimicrob Chemother. 2011;66(Suppl 3):iii33–44.
12. Shorr AF, Kollef M, Eckburg PB, Llorens L, Friedland HD. Assessment of ceftaroline fosamil in the treatment of community-acquired bacterial pneumonia due to Streptococcus pneumoniae: insights from two randomized trials. Diagn Microbiol Infect Dis. 2013;75(3):298–303.
13. File TM Jr, Low DE, Eckburg PB, Talbot GH, Friedland HD, Lee J, Llorens L, Critchley I, Thye D. Integrated analysis of FOCUS 1 and FOCUS 2: randomized, doubled-blinded, multicenter phase 3 trials of the efficacy and safety of ceftaroline fosamil versus ceftriaxone in patients with community-acquired pneumonia. Clin Infect Dis. 2010; 51(12):1395–405.
14. Zhong NS, Sun T, Zhuo C, D'Souza G, Lee SH, Lan NH, Chiang CH, Wilson D, Sun F, Iaconis J, Melnick D. Ceftaroline fosamil versus ceftriaxone for the treatment of Asian patients with community-acquired pneumonia: a randomised, controlled, double-blind, phase 3, non-inferiority with nested superiority trial. Lancet Infect Dis. 2015;15(2):161–71.
15. Arshad S, Hartman P, Perri MB, Moreno D, Zervos MJ. Ceftaroline Fosamil for treatment of methicillin-resistant Staphylococcus aureus hospital-acquired pneumonia and health care–associated pneumonia: a 5-year matched case-control evaluation of epidemiology and outcomes. Infect Dis Clin Pract. 2016; 24(2):87–91.
16. Guervil DJ, Kaye KS, Hassoun A, Cole P, Huang XY, Friedland HD. Ceftaroline fosamil as first-line versus second-line treatment for acute bacterial skin and skin structure infections (ABSSSI) or community-acquired bacterial pneumonia (CABP). J Chemother. 2016;28(3):180–6.
17. Udeani G, Evans J, Cole P, Friedland HD. Ceftaroline fosamil for the treatment of community-acquired bacterial pneumonia in elderly patients. Hosp Pract. 2014;42(3):109–15.
18. Ramani A, Udeani G, Evans J, Jandourek A, Cole P, Smith A, David FH. Contemporary use of ceftaroline fosamil for the treatment of community-acquired bacterial pneumonia: CAPTURE study experience. J Chemother. 2014;26(4):229–34.
19. Vazquez JA, Maggiore CR, Cole P, Smith A, Jandourek A, Friedland HD. Ceftaroline Fosamil for the treatment of Staphylococcus aureus bacteremia secondary to acute bacterial skin and skin structure infections or community-acquired bacterial pneumonia. Infect Dis Clin Pract. 2015;23(1):39–43.
20. Casapao AM, Davis SL, Barr VO, Klinker KP, Goff DA, Barber KE, Kaye KS, Mynatt RP, Molloy LM, Pogue JM, Rybak MJ. Large retrospective evaluation of the effectiveness and safety of ceftaroline fosamil therapy. Antimicrob Agents Chemother. 2014;58(5):2541–6.
21. Kaye KS, Udeani G, Cole P, Friedland HD. Ceftaroline fosamil for the treatment of hospital-acquired pneumonia and ventilator-associated pneumonia. Hosp Pract. 2015;43(3):144–9.
22. Eckburg PB, Friedland HD, Llorens L, Smith A, Witherell GW, Laudano JB, Thye D. Day 4 clinical response of Ceftaroline Fosamil versus ceftriaxone for community-acquired bacterial pneumonia. Infect Dis Clin Pract. 2012;20(4): 254–60.

Measurements

DNA methylation levels in whole blood were determined with the Illumina Infinium Human Methylation 450 K array. After quality control, the final dataset contained DNA methylation data presented as beta values for 420,938 CpG probes [18] (See supplementary methods for sample processing and quality control).

Statistical analyses

Epigenome-wide association analysis (EWAS) in whole blood We assessed the association between pack years in current smokers and epigenome-wide DNA methylation in whole blood. We performed robust linear regression using the *MASS* package in R and adjusted the model for the potential confounders age and gender. To adjust for technical variation, principal components were calculated using the 220 control probes incorporated in the Illumina 450 K chip. The principal components that explain >1% of the technical variation ($N = 7$) were included in the analysis. To adjust for the cellular heterogeneity of the whole blood samples, we included proportional white blood cell counts of mononuclear cells, lymphocytes, neutrophils and eosinophils obtained by standard laboratory techniques.

Mediation analysis To assess if the CpG-sites identified in the EWA study were also associated with lung function levels, we performed mediation analysis using the R-package *Mediation* [19]. For every individual CpG-site, the Average Causal Mediation Effect (ACME), Average Direct Effect (ADE), Total Effect and Proportion Mediated was calculated. When the p-value of ACME was below 0.05 for a particular CpG-site (tested 2-sided), this CpG-site was considered to be significantly associated with lung function levels.

Study II: Validation study in lung tissue

Study population

DNA methylation in lung tissue was studied in patients undergoing lung resection, lung volume reduction or transplant surgery in the University Medical Center Groningen as previously described [20]. If resection surgery was conducted for tumor removal, macroscopically normal lung tissue was taken far distant form the tumor. All samples were histologically checked for abnormalities using standard haematoxylin and eosin staining. To reach a power of 90% with an alpha of 5%, we selected a total of 47 subjects, being 16 never smokers, 15 ex-smokers and 16 current smokers. The power analysis can be found in the online supplement. All ex- and current smokers had a smoking history of >5 pack years and all ex-smokers quitted smoking for at least 1 year.

We studied gene expression in 36 of the 47 selected subjects included in our lung tissue validation study [20].

Measurements

DNA methylation in lung tissue DNA methylation in lung tissue was determined with the PyroMark Q48 Autoprep System. Quality of the pyrosequencing was assessed for every CpG-site in all the subjects individually and the subject was excluded for a particular CpG-site if the default software quality control was not passed. Primers for cg01940273 did not match with the original sequence and cg01940273 was excluded from the validation study. Primer sequences are shown in the online supplement.

Gene expression in lung tissue Total RNA was extracted from lung tissue at Rosetta Inpharmatics Gene Expression Laboratory (Seattle, WA, USA). mRNA profiling was performed using a custom-made Affymetrix HU133 array (GPL 10379) containing 751 controls probe sets and 51,627 non-control probe sets. Gene expression was normalized with the Robust Multichip Average method implemented in the Affymetrix Power Tools software [20].

Statistical analysis

DNA methylation in lung tissue The association between smoking status and DNA methylation in lung tissue was studied using linear regression analysis using R. The analyses were adjusted for the potential confounders age and gender.

Expression quantitative trait methylation (eQTM) analysis in lung tissue For the CpG-sites that were differentially methylated in lung tissue, we tested the association between DNA methylation levels and gene expression, i.e. expression quantitative trait methylation (eQTM) analysis. Per CpG-site, all the gene expression probe sets within 1 MB on either side were selected. An association was considered significant when the p-value was lower than the Bonferroni adjusted p-value (=0.05 / the number of probe sets within a 2 MB window of the indicated CpG-site).

Results

Study I: Epigenome-wide association study (EWAS) in whole blood

Study population

Population characteristics are shown in Table 1. Notably, the study population was non-random, i.e. selected based on the presence or absence of airway obstruction.

Epigenome-wide association analysis (EWAS) in whole blood

The EWAS in whole blood identified 15 CpG-sites that were significantly (Bonferroni corrected p-value $< 0.05/420938 = 1.19 \times 10^{\wedge -7}$) associated with pack years (Fig. 2). Higher number of pack years was associated with lower levels of DNA methylation in 13 of the 15 identified CpG-sites (see Table 2). We identified two novel CpG-sites, cg22994830

Table 1 Population characteristics

	LifeLines Cohort
Number	658
Males, N (%)	375 (57,0)
Age, years (range)	46 (22–79)
Pack year, years, mean (range)	20,6 (5–100)
FEV_1/FVC (%), mean (range)	71,7 (40,1 - 92,4)
FEV_1(%pred)*, mean (range)	94,4 (47,7 - 138,4)
COPD cases, N (%)	279 (42,4)
GOLD COPD Stage ≥ 2†, N (%)	102 (15,6)

* Calculated with GLI-2012 if possible
† COPD GOLD stage > 2 (FEV_1/FVC < 70% and FEV_1 between 50 and 80% of predicted)
COPD, Chronic Obstructive Pulmonary Disease; FEV_1, Forced Expiratory Volume in 1 s; FVC, Forced Vital Capacity

annotated to Protein Kinase CAMP-Dependent Type 1 Regulatory Subunit Beta *(PRKAR1B)* and cg20451986 located in the intergenic region of *11q25* between the genes *loc100126239* and Junctional Adhesion Molecule 3 (*JAM3*). As indicated in Table 2, we identified several CpG-sites to be related to pack years, that were described in earlier studies in association with smoking status [12, 21–24]. An overview of all significant CpG sites at nominal p-value < 0.05 can be obtained upon request by the corresponding author.

Mediation analysis
The mediation analysis revealed that 10 CpG-sites were significantly associated with lung function levels (Additional file 2).

Study II: Validation study in lung tissue
Study population
We validated DNA methylation levels in lung tissue of 47 subjects, divided into 3 equal groups based on smoking status (see Additional file 3 for subject characteristics).

DNA methylation in lung tissue
Figure 3 shows that the current smokers had significant lower DNA methylation levels at 4 out of the 9 CpG sites than never smokers (Bonferroni corrected p-value of 0.05/9=0.00556). For cg21566642, the DNA methylation levels were significantly different between current and never smokers at a nominal p-value of 0.05. An overview of the complete analysis can be found in the online supplement (Additional file 4).

Expression quantitative trait methylation (eQTM) analysis in lung tissue
DNA methylation at cg05575921 and cg21161138 (the two CpG-sites annotated to *AHRR)* was significantly associated with gene expression levels of *AHRR* in lung tissue (Fig. 4a and c). As indicated in Fig. 4b and d, current smokers showed lower DNA methylation levels together with higher expression levels compared to ex- and never smokers. For the other 3 differentially methylated CpG-sites in lung tissue, we found novel significant associations with gene expression levels. DNA methylation levels at cg05951221 and cg21566642, located in the intergenic region on chromosome 2, were associated with gene expression levels of the genes Autophagy Related 16 Like1 (*ATG16L1*) and DIS3 Like 3′-5′Exoribonuclease (*DIS3L2*) (Fig. 5a-d). DNA methylation levels at cg06126421, located in the intergenic region on chromosome 6, were associated with gene expression levels of the genes Mucin 21 (*MUC21*) and Tubulin Beta Class I (*TUBB*) (Fig. 5e-f). A complete overview of the eQTM analysis can be found in Additional file 5.

Discussion
In this study, we showed that DNA methylation at 15 CpG-sites was significantly associated with pack years. Next to previously described CpG-sites, we identified 2 novel CpG-sites: cg22994830, annotated to *PRKAR1B*,

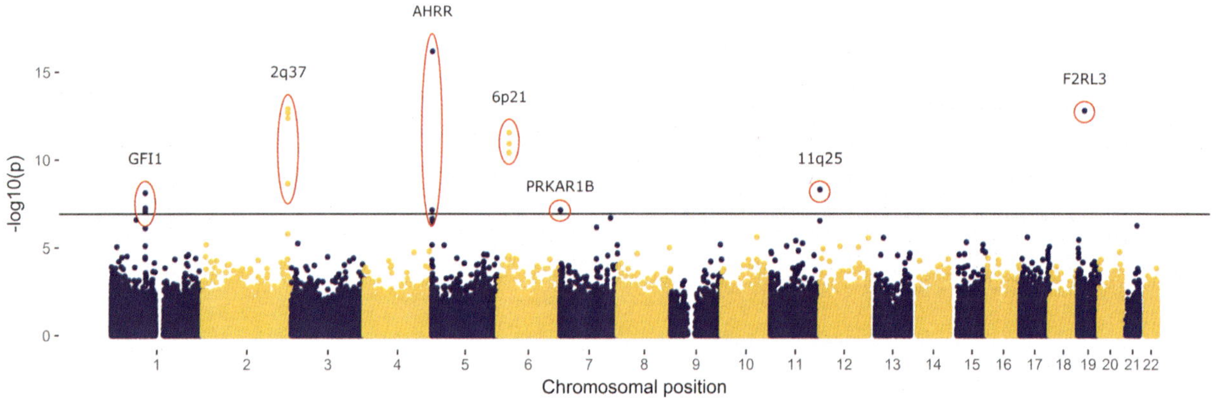

Fig. 2 *Manhattan plot of the EWAS on pack years in current smokers.* Every dot represents an individual CpG-site. Location on the X-axis indicates the chromosomal position and location on the Y-axis indicates the inversed log [10] p-value. Horizontal line indicates genome wide significance ($p < 1.19 \times 10^{-7}$)

Table 2 Genome-wide significant results of EWAS in whole blood

CpG-site	B	SE	*P*-value	Adj. *P*-value	Gene annotation	Gene function[#]
cg05575921*	– 0.00360	0.00043	6.80E-17	2.86E-11	AHRR	Repressor of AHR, important in dioxin toxicity and involved in regulation of cell growth and differentiation
cg21566642*	– 0.00176	0.00024	1.21E-13	5.09E-08	*NA*	*NA*
cg03636183*	– 0.00211	0.00029	1.55E-13	6.53E-08	F2RL3	Plays a role in platelet activation and hypomethylation may be associated with human lung cancer
cg05951221*	– 0.00130	0.00018	2.01E-13	8.48E-08	*NA*	*NA*
cg01940273*	– 0.00143	0.00020	4.20E-13	1.77E-07	*NA*	*NA*
cg06126421*	– 0.00230	0.00033	2.75E-12	1.16E-06	*NA*	*NA*
cg15342087*	– 0.00092	0.00014	1.23E-11	5.19E-06	*NA*	*NA*
cg24859433*	– 0.00089	0.00014	3.91E-11	1.65E-05	*NA*	*NA*
cg27241845*	– 0.00110	0.00018	2.21E-09	9.30E-04	*NA*	*NA*
cg20451986	0.00104	0.00018	4.85E-09	2.04E-03	*NA*	*NA*
cg12876356*	– 0.00244	0.00042	7.55E-09	3.18E-03	GFI1	Transcription repressor essential for hematopoiesis
cg09935388*	– 0.00218	0.00040	5.42E-08	2.28E-02	GFI1	Transcription repressor essential for hematopoiesis
cg21161138*	– 0.00106	0.00020	7.10E-08	2.99E-02	AHRR	Repressor of AHR, important in dioxin toxicity and involved in regulation of cell growth and differentiation
cg22994830	0.00102	0.00019	7.17E-08	3.02E-02	PRKAR1B	Involved in cAMP signaling in cells
cg18146737*	– 0.00256	0.00048	8.19E-08	3.45E-02	GFI1	Transcription repressor essential for hematopoiesis

*Associated with smoking status in previous studies
[#]Gene function obtained by www.genecards.org

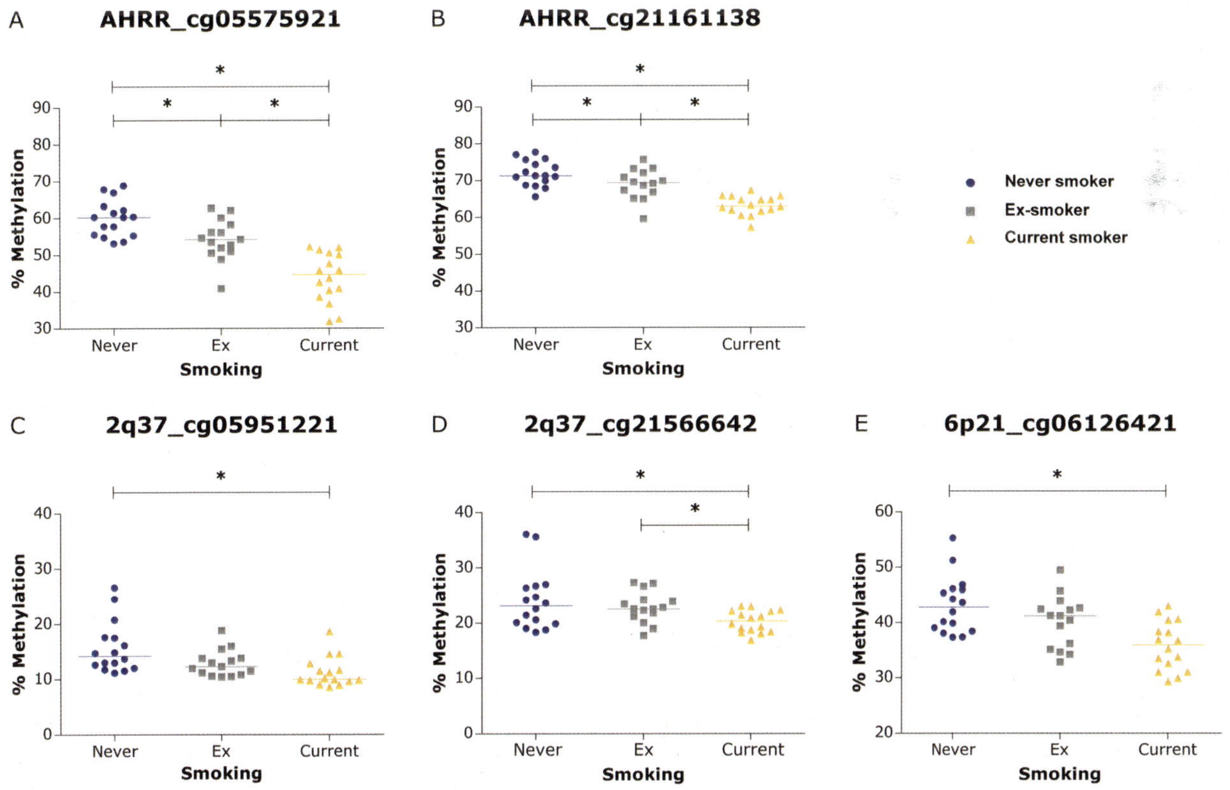

Fig. 3 *DNA methylation levels in lung tissue.* CpG-sites that differ in DNA methylation levels between never smokers (blue circles), ex-smokers (gray squares) and current smokers (yellow triangles) are shown

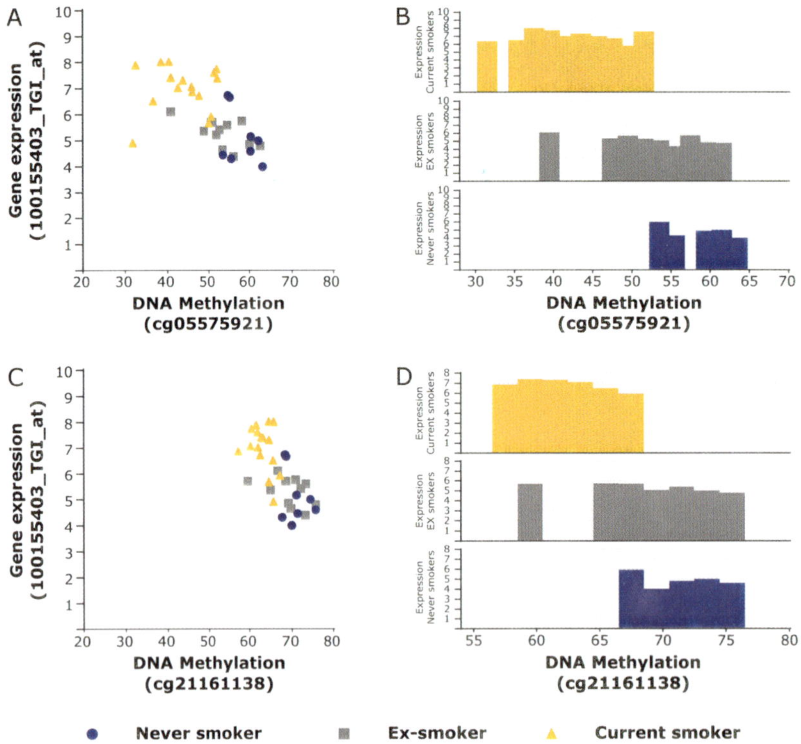

Fig. 4 *Association between DNA methylation levels and gene expression of AHRR in lung tissue.* **a** and **c**) DNA methylation levels are presented on the X-axis and the normalized gene expression levels are shown on the Y-axis. Blue circles = never smokers, gray squares = ex-smokers and yellow triangles = current smoker. **b** and **d**) DNA methylation levels are presented on the X-axis and the average of the normalized gene expression levels distributed per 2% DNA methylation are shown on the Y-axis. The upper part with yellow bars represents current smokers, the middle part with gray bars represents ex-smokers and the lower part with blue bars represent never smokers

and cg20451986, located in the intergenic region of chromosome 11. 10 CpG-sites were additionally associated with lung function levels and we validated 5 of these CpG-sites in lung tissue. We found several significant associations between DNA methylation and gene expression in lung tissue. Moreover, we found novel associations for the CpG-sites located in the intergenic regions of chromosome 2 and 6 and biological plausible genes in lung tissue.

In our EWA study, we identified 2 novel CpG-sites associated with pack years. One of them, cg22994830, is located in the body of *PRKAR1B*. As a regulatory subunit of cyclic AMP-dependent protein kinase A, this gene is involved in several cellular events including ion transport, metabolism and transcription. *PRKAR1B* has shown to be implicated in neurodegenerative disorders, however, a role for *PRKAR1B* in pulmonary diseases is currently unknown [25]. The other novel CpG-site cg20451986 has not been annotated to a gene yet. The gene that is closest to this CpG-site, at approximately 10,000 base pairs, is *JAM3*, a gene involved in cell-cell adhesion. While we performed an EWA study on the association between DNA methylation and pack years as a cumulative measurement of exposure to cigarette smoke, as reviewed by *Gao* et al, earlier studies investigated differences in DNA methylation levels between never and current smokers [22]. Nevertheless, we identified several CpG-sites that have been described before. Our third most significant CpG-site cg03636183 located in the gene *F2RL3*, was one of the first sites that was found to be associated with smoking status [23]. In addition, a study by *Zeilinger* et al showed associations of CpG-sites located in the genes *AHRR, GFI1, F2RL3* and the unknown intergenic regions at chromosome 2 and 6 with smoking status [12]. Nine of our identified CpG-sites were identical to the CpG-sites discovered by Zeilinger's study.

A major strength of our study is that we validated our findings in lung tissue, the actual tissue of interest. This is in contrast to previous studies in which the most significant CpG-sites from the EWAS were validated by replication in whole blood of other populations [12, 13, 23]. In our study, DNA methylation at one of the CpG-sites located in the body of *AHRR*, cg21161138, was significantly lower in current smokers compared to never smokers in lung tissue, in line with previous findings by *Shenker* et al [24]. In addition, the association

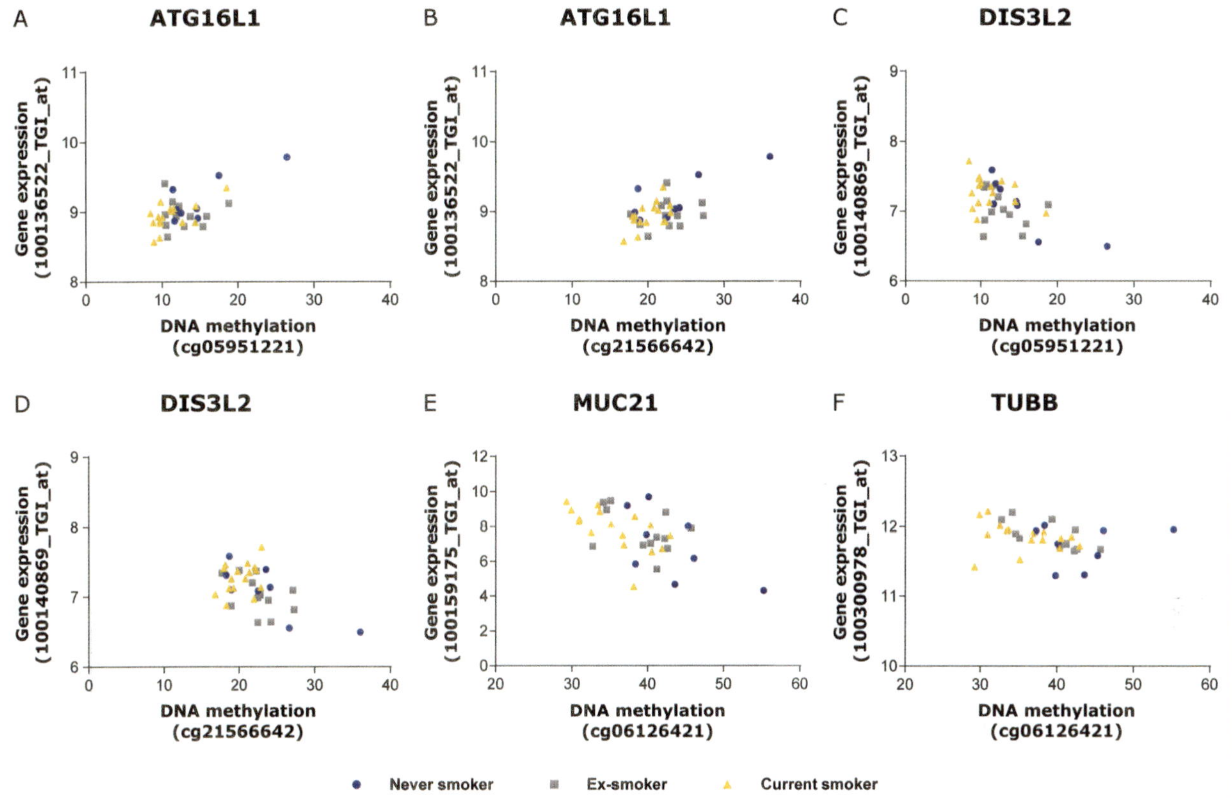

Fig. 5 *eQTM analysis for CpG-sites at the intergenic regions on chromosome 2 and 6.* DNA methylation levels are presented on the X-axis en the normalized gene expression levels are shown on the Y-axis. Blue circles = never smokers, gray squares = ex-smokers and yellow triangles = current smokers

between DNA methylation of cg21161138 and lower gene expression of *AHRR* in lung tissue also confirms findings of that earlier study. However, we were able to validate 4 additional CpG-sites in lung tissue. The fact that we could confirm a total of 5 CpG-sites, identified in whole blood, in lung tissue suggests that changes in DNA methylation in response to cigarette smoking directly occur at the local level in the lung. For cg03636183 located in the body of *F2RL3,* we neither found differences upon smoking in lung tissue nor an association between DNA methylation levels and gene expression. Since the intensities of the nucleotide peaks in the pyrosequence run of cg03636183 were low compared to other assays, despite the use of several different primers sets, we cannot exclude that actual differences in DNA methylation in lung tissue are masked by technical issues.

Several cross-sectional studies strongly suggest that DNA methylation in whole blood can be partially normalized upon smoking cessation [21, 26, 27]. In our study, we found that DNA methylation levels of ex-smokers are between the levels of never and current smokers for the 5 CpG-sites that are differentially methylated upon smoking. Moreover, with the eQTM analysis, we showed that for *AHRR* both DNA methylation and gene expression levels of ex-smokers tends more towards the levels observed for never smokers compared to current smokers. Even though this is cross-sectional data, it implies a reversible character of DNA methylation.

After identification and validation of CpG-sites that are associated with exposure to cigarette smoke in lung tissue, an important next step is to assess the functional relevance of the CpG-sites. For *AHRR,* the function is well studied. Briefly, *AHRR* inhibits the aryl hydrocarbon receptor pathway, which is involved in the removal of harmful environmental chemicals, including cigarette smoke. Cigarette smoking results in decreased DNA methylation and this decreased DNA methylation subsequently increases the expression of *AHRR.* This leads to reduced removal of harmful compounds and thereby thus potentially increasing the damage caused by these compounds [28]. In contrast, the other 3 CpG-sites that are different with smoking status in lung tissue have not yet been annotated to a gene, making it impossible to assess the potential function of DNA methylation at these sites. By performing an eQTM analysis, we tried to identify the genes that are regulated by these CpG-sites. For the 2 CpG-sites at chromosome 2, we found associations with gene expression of *ATG16L1* and *DIS3L2*. *ATG16L1* is an essential component of the autophagy pathway and mutations in this gene have been associated with inflammatory bowel disease. Since proper function of *ATG16L1* is necessary for host-defense responses against micro-organisms and inflammatory responses in Crohn's disease, this gene might be relevant in the respiratory system as well [29]. *DIS3L2* belongs to the family of exo-ribonucleases, key enzymes involved in the control of messenger RNA stability. *DIS3L2* has been associated with human diseases such as Perlman syndrome and Wilm's tumor, but a role in pulmonary diseases has not been described [30]. For cg06126421 located at the intergenic region of chromosome 6, we found an association between DNA methylation levels and the expression of the genes *TUBB* and *MUC21*. *TUBB* encodes a beta tubulin protein of the microtubule cytoskeleton and has shown to be involved in microcephaly with structural brain abnormalities in humans. A role for *TUBB* in lung-related pathologies, however, is currently unknown [31]. *MUC21* belongs to group of 22 mucin proteins, the major glycoprotein components of mucus, which forms the protective layer of the epithelial surface. Since overproduction of mucins is associated with common respiratory diseases including COPD, asthma and cystic fibrosis [32], *MUC21* is a biological plausible gene and further investigations into the inverse association between DNA methylation at cg06126421 and the expression of *MUC21* are warranted.

While our study is one of the first studies to validate a large panel of CpG-sites in actual lung tissue, we have to consider some limitations of our study. First, the results of the mediation analysis should be interpreted with caution. In our study, we used mediation analysis to select CpG-sites that were associated with lung function levels rather than implying biological mediation. We used pack years as cumulative measurement of the exposure to cigarette smoke to assess the association between cigarette smoking and DNA methylation. However, the number of pack years is estimated from self-reported information obtained from questionnaires of the LifeLines population-based cohort study. It has been suggested that self-reported estimations of smoking may underestimate the true smoking prevalence, since cigarette smoking is often interpreted as socially undesirable behavior [33]. Moreover, it has been stated that DNA methylation levels at specific CpG-sites in the genes *AHRR* and *F2RL3* are a better estimate for the exposure to cigarette smoke than pack years derived from self-report [34]. Within the mediation analysis, this potential misclassification of exposure to cigarette smoke may lead to overestimation of the mediation effect [35]. Furthermore, with the cross-sectional design of our study, we cannot infer causality from the mediation analysis. A second potential limitation of our study is that most of the lung tissue was obtained from tumor resection surgery. Although all the tissue has been histologically checked for abnormalities, DNA methylation might be affected by the tumor and potential metastases. However, since this holds for all groups under study, we assume that it will not lead to differences in DNA methylation between the groups.

Conclusions

We identified 15 CpG-sites that were associated with pack years, of which 2 CpG-sites were novel. From the 10 CpG-sites that were also associated with lung function levels, 5 CpG-sites could be validated in lung tissue. Significant associations with expression levels of biological plausible genes suggest a functional role for DNA methylation in lung tissue. Overall, our study showed for the first time that a panel of CpG-sites associated with cigarette smoking and lung function levels identified in whole blood is also associated with exposure to cigarette smoke in the tissue of interest, i.e. the lung. Further research should reveal the functional relevance of these CpG-sites in the lung and their role in the etiology of COPD.

Additional files

Additional file 1: Online supplement. (DOCX 158 kb)

Additional file 2: Overview of the results of the mediation analysis. (DOCX 23 kb)

Additional file 3: Subject characteristics lung tissue cohort. (DOCX 17 kb)

Additional file 4: Overview results of the association between DNA methylation and smoking status in lung tissue. (DOCX 19 kb)

Additional file 5: Overview results of the eQTM analysis. (PDF 553 kb)

Acknowledgements

Part of the data presented in this manuscript is from the Merck-Laval-UBC-Groningen Lung eQTL consortium. We thank the principal investigators of this consortium including Peter Paré, Wim Timens, Yohan Bossé, Maarten van den Berge, Don D. Sin, Philippe Joubert, Ke Hao, and David Nickle.

Funding

This work was supported by consortium grant number 4.1.13.007 of the Lung foundation Netherlands and a research grant of Stichting Astmabestrijding (2017/015). The LifeLines initiative has been made possible by funds from FES (Fonds Economische Structuurversterking), SNN (Samenwerkingsverband Noord Nederland) and REP (Ruimtelijk Economisch Programma).

Authors contributions

M.d.V., D.A.v.d.P., I.N., N.A., C.M.v.D., D.S.P., C.A.B., C.C.v.D., J.M.V. and H.M.B were involved in the conception and design of the research; M.d.V., D.A.v.d.P., R.N.V.S. and W.K. performed the analyses and experiments; M.d.V. and H.M.B. interpreted the results. M.d.V. prepared figures and drafted the manuscript. H.M.B. critically reviewed and revised the manuscript; all authors read and approved the final version of the manuscript.

Ethics approval and consent to participate

LifeLines Groningen.

Written informed consents was provided by all included subjects and the study was approved by the Medical Ethics Committee of the University Medical Center Groningen (2007/152).
Lung tissue cohort.
Lung tissue was collected from patients undergoing lung resection, lung volume reduction or transplant surgery in Groningen (The Netherlands) in accordance with the Research Code of the University Medical Center Groningen and Dutch national ethical and professional guidelines.

Competing interests
The authors declare that they have no competing interests.

Author details
[1]University of Groningen, University Medical Center Groningen, Department of Epidemiology, Hanzeplein 1, Groningen 9713, GZ, The Netherlands. [2]University of Groningen, University Medical Center Groningen, Groningen Research Institute for Asthma and COPD (GRIAC), Groningen, The Netherlands. [3]Department of Epidemiology, Erasmus Medical Center, Rotterdam, The Netherlands. [4]University of Groningen, University Medical Center Groningen, Department of Obstetrics and Gynaecology, Groningen, The Netherlands. [5]University of Groningen, University Medical Center Groningen, Department of Pathology and Medical Biology, Groningen, The Netherlands. [6]University of Groningen, University Medical Center Groningen, Department of Genetics, Groningen, The Netherlands.

References
1. From the Global Strategy for the Diagnosis, Management and Prevention of COPD, Global Initiative for Chronic Obstructive Lung Disease (GOLD) 2015. Available from: http://www.goldcopd.org/.
2. Adeloye D, Chua S, Lee C, Basquill C, Papana A, Theodoratou E, et al. Global and regional estimates of COPD prevalence: systematic review and meta-analysis. J Glob Health. 2015;5(2):020415.
3. van der Plaat DA, de Jong K, Lahousse L, Faiz A, Vonk JM, van Diemen CC, et al. Genome-wide association study on the FEV1/FVC ratio in never-smokers identifies HHIP and FAM13A. J Allergy Clin Immunol. 2016:6.
4. Bosse Y. Updates on the COPD gene list. Int J Chron Obstruct Pulmon Dis. 2012;7:607–31.
5. Hobbs BD, de Jong K, Lamontagne M, Bosse Y, Shrine N, Artigas MS, et al. Genetic loci associated with chronic obstructive pulmonary disease overlap with loci for lung function and pulmonary fibrosis. Nat Genet. 2017;49(3):426–32.
6. de Jong K, Boezen HM, Kromhout H, Vermeulen R, Postma DS, Vonk JM. Association of occupational pesticide exposure with accelerated longitudinal decline in lung function. Am J Epidemiol. 2014;179(11):1323–30.
7. de Jong K, Vonk JM, Timens W, Bosse Y, Sin DD, Hao K, et al. Genome-wide interaction study of gene-by-occupational exposure and effects on FEV1 levels. J Allergy Clin Immunol. 2015;136(6):1664–72.e1–14.
8. Kheirallah AK, Miller S, Hall IP, Sayers I. Translating lung function genome-wide association study (GWAS) findings. New Insights for Lung Biology Adv Genet. 2016;93:57–145.
9. Madrigano J, Baccarelli A, Mittleman MA, Wright RO, Sparrow D, Vokonas PS, et al. Prolonged exposure to particulate pollution, genes associated with glutathione pathways, and DNA methylation in a cohort of older men. Environ Health Perspect. 2011;119(7):977–82.
10. Yang IV, Lozupone CA, Schwartz DA. The environment, epigenome, and asthma. J Allergy Clin Immunol. 2017;140(1):14–23.
11. Jones PA. Functions of DNA methylation: islands, start sites, gene bodies and beyond. Nat Rev Genet. 2012;13(7):484–92.
12. Zeilinger S, Kuhnel B, Klopp N, Baurecht H, Kleinschmidt A, Gieger C, et al. Tobacco smoking leads to extensive genome-wide changes in DNA methylation. PLoS One. 2013;8(5):e63812.
13. Qiu W, Baccarelli A, Carey VJ, Boutaoui N, Bacherman H, Klanderman B, et al. Variable DNA methylation is associated with chronic obstructive pulmonary disease and lung function. Am J Respir Crit Care Med. 2012;185(4):373–81.
14. Panni T, Mehta AJ, Schwartz JD, Baccarelli AA, Just AC, Wolf K, et al. Genome-wide analysis of DNA methylation and fine particulate matter air pollution in three study populations: KORA F3, KORA F4, and the normative aging study. Environ Health Perspect. 2016;124(7):983–90.
15. Kohansal R, Martinez-Camblor P, Agusti A, Buist AS, Mannino DM, Soriano JB. The natural history of chronic airflow obstruction revisited: an analysis of the Framingham offspring cohort. Am J Respir Crit Care Med. 2009;180(1):3–10.
16. Mohamed Hoesein FA, Zanen P, Boezen HM, Groen HJ, van Ginneken B, de Jong PA, et al. Lung function decline in male heavy smokers relates to baseline airflow obstruction severity. Chest. 2012;142(6):1530–8.
17. Scholtens S, Smidt N, Swertz MA, Bakker SJ, Dotinga A, Vonk JM, et al. Cohort profile: LifeLines, a three-generation cohort study and biobank. Int J Epidemiol. 2015;44(4):1172–80.
18. van der Plaat DA, de Jong K, de Vries M, van Diemen CC, Nedeljkovic I, Amin N, et al. Occupational exposure to pesticides is associated with differential DNA methylation. Occup Environ Med. 2018;75(6):427–35.
19. Tingley D, Yamamoto T, Hirose K, Keele L, Imai K. Mediation: R package for causal mediation analysis. J Stat Softw. 2014;59(5).
20. Hao K, Bosse Y, Nickle DC, Pare PD, Postma DS, Laviolette M, et al. Lung eQTLs to help reveal the molecular underpinnings of asthma. PLoS Genet. 2012;8(11):e1003029.
21. Wan ES, Qiu W, Baccarelli A, Carey VJ, Bacherman H, Rennard SI, et al. Cigarette smoking behaviors and time since quitting are associated with differential DNA methylation across the human genome. Hum Mol Genet. 2012;21(13):3073–82.
22. Gao X, Jia M, Zhang Y, Breitling LP, Brenner H. DNA methylation changes of whole blood cells in response to active smoking exposure in adults: a systematic review of DNA methylation studies. Clin Epigenetics. 2015;7:113-015-0148-3 eCollection 2015.
23. Breitling LP, Yang R, Korn B, Burwinkel B, Brenner H. Tobacco-smoking-related differential DNA methylation: 27K discovery and replication. Am J Hum Genet. 2011;88(4):450–7.
24. Shenker NS, Polidoro S, van Veldhoven K, Sacerdote C, Ricceri F, Birrell MA, et al. Epigenome-wide association study in the European prospective investigation into Cancer and nutrition (EPIC-Turin) identifies novel genetic loci associated with smoking. Hum Mol Genet. 2013;22(5):843–51.
25. Wong TH, Chiu WZ, Breedveld GJ, Li KW, Verkerk AJ, Hondius D, et al. PRKAR1B mutation associated with a new neurodegenerative disorder with unique pathology. Brain. 2014;137(Pt 5):1361–73.
26. Guida F, Sandanger TM, Castagne R, Campanella G, Polidoro S, Palli D, et al. Dynamics of smoking-induced genome-wide methylation changes with time since smoking cessation. Hum Mol Genet. 2015;24(8):2349–59.
27. Tsaprouni LG, Yang TP, Bell J, Dick KJ, Kanoni S, Nisbet J, et al. Cigarette smoking reduces DNA methylation levels at multiple genomic loci but the effect is partially reversible upon cessation. Epigenetics. 2014;9(10):1382–96.
28. Lee KW, Pausova Z. Cigarette smoking and DNA methylation. Front Genet. 2013;4:132.
29. Salem M, Ammitzboell M, Nys K, Seidelin JB, Nielsen OH. ATG16L1: a multifunctional susceptibility factor in Crohn disease. Autophagy. 2015;11(4):585–94.
30. Pashler AL, Towler BP, Jones CI, Newbury SF. The roles of the exoribonucleases DIS3L2 and XRN1 in human disease. Biochem Soc Trans. 2016;44(5):1377–84.
31. Ngo L, Haas M, Qu Z, Li SS, Zenker J, Teng KS, et al. TUBB5 and its disease-associated mutations influence the terminal differentiation and dendritic spine densities of cerebral cortical neurons. Hum Mol Genet. 2014;23(19):5147–58.
32. Evans CM, Koo JS. Airway mucus: the good, the bad, the sticky. Pharmacol Ther. 2009;121(3):332–48.
33. Connor Gorber S, Schofield-Hurwitz S, Hardt J, Levasseur G, Tremblay M. The accuracy of self-reported smoking: a systematic review of the relationship between self-reported and cotinine-assessed smoking status. Nicotine Tob Res. 2009;11(1):12–24.
34. Lee DH, Hwang SH, Lim MK, Oh JK, Song DY, Yun EH, et al. Performance of urine cotinine and hypomethylation of AHRR and F2RL3 as biomarkers for smoking exposure in a population-based cohort. PLoS One. 2017;12(4):e0176783.
35. Valeri L, Reese SL, Zhao S, Page CM, Nystad W, Coull BA, et al. Misclassified exposure in epigenetic mediation analyses. Does DNA methylation mediate effects of smoking on birthweight? Epigenomics. 2017;9(3):253–65.

12

The utility of biomarkers in diagnosis of aspirin exacerbated respiratory disease

Suzy A. A. Comhair[1*], Grazyna Bochenek[2], Sara Baicker-McKee[1], Zeneng Wang[1], Tomasz Stachura[2], Marek Sanak[2], Jeffrey P. Hammel[1], Stanley L. Hazen[1], Serpil C. Erzurum[1,3] and Ewa Nizankowska-Mogilnicka[2]

Abstract

Background: Aspirin-exacerbated respiratory disease (AERD) is a distinct eosinophilic phenotype of severe asthma with accompanying chronic rhinosinusitis, nasal polyposis, and hypersensitivity to aspirin. Urinary 3-bromotyrosine (uBrTyr) is a noninvasive marker of eosinophil-catalyzed protein oxidation. The lack of in vitro diagnostic test makes the diagnosis of AERD difficult. We aimed to determine uBrTyr levels in patients with AERD ($n = 240$) and aspirin-tolerant asthma (ATA) ($n = 226$) and to assess whether its addition to urinary leukotriene E_4 ($uLTE_4$) levels and blood eosinophilia can improve the prediction of AERD diagnosis.

Methods: Clinical data, spirometry and blood eosinophilis were evaluated. UBrTyr and $uLTE_4$ levels were measured in urine by HPLC and ELISA, respectively.

Results: Both groups of asthmatics (AERD, n = 240; ATA, n = 226) had significantly higher uBrTyr, $uLTE_4$ levels, and blood eosinophils than healthy controls (HC) ($n = 71$) ($p < 0.05$). $ULTE_4$ levels and blood eosinophils were significantly higher in AERD as compared to ATA ($p = 0.004$, $p < 0.0001$, respectively). whereas uBrTyr levels were not significantly different between both asthma phenotypes ($p = 0.34$). Asthmatics with high levels of uBrTyr (> 0.101 ng/mg Cr), $uLTE_4$ levels (> 800 pg/mg Cr) and blood eosinophils (> 300 cells/ul) were 7 times more likely to have AERD.. However, uBrTyr did not increase the benefit for predicting AERD when $uLTE_4$ and blood eosinophils were already taken into account ($p = 0.57$).

Conclusion: UBrTyr levels are elevated both in AERD and ATA as compared to HC, but they could not differentiate between these asthma phenotypes suggesting a similar eosinophilic activation. The addition of uBrTyr to elevated uLTE4 levels and blood eosinophils did not statistically enhance the prediction of AERD diagnosis.

Keywords: Asthma, BromoTyrosine, Leukotriene, AERD

Background

Around 7% of asthmatics are hypersensitive to aspirin and other non-steroidal anti-inflammatory drugs (NSAIDs) [1]. This asthma phenotype, referred to as Aspirin-Exacerbated Respiratory Disease (AERD), is characterized by the presence of usually severe asthma, chronic rhinosinusitis with nasal polyposis, and acute asthma attacks with naso-ocular symptoms after ingestion of aspirin and other NSAIDs [2]. Previous studies have shown that patients with AERD have increased emergency department visits, hospitalizations, and corticosteroid bursts compared to those with aspirin-tolerant asthma (ATA) [3, 4]. About half of AERD patients have severe asthma that requires chronic treatment with high dose of inhaled corticosteroids or oral corticosteroids to control the disease [4, 5].

AERD is an inflammatory condition of the upper and lower airway characterized by increased eosinophils and mast cells. Mechanistic studies have shown that AERD is linked to abnormalities/dysregulation of the cyclooxygenase (COX) and lipooxygenase (LOX) pathway [2, 6]. It has been suggested that abnormal regulation of 5-LOX and leukotriene C_4 synthase (LTC4S) pathways that results in increased production of cysteinyl leukotrienes (CysLTs) leads to asthmatic attacks [2, 7, 8]. Urinary leukotriene E_4 ($uLTE_4$), a stable CysLTs metabolite, is used to measure their systemic production [9] and can

* Correspondence: comhais@ccf.org
[1]Cleveland Clinic, Lerner Research Institute, 9500 Euclid Avenue, NB2-40, Cleveland, OH 44195, USA
Full list of author information is available at the end of the article

be helpful in differentiating AERD from ATA [10, 11]. Sources of LTE_4 include many cells of the upper and lower airways such as eosinophils, mast cells, basophils, as well as macrophages, platelets, and neutrophils [12].

Eosinophils are important effector cells in asthma and even more so in AERD. Blood eosinophilia is well-recognized biomarker of active inflammation in asthma [13, 14]. Activated eosinophils degranulate to release among others eosinophil peroxidase (EPO), which is unique in its ability to convert respiratory burst-generated hydrogen peroxide into hypobromous acid, a reactive brominating oxidant that modifies protein tyrosine residues, forming 3-bromotyrosine (BrTyr) [15, 16]. BrTyr, a biochemical fingerprint of eosinophil activation as a highly stable product can be detected in urine.

Currently, oral aspirin challenge is the gold standard to confirm the diagnosis of AERD [17, 18]. However, this test is time-consuming, can cause adverse reactions, and is unsuitable in severe asthma patients [17]. Therefore, noninvasive methods that could assist in diagnosis are urgently needed.

To our knowledge, there is no generally recognized, clinically available in vitro test or biomarker to determine the presence of AERD.

The purpose of this study was to determine uBrTyr levels in patients with AERD and ATA and to explore if uBrTyr might predict AERD. Moreover, we wanted to test whether adding elevated uBrTyr levels to elevated $uLTE_4$ levels and blood eosinophil counts could improve the prediction of AERD.

Methods

Study population

Patients with asthma were recruited from the outpatient clinic of the Department of Internal Medicine, Jagiellonian University Medical College, Krakow. All patients were clinically stable without any asthma exacerbations within the 6 weeks preceding the study. All data and sample collection have been previously described [11].

The diagnosis of AERD was determined through typical clinical presentation and at least 1 asthma attack after ingestion of aspirin or another NSAID in the past. This diagnosis was confirmed by a positive aspirin challenge in the majority of patients. However, clinical safety limitation prohibited a small group of AERD patients (16.7%, $n = 40$)) with very severe asthma to undergo aspirin challenge. Their aspirin hypersensitivity was confirmed based on their medical history with previous reactions related to ingestion of NSAIDs well documented in medical records. Removal of these severe asthmatics could introduce additional bias in characteristics of AERD phenotype, for which severe steroid dependent asthma is very typical.

All ATA patients had used aspirin without any adverse effects. Healthy control subjects (HC) without history of asthma, allergy, and any hypersensitivity reactions to NSAIDs were enrolled for comparison of baseline values of inflammatory biomarkers.

Written informed consent was obtained from all participants under a protocol approved by the Jagiellonian University Ethics Review Committee.

Evaluation of asthma was determined by the National Asthma Education and Prevention Program (NAEPP) EPR-3 guidelines [19].

Asthma control was assessed by the Asthma Control Test (ACT) [20].

Study procedures

Spirometry (MasterScreen, Jaeger, Wurzburg, Germany) was carried out at baseline and after administration of 4 puffs of salbutamol. The best of 3 repeatable forced expiratory maneuvers was recorded. The percent predicted values of FEV_1 and FEV_1/FVC were automatically calculated.

Blood eosinophil counts were calculated using a Fuchs-Rosenthal chamber.

Urine analysis

Morning urine samples were collected after a 2 h accumulation of urine in the bladder which allows for less variation in urine creatinine levels [10].

Urine creatinine was measured by enzymatic method using automated chemical analyzer COBAS Integra 400 plus (Roche Diagnostics USA, Indianapolis, IN).

Urinary BrTyr was assayed using stable isotope dilution High Performance Liquid Chromatography (HPLC) with on-line electrospray ionization tandem mass spectrometry. First, a solid phase extraction was performed. Briefly 20 μl internal standard composed of 0.5 μM synthetic [$^{13}C_6$]-3-bromotyrosine, 1 mM [$^{13}C_9$, ^{15}N] tyrosine, and 1 mM creatinine-d_3 (Cambridge Isotope Laboratories) was spiked into 200 μl urine followed by acidification with 1 ml 0.1% formic acid. The acidified urine was loaded to a Biotage® auto solid phase extraction system with 3 ml DSC- 18 column used. DSC-18 column was balanced with 2 × 3 ml methanol and then 2 × 3 ml 0.1% formic acid, washed with 2 × 3 ml 0.1% formic acid, and the product was eluated with 3 ml 0.1% formic acid in 30% methanol. The product was dried under SpeedVacuum, and then resuspended in 100 μl H_2O. Secondly, LC/MS/MS was used to quantify urinary BrTyr. Five microliters of the extraction was analyzed by injection onto a Titan™ C18 UHPLC Column (1.9 μm particle size, L × I.D. 10 cm × 2.1 mm, Supelco) at a flow rate of 0.4 ml min^{-1} using a 2 Shimadzu LC-20 AD Nexera CL pump system, SIL-30 AC MP CL autosampler interfaced with an Shimadzu 8050 mass spectrometer. A discontinuous gradient was generated to resolve the analytes by mixing solvent A (0.2% formic acid in water) with solvent B (0.2% formic acid in methanol) at different ratios starting from 0% B for 3 min, then linearly to 100% B over 3.5 min, then hold for 3 min, and then back to 0% B. [$^{13}C_9$, $^{15}N_1$]-tyrosine was included to simultaneously monitor for potential artificial generation of analyte. 3-bromotyrosine, creatinine, and their respective internal standards [$^{13}C_6$]-3-bromotyrosine and creatinine-d_3 were monitored using electrospray ionization in positive-ion mode with multiple reaction monitoring (MRM) of precursor and characteristic product-ion transitions of m/z 260 → 135, 114 → 44, 266 → 141 and 117 → 47 amu, respectively. The parameters for the ion monitoring were optimized automatically. Nitrogen (99.95% purity) was used as the source, and helium was used as collision gas. Various concentrations of nonisotopically-labeled 3-bromotyrosine were spiked into control urine to prepare the calibration curves for quantification of 3-bromotyrosine. The internal standard [$^{13}C_6$]-3-bromotyrosine was used for quantification as well as to calculate recovery rate of TMAO (which was > 80% based on separate control studies). Under the conditions employed for the assay, no artificial bromination was detected. Results of urinary BrTyr were expressed in nanograms per mg of creatinine.

$ULTE_4$ was measured in unpurified urine samples by direct enzyme immunoassay (Cayman Chemical, Ann Arbor, MI). Supernatants of freshly collected spot urine samples were stored at – 80°Celsius for not longer than 6 months. After thawing at 4 °C, urine was diluted in phosphate buffered saline (1:10). The measurement was repeated using 1:30 dilution of urine for samples in which the LTE_4 concentration exceeded the uppermost calibrator concentration of the assay (1000 pg/mL). Results of urinary LTE_4 measurements were expressed in picograms per mg of creatinine.

Statistical analyses

Quantitative characteristics of the study population were described using mean and standard error, while categorical characteristics were described using means and percents. Groups were compared with respect to baseline quantitative characteristics and marker levels among the groups with t-tests and analyses of variance for approximately normally distributed variables, while the Wilcoxon rank-sum test was used with respect to variables demonstrating non-normal distributions. Groups were compared using the likelihood-ratio χ^2 test with respect to categorical variables. To evaluate uBrTyr, $uLTE_4$, and blood eosinophils as biomarkers for AERD diagnosis, cut-points were used. A receiver operating characteristic (ROC) analysis was used to identify an optimal cut-point for uBrTyr and $uLTE_4$. A cut-point for blood eosinophils > 300 cells/μL was based on published data [21, 22]. Logistic regression was used to estimate odds ratios for the identification of AERD (vs ATA) with respect to the dichotomized forms of the biomarkers. The logistic regression analyses were also performed with covariate adjustment for baseline FEV_1%, chronic rhinosinusitis, and any steroid use was performed with the logistic regression modeling. The incremental predictive ability of each marker in the regression model was assessed using areas under the ROC curves estimated with 10-fold cross-validation for the full model and for models excluding markers individually. Correlations among quantitative variables were assessed using Spearman's rank-sum correlation coefficients, which are suitable for data with any distribution. A p-value less than or equal to 0.05 was defined as statistically significant.

Results

Subject characteristics

The study included 240 patients with AERD, 226 patients with ATA, and 71 HC. Almost the same population has been previously described [11]. The clinical characteristics of the study subjects are shown in Table 1. Age and gender were distributed significantly differently in asthmatics, i.e., AERD and ATA when compared to (HC), but no difference between AERD and ATA was found. (Table 1). The AERD subjects had worse lung functions and significantly longer asthma duration than the ATA subjects (Table 1). Medication use was different between the AERD and the ATA groups. No difference was found with respect to the ACT scores (Table 1).

Asthma biomarkers

Both AERD and ATA groups had significantly higher levels of uBrTyr, $uLTE_4$, and blood eosinophils than HC (Fig. 1). Furthermore, $uLTE_4$ levels and blood eosinophils were significantly higher in AERD as compared to ATA ($p < 0.0001$, $p = 0.004$, respectively), whereas uBrTyr levels were not significantly different between these two asthmatic phenotypes ($p = 0.3406$) (Fig. 1).

UBrTyr and $uLTE_4$ levels correlated with each other both in the AERD [$R = 0.160$, $p = 0.01$] and the ATA [$R = 0.151$, $p = 0.02$] groups. Blood eosinophils correlated significantly with $uLTE_4$ levels in both asthma phenotypes [ATA: $R = 0.165$, $p = 0.01$; AERD: $R = 0.276$, $p < 0.0001$], whereas no such correlation was found with eosinophil counts and uBrTyr levels.

Both uBrTyr and $uLTE_4$ levels did not correlate with severity of airway obstruction measured by FEV_1% predicted and FEV_1%FVC in either asthma phenotype, while only a borderline correlation was found between FEV_1%FVC and $uLTE_4$ in ATA [$R = 0.140$, $p = 0.05$].

To evaluate if studied biomarkers have the ability to predict an AERD diagnosis, values for each biomarker

Table 1 Participant characteristics

	AERD [*n* = 240]	ATA [*n* = 226]	Control [*n* = 71]	*p*-value (ANOVA)	T-Test
Demographics					
Age (yrs)	49.3 [0.8]	49.7 [1.0]	44.3 [1.6]	0.008	
Gender [M/F]	74/166	68/158	35/36	0.007	
BMI (kg/m^2)	26.7 [0.3]	27.1 [0.4]	25.6 [1.0]		
Duration of asthma (yrs)	18.8 [0.8]	15.2 [1.0]	n/a		< 0.0001
ACT; uncontrolled, n [%]	108 [46]	98 [46]	n/a		
Medication use					
High dose ICS/Oral CS, n (%)	63 (26)	37 (18)	n/a		0.03
High dose ICS > 500 (μg/d), n (%)	62 (26)	52 (25.5)	n/a		
Low dose ICS ≤500 (μg/d), n (%)	78 (33)	92 (44.7)	n/a		0.008
No ICS or Oral CS, n (%)	3 (14)	25 (12.4)	n/a		
Lung functions					
FEV_1% predicted	79.8 [1.3]	86.6 [1.4]	n/a		0.0003
FEV_1 %FVC	68.8 [0.7]	74.8 [0.7]	n/a		< 0.0001

Mean (SEM); Definition of abbreviations: *AERD* Aspirin-Exacerbated Respiratory Disease, *ATA* Aspirin Tolerant Asthma, *M* Male, *F* Female, *BMI* Body mass index, *FEV_1* Forced expiratory volume in 1 s, *FVC* Forced vital capacity, *CS* Corticosteroidsm, *ICS* Inhaled Corticosteroids

were dichotomized at cutoffs derived from ROC curve analyses. The cutoff value for uBrTyr was 0.101 ng/mg Cr (specificity 37%, sensitivity 70%), and the cutoff value for $uLTE_4$ was 800 pg/mg Cr (specificity 81%, sensitivity 50%). A high level of uBrTyr did not confer greater odds of having AERD (OR 1.3; 95% Cl 0.9–2.0, $p = 0.15$) (Fig. 2). The odds ratio for predicting AERD with respect to blood eosinophils > 300 cells/uL was 1.8 (95% CI 1.2–2.6, $p = 0.003$) (Fig. 2). A high level of $uLTE_4 > 800$ pg/mg Cr conferred 4.1-fold odds of having AERD (95% CI 2.7–6.3; $p < 0.0001$). The combination of high blood eosinophils together with high $uLTE_4$ levels increased the odds for AERD diagnosis 6.0-fold (95% CI 3.4–10.9, $p < 0.0001$), with frequency of AERD of 79.6% (74/93) among asthmatics with both characteristics versus 39.5% (77/195) among patients with neither characteristic. Asthmatics with a combination of high blood eosinophil counts, $uLTE_4$ levels, and uBrTyr levels had 7.1 times greater odds to have AERD than patients with none of the biomarkers elevated (95% CI 3.4–15.8, $p < 0.0001$) (Fig. 2), with frequency of AERD of 83.1% (59/71) among asthmatics with all three characteristics versus 41.0% (32/78) among patients with none of the characteristics. In the multivariable model with all 3 biomarkers, uBrTyr did not show

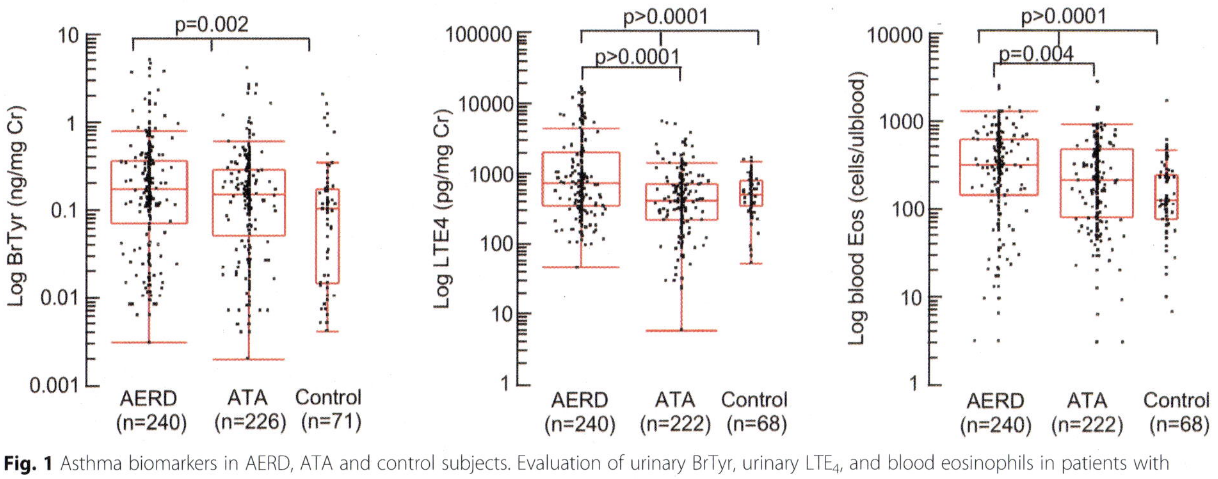

Fig. 1 Asthma biomarkers in AERD, ATA and control subjects. Evaluation of urinary BrTyr, urinary LTE_4, and blood eosinophils in patients with Aspirin-Exacerbated Respiratory Disease (AERD) ($n = 240$), patients with Aspirin-Tolerant Asthma (ATA) ($n = 222$), and control subjects ($n = 68$). All markers were significantly different between the three groups (ANOVA, $p < 0.05$). Urinary BrTyr was the only biomarker not significantly different between ATA and AERD ($p > 0.05$)

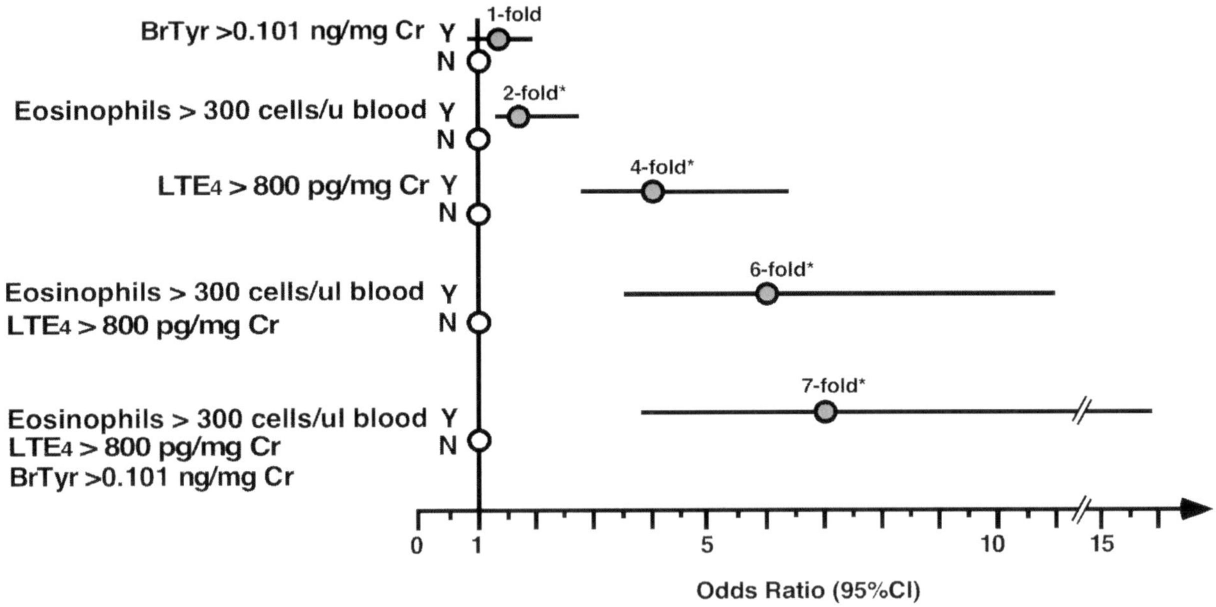

Fig. 2 Odds ratios and 95% confidence intervals for the association between the presence of elevated marker levels, individually and in combination, versus the diagnosis of AERD. Results shown represent the ORs *(filled circles)* and 95% CI *(lines)* of having AERD versus ATA *(open circles)* for participants with high levels of urinary BrTyr and/or high levels of blood eosinophils, and/or high levels of urinary LTE4 compared with participants with low levels of these markers. *Asterisk* indicates $P < 0.05$

statistically significant evidence of an additive benefit for predicting AERD when $uLTE_4$ and blood eosinophils were already taken into account [adjusted odds ratio 1.1, 95% CI 0.8–1.7, $p = 0.57$].

When performing further covariate adjustment for baseline $FEV_1\%$, chronic rhinosinusitis, and steroid use, the combination of high blood eosinophils together with high $uLTE_4$ levels increased the odds for AERD diagnosis 3.5-fold (95% CI 1.7–7.4, $p = 0.0007$), which was smaller than the 6.0-fold estimate without the additional covariate adjustments. Asthmatics with a combination of high blood eosinophil counts, $uLTE_4$ levels, and uBrTyr levels had covariate-adjusted 7.7 times greater odds to have AERD than patients with none of the biomarkers elevated (95% CI 2.8–24.7, $p = 0.0002$), which was slightly higher than the 7.1-fold estimate obtained without the additional covariate adjustments. The additive benefit of uBrTyr for predicting AERD when $uLTE_4$ and blood eosinophils were already taken into account also jumped upward a bit [adjusted odds ratio 1.5, 95% CI 0.9–2.5, $p = 0.09$] when adjusting for the additional covariates, compared to the 1.1-fold increase estimated without the additional adjustments. The adjustment for steroid use was also performed with respect to only high dose steroid use, but the odds ratio estimates for the biomarkers was virtually identical to those obtained with the adjustment for any steroid use. Using ROC curves, 10-fold cross-validated AUC estimates were 0.82 for the full model and for models excluding either uBrTyr or blood eosinophils, while the exclusion of $uLTE_4$ yielded an estimate of 0.79. This is not surprising given that among the biomarkers, only $uLTE_4$ levels yielded a statistically significant association with AERD when adjusting for the other biomarkers and the selected covariates.

The cutpoint for uBrTyr level to predict asthma regardless of phenotype was > 0.17 ng/mg Cr (specificity, 79%; sensitivity, 45%). Subjects with baseline uBrTyr levels > 0.17 ng/mg Cr were 3.1 times (95% CI 1.7–5.8], $p > 0.0002$) as likely to have asthma.

Discussion

Aspirin challenge is currently considered as the gold standard and the only reliable method for the diagnosis of AERD. However, due to certain limitations of this procedure, an intensive search for in vitro diagnostic biomarkers useful in identifying patients with AERD is underway.

Novel biomarkers such as serum periostin [23], plasma eosinophil-derived neurotoxin [24], serum levels of LTE_4, and LTE_4/PGF_2 alfa ratio [25] have been suggested but are not routinely done as in vitro diagnostic tests. They require verification in further studies.

As the imbalance of arachidonic acid metabolism and increased inflammation are important pathophysiologic features of AERD, we investigated if a panel of biomarkers reflecting these imbalances could be used for the prediction of this asthma phenotype. The current study confirmed previous reports that $uLTE_4$ levels and blood eosinophil counts are increased in AERD patients as compared with ATA patients [9, 11, 26–28]. Additionally, it revealed that both elevated blood eosinophil count and increased $uLTE_4$ levels separately enhanced the chance of AERD diagnosis 1.8-fold and 4.2-fold, respectively. The novel finding is that the combination of these two biomarkers powers that prediction 6.0-fold.

Recently, Bochenek et al. demonstrated that a set of clinical parameters comprising nasal polyps, upper airway symptoms, nasal corticosteroid treatment, asthma exacerbations, FEV_1% predicted, and age of asthma onset had a superior accuracy in the prediction of AERD diagnosis to the measurement of $uLTE_4$ level alone [11]. Addition of high $uLTE_4$ level to clinical parameters slightly enhanced the prediction of such diagnosis.

Ban et al. analyzed a metabolite profile that involved the arachidonic acid pathway for discriminating AERD from ATA and revealed that serum levels of LTE_4 and even more so $LTE_4/PGF_2\alpha$ ratio can be potential in vitro diagnostic biomarkers for AERD [25]. Thus, similarly to the current study, the combination of two biomarkers together improved the diagnostic value of the test.

Eosinophils and mast cells play an important role in the pathogenesis of AERD [7]. Studies have suggested that eosinophils in AERD are driving cysteinyl leukotrienes overproduction and eosinophils proteins, e.g. ECP increased following aspirin provocation fast [29, 30]. Previous findings showed that uBrTyr can be used as (1) a molecular fingerprint of eosinophil activation; (2) a predictor of asthma and asthma exacerbation; and (3) a biomarker for asthma severity and corticosteroid responsiveness [15, 16, 31–34]. Despite serving as a marker for eosinophil activation, uBrTyr levels did not correlate with the amount of blood eosinophils found in either the AERD or in the ATA group. The study by Mita et al. on very small groups of patients with AERD ($n = 12$), ATA ($n = 12$), and control subjects ($n = 18$) showed also that higher uBrTyr levels in asthmatics were not related to the presence of aspirin sensitivity, but rather to their asthma alone [35]. As shown previously with asthmatic adult and pediatric populations [31, 32, 35], in our cohort of adult asthmatics uBrTyr levels were also increased in asthma when compared with HC and could be used as a biomarker of asthma. However, a higher uBrTyr level alone cannot distinguish patients with AERD from patients with ATA, and thus it cannot be used as a single parameter helpful in the diagnosis of AERD. The multivariable modeling conducted presently demonstrates a slight predictive benefit of uBrTyr level in addition to the use of elevated blood eosiniphils and elevated $uLTE_4$ that is enhanced with covariate adjustment for FEV_1%, chronic rhinosinusitis, and steroid use, though not reaching a magnitude of statistical significance ($p = 0.09$).

Conclusion

This study reveals that uBrTyr levels are increased both in AERD and in ATA but cannot identify AERD. This suggested that the activation and the role of eosinophils in the controlled asthma is similar regardless aspirin hypersensitivity. The addition of uBrTyr to elevated uLTE4 levels and blood eosinophils did not statistically enhance the prediction of AERD diagnosis.14.

Abbreviations

AERD: Aspirin-exacerbated respiratory disease; ATA: Aspirin-tolerant asthma; COX: Cyclooxygenase; CysLTs: Cysteinyl leukotrienes; HC: Healthy controls; HPLC: High Performance Liquid Chromatography; LOX: Lipoxygenase; LTC4S: Leukotriene C_4 synthase; UBrTyr: Urinary 3-bromotyrosine; $ULTE_4$: Urinary $leukotriene_4$ E

Acknowledgements

Not applicable

Funding

National Institutes of Health (HL103453, HL081064), the Alfred Lerner Memorial Chair in Innovative Biomedical Research. Mass spectrometry studies were performed on instruments housed in a facility partially supported by a Center of Innovation Award by AB SCIEX. Grant from the Jagiellonian University Medical College (K/ZDS/002794). "The funders had no role in study design, data collection and analysis, decision to publish, or preparation of the manuscript."

Authors' contributions

SAAC, SLH and SCE, literature search, data analysis/interpretation, figures, and writing; ENM, GB, study design, data collection /interpretation, figures, writing; TS and MS- study design, data collection, SBM and ZW- data collection; JPH, statistical analysis. All authors read and approved the final manuscript.

Competing interests

SLH is named as co-inventor on pending and issued patents held by the Cleveland Clinic relating to cardiovascular diagnostics and asthmatic therapeutics, and has the right to receive royalty payment for inventions or discoveries both related tocardiovascular and asthmatic diagnostics or therapeutics from the Cleveland Clinic, Quest Diagnostics and Proctor & Gamble. SLH also reports having been paid as a Consultant from Proctor & Gamble, and having received research funds from Proctor & Gamble and Roche.DD.

Author details

[1]Cleveland Clinic, Lerner Research Institute, 9500 Euclid Avenue, NB2-40, Cleveland, OH 44195, USA. [2]Department of Internal Medicine, Faculty of Medicine, Jagiellonian University Medical College, Krakow, Poland. [3]Respiratory Institute, Cleveland Clinic, Cleveland, USA.

References

1. Rajan JP, Wineinger NE, Stevenson DD, White AA. Prevalence of aspirin-exacerbated respiratory disease among asthmatic patients: a meta-analysis of the literature. J Allergy Clin Immunol. 2015;135(3):676–81 e671.
2. Stevenson DD, Szczeklik A. Clinical and pathologic perspectives on aspirin sensitivity and asthma. J Allergy Clin Immunol. 2006;118(4):773–86 quiz 787-778.
3. Moon JY, Kim SH, Kim TB, et al. Aspirin-intolerant asthma in the Korean population: prevalence and characteristics based on a questionnaire survey. Respir Med. 2013;107(2):202–8.
4. Szczeklik A, Nizankowska E, Duplaga M. Natural history of aspirin-induced asthma. AIANE investigators. European network on aspirin-induced asthma. Eur Respir J. 2000;16(3):432–6.
5. Bochenek G, Szafraniec K, Kuschill-Dziurda J, Nizankowska-Mogilnicka E. Factors associated with asthma control in patients with aspirin-exacerbated respiratory disease. Respir Med. 2015;109(5):588–95.
6. Szczeklik A, Gryglewski RJ, Czerniawska-Mysik G. Relationship of inhibition of prostaglandin biosynthesis by analgesics to asthma attacks in aspirin-sensitive patients. Br Med J. 1975;1(5949):67–9.
7. Cowburn AS, Sladek K, Soja J, et al. Overexpression of leukotriene C4 synthase in bronchial biopsies from patients with aspirin-intolerant asthma. J Clin Invest. 1998;101(4):834–46.
8. Israel E, Fischer AR, Rosenberg MA, et al. The pivotal role of 5-lipoxygenase products in the reaction of aspirin-sensitive asthmatics to aspirin. Am Rev Respir Dis. 1993;148(6 Pt 1):1447–51.
9. Kumlin M, Dahlen B, Bjorck T, Zetterstrom O, Granstrom E, Dahlen SE. Urinary excretion of leukotriene E4 and 11-dehydro-thromboxane B2 in response to bronchial provocations with allergen, aspirin, leukotriene D4, and histamine in asthmatics. Am Rev Respir Dis. 1992;146(1):96–103.
10. Divekar R, Hagan J, Rank M, et al. Diagnostic utility of urinary LTE4 in asthma, allergic rhinitis, chronic rhinosinusitis, nasal polyps, and aspirin sensitivity. J Allergy Clin Immunol Pract. 2016;4(4):665–70.
11. Bochenek G, Stachura T, Szafraniec K, et al. Diagnostic accuracy of urinary LTE4 measurement to predict aspirin-exacerbated respiratory disease in patients with asthma. J Allergy Clin Immunol Pract. 2018;6(2):528–35. https://doi.org/10.1016/j.jaip.2017.07.001.
12. Laidlaw TM, Kidder MS, Bhattacharyya N, et al. Cysteinyl leukotriene overproduction in aspirin-exacerbated respiratory disease is driven by platelet-adherent leukocytes. Blood. 2012;119(16):3790–8.
13. Bousquet J, Chanez P, Lacoste JY, et al. Eosinophilic inflammation in asthma. N Engl J Med. 1990;323(15):1033–9.
14. Wenzel SE. Asthma phenotypes: the evolution from clinical to molecular approaches. Nat Med. 2012;18(5):716–25.
15. MacPherson JC, Comhair SA, Erzurum SC, et al. Eosinophils are a major source of nitric oxide-derived oxidants in severe asthma: characterization of pathways available to eosinophils for generating reactive nitrogen species. J Immunol. 2001;166(9):5763–72.
16. Wu W, Samoszuk MK, Comhair SA, et al. Eosinophils generate brominating oxidants in allergen-induced asthma. J Clin Invest. 2000;105(10):1455–63.
17. Nizankowska-Mogilnicka E, Bochenek G, Mastalerz L, et al. EAACI/GA2LEN guideline: aspirin provocation tests for diagnosis of aspirin hypersensitivity. Allergy. 2007;62(10):1111–8.
18. Macy E, Bernstein JA, Castells MC, et al. Aspirin challenge and desensitization for aspirin-exacerbated respiratory disease: a practice paper. Ann Allergy Asthma Immunol. 2007;98(2):172–4.
19. National Asthma Education and Prevention Programme. Expert Panel Report 3: guidelines for the diagnosis and management of asthma. https://www.nhlbi.nih.gov/health-pro/guidelines/current/asthma-guidelines2007.
20. Nathan RA, Sorkness CA, Kosinski M, et al. Development of the asthma control test: a survey for assessing asthma control. J Allergy Clin Immunol. 2004;113(1):59–65.
21. Katz LE, Gleich GJ, Hartley BF, Yancey SW, Ortega HG. Blood eosinophil count is a useful biomarker to identify patients with severe eosinophilic asthma. Ann Am Thorac Soc. 2014;11(4):531–6.
22. Price DB, Rigazio A, Campbell JD, et al. Blood eosinophil count and prospective annual asthma disease burden: a UK cohort study. Lancet Respir Med. 2015; 3(11):849–58.
23. Kim MA, Izuhara K, Ohta S, et al. Association of serum periostin with aspirin-exacerbated respiratory disease. Ann Allergy Asthma Immunol. 2014;113(3): 314–20.
24. Shin SW, Park JS, Park CS. Elevation of eosinophil-derived neurotoxin in plasma of the subjects with aspirin-exacerbated respiratory disease: a possible peripheral blood protein biomarker. PLoS One. 2013;8(6):e66644.
25. Ban GY, Cho K, Kim SH, et al. Metabolomic analysis identifies potential diagnostic biomarkers for aspirin-exacerbated respiratory disease. Clin Exp Allergy. 2017;47(1):37–47.
26. Christie PE, Tagari P, Ford-Hutchinson AW, et al. Urinary leukotriene E4 concentrations increase after aspirin challenge in aspirin-sensitive asthmatic subjects. Am Rev Respir Dis. 1991;143(5 Pt 1):1025–9.
27. Smith CM, Hawksworth RJ, Thien FC, Christie PE, Lee TH. Urinary leukotriene E4 in bronchial asthma. Eur Respir J. 1992;5(6):693–9.
28. Higashi N, Taniguchi M, Mita H, et al. Clinical features of asthmatic patients with increased urinary leukotriene E4 excretion (hyperleukotrienuria): involvement of chronic hyperplastic rhinosinusitis with nasal polyposis. J Allergy Clin Immunol. 2004;113(2):277–83.
29. Choi GS, Kim JH, Shin YS, Ye YM, Kim SH, Park HS. Eosinophil activation and novel mediators in the aspirin-induced nasal response in AERD. Clin Exp Allergy. 2013;43(7):730–40.
30. Steinke JW, Payne SC, Borish L. Eosinophils and mast cells in aspirin-exacerbated respiratory disease. Immunol Allergy Clin N Am. 2016;36(4): 719–34.
31. Wedes SH, Khatri SB, Zhang R, et al. Noninvasive markers of airway inflammation in asthma. Clin Transl Sci. 2009;2(2):112–7.
32. Wedes SH, Wu W, Comhair SA, et al. Urinary bromotyrosine measures asthma control and predicts asthma exacerbations in children. J Pediatr. 2011;159(2):248–55 e241.
33. Wu W, Chen Y, d'Avignon A, Hazen SL. 3-Bromotyrosine and 3,5-dibromotyrosine are major products of protein oxidation by eosinophil peroxidase: potential markers for eosinophil-dependent tissue injury in vivo. Biochemistry. 1999;38(12):3538–48.
34. Wu W, Chen Y, Hazen SL. Eosinophil peroxidase nitrates protein tyrosyl residues. Implications for oxidative damage by nitrating intermediates in eosinophilic inflammatory disorders. J Biol Chem. 1999;274(36):25933–44.
35. Mita H, Higashi N, Taniguchi M, Higashi A, Kawagishi Y, Akiyama K. Urinary 3-bromotyrosine and 3-chlorotyrosine concentrations in asthmatic patients: lack of increase in 3-bromotyrosine concentration in urine and plasma proteins in aspirin-induced asthma after intravenous aspirin challenge. Clin Exp Allergy. 2004;34(6):931–8.

13

Efficacy and safety of nintedanib in advanced idiopathic pulmonary fibrosis

Hee-Young Yoon, Sojung Park, Dong Soon Kim and Jin Woo Song*

Abstract

Background: Phase 3 trials have shown that nintedanib reduces the decline in forced vital capacity (FVC) in patients with mild-to-moderate idiopathic pulmonary fibrosis (IPF) with acceptable safety profiles; however, its effects on advanced IPF are unclear. We investigated the efficacy and safety of nintedanib in patients with advanced IPF.

Methods: Prospective data were obtained from 108 IPF patients administered at least one dose of nintedanib. Of these patients, 47.2% had advanced IPF (FVC < 50% predicted, or diffusing capacity < 30% predicted).

Results: The median treatment duration was 42.2 weeks. Nintedanib significantly reduced the decline rate in both FVC (− 0.55% [before] vs. -0.32% [after] predicted/month, $p = 0.020$) and total lung capacity (TLC) (− 0.35% vs. -0.06% predicted/month, $p < 0.001$) in all patients. A significant improvement in FVC decline rate after treatment was also observed in the advanced group (− 0.77% vs. -0.22% predicted/month, $p = 0.003$), but not in the non-advanced group (− 0.41% vs. -0.33% predicted/month, $p = 0.564$). Adverse events occurred in 97.2% of the cohort, including diarrhoea (50.0%) and anorexia (45.4%). Following adjustment for treatment duration, no inter-group difference in odds ratio was observed for the occurrence of adverse events. However, the advanced group showed a higher frequency of treatment interruption (68.0% vs. 40.0%), mainly as a result of disease progression (47.1% vs. 36.4%).

Conclusions: The efficacy and safety profiles of nintedanib in the advanced group were comparable to those in the non-advanced group except for a higher frequency of discontinuation, which may be due to the advanced status itself.

Keywords: Idiopathic pulmonary fibrosis, Respiratory function tests, Nintedanib, Treatment outcome, Adverse effects

Background

Idiopathic pulmonary fibrosis (IPF) is a chronic, progressive, fibrosing interstitial pneumonia characterized by poor prognosis [1, 2]. The pathogenesis of IPF is suggested to involve several profibrotic mediators, such as fibroblast growth factors (FGFs), platelet-derived growth factors (PDGFs), and transforming growth factor beta [3, 4]. Nintedanib, an intracellular tyrosine kinase inhibitor that targets vascular endothelial growth factor, FGFs, and PDGF receptors, has shown anti-fibrotic and anti-inflammatory activity in a preclinical study [5, 6]. Recent randomised controlled trials of patients with mild-to-moderate IPF revealed that nintedanib reduced the rate of decline of forced vital capacity (FVC) and disease progression, and that adverse events (AEs) were well tolerated [7, 8].

Limited data have suggested that nintedanib may also stabilise the decline in lung function in patients with advanced IPF [9]. Post-hoc subgroup analyses of pooled data from two phase 3 trials, in which patients with IPF were classified according to baseline FVC % predicted (≤ 70%, > 70%; ≤ 80%, > 80%; or ≤ 90%, > 90%), showed no statistically significant inter-group differences in the effect of nintedanib on the annual rate of decline in FVC [10–12]. In an exploratory subgroup analysis of the open-label extension trial, INPULSIS-ON, in which patients were classified according to baseline FVC % predicted (≤ 50%, > 50%), the decline in FVC in both subgroups was similar to that observed in the phase 3 trials. However, the number of patients with FVC ≤ 50% predicted was small ($n = 24$), and the efficacy and safety analyses were only descriptive [9].

* Correspondence: jwsong@amc.seoul.kr
Department of Pulmonary and Critical Care Medicine, Asan Medical Centre, University of Ulsan College of Medicine, Olympic-Ro 43-Gil, Songpa-Gu, Seoul 05505, Republic of Korea

The aim of the present study was to compare the efficacy and safety of nintedanib in patients with advanced and non-advanced IPF.

Methods

Study subjects

Between August 2014 and December 2016, a total of 108 patients with IPF who received nintedanib through the named patient use programme at Asan Medical Centre, Seoul, Republic of Korea, were recruited for this study (Fig. 1). The inclusion and exclusion criteria of the named patient use programme are shown in Additional file 1: Table S1. IPF was confirmed in 42.7% of the 108 patients via biopsy (37.4% in the advanced group and 45.6% in the non-advanced group). All patients fulfilled the IPF diagnostic criteria of the American Thoracic Society (ATS)/European Respiratory Society/Japanese Respiratory Society/Latin American Thoracic Association [1]. Patients with baseline FVC < 50% predicted, or diffusing capacity for carbon monoxide (DLco) < 30% predicted, were classified as advanced IPF cases. The study was approved by the Institutional Review Board of the Asan Medical Centre (2014–0805) and all patients provided written informed consent prior to inclusion.

Clinical variables

The data on baseline demographics, lung function tests, and the 6 min walk test (6MWT) were obtained at the time of nintedanib initiation. Spirometry to measure FVC, plethysmography to measure total lung capacity (TLC) and evaluation of DLco were performed at 3 month intervals, in accordance with the recommendations of ERS/ATS [13–15]. The results were expressed as percentages of normal predicted values. The 6MWT was performed in accordance with ATS guidelines at the time of initiation of nintedanib with the following minor modification: the technician continually monitored the oxygen saturation levels of the patient with no additional remark or encouragement [16].

Evaluation of efficacy

Efficacy was evaluated in all patients who were treated with at least one dose of nintedanib and underwent pulmonary function tests at least three times in each pre- and post-treatment period. The decline rate of lung function, which was estimated by the mixed-effects model, was compared between before and after treatment, or between the advanced and non-advanced group. The adjusted lung function values at each time point in the pre- and post-treatment periods were compared with baseline values. For categorical comparisons, disease progression was defined as a ≥ 10% absolute decline in FVC over 12 months ($FVC_{after\ 12\ months} - FVC_{baseline}$).

Evaluation of safety

Safety was assessed in all patients who received at least one dose of nintedanib. AEs were monitored from the initiation of treatment to 28 days after the final dose of nintedanib and assessed at each follow-up visit by physician's examination. The time of occurrence and termination was recorded. The AE terms were classified in accordance with the *Medical Dictionary for Regulatory Affairs*. Acute exacerbation was defined as an acute, clinically significant deterioration of unidentifiable cause in a patient with IPF [17]. Serious AEs (SAEs) were defined as adverse drug events occurring at any dose that resulted in one of the following outcomes: 1) death; 2) life-threatening hospitalization; 3) disability or permanent damage; 4) any

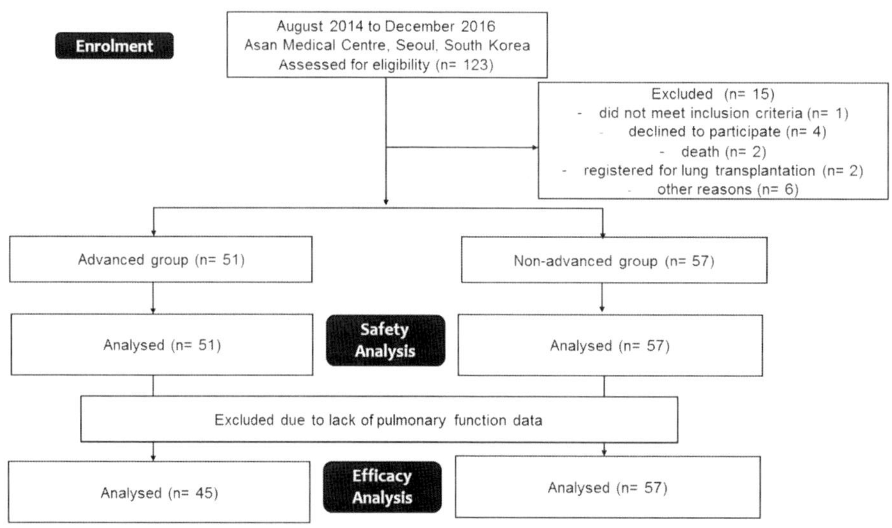

Fig. 1 Enrolment of the study subjects

event that required intervention to prevent permanent impairment or damage; or 5) any other serious medical event.

Statistical analysis

Continuous variables are expressed as the mean ± standard deviation (SD) or median with interquartile range (IQR) and the categorical variables are expressed as percentages. Continuous variables were analysed by using Student's *t*-test or the Mann-Whitney *U* test. Categorical variables were analysed by using Pearson chi-square test or the Fisher exact test. A mixed-effects model was used to examine the rate of decline of lung function and the adjusted mean changes from baseline, using age, sex, body mass index (BMI), and smoking status as fixed effects, and time-by-person (slope) as a random effect. To compare the efficacy between the advanced and non-advanced groups, or between the pre- and post-treatment periods, the time-by-group or time-by-treatment period was used as fixed effects in addition to the mixed-effects model. The odds ratio (OR) and 95% confidence interval (CI) for the occurrence of AEs in the advanced group compared with that in the non-advanced group were adjusted for treatment duration by using binary logistics regression analysis. All tests for significance were two-sided, and variables with p-values of < 0.05 were considered to indicate statistical significance. All statistical analyses were computed by using SPSS version 23.0 (SPSS Inc., Chicago, IL, USA).

Results

Baseline characteristics of the cohort

The median follow-up duration was 43.7 weeks (IQR: 22.9–70.0 weeks). The mean age of patients was 66.7 years; 79.6% of the patients were men and 47.2% were classified into the advanced group (Table 1). The median duration of exposure to nintedanib was 42.2 weeks (IQR: 18.9–66.8 weeks; 26.7 weeks in the advanced group and 57.0 weeks in the non-advanced group, $p < 0.001$). Compared with the patients in the non-advanced group, those in the advanced group were less likely to be current smokers, and tended to have a lower BMI, poorer lung function and exercise capacity, higher mean estimated systolic pulmonary arterial pressure, and more frequent use of steroids (Table 1).

Lung function decline rates

The efficacy was evaluated in 102 patients (45 in the advanced IPF group and 57 in the non-advanced IPF group) and the median treatment duration was 44.1 weeks (29.1 weeks in the advanced group and 57.0 weeks in the non-advanced group, $p < 0.001$).

In all patients, the decline rate in FVC was significantly reduced after treatment (– 0.55% ± 0.08% [before] vs. -0.32% ± 0.09% [after] predicted/month, $p = 0.020$; Fig. 2). Similar trends were observed for TLC. In contrast, the decline rate in DLco was not changed after treatment (– 1.60 ± 0.15% vs. -0.78 ± 0.19% predicted/month, $p = 0.921$).

In the advanced IPF group, the decline rate in FVC decreased after treatment (– 0.77% ± 0.13% [before] vs. -0.22% ± 0.13% [after] predicted/month, $p = 0.003$; Fig. 2). However, only a numerical improvement in FVC decline rate after treatment was observed in the non-advanced group (– 0.41% ± 0.09% vs. -0.33% ± 0.11% predicted/month, $p = 0.564$). There was a significant difference in FVC decline rate between the advanced and non-advanced groups before treatment (– 0.77% ± 0.13% [advanced] vs. -0.41% ± 0.09% [non--advanced] predicted/month, $p = 0.018$), but not after treatment (– 0.22% ± 0.13% vs. -0.33% ± 0.11% predicted/month, p = 0.564). In both groups, the decline rate in TLC was significantly reduced after treatment, which was not the case for DLco.

Lung function changes

The adjusted mean FVC changes from baseline were significant before treatment (ΔFVC: – 6.4% ± 0.9% predicted, $p < 0.001$ [12 months]; – 3.0% ± 0.6% predicted, $p < 0.001$ [6 months]), but were not significant after treatment (ΔFVC: – 1.4% ± 1.2% predicted, $p = 0.227$ [6 months]; – 3.0% ± 1.5% predicted, $p = 0.055$ [12 months]; Fig. 3). The adjusted differences in TLC showed a trend similar to that of FVC; however, the differences in DLco from baseline were significant before and after treatment.

In the advanced group, the adjusted mean FVC changes from baseline were significant before treatment (ΔFVC: – 9.5% ± 1.3% predicted, $p < 0.001$ [12 months]; – 3.4% ± 0.9% predicted, $p < 0.001$ [6 months]), but not after treatment (ΔFVC: – 1.7% ± 1.3% predicted, $p = 1.000$ [6 months]; – 1.4% ± 1.5% predicted, $p = 0.403$ [12 months]; Fig. 3). The results for the non-advanced group were comparable; however, the changes in FVC at 12 months after treatment were significant (– 3.5% ± 1.7% predicted, $p = 0.043$). The adjusted differences in TLC showed a trend similar to that of FVC in both groups; however, the differences in DLco from baseline were significant before and after treatment.

Disease progression

In the total cohort, a significant reduction in the rate of disease progression was observed after treatment (61.1% [before] vs. 33.3% [after], $p = 0.008$; Fig. 4). Similar trends were observed in the advanced group (78.9% vs. 9.1%, $p < 0.001$); however, a numerical improvement after treatment was only observed in the non-advanced group (51.4% vs. 41.2%, $p = 0.472$). Compared with the non-advanced group, the rate of disease progression in the advanced group was significantly higher (78.9% [advanced] vs. 51.4% [non-advanced], $p = 0.048$) before

Table 1 Comparison of the baseline characteristics between the advanced and non-advanced idiopathic pulmonary fibrosis groups

Characteristic	Total	Advanced	Non-advanced	*P*-value
Number of patients	108	51	57	
Age, years	66.7 ± 7.9	66.4 ± 8.6	68.2 ± 7.2	0.236
Male	86 (79.6)	39 (76.5)	47 (82.5)	0.441
Smoking status				0.027
Never smoker	25 (23.1)	16 (31.4)	9 (15.8)	
Former smoker	79 (73.1)	35 (68.6)	44 (77.2)	
Current smoker	4 (3.7)	0 (0.0)	4 (7.0)	
Body mass index, kg/m^2	23.3 ± 3.2	22.7 ± 3.4	24.2 ± 2.7	0.018
Time since diagnosis, months	39.7 ± 32.0	41.2 ± 35.3	38.9 ± 29.1	0.709
Comorbidities				
Diabetes mellitus	22 (20.4)	9 (17.6)	13 (22.8)	0.506
Cardiovascular disease	11 (10.2)	4 (7.8)	7 (12.3)	0.447
Cerebrovascular disease	4 (3.7)	3 (5.9)	1 (1.8)	0.642
Chronic liver disease	3 (2.8)	2 (3.9)	1 (1.8)	0.601
Pulmonary function test				
FVC, % predicted	56.2 ± 15.1	46.8 ± 9.5	65.3 ± 13.5	< 0.001
DLco, % predicted	35.7 ± 12.6	27.1 ± 9.8	43.6 ± 9.4	< 0.001
TLC, % predicted	58.0 ± 12.2	50.8 ± 7.6	65.0 ± 11.5	< 0.001
6MWT				
Distance, m	341.2 ± 122.5	275.0 ± 107.4	411.9 ± 96.4	< 0.001
Lowest SaO_2, %	84.2 ± 5.3	82.8 ± 4.8	87.4 ± 4.8	< 0.001
SPAP, mmHg[a]	36.4 ± 1.1	38.8 ± 13.0	34.2 ± 9.2	0.039
Previous treatment				
Pirfenidone	20 (18.5)	10 (19.3)	10 (17.5)	0.783
Prednisolone	17 (15.7)	13 (25.5)	4 (7.0)	0.008
Immunosuppressants	11 (10.2)	9 (17.6)	2 (3.5)	0.015
N-Acetylcysteine	5 (4.6)	0 (0.0)	5 (8.8)	0.059
None	66 (60.6)	26 (51.0)	40 (70.2)	0.041

Data are presented as mean ± standard deviation or number (%), unless otherwise indicated
FVC Forced vital capacity, *DLco* Diffusing capacity of the lung for carbon monoxide, *TLC* Total lung capacity, *6MWT* 6 min walk test, *SaO_2* Saturation of oxygen, *SPAP* Estimated systolic pulmonary arterial pressure
[a]Measured by echocardiography

treatment and lower (9.1% vs. 41.2%, $p = 0.050$) after treatment.

Adverse events

Of the 108 patients who received at least one dose of nintedanib, 97.2% experienced AEs (Table 2). The most frequent AE was diarrhoea (50.0%), followed by anorexia (45.4%), nausea/vomiting (24.1%), dyspepsia (18.5%) and cough (18.5%). No difference in the incidence of AEs was observed between the advanced and non-advanced groups (98.0% vs. 95.5%, $p = 1.000$). The advanced group had a lower frequency of diarrhea (37.3% vs. 61.4%, $p = 0.012$) and a higher frequency of nausea/vomiting (33.3% vs. 15.8%, $p = 0.033$) than the non-advanced group; however, no inter-group differences were found in terms of the OR in the occurrence of AEs after adjustment for treatment duration (Additional file 1: Table S2). The median time-of-onset for AEs was 4.3 weeks (IQR: 1.6–11.7 weeks), and no inter-group difference was observed between the advanced and non-advanced groups (3.9 vs. 4.9 weeks, $p = 0.373$), except for anorexia (5.0 weeks vs. 17.6 weeks, $p = 0.042$; Additional file 1: Table S3).

Serious adverse events

SAEs were reported in 54.6% of patients in the cohort. The most common SAE was pneumonia (27.8%; Table 3). Cardiac disorders occurred in three patients (2.8%): acute myocardial infarction, stable angina, and atrial fibrillation. No inter-group differences in the incidence of SAEs (62.7% [advanced] vs. 47.4% [non-advanced], $p = 0.109$)

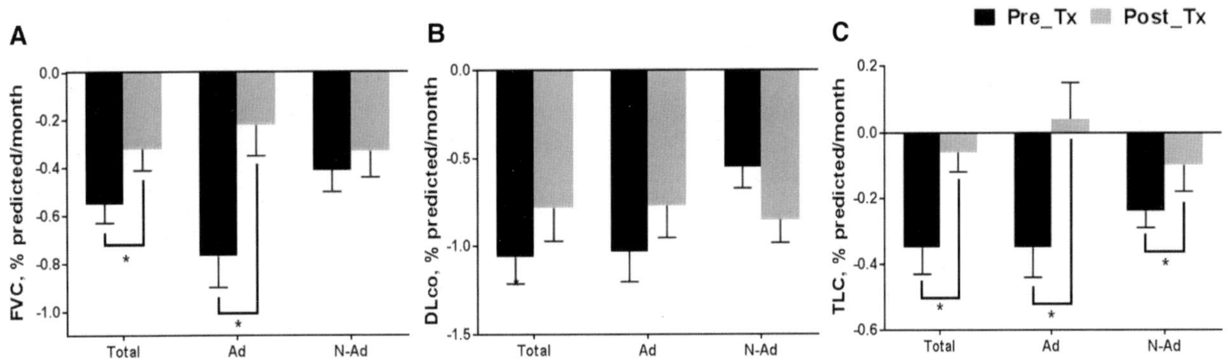

Fig. 2 Rate of decline in lung function before and after treatment. **a** The rate of decline in FVC before and after treatment. **b** The rate of decline in DLco before and after treatment. **c** The rate of decline in TLC before and after treatment. Each bar and line represent the mean and standard deviation. *$p < 0.05$. Total, total patients; Ad, advanced group; N-Ad, non-advanced group; Pre_Tx, before treatment; Post_Tx, after treatment; FVC, forced vital capacity; DLco, diffusing capacity of the lung for carbon monoxide; TLC, total lung capacity

and the adjusted OR for SAEs were observed. However, the patients in the advanced subgroup had a tendency for a higher risk of pneumothorax (OR: 8.611, 95% CI: 0.851–87.135, $p = 0.068$; Additional file 1: Table S4).

Treatment discontinuation

Of the 105 patients who experienced AEs, 53.3% permanently discontinued treatment because of AEs (Table 4). Of all the patients who experienced AEs, 33.3% maintained treatment at the same dosage, 4.8% received a transient dose reduction, and 8.6% received a permanent dose reduction. The most frequent reasons for permanent discontinuation were disease progression (42.9%), anorexia (16.1%), and weight loss (10.7%; Table 5). The number of patients who permanently discontinued treatment as a result of AEs was significantly higher in the advanced group than in the non-advanced group (68.0% vs. 40.0%, $p = 0.004$; Table 4). However, with the exception of a high rate of anorexia in the advanced group (23.5% vs. 4.5%, $p = 0.074$; Table 5), no inter-group differences were found in the reasons for permanent discontinuation.

Discussion

In the present study, nintedanib reduced the lung function decline in patients with IPF in a real-world setting. A comparable reduction in the decline of lung function was observed in the advanced and non-advanced groups. The majority of patients experienced AEs, and thus, half of these individuals were discontinued from treatment. In most cases, this was a result of disease progression. The frequency of AEs in the advanced group was similar to that in the non-advanced group. However, a higher frequency of treatment interruption was observed in the advanced group, mainly as a result of disease progression.

Data from phase 3 trials have indicated that nintedanib may be effective for the treatment of IPF, regardless of lung function [10–12]. However, these trials excluded patients with severely impaired lung function (FVC < 50% predicted or DLco < 30% predicted) [8] and the updated guidelines suggested that future trials should focus on this group of patients [1]. The present results showed that nintedanib delayed the decline in the lung function of patients with advanced IPF to an extent comparable with that observed in non-advanced cases. This is consistent with the results of previous studies [9, 18]. In a subgroup analysis of INPULSIS-ON, the absolute mean change in FVC from baseline to week 48 in patients ($n = 24$) with baseline FVC ≤ 50% predicted was similar to that in those ($n = 558$) with baseline FVC > 50% predicted (– 62.3 vs. -87.9 mL), which suggested that nintedanib may have a similar effect on disease progression in patients with advanced disease and those with less advanced disease [9]. A recent retrospective observational study, in 94 patients with IPF treated with nintedanib, also showed that median changes in FVC after 12 months were not different (Δ FVC: -6.52 vs. -2.60% predicted, $p = 0.56$) between patients with baseline FVC < 50% predicted ($n = 9$) and > 50% predicted ($n = 48$) [18]. However, the number of patients with advanced IPF was small [9, 18] and the efficacy analysis was descriptive [9]. The present study has therefore generated more robust evidence for the significant stabilising effect of nintedanib on the decline in lung function in patients with advanced IPF.

The present data indicated that nintedanib may be more effective for patients in the advanced group than for those in the non-advanced group. The rate of decline of FVC was significantly higher in the advanced group than in the non-advanced group before treatment, but this difference was not observed after treatment. A significant stabilisation of the FVC decline rate and a reduction in the rate of disease progression after treatment

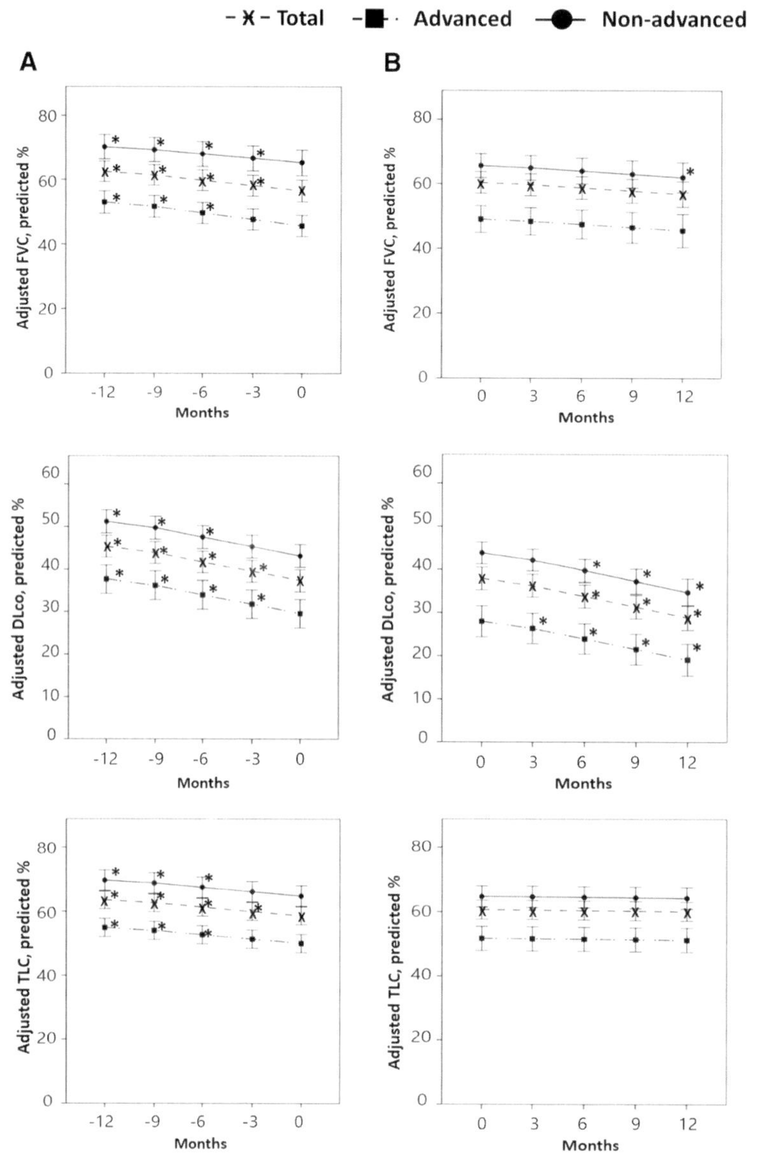

Fig. 3 Adjusted changes in lung function before and after treatment. **a** Serial adjusted changes in FVC, DLco, and TLC before treatment. **b** Serial adjusted changes in FVC, DLco, and TLC after treatment. Each dot and error bar represent the mean and 95% confidence interval. *$p < 0.05$ (compared with baseline values). Total, total patients; FVC, forced vital capacity; DLco, diffusing capacity of the lung for carbon monoxide; TLC, total lung capacity

were also observed in the advanced group, but not in the non-advanced group. Previous reports supported our findings [10, 18]. In a pooled analysis of the INPULSIS trial, the results of the prespecified subgroup analyses (baseline FVC ≤ 70% predicted vs. > 70% predicted) suggested a more profound effect of the treatment in the advanced group for acute exacerbation (hazard ratio: 0.52 [≤ 70% predicted] vs. 1.00 [> 70% predicted], $p = 0.175$) and change from baseline in St. George's Respiratory Questionnaire (difference in the adjusted changes between nintedanib and placebo: − 3.34 vs. -0.34, $p = 0.063$). Tzouvelekis et al. also demonstrated that the change in FVC after 12 months of treatment was significantly lower in patients with baseline FVC < 80% predicted than in those without (Δ FVC: 1.42% vs. -10.11% predicted, $p = 0.03$) [18]. In addition, previous studies suggested that pirfenidone, another antifibrotic agent used in the treatment of IPF, may be more effective in patients with a greater impairment of lung function, because they cause a greater decline in lung function before treatment [19–21]. Therefore, the absence of a significant reduction in the rate of decline of FVC or disease progression in the non-advanced group may be a result of the modest decrease in FVC before treatment; however, the rate of decline in TLC and the adjusted mean changes from baseline in FVC and

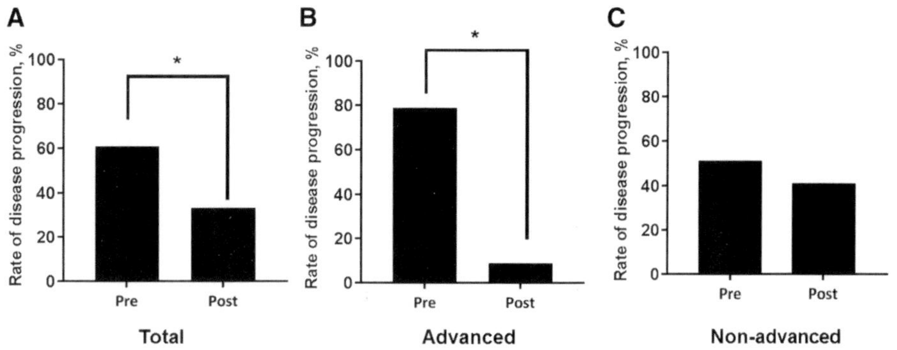

Fig. 4 Categorical changes in lung function before and after treatment. **a** Total cohort; **b** Advanced group; **c** Non-advanced group. Disease progression was defined as a ≥ 10% absolute decline in FVC over 12 months. Pre, pre-treatment; Post, post-treatment

TLC was significantly reduced after treatment in this group.

Although a significant reduction in the decline of FVC and TLC was observed in the present cohort, no such reduction was observed for DLco. The decline in DLco is an indicator of poor prognosis in IPF [2, 22]. However, DLco is also associated with pulmonary hypertension [22, 23]. Pulmonary hypertension is prevalent in patients with advanced IPF [24, 25]. Compared with the previous cohorts [8], patients in the present study had poor lung function (FVC: 79.5–80.0% vs. 56.2% predicted, DLco: 47–47.8% vs. 35.7% predicted), and one-third of the patients had suspected pulmonary hypertension (Table 1).

The incidence of AEs in the present cohort was similar to that reported in previous research (95.3% vs. 94.5–96.4%) [8]. Comparable rates were found for diarrhoea (61.5% vs. 61.5–63.2%), nausea (24.3% vs. 22.7–26.1%) and upper respiratory infection (9.0% vs. 9.1%). However, anorexia was more frequent in the present study (45.4% vs. 8.4–12.4%). Our findings reflect the real-world experience, and other studies of patients with IPF treated with nintedanib within a compassionate use programme have generated similar results (19.1–38.7%) [18, 26, 27]. Real-world studies [18, 26] usually include patients with more severely impaired lung function (FVC: 64–68% vs. 79.5–80.0% predicted) than phase 3 trials [8]. A previous study suggested that a high Gender-Age-Physiology score and a

Table 2 Comparison of adverse events between the advanced and non-advanced idiopathic pulmonary fibrosis groups

Characteristic	Total	Advanced	Non-advanced	*P*-value
Number of patients	108	51	57	
Adverse events	105 (97.2)	50 (98.0)	55 (95.5)	1.000
Diarrhoea	54 (50.0)	19 (37.3)	35 (61.4)	0.012
< 4 times/day	38 (35.2)	15 (29.4)	23 (4.0)	0.264
4–6 times/day	13 (12.0)	2 (3.9)	11 (19.3)	0.014
> 6 times/day	3 (2.8)	2 (3.9)	1 (1.8)	0.601
Anorexia	49 (45.4)	27 (52.9)	22 (38.6)	0.135
Nausea/vomiting	26 (24.1)	17 (33.3)	9 (15.8)	0.033
Dyspepsia	20 (18.5)	8 (15.7)	12 (21.1)	0.541
Cough	20 (18.5)	9 (17.6)	11 (19.3)	0.825
Dyspnoea	16 (14.8)	10 (19.6)	6 (10.5)	0.185
Weight loss	16 (14.8)	8 (15.7)	8 (14.0)	0.809
General weakness	14 (13.0)	9 (17.6)	5 (8.8)	0.170
Upper respiratory infection	11 (10.2)	4 (7.8)	7 (12.3)	0.447
Hepatotoxicity				
> 3× ULN	9 (8.3)	6 (11.8)	3 (5.3)	0.302
> 5× ULN	4 (3.7)	3 (5.9)	1 (1.8)	0.342

Data are presented as numbers (%), unless otherwise indicated
ULN Upper limit of normal

Table 3 Comparison of serious adverse events between the advanced and non-advanced idiopathic pulmonary fibrosis groups

Characteristic	Total	Advanced	Non-advanced	*P*-value
Number of patients	108	51	57	
Serious adverse events	59 (54.6)	32 (62.7)	27 (47.4)	0.109
Pneumonia	30 (27.8)	16 (31.4)	14 (24.6)	0.430
Acute exacerbation	9 (8.3)	5 (9.8)	4 (7.0)	0.732
Pneumothorax	6 (5.6)	5 (9.8)	1 (1.8)	0.098
Lung cancer	4 (3.7)	1 (2.0)	3 (5.3)	0.620
Pulmonary thromboembolism	3 (2.8)	1 (2.0)	2 (3.5)	1.000
Cardiac disorders[a]	3 (2.8)	1 (2.0)	2 (3.5)	1.000
Cerebral vascular disease	1 (0.9)	1 (2.0)	0 (0.0)	0.472
Death	18 (16.7)	11 (21.6)	7 (12.3)	0.196
Pneumonia	10 (9.3)	7 (13.7)	3 (5.3)	0.186
Acute exacerbation	2 (1.9)	0 (0.0)	2 (1.9)	0.497
Severe liver injury[b]	1 (0.9)	0 (0.0)	1 (1.8)	1.000
Cancer progression	1 (0.9)	1 (2.0)	0 (0.0)	0.472
Myocardial infarction	1 (0.9)	0 (0.0)	1 (1.8)	1.000
Unknown	3 (2.8)	1 (2.0)	2 (3.5)	1.000

Data are presented as numbers (%), unless otherwise indicated
[a]Includes acute myocardial infarction, stable angina and atrial fibrillation
[b]Defined as an aspartate transaminase or alanine transaminase level of > 5× the upper normal limit or presence of hepatic failure

lower performance status were associated with the development of nausea or anorexia during the treatment of patients with IPF with nintedanib [28]. Concurrent medication may also contribute to the more frequent occurrence of anorexia in the real-world setting.

In the present study, the rate of diarrhea was higher in the non-advanced group than in the advanced group. This finding may be attributable to the higher exposure to nintedanib in the non-advanced group, which included more patients without dose modification and administered a longer duration of treatment. To minimize the difference in treatment duration between the two groups, we estimated adjusted ORs for AEs, and no significant difference in the risk of AEs was observed between the advanced and non-advanced groups. This finding was consistent with that of a previous report, which showed no significant difference in the rate of adverse reactions to nintedanib between advanced (FVC < 50% predicted or diffusing capacity < 30% predicted) and non-advanced groups [29].

Pneumonia was the most common serious adverse event in the present study, but the frequency was not different between the advanced and non-advanced groups. In the INPULSIS trials, the frequency of infection (56.3% [nintedanib] vs. 53.9% [placebo]) was also similar in both the nintedanib and placebo groups, which suggested that nintedanib was not associated with pneumonia [30]. In our study, the frequency of pneumonia was higher than in other study (27.8% vs. 3.1%) [31]. This result may be due to lower BMI of the patients in our study (BMI: 23.3 vs. 27.5 kg/m^2) [31], and being underweight is generally associated with an increased risk of community acquired pneumonia (odds ratios 1.04–2.20) [32]. No inter-group difference was found in the risk of SAEs. However, the advanced group showed a

Table 4 Comparison of treatment interruption due to adverse events between the advanced and non-advanced idiopathic pulmonary fibrosis groups

Characteristic	Total	Advanced	Non-advanced	*P*-value
Number of patients	105	50	55	
Administration without dose reduction	35 (33.3)	10 (20.0)	25 (45.5)	0.006
AEs leading to transient dose reduction	5 (4.8)	0 (0.0)	5 (4.8)	0.058
AEs leading to permanent dose reduction	9 (8.6)	6 (12.0)	3 (5.5)	0.304
AEs leading to permanent discontinuation	56 (53.3)	34 (68.0)	22 (40.0)	0.004

Data are presented as number (%), unless otherwise indicated
AEs Adverse events

Table 5 Comparison of reasons for drug interruption due to adverse events between the advanced and non-advanced idiopathic pulmonary fibrosis groups

Characteristic	Total	Advanced	Non-advanced	*P*-value
Number of patients	56 (100.0)	34 (100.0)	22 (100.0)	
Disease progression[a]	24 (42.9)	16 (47.1)	8 (36.4)	0.430
Anorexia	9 (16.1)	8 (23.5)	1 (4.5)	0.074
Weight loss	6 (10.7)	2 (5.9)	4 (18.2)	0.198
General weakness	6 (10.7)	5 (14.7)	1 (4.5)	0.386
Diarrhoea	5 (8.9)	2 (5.9)	3 (13.6)	0.371
Nausea/vomiting	5 (8.9)	2 (5.9)	3 (13.6)	0.371
Pulmonary thromboembolism	3 (5.4)	1 (2.9)	2 (9.1)	0.555
Pneumonia	2 (3.6)	2 (5.9)	0 (0.0)	0.514

Data are presented as numbers (%), unless otherwise indicated
[a]Includes disease worsening, acute exacerbation and death

tendency for a higher risk of pneumothorax (OR: 8.611; $p = 0.068$). In a recent study, pneumothorax in patients with IPF was associated with disease severity (presence of extensive reticular abnormalities) and poor outcome (hazard ratio, 2.85; $p = 0.006$) [33].

Compared with previous studies [8, 29, 34], the rate of discontinuation because of AEs in the present cohort was high (19–26.3% vs. 53.0%), which may be attributable to the severe disease status of a large proportion of the cohort. This was also consistent with the finding that disease progression was the most common cause of drug discontinuation. Diarrhea led to premature discontinuation in 4.6% of patients, which was consistent with findings from other phase 3 trials (4.3–4.5%). However, discontinuation owing to anorexia occurred more frequently in the present cohort (8.3% vs. 1.2–1.6%) [8]. The high discontinuation rate owing to anorexia in Asian patients in the INPULSIS trials (3.1% vs. 1.2–1.6%) [35] is an indication that racial or cultural differences may contribute to these findings. The number of patients that were permanently discontinued from the study owing to AEs was significantly higher in the advanced group than in the non-advanced group. This was consistent with a previous report, which found that a higher proportion of patients with FVC ≤ 50% predicted discontinued treatment owing to AEs (41.5% vs. 22.5%) and disease progression (17.1% vs. 5.4%) than patients with FVC > 50% predicted [9]. Low body weight is a factor that increases the exposure to nintedanib at equal doses [36]; therefore, the high treatment discontinuation rate in the advanced group may be related to this factor.

The present study has some limitations. First, the study was performed at a single center and included patients with varying disease severities and comorbidities. However, the demographic features and lung function of the cohort were comparable with those of other studies, and systematic history collection, physical examination and blood tests for possible AEs were performed on all patients at follow-up visits. Second, the number of patients was relatively small and patients in the advanced group were more frequently excluded from the efficacy analysis than those in the non-advanced group. Thus, there is a possibility of selection bias because the remaining patients might be better responders to treatment after the exclusion of patients who had difficulties performing pulmonary function tests or died. However, because the number of patients excluded was not large ($n = 6$), these effects would not have a significant impact on the overall results. Third, the study lacked a control group. However, a previous randomised placebo-controlled trial showed that nintedanib effectively reduced lung function decline in patients with non-advanced IPF [8].

Conclusions

In conclusion, the present data suggest that nintedanib may stabilise lung function decline in patients with IPF treated in the real-world setting, irrespective of baseline lung function. The efficacy and safety profiles of nintedanib in the advanced group were comparable to those in the non-advanced group. Nintedanib could therefore represent a treatment option for patients with advanced IPF, especially those who are not candidates for lung transplantation. Further large-scale studies are warranted to confirm the present findings.

Additional file

Additional file 1: Table S1. Inclusion and exclusion criteria of the named patient use programme for nintedanib. IPF, idiopathic pulmonary fibrosis; ATS, American Thoracic Society; ERS, European Respiratory Society; JRS, Japanese Respiratory Society; ALAT, Latin American Thoracic Association; AST, aspartate aminotransferase; ALT, alanine aminotransferase; INR, international normalised ratio. **Table S2.** Odds ratios for the development of adverse events, adjusted for treatment duration, in the advanced group compared with the non-advanced idiopathic pulmonary fibrosis group. OR, odds ratio; CI, confidence interval. * Compared with the non-advanced group. **Table S3.** Comparison of time-to-occurrence of adverse events between the advanced and non-advanced idiopathic pulmonary fibrosis groups. Data are presented as median [interquartile range, weeks], unless otherwise indicated. URI, upper respiratory infection. **Table S4.** Odds ratios for the development of serious adverse events, adjusted for treatment duration, in the advanced group compared with the non-advanced idiopathic pulmonary fibrosis group. OR, odds ratio; CI, confidence interval. * Compared with the non-advanced group. (DOCX 24 kb)

Abbreviations

AEs: Adverse events; ATS: American Thoracic Society; BMI: Body mass index; CI: Confidence interval; DLco: Diffusing capacity of the lung for carbon monoxide; FGFs: Fibroblast growth factors; FVC: Forced vital capacity; IPF: Idiopathic pulmonary fibrosis; IQR: Interquartile range; OR: Odds ratio; PDGFs: Platelet-derived growth factors; SAEs: Serious AEs; SD: Standard deviation; TLC: Total lung capacity

Funding

This study was supported by a grant of the Basic Science Research Program through the National Research Foundation of Korea (NRF) funded by the Ministry of Science and ICT (NRF-2016R1A2B4016318). The funding sources were not involved in the study design, analysis or interpretation of data, or the decision to submit the manuscript for publication.

Authors' contributions

HYY and JWS accept full responsibility for the content of the manuscript, including the data and the analyses. JWS made substantial contributions to the conception and design of the study. HYY, SJP, and JWS made substantial contributions to the analysis and interpretation of the data. HYY, SJP, and JWS drafted the initial manuscript. All authors have discussed the results, reviewed, and approved the final manuscript.

Competing interests

The authors declare that they have no competing interests.

References

1. Raghu G, Collard HR, Egan JJ, Martinez FJ, Behr J, Brown KK, Colby TV, Cordier J-F, Flaherty KR, Lasky JA. An official ATS/ERS/JRS/ALAT statement: idiopathic pulmonary fibrosis: evidence-based guidelines for diagnosis and management. Am J Respir Crit Care Med. 2011;183:788–824.
2. Ley B, Collard HR, King TE. Clinical course and prediction of survival in idiopathic pulmonary fibrosis. Am J Respir Crit Care Med. 2011;183:431–40.
3. Coward WR, Saini G, Jenkins G. The pathogenesis of idiopathic pulmonary fibrosis. Ther Adv Respir Dis. 2010;4:367–88.
4. Allen JT, Spiteri MA. Growth factors in idiopathic pulmonary fibrosis: relative roles. Respir Res. 2001;3:1.
5. Hilberg F, Roth GJ, Krssak M, Kautschitsch S, Sommergruber W, Tontsch-Grunt U, Garin-Chesa P, Bader G, Zoephel A, Quant J. BIBF 1120: triple angiokinase inhibitor with sustained receptor blockade and good antitumor efficacy. Cancer Res. 2008;68:4774–82.
6. Wollin L, Wex E, Pautsch A, Schnapp G, Hostettler KE, Stowasser S, Kolb M. Mode of action of nintedanib in the treatment of idiopathic pulmonary fibrosis. Eur Respir J. 2015. https://doi.org/10.1183/09031936.00174914.
7. Richeldi L, Costabel U, Selman M, Kim DS, Hansell DM, Nicholson AG, Brown KK, Flaherty KR, Noble PW, Raghu G. Efficacy of a tyrosine kinase inhibitor in idiopathic pulmonary fibrosis. N Engl J Med. 2011;365:1079–87.
8. Richeldi L, du Bois RM, Raghu G, Azuma A, Brown KK, Costabel U, Cottin V, Flaherty KR, Hansell DM, Inoue Y. Efficacy and safety of nintedanib in idiopathic pulmonary fibrosis. N Engl J Med. 2014;370:2071–82.
9. Wuyts WA, Kolb M, Stowasser S, Stansen W, Huggins JT, Raghu G. First data on efficacy and safety of Nintedanib in patients with idiopathic pulmonary fibrosis and forced vital capacity of≤ 50% of predicted value. Lung. 2016;194:739–43.
10. Costabel U, Inoue Y, Richeldi L, Collard HR, Tschoepe I, Stowasser S, Azuma A. Efficacy of Nintedanib in idiopathic pulmonary fibrosis across Prespecified subgroups in INPULSIS. Am J Respir Crit Care Med. 2016;193:178–85.
11. Maher TM, Flaherty KR, Noble PW, Vancheri C, Wuyts WA, Kimura T, Hallmann C, Stowasser S, Richeldi L. Effect of baseline FVC on lung function decline with nintedanib in patients with IPF. Eur Respir J. 2015;46:OA4499.
12. Kolb M, Richeldi L, Behr J, Maher TM, Tang W, Stowasser S, Hallmann C, du Bois RM. Nintedanib in patients with idiopathic pulmonary fibrosis and preserved lung volume. Thorax. 2017;72(4):340–6.
13. Miller MR, Hankinson J, Brusasco V, Burgos F, Casaburi R, Coates A, Crapo R, Enright P, Van Der Grinten C, Gustafsson P. Standardisation of spirometry. Eur Respir J. 2005;26:319–38.
14. Macintyre N, Crapo R, Viegi G, Johnson D, Van Der Grinten C, Brusasco V, Burgos F, Casaburi R, Coates A, Enright P. Standardisation of the single-breath determination of carbon monoxide uptake in the lung. Eur Respir J. 2005;26:720–35.
15. Miller MR, Hankinson J, Brusasco V, Burgos F, Casaburi R, Coates A, Crapo R, Enright P, van der Grinten CP, Gustafsson P, et al. Standardisation of spirometry. Eur Respir J. 2005;26:319–38.
16. the ATS Committee on Proficiency Standards for Clinical Pulmonary Function Laboratories. ATS statement: guidelines for the six-minute walk test. Am J Respir Crit Care Med. 2002;166:111–7.
17. Collard HR, Moore BB, Flaherty KR, Brown KK, Kaner RJ, King TE, Lasky JA, Loyd JE, Noth I, Olman MA, et al. Acute exacerbations of idiopathic pulmonary fibrosis. Am J Respir Crit Care Med. 2007;176:636–43.
18. Tzouvelekis A, Karampitsakos T, Kontou M, Granitsas A, Malliou I, Anagnostopoulos A, Ntolios P, Tzilas V, Bouros E, Steiropoulos P, et al. Safety and efficacy of nintedanib in idiopathic pulmonary fibrosis: a real-life observational study in Greece. Pulm Pharmacol Ther. 2018;49:61–6.
19. Harari S, Caminati A, Albera C, Vancheri C, Poletti V, Pesci A, Luppi F, Saltini C, Agostini C, Bargagli E, et al. Efficacy of pirfenidone for idiopathic pulmonary fibrosis: an Italian real life study. Respir Med. 2015;109:904–13.
20. Okuda R, Hagiwara E, Baba T, Kitamura H, Kato T, Ogura T. Safety and efficacy of pirfenidone in idiopathic pulmonary fibrosis in clinical practice. Respir Med. 2013;107:1431–7.
21. Tzouvelekis A, Ntolios P, Karampitsakos T, Tzilas V, Anevlavis S, Bouros E, Steiropoulos P, Koulouris N, Stratakos G, Froudarakis M, Bouros D. Safety and efficacy of pirfenidone in severe idiopathic pulmonary fibrosis: a real-world observational study. Pulm Pharmacol Ther. 2017;46:48–53.
22. Hamada K, Nagai S, Tanaka S, Handa T, Shigematsu M, Nagao T, Mishima M, Kitaichi M, Izumi T. Significance of pulmonary arterial pressure and diffusion capacity of the lung as prognosticator in patients with idiopathic pulmonary fibrosis. Chest. 2007;131:650–6.
23. Nathan SD, Shlobin OA, Ahmad S, Urbanek S, Barnett SD. Pulmonary hypertension and pulmonary function testing in idiopathic pulmonary fibrosis. Chest. 2007;131:657–63.
24. Nathan SD, Shlobin OA, Ahmad S, Koch J, Barnett SD, Ad N, Burton N, Leslie K. Serial development of pulmonary hypertension in patients with idiopathic pulmonary fibrosis. Respiration. 2008;76:288–94.
25. Nadrous HF, Pellikka PA, Krowka MJ, Swanson KL, Chaowalit N, Decker PA, Ryu JH. The impact of pulmonary hypertension on survival in patients with idiopathic pulmonary fibrosis. Chest. 2005;128:616s–7s.
26. Bonella F, Kreuter M, Hagmeyer L, Neurohr C, Keller C, Kohlhaeufl MJ, Muller-Quernheim J, Milger K, Prasse A. Insights from the German compassionate use program of Nintedanib for the treatment of idiopathic pulmonary fibrosis. Respiration. 2016;92:98–106.
27. Toellner H, Hughes G, Beswick W, Crooks MG, Donaldson C, Forrest I, Hart SP, Leonard C, Major M, Simpson AJ, Chaudhuri N. Early clinical experiences with nintedanib in three UK tertiary interstitial lung disease centres. Clin Transl Med. 2017;6:41.

28. Kato M, Kono K, Yamada T, Kanemaru R, Ihara H, Sato T, Harada N, Togo S, Nagaoka T, Takahashi F, et al. Risk factors of nausea or anorexia following nintedanib administration in patients with idiopathic pulmonary fibrosis. In: A42 ILD SCIENTIFIC ABSTRACTS: TREATMENT AND ACUTE EXACERBATION; 2018. p. A1643.
29. Galli JA, Pandya A, Vega-Olivo M, Dass C, Zhao H, Criner GJ. Pirfenidone and nintedanib for pulmonary fibrosis in clinical practice: tolerability and adverse drug reactions. Respirology. 2017;22:1171–8.
30. Corte T, Bonella F, Crestani B, Demedts MG, Richeldi L, Coeck C, Pelling K, Quaresma M, Lasky JA. Safety, tolerability and appropriate use of nintedanib in idiopathic pulmonary fibrosis. Respir Res. 2015;16:116.
31. Brunnemer E, Walscher J, Tenenbaum S, Hausmanns J, Schulze K, Seiter M, Heussel CP, Warth A, Herth FJF, Kreuter M. Real-world experience with Nintedanib in patients with idiopathic pulmonary fibrosis. Respiration. 2018; 95:301–9.
32. Torres A, Peetermans WE, Viegi G, Blasi F. Risk factors for community-acquired pneumonia in adults in Europe: a literature review. Thorax. 2013; 68:1057–65.
33. Nishimoto K, Fujisawa T, Yoshimura K, Enomoto Y, Enomoto N, Nakamura Y, Inui N, Sumikawa H, Johkoh T, Colby TV, Suda T. The prognostic significance of pneumothorax in patients with idiopathic pulmonary fibrosis. Respirology. 2018;23(5):519–25.
34. Hughes G, Toellner H, Morris H, Leonard C, Chaudhuri N. Real world experiences: Pirfenidone and Nintedanib are effective and well tolerated treatments for idiopathic pulmonary fibrosis. J Clin Med. 2016;5. https://doi.org/10.3390/jcm5090078.
35. Taniguchi H, Xu Z, Azuma A, Inoue Y, Li H, Fujimoto T, Bailes Z, Schlenker-Herceg R, Kim DS. Subgroup analysis of Asian patients in the INPULSIS((R)) trials of nintedanib in idiopathic pulmonary fibrosis. Respirology. 2016;21:1425–30.
36. Schmid U, Doege C, Dallinger C, Freiwald M. Population pharmacokinetics of nintedanib in patients with idiopathic pulmonary fibrosis. Pulm Pharmacol Ther. 2018;48:136–43.

14

Modulation of airway hyperresponsiveness by rhinovirus exposure

Dennis Lo[1], Joshua L. Kennedy[2], Richard C. Kurten[3], Reynold A. Panettieri Jr[1] and Cynthia J. Koziol-White[1*]

Abstract

Rhinovirus (RV) exposure has been implicated in childhood development of wheeze evoking asthma and exacerbations of underlying airways disease. Studies such as the Copenhagen Prospective Studies on Asthma in Childhood (COPSAC) and Childhood Origins of ASThma (COAST) have identified RV as a pathogen inducing severe respiratory disease. RVs also modulate airway hyperresponsiveness (AHR), a key characteristic of such diseases. Although potential factors underlying mechanisms by which RV induces AHR have been postulated, the precise mechanisms of AHR following RV exposure remain elusive.

A challenge to RV-related research stems from inadequate models for study. While human models raise ethical concerns and are relatively difficult in terms of subject recruitment, murine models are limited by susceptibility of infection to the relatively uncommon minor group (RV-B) serotypes, strains that are generally associated with infrequent clinical respiratory virus infections. Although a transgenic mouse strain that has been developed has enhanced susceptibility for infection with the common major group (RV-A) serotypes, few studies have focused on RV in the context of allergic airways disease rather than understanding RV-induced AHR. Recently, the receptor for the virulent RV-C CDHR3, was identified, but a dearth of studies have examined RV-C-induced effects in humans. Currently, the mechanisms by which RV infections modulate airway smooth muscle (ASM) shortening or excitation-contraction coupling remain elusive. Further, only one study has investigated the effects of RV on bronchodilatory mechanisms, with only speculation as to mechanisms underlying RV-mediated modulation of bronchoconstriction.

Keywords: Rhinovirus, Airway Hyperresponsiveness, Airway smooth muscle, Inflammation

Background

In vitro studies - mechanisms of airway hyperresponsiveness

Airway hyperresponsiveness (AHR) is characterized by inflammation and bronchoconstriction in response to nonspecific stimuli [1] and is a key characteristic of chronic lung disorders such as asthma and chronic obstructive pulmonary disease (COPD). Exposure to environmental toxins has been an important area of study with respect to AHR. For instance, findings by Jude et al. [2] suggested that formaldehyde, an air pollutant, induced AHR in human airway smooth muscle (HASM) cells by altering contractile pathways in the cell. Ozone, another common pollutant, can induce AHR in human lung explants and ASM cells [3–5]. After toxicant exposure, cytokines liberated from airway structural cells or trafficking leukocytes modulate bronchomotor tone. Cooper et al. [6] demonstrated that human lung explants incubated with interleukin (IL)-13 exhibited AHR; other studies similarly found enhanced contractility after IL-13 exposure in HASM [7–9]. Studies by Amrani et al. [10] and Hotta et al. [11] have also implicated tumor necrosis factor-α (TNF-α) in the induction of enhanced ASM contractility. Respiratory pathogens have also gained attention as inducers of AHR. However, unlike for inflammatory cytokines, mechanisms whereby viral infection, specifically rhinovirus (RV), does this is subject to debate and largely have not been elucidated.

Evidence of RV-induced AHR

Over the past few decades, RVs, the viruses precipitating the common cold, have been recognized as important pathogens in the development of wheeze leading to asthma and exacerbation of chronic respiratory disease.

* Correspondence: cjk167@rbhs.rutgers.edu
[1]Department of Medicine, Rutgers Institute for Translational Medicine and Science, Rutgers University, New Brunswick, NJ, USA
Full list of author information is available at the end of the article

Evidence supports that RVs are the most prevalent respiratory viruses among patients with wheeze and asthma, especially in children [12–14]. Additionally, data from the Childhood Origins of ASThma (COAST) and Copenhagen Prospective Studies on Asthma in Childhood (COPSAC), which are high-risk birth cohort studies, established a link between RV-induced wheeze in children and risk/development of asthma [15, 16]. RV infections have also been implicated in exacerbations of asthma [17–20]. RV infection in vivo induces AHR, which is characterized by bronchoconstriction and inflammation of the airways [21–25]. Accordingly, investigators have pursued studies of AHR in non-diseased and asthma/COPD subjects after RV exposure.

Studying molecular mechanisms underlying RV-induced AHR

Current models of RV-induced AHR include murine, single cell culture, cellular co-culture, and human models. Most studies have focused on in vitro systems to characterize inflammatory responses to RV. Infections of epithelial cell monolayers are useful for studying a single cell type, and epithelial cell co-cultures with other cell types have been successfully used to study the immune response [26]. However, even both approaches are incapable of capturing an integrated ex vivo model of cell-cell interaction critical to modeling infection and AHR that have been observed in vivo.

Murine studies provide a platform to study RV infections and AHR, but these studies are limited by species selectivity to minor group RV serotypes. Despite the development of a mouse strain expressing a chimeric intercellular adhesion molecule 1 (ICAM-1) for mouse recognition of RV-A16 [27, 28], what little experimental data exists is framed within the context of an allergic airways disease model rather than focusing on the direct effects of RV-A16 on AHR.

Obtaining approval for experimental RV studies in humans has been challenging, and disease context for asthma is limited to mild severity, leaving many questions left unanswered. Several prospective cross-sectional studies have shown associations between RV infection and asthma inception and exacerbations. However, these studies are limited in their ability to provide mechanisms that lead to AHR. Experimental challenge models in humans provide some opportunity to study AHR in the correct host and in the context of disease. In this review, we will discuss the current models and approaches to evaluate AHR during viral infection and speculate on potential mechanisms of RV-induced AHR as outlined in the known literature to date.

Models of RV-induced AHR

Animal models of RV infection

While human models of RV infection are most relevant, ethical concerns and practical limitations exist where investigators have chosen to use animal models. Yin and Lomax [29] developed a murine model of RV infection that mimics the effects of RV regarding inflammation, AHR, and exacerbations of allergic airways disease. Notable advantages to this model include an intact immune system, ability to genetically manipulate aspects of the immune response to determine the specific role in response to RV, and easy handling [30]. However, limitations lie in the inability to sustain RV titers after 24 h, as well as lack of responsiveness of murine ASM to a variety of bronchoconstrictors [31]. Additionally, many studies regarding acute RV-induced effects in vivo examine RV-B serotypes in mice since RV-A serotypes do not bind mouse ICAM-1 [27, 32] due to lack of homology with human ICAM-1. Studies on RV-B serotypes, however, are not may not be readily translational to human disease given that RV-A and RV-C serotypes have been associated with more severe symptoms in comparison to RV-B serotypes [33–36] and that many clinical studies of RV infection are proportionally skewed towards greater detection of RV-A and RV-C serotypes [20, 37–40].

In 2003, Tuthill et al. [28] developed an in vitro murine model suitable for major group RV (including RV-A16) infection. They achieved infection and replication of RV-A16 in a murine lower epithelial cell line expressing chimeric ICAM-1 with human domains for EC1 and 2. Similarly, Bartlett et al. [27] developed a BALB/c mouse strain transgenic for EC1 and 2 of human ICAM-1 that supports RV-A16 infection, thereby serving as a model that supports both RV-A and RV-B infection [41]. After viral infection, the transgenic mice exhibited replication-dependent features similar to those seen following RV-1B exposure, including airway inflammation, mucin production, and cytokine induction. Further, OVA-sensitized and challenged mice infected with RV-1B showed enhanced airway inflammation and hyper-responsiveness, serving as a murine model for RV-1B-induced allergic asthma exacerbations. A murine model for RV-induced COPD exacerbation was also developed by Singanayagam et al. [42]. Increases in TNF-α, interferon-γ-induced protein-10 (IP-10), and regulated on activation, normal T cell expressed and secreted (RANTES) expression were observed after a single elastase treatment followed by RV-1B infection. However, the translation of these models to human disease is tenuous.

While murine models are useful in elucidating some RV-induced effects in vivo, numerous immunologic differences exist between mice and humans that include differences in proportions of neutrophils and lymphocytes in peripheral blood and differences in Th_1 differentiation [43]. Others have elegantly described the difference between murine and human lymphocytes: human lymphocytes demonstrate greater overlap in Th_1 and Th_2 cytokine profiles compared to murine lymphocytes [44]. Irvin and Bates [45] described anatomical differences between the murine and human lung, including those in lung branching pattern, airway caliber, thickness of epithelium, presence of submucosal glands, etc. Such factors could play a significant role in interpretation and extrapolation of results obtained from murine RV studies to RV studies in humans, making the findings of these studies challenging to translate to humans.

Recently, a cell culture system for RV-C serotypes was developed [46] and the receptor for RV-C serotypes, cadherin-related family member 3 (CDHR3), was identified [47]. The next step is exploring the pathogenic mechanism of RV-C infection in a murine model, possibly through transgenic mice expressing CDHR3. This new model may offer new opportunities in the study of virus-induced AHR.

Airway cell co-culture models of RV infection

Studies have utilized an epithelial cell/airway smooth muscle co-culture model to examine cell-cell interactions in precipitating AHR. Damera et al. [48] found enhanced prostaglandin E_2 in a co-culture of differentiated human airway epithelial and HASM cells after ozone exposure. Others found a 2.5-fold increase in HASM cell numbers in a co-culture with human airway epithelial cells (HAEC) compared to the HASM monolayer [49]. Although these single cell cultures are suitable for investigating secretion of inflammatory or contractile mediators, the monolayer model fails to reproduce the complex interactions of different airway cells in vivo. A co-culture cell model offers perhaps a more appropriate experimental design to study AHR.

Few studies have explored airway co-culture models to study RV infection (Table 1). However, the effects of RV-conditioned media on airway cells has been studied. Van Ly et al. [50] infected primary HAECs with RV for 24 h and observed β_2 adrenoceptor (β_2AR) desensitization in primary HASM after exposure to the RV-induced medium. Similarly, Rajan et al. [51] co-cultured human peripheral blood mononuclear cells (PBMCs) and RV-infected HAEC in a two-chamber trans-well tissue culture system and found increased levels of interferon (IFN) λ2 (also known as IL-28A), IFN-α, monocyte chemoattractant protein (MCP)-2, and macrophage inflammatory protein (MIP)-1β. The synergistic effects of the co-culture model showed elevated levels of IP-10 and MCP-1 in a primary HAEC/human monocyte co-culture after RV exposure [52]. Shariff et al. [53] identified that exposure of medium from RV-infected primary HAECs led to primary ASM chemotaxis, primarily modulated by RANTES. However, the number of studies using

Table 1 Rhinovirus Studies

Method/Study	Advantages	Disadvantages	References
ASM cells	Primary cell modulating AHR and airway tone	Direct infection with RV not likely given architecture of the lung	Hakonarson 1998 [73]; Van Ly 2013 [50], Shariff 2017 [53];
Co-cultures of airway cells	Integrated response of multiple cell types	Few studies elucidating modulation of RV-induced AHR	Korpi-Steiner 2010 [52]; Van Ly 2013 [50]; Rajan 2013 [51]
Clinical isolates	Tissue from infected patients with and without asthma/COPD	Inconsistent findings with respect to susceptibility to infection/ symptoms	Marin 2000 [94]; Corne 2002 [95]; Greene 2002; de Kluijver 2003 [108]; DeMore 2009 [109]; Schneider 2010 [96]; Kennedy 2014 [18]
PCLS	Intact architecture of the lung tissue/airways	No circulating immune cells	Kennedy and Koziol-White 2018 [24]
Murine studies	Easy to manipulate genetically to understand mechanisms of RV-induced AHR	Only susceptible to RV-B infection, a serotype not associated severe RV infections/symptoms. Model with human ICAM-1 limited to RV infection in the context of allergic airways disease.	Tuthill 2003 [28]; Bartlett 2008 [27]; Meurs 2008 [31]; Calvo 2009 [34]; Lau 2009 [35]; Miller 2009 [36]; Bizzintino 2011 [33]
Pediatric in vivo studies	• Correlation between RV exposure and wheeze in a large population of pediatric subjects. • Identification of potential targets for abrogation of RV-induced AHR/development of asthma. • Experimental RV challenge to study relationship between IgE levels and exacerbation severity.	• Primarily performed in subjects with European ethnic background. • Little extrapolation to other ethnic groups due to prevalency of polymorphism associated with wheeze.	Lemanske 2002 [16]; Kotaniemi-Syrjänen 2003 [80]; Zambrano 2003 [25]; Bisgaard 2004 [15]; Jackson 2008 [64]; Calişkan 2013 [89]

co-cultures to study airways disease has been limited due to the necessity of air-liquid interface culture as well as primary HAECs. A study by Pezzulo et al. [54] confirmed that the transcriptional profile of differentiated HAECs more closely resembles the human airway epithelium than transformed airway epithelial cell lines. Therefore, the use of primary epithelial cells in co-cultures rather than utilizing transformed epithelial cell lines is the most physiologically relevant system to study the effects of RV.

Ex vivo tissue models of AHR and respiratory virus exposure

Primary airway cell culture and precision cut lung slices (PCLS) are currently used to study effects of a number of lung insults ex vivo (Table 1). While primary cell culture and in vitro co-culture consist of only a few cell types, human PCLS prepared from organ donors consist of many relevant cell types of the respiratory tract situated within their native micro-anatomical environment. Maintaining the in vivo properties of the cultured cells, such as structure, promotes PCLS as an especially suitable model for studying airways disease [26]. For instance, this system also maintains ciliary motility and responsiveness to contractile agonists, including carbachol (CCh), a cholinergic agonist much like methacholine. Kennedy et al. [24] assessed carbachol responsiveness after infection with RV39 in PCLS from donors with a history of asthma. Other viruses have also been studied using this approach. Sun et al. [55] studied the human respiratory syncytial virus (RSV) and found a response to RSV immunostimulatory defective viral genomes (iDVG) in PCLS. Avgousti et al. [56] found that protein VII, a highly basic cellular histone-like protein encoded by adenoviruses, alters cellular chromatin in human PCLS. Furthermore, Kim et al. [57] found that deficiency in melanoma differentiation-associated protein (MDA)-5, a protein that detects motifs in viral oligonucleotides, enhanced constriction in mruine PCLS after infection with Sendai virus. Another study showed incubation of human PCLS with high-concentration poly (I:C) had little effect on contractility but induced secretion of cytokines and chemokines [6].

Despite the relevance of the human PCLS in studying RV-induced AHR, the limited availability of human lung tissue makes animal PCLS a viable alternative. Ressmeyer et al. [58] studied bronchoconstriction in guinea pig PCLS and found similar responsiveness to endogenous mediators when compared to humans. Henjakovic et al. [59] reported that murine PCLS exposed to trimellitic anhydride and DNCB, two allergenic sensitizers, exhibited the same effects as observed in vivo. Furthermore, Fox [60] observed that porcine PCLS shared similar contractile agonist sensitivity with human airways and studied inflammatory mediator secretion by PCLS from the murine model of allergic airways disease.

Clinical models of RV infection

A number of studies have investigated the clinical effects of RV exposure in human subjects in both cross-sectional studies and in human challenge models (Table 1). An early RV challenge study by Grunberg et al. [22] found a decrease in the provocation concentration for a 20% decrease in forced expiratory volume in 1 s (FEV_1) and increases in IL-8 levels in atopic asthmatic subjects with RV-A16. A cross-sectional clinical study found increased AHR to methacholine in children (ages 7–12 with intermittent asthma) with RV-induced asthma during the course of reported colds [61]. These studies confirmed the findings of earlier work by Zambrano et al. [25], which showed increased methacholine sensitivity in highly atopic individuals (ages 18–30, total IgE > 371 IU/mL) during RV-A16 experimental challenge. Proud et al. [62] found significantly increased symptom scores in RV-infected subjects compared to sham-infected controls (in 20 year old subjects), and others have shown increased IL-25 and IL-33 in human subjects (ages 26–36, and ages birth to 6 years old) after experimental RV-A16 infection [63, 64]. Since majority of studies have investigated RV in the context of underlying airways disease, the fundamental mechanisms through which RV modulates AHR remains elusive.

There is evidence for neurogenic inflammation playing a part in both asthma and rhinitis, a hallmark of respiratory tract infections with virus. Such findings suggest that neurokinins and innervation of the airways may play a role in modulating RV-induced AHR via changing the responses of nerves in the airways [65, 66]. A single study of five subjects with colds noted that inhalation of substance P, which stimulates cough responses in guinea pigs following release from the nerves [67], induced cough in normal subjects infected with RV but had little effect on subjects without RV infection [68]. The therapeutic that was effective at diminishing these effects was procaterol, a β_2 adrenergic receptor agonist, which mainly targets airway smooth muscle to induce bronchodilation of the airways. However, this study did not directly test the idea that RV infection induces release of neurokinins into the airways to induce AHR. Thus far, there have been no studies linking neurokinin receptor agonists like substance P to RV-induced AHR, only a putative role for receptors for these agents in respiratory syncytial virus infection in rats [69, 70]. A study by Abdullah et al. shows that RV upregulates transient receptor potential (TRP) channels, which are known to modulate neurogenic signals and have been implicated in cough [71], in neurons. To date no other studies have been performed to expand upon this study, so it is unclear as to whether TRP channels play a role in RV-induced AHR. Additionally, an experimental RV infection model in human subjects noted that RV infection enhanced responsiveness to histamine rather than bradykinin, thereby suggesting that airway sensory nerves may not play much of a role in RV-induced asthma exacerbations [22]. The findings of all of these studies that suggest a role for neurogenic inflammation in RV-induced AHR are difficult to use to establish clinical relevance for the paradigm because: (1) there is significant interspecies variation between human and animal models, and (2) there is a significant amount of afferent sensory innervation variability among human subjects [72].

Understanding mechanisms of RV-induced AHR and ASM cell function

Currently, there is limited understanding of mechanisms by which RV modulates airway contractility. Given that ASM is the pivotal cell modulating bronchomotor tone and hyperreactivity, modulation of contraction and relaxation of this tissue is a logical starting point to discover mechanisms of RV-induced AHR. Upon finding that RV enhanced airway contractile responsiveness and reduced β-agonist isoproterenol efficacy in isolated rabbit and human ASM, Hakonarson et al. [73] found diminished cAMP levels, increased $G_{\alpha i}$ expression, and enhanced ICAM-1 expression on the cell surface of ASM. While an increase in ICAM-1 density on the cell surface can enhance RV binding to improve infection rates, higher $G_{\alpha i}$ expression and lower cAMP level could then contribute to RV-induced airway hyperresponsiveness. As $G_{\alpha i}$ inhibits adenylyl cyclase, cAMP levels diminish and subsequently, Protein Kinase A (PKA) fails to inactivate myosin light chain kinase (MLCK) to induce bronchodilation. According to McGraw et al. [7], increased $G_{\alpha i}$ decreased β_2AR-mediated bronchodilation and M_3-muscarinic receptor (M_3R)-mediated bronchoconstriction in murine ASM. Interestingly, this finding translates to a protective effect with regard to bronchoconstriction in conjunction with reduced effect of $ß_2$AR-agonists. Others postulated that $G_{\alpha i}$ upregulation activates Rho via Rho guanine nucleotide exchange factors (GEFs), that then evokes actin polymerization in ASM (as described in [74–77]). Croxton et al. [78] found that modulation of $G_{\alpha i}$ contributes to Ca^{2+} sensitization in tracheal smooth muscle, thereby potentially increasing airway contractility.

RV-induced effects on ASM excitation-contraction (E-C) coupling

To date, few studies have been conducted examining mechanisms of RV-induced modulation of airway contractility. Hakonarson et al. [79] identified IL-1β to be involved in rabbit and HASM responsiveness following RV exposure. After pretreatment of rabbit tissue with an IL-1 recombinant human receptor antagonist, RV-induced changes in responsiveness were attenuated. Additionally, RV exposure induced IL-1β expression, which was ICAM-1 dependent. According to Van Ly et al. [50], HAECs exposed to RV secreted factors into the media that induced β_2AR desensitization in human ASM through TLR activation of cyclooxygenase-2-induced prostaglandins. Kennedy et al. [24] found that RV39 exposure of non-asthma-derived human precision cut lung slices failed to induce hyperresponsiveness to a contractile agonist, but exposure of asthma-derived lung slices induced hyperresponsiveness of the small airways. Overall some studies suggest potential mechanisms underlying RV-induced AHR; however, more work is needed to thoroughly examine mechanisms of this phenomenon.

Clinical studies: RV and the development of wheeze and AHR

Rhinoviruses have been implicated in the development of wheeze that evokes childhood asthma. Johnston et al. [13] identified RVs induce two thirds of upper respiratory viral infections in children (ages 9–11) with cough/wheeze through a community based longitudinal study. Similarly, RVs were detected in 33% of nasopharyngeal aspirates in children hospitalized for wheezing. In the same study, RV-positive cases were associated with development of asthma (OR = 4.14) while RV-negative cases were not [80]. Notably, it was reported that ~ 90% of children with RV wheezing illness in the third year had developed asthma by the sixth year [64]. The COAST birth cohort study revealed a significant role of RVs in pediatric wheezing illness and development of asthma [81–84]. RV was associated with asthma at 13 years as well as significantly reduced lung function measures compared to measures observed with exposure to other respiratory viruses. In another high-risk cohort study, a statistically significant association between wheezy lower respiratory infection by RV and current asthma, persistent wheeze, and current wheeze was reported [85]. Recently, findings from a meta-analysis confirmed a possible association between RV-induced wheeze in the first 3 years and development of wheeze or asthma [86]. Other factors may co-influence the association between RV and the inception of asthma. Lukkarinen and colleagues studied 127 steroid-naive children with a first episode of wheeze [87]. Subjects were enrolled around 11 months of age and re-evaluated for asthma at age 7 years. The authors found that 37 of these children maintained an asthma diagnosis and were atopic at the follow-up. The risk factors discovered at study enrollment for future atopic asthma included allergic sensitization (OR 12; $p < 0.001$), eczema (OR 4.8; $p = 0.014$), and wheezing with rhinovirus (OR 5.0; $p = 0.035$).

Although the above studies provide strong evidence for a relationship between RV and the development of wheeze/asthma, it was not possible to determine whether RV-induced wheezing precipitates asthma. While the causation relationship is a possibility, another plausible hypothesis is that RV-induced wheeze in infancy is only a sign of predisposition to development of asthma.

Atopy, RV, and wheezing

Atopy is a risk factor that has been implicated in the development of RV-induced exacerbations of asthma. A positive association between IgE sensitization and RV wheezing illness in hospitalized wheezing children was found [88]. In another study, RV-infected children sensitized to allergens exhibited higher odds of wheezing compared to controls [20]. A genetic predisposition toward developing wheeze leading to asthma has also been impugned. A susceptibility locus on the 17q21 chromosome in COAST and COPSAC cohorts was discovered [89]. The 17q21 genotypes were found to have significant association with children with RV wheezing illness but not with those without RV wheezing illness. Interestingly, previous studies (genome-wide association studies in particular) have identified the locus in the 17q21 chromosome to be linked to the development of asthma [90, 91]. However, since the birth cohort study encompassed subjects of primarily European descent, the findings may not be applicable to the general population. Bochkov et al. [47] similarly identified an asthma susceptibility gene product in CDHR3 and proposed that the Tyr_{529} variant at rs6967330 (rs6967330-A) in the *CDHR3* gene is a potential risk factor for RV-C wheezing illness. The $COPSAC_{2010}$ and COAST birth cohorts confirmed the association of the rs6967330-A variant with respiratory episodes with RV-C detection [92]. The 1000 Genomes Projects found rs6967330-A to be most predominant in African populations [92], which report high asthma incidence and morbidity [93].

RV-induced AHR in asthma, COPD, and healthy subjects

RVs have been found to play an important role in the context of chronic respiratory disease. Studies have demonstrated that although healthy patients respond to RV with respiratory symptoms, those with an underlying airways disorder respond to a greater degree when exposed to the same virus/amount of virus. RV RNA was detected in nasopharyngeal swabs of 32.4% of asymptomatic asthmatic children compared to none in controls, implying the persistent presence of RV in asthmatics [94]. Others found that subjects with asthma were not more susceptible to RV infection than controls but exhibited more severe and longer-lasting lower respiratory symptoms [95]. Similarly, elevated baseline cytokine levels in primary COPD-derived epithelial cells appeared to increase susceptibility of COPD epithelial cells to RV infection due to significantly increased viral titer and copy number post infection [96]. Thus, an important area of focus examines the effects of RV infection in normal compared to diseased subjects due to the role of RVs in the exacerbation of respiratory symptoms.

One key feature observed in RV-infected asthma subjects is the possibility of an impaired innate immune response in the host. In vitro studies by Wark et al. [97] found that apoptotic responses were impaired and IFN-β secretion was > 2.5 times lower in primary HAECs from asthmatic subjects compared to healthy controls. This clearly demonstrated the compromised host innate immune response in asthma and susceptibility to viral replication. Asthma subjects also exhibited eosinophilic inflammation in addition to significant reduction in FEV_1, peak expiratory flow, provocative concentration of histamine, and total blood lymphocytes after RV infection [98]. Such changes were associated with reduced production of Th_1 cytokines IFN-γ and IL-10 as well as increased production of Th_2 cytokines IL-4, IL-5, and IL-13. Similarly, Sykes et al. [99] determined significantly diminished concentrations of type I interferon proteins IFN-α, IFN-α2, and IFN-β in BAL cells of RV-infected asthmatic subjects. Additionally, deficient type I interferon production was associated with AHR and more positive skin prick test responses, and was associated with more severe childhood asthma [100–102]. Baraldo et al. [103] and Pritchard et al. [104] have also found diminished levels of type I interferons after RV infection in bronchial biopsies from asthmatic children and from media in which PBMCs from asthmatic subjects were cultured, respectively. It is important to mention that others have seen similar levels of type I interferons and IL-15 in asthmatics during RV-induced exacerbations of asthma [18, 105], suggesting that innate immune deficiency may only be relevant in specific patient subtypes.

A notable factor contributing to severity of RV-induced AHR is atopy, although there are conflicting findings. In a study of allergic and non-allergic subjects, Gern et al. [106] found that RV infection induced an increase in airway responsiveness to histamine in allergic subjects and no change in controls. Others found that allergic children experienced more upper respiratory symptoms and asthma exacerbations as well as prolonged duration of AHR compared to controls [61]. Furthermore, in a case-control study the combination of sensitization and exposure to allergen and detection of respiratory virus heightened the risk of hospitalization for asthma [107]. However, chronic low-dose house dust mite allergen exposure did not exert a synergistic effect with RV infection in mild to moderate allergic asthma [108]. Mild allergic subjects with asthma did not exhibit more severe symptoms compared to healthy subjects [109]. Interestingly, treatment with CNTO3157, an inhibitory monoclonal antibody to Toll-like receptor 3 (TLR3), failed to prevent an RV-induced fall in FEV_1 and airway symptoms in subjects with asthma but ameliorated symptoms in healthy subjects [110]. This finding implies that inflammation may be unchecked in asthma due to viral infection. Additionally, the use of non-specific anti-inflammatories like corticosteriods has been limited in its efficacy in certain subsets of RV-infected individuals. This is supported by evidence demonstrating that inhaled corticosteroids provide limited protection against virus-induced asthma exacerbations [111, 112].

Rhinovirus in the context of air pollution

Several studies have examined the effects of air pollutants on airway reactivity and inflammation, as well as the effects of cigarette smoke. However, there has been a paucity of studies examining the effects of air pollutants on RV-induced inflammation or AHR, or how RV infection impacts the effects of air pollutant exposure. Many of the studies have been in vitro studies of single cell types. Some studies of cigarette smoke (CS) exposure in the context of RV in airway epithelial cells note that RV replication is increased following CS exposure [113, 114], but others have found that there was little effect on viral titer [115, 116]. CS exposure has also been found to modulate RV-induced gene expression and inflammatory mediator release from airway cells, decreasing innate inflammatory gene expression and release of IP-10 [113–116] while increasing release of IL-8 from epithelial cells [117]. Capistrano et al. noted that exposure to biomass smoke had no effect on viral load, but enhanced RV-A16-induced IL-8 production but not IL-6 production from human lung fibroblasts [118]. Oxidant pollutant exposure, particularly NO_2 and O_3, alone can induce release of inflammatory mediators from airway epithelial cells. When combined with RV-A16 it was noted that IL-8 release from BEAS-2B cells was significantly augmented over RV-A16, NO_2, or O_3 alone [119]. However, a study of experimental RV exposure with exposure to O_3 following virus inoculation noted that there were no differences in the following parameters: RV titers, recruitment of neutrophils, interferon levels in nasal lavage, or changes in serum neutralizing antibody to RV [120]. The disconnect between the aforementioned studies could be due the different parameters that were studied, or could be due to an in vitro versus an in vivo study.

Exposure to particulate matter (PM2.5) alone induces wheezing and inflammation in individuals exposed to it. An observational study noted that there was a significant interaction between PM2.5 and RV infection in asthmatics that caused a significant decrease in both FEF_{25-75} and FEV1% predicted values compared to asthmatics with no RV infection [121]. Interestingly, a study in rat lung epithelial cells noted that exposure to diesel exhaust particles upregulated expression of ICAM-1 and LDL, both receptors for different RV serotypes [122], suggesting that exposure to diesel exhaust particles may serve to enhance sensitivity of the airways to RV infection. These findings suggest that the effect of air pollution on RV-induced AHR and inflammation appear to be dependent on the type of pollution that the individual is exposed to, and whether or not the individual has underlying lung disease. Overall, there seems to be an additive effect of air pollution on top of what RV infection already elicits.

Summary

Although significant work has been performed studying the effects of RV exposure/infection on modulation of lung inflammation alone, or in the context of asthma and COPD, molecular mechanisms underlying RV-induced AHR remain unclear. Additionally, whether alterations in these mechanisms in subjects with asthma or COPD is what drives more severe AHR and respiratory symptoms is also uncertain. New and novel models of the lung will provide insight into targets to abrogate RV-induced AHR in ASM, as well as to abrogate RV-induced exacerbations of underlying airways disease.

The use of antivirals in treatment of RV infection clinically has failed, and it is unlikely that a targeted RV therapy will be developed due to the large diversity of serotypes. Targeting structural cells of the airways presents a unique approach to abrogate RV effects on AHR and inflammation. Identification of inflammatory mediators inducing sustained AHR and novel pathways involved in alterations in contractility of the airways may serve as targets for therapeutics in subjects both with and without lung disease. Traditional therapy for RV-induced exacerbations, mainly the use of corticosteroids, has been shown to be ineffective in the treatment of RV-induced AHR and inflammation. Conversion of an exacerbation of asthma to nothing more than a common could would be a new paradigm that would decrease asthma morbidity and mortality. A more focused approach targeting soluble mediators that enhance excitation-contraction coupling in airway smooth muscle may provide a more precise approach in treatment of RV-induced exacerbations of asthma.

Abbreviations

AHR: Airway Hyperresponsiveness; ASM: Airway Smooth Muscle; cAMP: Cyclic Adenosine Monophosphate; Cch: Carbachol; CDHR3: Cadherin-related family member 3; COAST: Childhood Origins of ASThma; COPD: Chronic Obstructive Pulmonary Disease; COPSAC: Copenhagen Prospective Studies on Asthma in Childhood; E-C: Excitation-Contraction; FEV_1: Forced Expiratory Volume in 1 s; GEF: Guanine nucleotide Exchange Factors; HAEC: Human Airway Epithelial Cells; ICAM-1: Intracellular Adhesion Molecule 1; iDVG: Immunostimulatory Defective Viral Genomes; IFN: Interferon; IgE: Immunoglobulin E; IL: Interleukin; IP-10: Interferon gamma-induced protein 10; M_3R: Muscarinic Receptor 3; MCP: Monocyte Chemoattractant Protein; MIP: Macrophage Inhibitory Protein; OR: Odds Ratio; OVA: Ovalbumin; PBMC: Peripheral Blood Mononuclear Cells; PCLS: Precision Cut Lung Slices; RANTES: Regulated on activation, normal T cell expressed and secreted; RNA: Ribonucleic Acid; RSV: Respiratory Syncytial Virus; RV: Rhinovirus; Th: T helper cell; TNFα: Tumor Necrosis Factor α; TRP: Transient receptor potential; Tyr: Tyrosine; β_2AR: Beta 2 Adrenergic Receptor

Acknowledgements

Not applicable.

Funding

This review was supported by NIH P01-HL114471-03 (RAP and RCK) and 1K08A1121345-01A1, KL2TR000063, UL1TR000039, P20GM121293, and P20GM103625 (JLK).

Author's contributions

DL, JLK and CK-W conception and design of the manuscript, drafting of the manuscript; RAP, RCK and JLK critical review and editing of the manuscript. All authors read and approved the final manuscript.

Competing interests

The authors declare that they have no competing interests.

Author details

[1]Department of Medicine, Rutgers Institute for Translational Medicine and Science, Rutgers University, New Brunswick, NJ, USA. [2]Department of Pediatrics, Division of Allergy and Immunology, University of Arkansas for Medical Sciences, Little Rock, AR, USA. [3]Department of Physiology and Biophysics, University of Arkansas for Medical Sciences, Little Rock, AR, USA.

References

1. Postma DS, Kerstjens HA. Characteristics of airway hyperresponsiveness in asthma and chronic obstructive pulmonary disease. Am J Respir Crit Care Med. 1998;158:S187–92.
2. Jude J, Koziol-White C, Scala J, Yoo E, Jester W, Maute C, Dalton P, Panettieri R Jr. Formaldehyde induces rho-associated kinase activity to evoke airway Hyperresponsiveness. Am J Respir Cell Mol Biol. 2016;55:542–53.
3. Cho HY, Zhang LY, Kleeberger SR. Ozone-induced lung inflammation and hyperreactivity are mediated via tumor necrosis factor-alpha receptors. Am J Physiol Lung Cell Mol Physiol. 2001;280:L537–46.
4. Roux E, Guibert C, Crevel H, Savineau JP, Marthan R. Human and rat airway smooth muscle responsiveness after ozone exposure in vitro. Am J Phys. 1996;271:L631–6.
5. Seltzer J, Bigby BG, Stulbarg M, Holtzman MJ, Nadel JA, Ueki IF, Leikauf GD, Goetzl EJ, Boushey HA. O3-induced change in bronchial reactivity to methacholine and airway inflammation in humans. *J Appl Physiol (1985).* 1986;60:1321–6.
6. Cooper PR, Lamb R, Day ND, Branigan PJ, Kajekar R, San Mateo L, Hornby PJ, Panettieri RA Jr. TLR3 activation stimulates cytokine secretion without altering agonist-induced human small airway contraction or relaxation. Am J Physiol Lung Cell Mol Physiol. 2009;297:L530–7.
7. McGraw DW, Elwing JM, Fogel KM, Wang WC, Glinka CB, Mihlbachler KA, Rothenberg ME, Liggett SB. Crosstalk between Gi and Gq/Gs pathways in airway smooth muscle regulates bronchial contractility and relaxation. J Clin Invest. 2007;117:1391–8.
8. Risse PA, Jo T, Suarez F, Hirota N, Tolloczko B, Ferraro P, Grutter P, Martin JG. Interleukin-13 inhibits proliferation and enhances contractility of human airway smooth muscle cells without change in contractile phenotype. Am J Physiol Lung Cell Mol Physiol. 2011;300:L958–66.
9. Tliba O, Deshpande D, Chen H, Van Besien C, Kannan M, Panettieri RA Jr, Amrani Y. IL-13 enhances agonist-evoked calcium signals and contractile responses in airway smooth muscle. Br J Pharmacol. 2003;140:1159–62.
10. Amrani Y, Martinet N, Bronner C. Potentiation by tumour necrosis factor-alpha of calcium signals induced by bradykinin and carbachol in human tracheal smooth muscle cells. Br J Pharmacol. 1995;114:4–5.
11. Hotta K, Emala CW, Hirshman CA. TNF-alpha upregulates Gialpha and Gqalpha protein expression and function in human airway smooth muscle cells. Am J Phys. 1999;276:L405–11.
12. Freymuth F, Vabret A, Brouard J, Toutain F, Verdon R, Petitjean J, Gouarin S, Duhamel JF, Guillois B. Detection of viral, chlamydia pneumoniae and mycoplasma pneumoniae infections in exacerbations of asthma in children. J Clin Virol. 1999;13:131–9.
13. Johnston SL, Pattemore PK, Sanderson G, Smith S, Lampe F, Josephs L, Symington P, O'Toole S, Myint SH, Tyrrell DA, et al. Community study of role of viral infections in exacerbations of asthma in 9-11 year old children. BMJ. 1995;310:1225–9.
14. Miller EK, Lu X, Erdman DD, Poehling KA, Zhu Y, Griffin MR, Hartert TV, Anderson LJ, Weinberg GA, Hall CB, et al. Rhinovirus-associated hospitalizations in young children. J Infect Dis. 2007;195:773–81.
15. Bisgaard H. The Copenhagen prospective study on asthma in childhood (COPSAC): design, rationale, and baseline data from a longitudinal birth cohort study. Ann Allergy Asthma Immunol. 2004;93:381–9.
16. Lemanske RF Jr. The childhood origins of asthma (COAST) study. Pediatr Allergy Immunol. 2002;13(Suppl 15):38–43.
17. Heymann PW, Carper HT, Murphy DD, Platts-Mills TA, Patrie J, McLaughlin AP, Erwin EA, Shaker MS, Hellems M, Peerzada J, et al. Viral infections in relation to age, atopy, and season of admission among children hospitalized for wheezing. J Allergy Clin Immunol. 2004;114:239–47.
18. Kennedy JL, Shaker M, McMeen V, Gern J, Carper H, Murphy D, Lee WM, Bochkov YA, Vrtis RF, Platts-Mills T, et al. Comparison of viral load in individuals with and without asthma during infections with rhinovirus. Am J Respir Crit Care Med. 2014;189:532–9.
19. Rakes GP, Arruda E, Ingram JM, Hoover GE, Zambrano JC, Hayden FG, Platts-Mills TA, Heymann PW. Rhinovirus and respiratory syncytial virus in wheezing children requiring emergency care. IgE and eosinophil analyses. Am J Respir Crit Care Med. 1999;159:785–90.
20. Soto-Quiros M, Avila L, Platts-Mills TA, Hunt JF, Erdman DD, Carper H, Murphy DD, Odio S, James HR, Patrie JT, et al. High titers of IgE antibody to dust mite allergen and risk for wheezing among asthmatic children infected with rhinovirus. J Allergy Clin Immunol. 2012;129:1499–505 e1495.
21. de Kluijver J, Grunberg K, Sont JK, Hoogeveen M, van Schadewijk WA, de Klerk EP, Dick CR, van Krieken JH, Sterk PJ. Rhinovirus infection in nonasthmatic subjects: effects on intrapulmonary airways. Eur Respir J. 2002;20:274–9.
22. Grunberg K, Timmers MC, Smits HH, de Klerk EP, Dick EC, Spaan WJ, Hiemstra PS, Sterk PJ. Effect of experimental rhinovirus 16 colds on airway hyperresponsiveness to histamine and interleukin-8 in nasal lavage in asthmatic subjects in vivo. Clin Exp Allergy. 1997;27:36–45.
23. Grunstein MM, Hakonarson H, Whelan R, Yu Z, Grunstein JS, Chuang S. Rhinovirus elicits proasthmatic changes in airway responsiveness independently of viral infection. J Allergy Clin Immunol. 2001;108:997–1004.
24. Kennedy JL, Koziol-White CJ, Jeffus S, Rettiganti MR, Fisher P, Kurten M, Eze A, House S, Sikes JD, Askew E, et al. Effects of rhinovirus 39 infection on airway hyperresponsiveness to carbachol in human airways precision cut lung slices. J Allergy Clin Immunol. 2018;141:1887–90 e1881.
25. Zambrano JC, Carper HT, Rakes GP, Patrie J, Murphy DD, Platts-Mills TA, Hayden FG, Gwaltney JM Jr, Hatley TK, Owens AM, Heymann PW.

Experimental rhinovirus challenges in adults with mild asthma: response to infection in relation to IgE. J Allergy Clin Immunol. 2003;111:1008–16.
26. Mertens TCJ, Karmouty-Quintana H, Taube C, Hiemstra PS. Use of airway epithelial cell culture to unravel the pathogenesis and study treatment in obstructive airway diseases. Pulm Pharmacol Ther. 2017;45:101–13.
27. Bartlett NW, Walton RP, Edwards MR, Aniscenko J, Caramori G, Zhu J, Glanville N, Choy KJ, Jourdan P, Burnet J, et al. Mouse models of rhinovirus-induced disease and exacerbation of allergic airway inflammation. Nat Med. 2008;14:199–204.
28. Tuthill TJ, Papadopoulos NG, Jourdan P, Challinor LJ, Sharp NA, Plumpton C, Shah K, Barnard S, Dash L, Burnet J, et al. Mouse respiratory epithelial cells support efficient replication of human rhinovirus. J Gen Virol. 2003;84:2829–36.
29. Yin FH, Lomax NB. Establishment of a mouse model for human rhinovirus infection. J Gen Virol. 1986;67(Pt 11):2335–40.
30. Saturni S, Contoli M, Spanevello A, Papi A. Models of respiratory infections: virus-induced asthma exacerbations and beyond. Allergy Asthma Immunol Res. 2015;7:525–33.
31. Meurs H, Gosens R, Zaagsma J. Airway hyperresponsiveness in asthma: lessons from in vitro model systems and animal models. Eur Respir J. 2008; 32:487–502.
32. Register RB, Uncapher CR, Naylor AM, Lineberger DW, Colonno RJ. Human-murine chimeras of ICAM-1 identify amino acid residues critical for rhinovirus and antibody binding. J Virol. 1991;65:6589–96.
33. Bizzintino J, Lee WM, Laing IA, Vang F, Pappas T, Zhang G, Martin AC, Khoo SK, Cox DW, Geelhoed GC, et al. Association between human rhinovirus C and severity of acute asthma in children. Eur Respir J. 2011;37:1037–42.
34. Calvo C, Garcia ML, Pozo F, Reyes N, Perez-Brena P, Casas I. Role of rhinovirus C in apparently life-threatening events in infants, Spain. Emerg Infect Dis. 2009;15:1506–8.
35. Lau SK, Yip CC, Lin AW, Lee RA, So LY, Lau YL, Chan KH, Woo PC, Yuen KY. Clinical and molecular epidemiology of human rhinovirus C in children and adults in Hong Kong reveals a possible distinct human rhinovirus C subgroup. J Infect Dis. 2009;200:1096–103.
36. Miller EK, Edwards KM, Weinberg GA, Iwane MK, Griffin MR, Hall CB, Zhu Y, Szilagyi PG, Morin LL, Heil LH, et al. A novel group of rhinoviruses is associated with asthma hospitalizations. J Allergy Clin Immunol. 2009;123: 98–104 e101.
37. Iwane MK, Prill MM, Lu X, Miller EK, Edwards KM, Hall CB, Griffin MR, Staat MA, Anderson LJ, Williams JV, et al. Human rhinovirus species associated with hospitalizations for acute respiratory illness in young US children. J Infect Dis. 2011;204:1702–10.
38. Lee WM, Lemanske RF Jr, Evans MD, Vang F, Pappas T, Gangnon R, Jackson DJ, Gern JE. Human rhinovirus species and season of infection determine illness severity. Am J Respir Crit Care Med. 2012;186:886–91.
39. Linsuwanon P, Payungporn S, Samransamruajkit R, Posuwan N, Makkoch J, Theanboonlers A, Poovorawan Y. High prevalence of human rhinovirus C infection in Thai children with acute lower respiratory tract disease. J Inf Secur. 2009;59:115–21.
40. Xiang Z, Gonzalez R, Xie Z, Xiao Y, Liu J, Chen L, Liu C, Zhang J, Ren L, Vernet G, et al. Human rhinovirus C infections mirror those of human rhinovirus a in children with community-acquired pneumonia. J Clin Virol. 2010;49:94–9.
41. Bartlett NW, Singanayagam A, Johnston SL. Mouse models of rhinovirus infection and airways disease. Methods Mol Biol. 2015;1221:181–8.
42. Singanayagam A, Glanville N, Walton RP, Aniscenko J, Pearson RM, Pinkerton JW, Horvat JC, Hansbro PM, Bartlett NW, Johnston SL. A short-term mouse model that reproduces the immunopathological features of rhinovirus-induced exacerbation of COPD. Clin Sci (Lond). 2015;129:245–58.
43. Mestas J, Hughes CC. Of mice and not men: differences between mouse and human immunology. J Immunol. 2004;172:2731–8.
44. Borish L, Rosenwasser LJ. Update on cytokines. J Allergy Clin Immunol. 1996; 97:719–33 quiz 734.
45. Bates JH, Irvin CG. Measuring lung function in mice: the phenotyping uncertainty principle. *J Appl Physiol (1985)*. 2003;94:1297–306.
46. Hao W, Bernard K, Patel N, Ulbrandt N, Feng H, Svabek C, Wilson S, Stracener C, Wang K, Suzich J, et al. Infection and propagation of human rhinovirus C in human airway epithelial cells. J Virol. 2012;86:13524–32.
47. Bochkov YA, Watters K, Ashraf S, Griggs TF, Devries MK, Jackson DJ, Palmenberg AC, Gern JE. Cadherin-related family member 3, a childhood asthma susceptibility gene product, mediates rhinovirus C binding and replication. Proc Natl Acad Sci U S A. 2015;112:5485–90.
48. Damera G, Zhao H, Wang M, Smith M, Kirby C, Jester WF, Lawson JA, Panettieri RA Jr. Ozone modulates IL-6 secretion in human airway epithelial and smooth muscle cells. Am J Physiol Lung Cell Mol Physiol. 2009;296: L674–83.
49. Malavia NK, Raub CB, Mahon SB, Brenner M, Panettieri RA Jr, George SC. Airway epithelium stimulates smooth muscle proliferation. Am J Respir Cell Mol Biol. 2009;41:297–304.
50. Van Ly D, Faiz A, Jenkins C, Crossett B, Black JL, McParland B, Burgess JK, Oliver BG. Characterising the mechanism of airway smooth muscle beta2 adrenoceptor desensitization by rhinovirus infected bronchial epithelial cells. PLoS One. 2013;8:e56058.
51. Rajan D, Gaston KA, McCracken CE, Erdman DD, Anderson LJ. Response to rhinovirus infection by human airway epithelial cells and peripheral blood mononuclear cells in an in vitro two-chamber tissue culture system. PLoS One. 2013;8:e66600.
52. Korpi-Steiner NL, Valkenaar SM, Bates ME, Evans MD, Gern JE, Bertics PJ. Human monocytic cells direct the robust release of CXCL10 by bronchial epithelial cells during rhinovirus infection. Clin Exp Allergy. 2010;40:1203–13.
53. Shariff S, Shelfoon C, Holden NS, Traves SL, Wiehler S, Kooi C, Proud D, Leigh R. Human rhinovirus infection of epithelial cells modulates airway smooth muscle migration. Am J Respir Cell Mol Biol. 2017;56:796–803.
54. Pezzulo AA, Starner TD, Scheetz TE, Traver GL, Tilley AE, Harvey BG, Crystal RG, McCray PB Jr, Zabner J. The air-liquid interface and use of primary cell cultures are important to recapitulate the transcriptional profile of in vivo airway epithelia. Am J Physiol Lung Cell Mol Physiol. 2011;300:L25–31.
55. Sun Y, Jain D, Koziol-White CJ, Genoyer E, Gilbert M, Tapia K, Panettieri RA Jr, Hodinka RL, Lopez CB. Immunostimulatory defective viral genomes from respiratory syncytial virus promote a strong innate antiviral response during infection in mice and humans. PLoS Pathog. 2015;11:e1005122.
56. Avgousti DC, Herrmann C, Kulej K, Pancholi NJ, Sekulic N, Petrescu J, Molden RC, Blumenthal D, Paris AJ, Reyes ED, et al. A core viral protein binds host nucleosomes to sequester immune danger signals. Nature. 2016; 535:173–7.
57. Kim WK, Jain D, Sanchez MD, Koziol-White CJ, Matthews K, Ge MQ, Haczku A, Panettieri RA Jr, Frieman MB, Lopez CB. Deficiency of melanoma differentiation-associated protein 5 results in exacerbated chronic postviral lung inflammation. Am J Respir Crit Care Med. 2014;189:437–48.
58. Ressmeyer AR, Larsson AK, Vollmer E, Dahlen SE, Uhlig S, Martin C. Characterisation of Guinea pig precision-cut lung slices: comparison with human tissues. Eur Respir J. 2006;28:603–11.
59. Henjakovic M, Martin C, Hoymann HG, Sewald K, Ressmeyer AR, Dassow C, Pohlmann G, Krug N, Uhlig S, Braun A. Ex vivo lung function measurements in precision-cut lung slices (PCLS) from chemical allergen-sensitized mice represent a suitable alternative to in vivo studies. Toxicol Sci. 2008;106:444–53.
60. Fox J: Utility of the precision cut lung slice model to investigate airway smooth muscle contraction. University of Nottingham, 2011.
61. Xepapadaki P, Papadopoulos NG, Bossios A, Manoussakis E, Manousakas T, Saxoni-Papageorgiou P. Duration of postviral airway hyperresponsiveness in children with asthma: effect of atopy. J Allergy Clin Immunol. 2005;116:299–304.
62. Proud D, Turner RB, Winther B, Wiehler S, Tiesman JP, Reichling TD, Juhlin KD, Fulmer AW, Ho BY, Walanski AA, et al. Gene expression profiles during in vivo human rhinovirus infection: insights into the host response. Am J Respir Crit Care Med. 2008;178:962–8.
63. Beale J, Jayaraman A, Jackson DJ, Macintyre JDR, Edwards MR, Walton RP, Zhu J, Man Ching Y, Shamji B, Edwards M, et al. Rhinovirus-induced IL-25 in asthma exacerbation drives type 2 immunity and allergic pulmonary inflammation. *Sci Transl Med*. 2014;6:256ra134.
64. Jackson DJ, Gangnon RE, Evans MD, Roberg KA, Anderson EL, Pappas TE, Printz MC, Lee WM, Shult PA, Reisdorf E, et al. Wheezing rhinovirus illnesses in early life predict asthma development in high-risk children. Am J Respir Crit Care Med. 2008;178:667–72.
65. Barnes PJ. Neurogenic inflammation in the airways. Respir Physiol. 2001;125: 145–54.
66. Gentile DA, Skoner DP. Viral rhinitis. Curr Allergy Asthma Rep. 2001;1:227–34.
67. Kohrogi H, Graf PD, Sekizawa K, Borson DB, Nadel JA. Neutral endopeptidase inhibitors potentiate substance P- and capsaicin-induced cough in awake Guinea pigs. J Clin Invest. 1988;82:2063–8.
68. Katsumata U, Sekizawa K, Inoue H, Sasaki H, Takishima T. Inhibitory actions of procaterol, a beta-2 stimulant, on substance P-induced cough in normal subjects during upper respiratory tract infection. Tohoku J Exp Med. 1989; 158:105–6.

69. Hu C, Wedde-Beer K, Auais A, Rodriguez MM, Piedimonte G. Nerve growth factor and nerve growth factor receptors in respiratory syncytial virus-infected lungs. Am J Physiol Lung Cell Mol Physiol. 2002;283:L494–502.
70. Piedimonte G, Rodriguez MM, King KA, McLean S, Jiang X. Respiratory syncytial virus upregulates expression of the substance P receptor in rat lungs. Am J Phys. 1999;277:L831–40.
71. Abdullah H, Heaney LG, Cosby SL, McGarvey LP. Rhinovirus upregulates transient receptor potential channels in a human neuronal cell line: implications for respiratory virus-induced cough reflex sensitivity. Thorax. 2014;69:46–54.
72. Atkinson SK, Sadofsky LR, Morice AH. How does rhinovirus cause the common cold cough? BMJ Open Respir Res. 2016;3:e000118.
73. Hakonarson H, Maskeri N, Carter C, Hodinka RL, Campbell D, Grunstein MM. Mechanism of rhinovirus-induced changes in airway smooth muscle responsiveness. J Clin Invest. 1998;102:1732–41.
74. Billington CK, Penn RB. Signaling and regulation of G protein-coupled receptors in airway smooth muscle. Respir Res. 2003;4:2.
75. Chiba Y, Sakai H, Misawa M. Possible involvement of G(i3) protein in augmented contraction of bronchial smooth muscle from antigen-induced airway hyperresponsive rats. Biochem Pharmacol. 2001;61:921–4.
76. Hirshman CA, Emala CW. Actin reorganization in airway smooth muscle cells involves Gq and Gi-2 activation of rho. Am J Phys. 1999;277:L653–61.
77. van Unen J, Reinhard NR, Yin T, Wu YI, Postma M, Gadella TW, Goedhart J. Plasma membrane restricted RhoGEF activity is sufficient for RhoA-mediated actin polymerization. Sci Rep. 2015;5:14693.
78. Croxton TL, Lande B, Hirshman CA. Role of G proteins in agonist-induced Ca2+ sensitization of tracheal smooth muscle. Am J Phys. 1998;275:L748–55.
79. Hakonarson H, Carter C, Maskeri N, Hodinka R, Grunstein MM. Rhinovirus-mediated changes in airway smooth muscle responsiveness: induced autocrine role of interleukin-1beta. Am J Phys. 1999;277:L13–21.
80. Kotaniemi-Syrjanen A, Vainionpaa R, Reijonen TM, Waris M, Korhonen K, Korppi M. Rhinovirus-induced wheezing in infancy--the first sign of childhood asthma? J Allergy Clin Immunol. 2003;111:66–71.
81. Anderson HM, Lemanske RF Jr, Evans MD, Gangnon RE, Pappas T, Grindle K, Bochkov YA, Gern JE, Jackson DJ. Assessment of wheezing frequency and viral etiology on childhood and adolescent asthma risk. J Allergy Clin Immunol. 2017;139:692–4.
82. Guilbert TW, Singh AM, Danov Z, Evans MD, Jackson DJ, Burton R, Roberg KA, Anderson EL, Pappas TE, Gangnon R, et al. Decreased lung function after preschool wheezing rhinovirus illnesses in children at risk to develop asthma. *J Allergy Clin Immunol*. 2011;128:532–538 e531-510.
83. Lemanske RF Jr, Jackson DJ, Gangnon RE, Evans MD, Li Z, Shult PA, Kirk CJ, Reisdorf E, Roberg KA, Anderson EL, et al. Rhinovirus illnesses during infancy predict subsequent childhood wheezing. J Allergy Clin Immunol. 2005;116:571–7.
84. Rubner FJ, Jackson DJ, Evans MD, Gangnon RE, Tisler CJ, Pappas TE, Gern JE, Lemanske RF Jr. Early life rhinovirus wheezing, allergic sensitization, and asthma risk at adolescence. J Allergy Clin Immunol. 2017;139:501–7.
85. Kusel MM, de Klerk NH, Kebadze T, Vohma V, Holt PG, Johnston SL, Sly PD. Early-life respiratory viral infections, atopic sensitization, and risk of subsequent development of persistent asthma. J Allergy Clin Immunol. 2007;119:1105–10.
86. Liu L, Pan Y, Zhu Y, Song Y, Su X, Yang L, Li M. Association between rhinovirus wheezing illness and the development of childhood asthma: a meta-analysis. BMJ Open. 2017;7:e013034.
87. Lukkarinen M, Koistinen A, Turunen R, Lehtinen P, Vuorinen T, Jartti T. Rhinovirus-induced first wheezing episode predicts atopic but not nonatopic asthma at school age. J Allergy Clin Immunol. 2017;140:988–95.
88. Jartti T, Kuusipalo H, Vuorinen T, Soderlund-Venermo M, Allander T, Waris M, Hartiala J, Ruuskanen O. Allergic sensitization is associated with rhinovirus-, but not other virus-, induced wheezing in children. Pediatr Allergy Immunol. 2010;21:1008–14.
89. Caliskan M, Bochkov YA, Kreiner-Moller E, Bonnelykke K, Stein MM, Du G, Bisgaard H, Jackson DJ, Gern JE, Lemanske RF Jr, et al. Rhinovirus wheezing illness and genetic risk of childhood-onset asthma. N Engl J Med. 2013;368:1398–407.
90. Binia A, Khorasani N, Bhavsar PK, Adcock I, Brightling CE, Chung KF, Cookson WO, Moffatt MF. Chromosome 17q21 SNP and severe asthma. J Hum Genet. 2011;56:97–8.
91. Moffatt MF, Kabesch M, Liang L, Dixon AL, Strachan D, Heath S, Depner M, von Berg A, Bufe A, Rietschel E, et al. Genetic variants regulating ORMDL3 expression contribute to the risk of childhood asthma. Nature. 2007;448:470–3.
92. Bonnelykke K, Coleman AT, Evans MD, Thorsen J, Waage J, Vissing NH, Carlsson CJ, Stokholm J, Chawes BL, Jessen LE, et al. Cadherin-related family member 3 genetics and rhinovirus C respiratory illnesses. Am J Respir Crit Care Med. 2018;197:589–94.
93. Barnes KC, Grant AV, Hansel NN, Gao P, Dunston GM. African Americans with asthma: genetic insights. Proc Am Thorac Soc. 2007;4:58–68.
94. Marin J, Jeler-Kacar D, Levstek V, Macek V. Persistence of viruses in upper respiratory tract of children with asthma. J Inf Secur. 2000;41:69–72.
95. Corne JM, Marshall C, Smith S, Schreiber J, Sanderson G, Holgate ST, Johnston SL. Frequency, severity, and duration of rhinovirus infections in asthmatic and non-asthmatic individuals: a longitudinal cohort study. Lancet. 2002;359:831–4.
96. Schneider D, Ganesan S, Comstock AT, Meldrum CA, Mahidhara R, Goldsmith AM, Curtis JL, Martinez FJ, Hershenson MB, Sajjan U. Increased cytokine response of rhinovirus-infected airway epithelial cells in chronic obstructive pulmonary disease. Am J Respir Crit Care Med. 2010;182:332–40.
97. Wark PA, Johnston SL, Bucchieri F, Powell R, Puddicombe S, Laza-Stanca V, Holgate ST, Davies DE. Asthmatic bronchial epithelial cells have a deficient innate immune response to infection with rhinovirus. J Exp Med. 2005;201:937–47.
98. Message SD, Laza-Stanca V, Mallia P, Parker HL, Zhu J, Kebadze T, Contoli M, Sanderson G, Kon OM, Papi A, et al. Rhinovirus-induced lower respiratory illness is increased in asthma and related to virus load and Th1/2 cytokine and IL-10 production. Proc Natl Acad Sci U S A. 2008;105:13562–7.
99. Sykes A, Edwards MR, Macintyre J, del Rosario A, Bakhsoliani E, Trujillo-Torralbo MB, Kon OM, Mallia P, McHale M, Johnston SL. Rhinovirus 16-induced IFN-alpha and IFN-beta are deficient in bronchoalveolar lavage cells in asthmatic patients. J Allergy Clin Immunol. 2012;129:1506–14 e1506.
100. Arroyave WD, Rabito FA, Carlson JC, Sever ML, Lefante J. Asthma severity, not asthma control, is worse in atopic compared with nonatopic adolescents with asthma. Ann Allergy Asthma Immunol. 2016;116:18–25.
101. Carroll WD, Lenney W, Child F, Strange RC, Jones PW, Whyte MK, Primhak RA, Fryer AA. Asthma severity and atopy: how clear is the relationship? Arch Dis Child. 2006;91:405–9.
102. Sarria EE, Mattiello R, Yao W, Chakr V, Tiller CJ, Kisling J, Tabbey R, Yu Z, Kaplan MH, Tepper RS. Atopy, cytokine production, and airway reactivity as predictors of pre-school asthma and airway responsiveness. Pediatr Pulmonol. 2014;49:132–9.
103. Baraldo S, Contoli M, Bazzan E, Turato G, Padovani A, Marku B, Calabrese F, Caramori G, Ballarin A, Snijders D, et al. Deficient antiviral immune responses in childhood: distinct roles of atopy and asthma. J Allergy Clin Immunol. 2012;130:1307–14.
104. Pritchard AL, White OJ, Burel JG, Carroll ML, Phipps S, Upham JW. Asthma is associated with multiple alterations in anti-viral innate signalling pathways. PLoS One. 2014;9:e106501.
105. Miller EK, Hernandez JZ, Wimmenauer V, Shepherd BE, Hijano D, Libster R, Serra ME, Bhat N, Batalle JP, Mohamed Y, et al. A mechanistic role for type III IFN-lambda1 in asthma exacerbations mediated by human rhinoviruses. Am J Respir Crit Care Med. 2012;185:508–16.
106. Gern JE, Calhoun W, Swenson C, Shen G, Busse WW. Rhinovirus infection preferentially increases lower airway responsiveness in allergic subjects. Am J Respir Crit Care Med. 1997;155:1872–6.
107. Green RM, Custovic A, Sanderson G, Hunter J, Johnston SL, Woodcock A. Synergism between allergens and viruses and risk of hospital admission with asthma: case-control study. BMJ. 2002;324:763.
108. de Kluijver J, Evertse CE, Sont JK, Schrumpf JA, van Zeijl-van der Ham CJ, Dick CR, Rabe KF, Hiemstra PS, Sterk PJ. Are rhinovirus-induced airway responses in asthma aggravated by chronic allergen exposure? Am J Respir Crit Care Med. 2003;168:1174–80.
109. DeMore JP, Weisshaar EH, Vrtis RF, Swenson CA, Evans MD, Morin A, Hazel E, Bork JA, Kakumanu S, Sorkness R, et al. Similar colds in subjects with allergic asthma and nonatopic subjects after inoculation with rhinovirus-16. *J Allergy Clin Immunol*. 2009;124:245–52 252 e241–243.
110. Silkoff PE, Flavin S, Gordon R, Loza MJ, Sterk PJ, Lutter R, Diamant Z, Turner RB, Lipworth BJ, Proud D, et al. Toll-like receptor 3 blockade in rhinovirus-induced experimental asthma exacerbations: a randomized controlled study. J Allergy Clin Immunol. 2018;141:1220–30.
111. Grunberg K, Sharon RF, Hiltermann TJ, Brahim JJ, Dick EC, Sterk PJ, Van Krieken JH. Experimental rhinovirus 16 infection increases intercellular

adhesion molecule-1 expression in bronchial epithelium of asthmatics regardless of inhaled steroid treatment. Clin Exp Allergy. 2000;30:1015–23.
112. Grunberg K, Sharon RF, Sont JK, In't Veen JC, Van Schadewijk WA, De Klerk EP, Dick CR, Van Krieken JH, Sterk PJ. Rhinovirus-induced airway inflammation in asthma: effect of treatment with inhaled corticosteroids before and during experimental infection. Am J Respir Crit Care Med. 2001; 164:1816–22.
113. Eddleston J, Lee RU, Doerner AM, Herschbach J, Zuraw BL. Cigarette smoke decreases innate responses of epithelial cells to rhinovirus infection. Am J Respir Cell Mol Biol. 2011;44:118–26.
114. Logan J, Chen L, Gangell C, Sly PD, Fantino E, Liu K. Brief exposure to cigarette smoke impairs airway epithelial cell innate anti-viral defence. Toxicol in Vitro. 2014;28:1430–5.
115. Hudy MH, Traves SL, Wiehler S, Proud D. Cigarette smoke modulates rhinovirus-induced airway epithelial cell chemokine production. Eur Respir J. 2010;35:1256–63.
116. Proud D, Hudy MH, Wiehler S, Zaheer RS, Amin MA, Pelikan JB, Tacon CE, Tonsaker TO, Walker BL, Kooi C, et al. Cigarette smoke modulates expression of human rhinovirus-induced airway epithelial host defense genes. PLoS One. 2012;7:e40762.
117. Hudy MH, Proud D. Cigarette smoke enhances human rhinovirus-induced CXCL8 production via HuR-mediated mRNA stabilization in human airway epithelial cells. Respir Res. 2013;14:88.
118. Capistrano SJ, Zakarya R, Chen H, Oliver BG. Biomass smoke exposure enhances rhinovirus-induced inflammation in primary lung fibroblasts. Int J Mol Sci. 2016;17.
119. Spannhake EW, Reddy SP, Jacoby DB, Yu XY, Saatian B, Tian J. Synergism between rhinovirus infection and oxidant pollutant exposure enhances airway epithelial cell cytokine production. Environ Health Perspect. 2002;110: 665–70.
120. Henderson FW, Dubovi EJ, Harder S, Seal E Jr, Graham D. Experimental rhinovirus infection in human volunteers exposed to ozone. Am Rev Respir Dis. 1988;137:1124–8.
121. Vempilly J, Abejie B, Diep V, Gushiken M, Rawat M, Tyner TR. The synergetic effect of ambient PM2.5 exposure and rhinovirus infection in airway dysfunction in asthma: a pilot observational study from the Central Valley of California. Exp Lung Res. 2013;39:434–40.
122. Ito T, Okumura H, Tsukue N, Kobayashi T, Honda K, Sekizawa K. Effect of diesel exhaust particles on mRNA expression of viral and bacterial receptors in rat lung epithelial L2 cells. Toxicol Lett. 2006;165:66–70.

15

Therapeutic potential of products derived from mesenchymal stem/stromal cells in pulmonary disease

Arezoo Mohammadipoor[1,2*], Ben Antebi[1], Andriy I. Batchinsky[1,3] and Leopoldo C. Cancio[1]

Abstract

Multipotent mesenchymal stem/stromal cells (MSCs) possess robust self-renewal characteristics and the ability to differentiate into tissue-specific cells. Their therapeutic potential appears promising as evident from their efficacy in several animal models of pulmonary disorders as well as early-phase clinical trials of acute respiratory distress syndrome (ARDS) and chronic obstructive pulmonary disease (COPD). Such therapeutic efficacy might be attributed to MSC-derived products (the "secretome"), namely conditioned media (CM) and extracellular vesicles (EVs), which have been shown to play pivotal roles in the regenerative function of MSCs. Importantly, the EVs secreted by MSCs can transfer a variety of bioactive factors to modulate the function of recipient cells via various mechanisms, including ligand-receptor interactions, direct membrane fusion, endocytosis, or phagocytosis.

Herein, we review the current state-of-the-science of MSC-derived CM and EVs as potential therapeutic agents in lung diseases. We suggest that the MSC-derived secretome might be an appropriate therapeutic agent for treating aggressive pulmonary disorders because of biological and logistical advantages over live cell therapy. Nonetheless, further studies are warranted to elucidate the safety and efficacy of these components in combating pulmonary diseases.

Keywords: Mesenchymal stem cells, Extracellular vesicles, Conditioned media, Lung disease, Acute respiratory distress syndrome, Acute lung injury, Chronic obstructive pulmonary disease, Pulmonary fibrosis, Bronchopulmonary dysplasia

Background

The increasingly high rates of morbidity and mortality due to acute and chronic lung diseases have emerged as one of the major public health issues globally. Pulmonary diseases are mainly caused by trauma, air pollution, smoking, and various pathogens and exert a devastating effect on quality of life [1]. Acute respiratory distress syndrome (ARDS), recognized as the most severe form of acute lung injury (ALI), is a life-threatening condition featuring acute hypoxemic respiratory failure, bilateral consolidation on chest radiograph, and absence of left atrial hypertension [2, 3]. ARDS most commonly occurs due to sepsis, smoke inhalation injury, near-drowning, severe pneumonia, or pulmonary contusion [3–6]. Mechanistic studies reveal that dysregulated inflammatory/immune responses, uncontrolled activation of coagulation pathways, and increased permeability of alveolar endothelial/epithelial barrier play pivotal roles in the pathogenesis of ARDS [3]. ARDS continues to be associated with a mortality rate of 30% to 40% despite advances in modern supportive care [2, 4, 7–9].

Among many destructive chronic lung diseases, such as idiopathic pulmonary fibrosis (IPF) and pulmonary hypertension, chronic obstructive pulmonary disease (COPD) is thought to be one of the leading causes of death worldwide. Approximately 20% of COPD patients present with emphysema, which is characterized by destruction of terminal bronchioles and alveolar walls causing overdistension of air spaces due to air trapping. Despite advances in the symptomatic treatment of emphysema, a cure remains obscure [1].

Stem-cell-based therapy is an attractive approach for treating both acute and chronic lung diseases, such as ARDS and COPD, mainly because the cells can simultaneously target multiple pathological processes to

* Correspondence: arezoo.mohammadipoor.ctr@mail.mil; Arezoo.mohammadipoor.ctr@mail.mil
[1]Multi-Organ Support Technology (MOST) Task Area, US Army Institute of Surgical Research, Fort Sam Houston, TX, USA
[2]Oak Ridge Institute for Science and Education, Oak Ridge, TN, USA
Full list of author information is available at the end of the article

protect lung function. Among the various types of stem cells, the therapeutic potential of mesenchymal stem/stromal cells (MSCs) has been extensively demonstrated in several animal models of pulmonary disorders [10–15], and is now being evaluated in phase II clinical trials for ARDS [16]. It is well established that MSCs impart their therapeutic effect via secretion of bioactive products, namely the secretome [17, 18]. Although not fully defined, the MSC secretome is comprised of an extended array of bioactive molecules that include cytokines, chemokines, growth factors, angiogenic factors, and extracellular vesicles (EVs), thus potentially contributing to the therapeutic benefits of the cells as evident from preclinical studies [19–23]. MSC secretome is readily available in the conditioned media (CM) of MSC cultures (MSC-CM) and, subsequently, MSC-derived EVs are isolated from the CM. The major advantage of MSC-derived secretome therapy over live-cell transplantation approach can be attributed to the inherent risks associated with live-cell transplants. Consequently, the MSC secretome is emerging as a viable option to replace the cells for the treatment of several lung disorders.

In this review, we describe the characteristics of MSC-CM and MSC-EVs as well as the methods of their isolation. Next, we summarize the current state-of-the-science relating to their therapeutic potential for various lung diseases. Finally, we will discuss the advantages and limitations of these products in clinical settings.

MSC-derived products: Light at the end of the tunnel

Mesenchymal stem/stromal cells at a glance

In 1968, Friedenstein and colleagues first discovered MSCs as a component of bone-marrow stromal tissue [24]. Subsequently, MSCs have been isolated from various tissues, such as adipose tissue, umbilical cord (UC) blood/tissue, placental tissue, and exfoliated deciduous teeth [25–29]. Since no unique surface marker(s) can exclusively identify these cells, in 2006, the Mesenchymal and Tissue Stem Cell Committee of the International Society for Cellular Therapy proposed the following criteria as minimal criteria to be satisfied for defining human MSCs. First, the cells must be plastic-adherent when maintained in standard culture conditions. Second, MSCs must express surface antigens such as CD105, CD73, and CD90 but should lack the expression of the following hematopoietic antigens: CD45, CD34, CD14 or CD11b, CD79a or CD19, and human leukocyte antigen (HLA)-DR. Third, MSCs must be capable of differentiating into osteoblasts, adipocytes, and chondroblasts in vitro [30]. That MSCs are easy to isolate and expand in culture is a major advantage from a logistical/feasibility standpoint. More importantly, MSCs have evolved as one of the mainstream cell-based therapeutic tools for regenerative medicine because of their inherent low immunogenicity and limited risk of tumorigenicity [29, 31, 32].

The initial motive for exploring their therapeutic benefits stemmed from the capability of MSCs to repair injured tissues by engrafting and replacing damaged cells through differentiation [29]. An array of other observations, however, suggests that MSCs could repair injured tissues and improve function without significant engraftment or differentiation. In fact, emerging evidence suggests that the therapeutic benefits of MSCs are derived from their secretome, and the subsequent paracrine action [29, 31–34].

MSC Secretome

The MSC-derived secretome is released into CM in vitro [19–22, 32, 35–41]. MSCs respond to environmental changes and stress signals from injured tissues by secreting a myriad of soluble factors (Table 1); for instance, early reports by Prockop and others showed that in response to hypoxia, MSCs correlatively increase the production of several angiogenic and anti-apoptotic factors, such as interleukin-6 (IL-6), vascular endothelial growth factor (VEGF), monocyte chemotactic protein (MCP-1), also known as chemokine [C-C motif] ligand 2 (CCL2)), and stanniocalcin-1 (STC-1) [36, 37]. In line with these findings, further studies revealed that the stimulation of MSCs with different insults and inflammatory cytokines, including lipopolysaccharide (LPS), tumor necrosis factor alpha (TNF-α), IL-1β, interferon gamma (IFN-γ), and serum from ARDS patients can induce the secretion of a variety of anti-inflammatory mediators, such as TNF-stimulating gene 6 protein (TSG-6), prostaglandin E2 (PGE2), indoleamine 2,3-dioxygenase (IDO), IL-10, and IL-1 receptor antagonist (IL-1ra) [39, 42–44].

Recent efforts have focused on the paracrine effects of MSCs both in vitro and in vivo [45–52]. MSC bioactive factors have been reported to mediate several known functions of MSCs, including the modulation of immune/inflammatory responses, reduction of oxidative stress, fibrosis, and apoptosis. They also promote angiogenesis, bacterial clearance, and regeneration. In addition to their soluble factors, MSCs also secrete different types of EVs contributing to the overall therapeutic response [19–23, 40, 41].

Structurally, EVs are nano- to micro-sized particles surrounded by a phospholipid bilayer. Most eukaryotes and prokaryotes have been shown to secrete a heterogeneous population of EVs. The presence of these vesicles can be detected in physiological fluids, such as plasma, urine, cerebrospinal fluid, milk as well as in the supernatant of cell cultures in vitro [53–55]. Of note, EVs were considered as cell debris [53, 55–57] till 1996 when Raposo et al. [58] presented evidence of their biological function. They demonstrated that EVs secreted by B

Table 1 Bioactive factors secreted by MSCs directly in CM or via EVs

Angiogenesis	Anti-apoptosis	Anti-fibrosis	Anti-oxidation	Chemo-attraction	Immuno- modulation	Proliferation
Ang1	FGF	Ang-1	HO-1	CCLs	HO-1	FGF
FGF	GM-CSF	FGF	IL-1β	CXCLs	IDO	HGF
HGF	HGF	HGF	STC-1	G-CSF	IL-1ra	IGF-1
IGF-1	IGF-1	KGF		LIF	IL-6	KGF
IL-6	IL-6	MMPs		M-CSF	IL-10	PDGF
MCP-1	STC-1	TIMP-1		MCP-1	LIF	VEGF
PDGF				SDF-1	PGE2	
VEGF					STC-1	
					TGF-β	
					TSG-6	

Ang-1 – angiopoietin 1, *CCL* – chemokine ligand, *CXCL* – chemokine (C-X-C motif) ligand, *FGF* – fibroblast growth factor, *GM-CSF* – granulocyte monocyte colony stimulating factor, *HGF* – hepatocyte growth factor, *HO-1* – hemeoxygenase 1, *IDO* – indoleamine 2,3-dioxygenase, *IGF-1* – insulin like growth factor 1, *IL* – interleukin, *IL-1ra* – IL-1 receptor antagonist, *KGF* – keratinocyte growth factor, *LIF* – leukemia inhibitory factor, *LL-37* – human cathelicidin, *MMP* – metalloproteinase, *MCP-1* – monocyte chemoattractant protein 1, *PDGF* – platelet derived growth factor, *PGE2* – prostaglandin E2, *SDF-1* – stem cell-derived factor 1, *STC-1* – stanniocalcin 1, *TIMP-1* – tissue inhibitor of metalloproteinase 1, *TGF-β* – transforming growth factor beta, *TSG-6* – tumor necrosis factor-stimulated gene 6, *VEGF* – vascular endothelial growth factor

lymphocytes can induce antigen-specific T lymphocyte responses in vitro. The pioneering observation by these authors prompted elaborate studies to establish the role of EVs as critical mediators in cell-to-cell communication [53, 57, 59–61]. Cumulative studies in the field reveal that upon their release into the extracellular milieu, EVs can interact with recipient cells by ligand-receptor interaction or by internalization via endocytosis, phagocytosis, and direct membrane fusion (Fig. 1). Targeted delivery of EVs to specific cells/tissues is facilitated by several types of membrane molecules that are embedded in the lipid bilayers. Interestingly, several studies reported the ability of EVs to regulate a variety of biological responses in recipient cells via transfer of an array of bioactive factors that include proteins, lipids, nucleic acids (mRNA, microRNA, transfer RNA, and double-stranded DNAs), as well as cellular organelles [41, 53, 57]. At present, based on their cellular origin, secretory mechanism, size, and surface markers, EVs are classified into 3 main categories 1) exosomes; 2) microvesicles; and 3) apoptotic bodies.

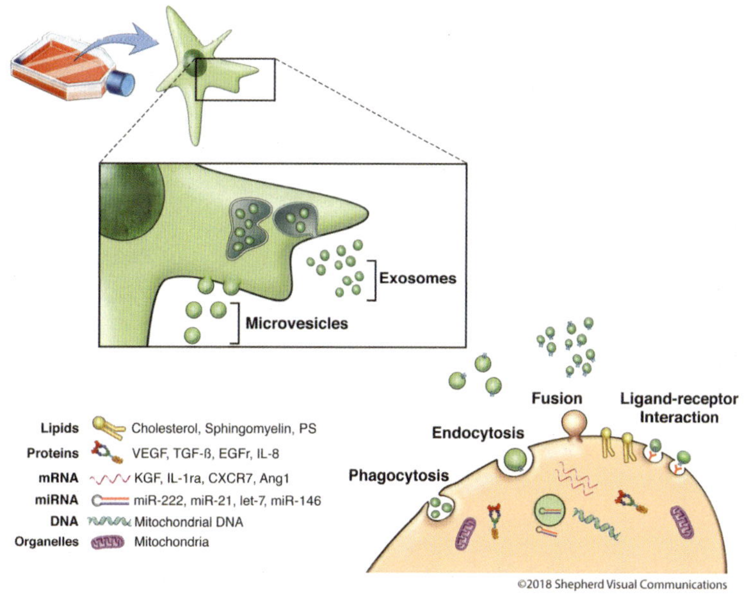

Fig. 1 Extracellular vesicles secreted by mesenchymal stem cells transfer their cargo to the recipient cells. In culture mesenchymal stem cells secrete exosomes and microvesicles that can transfer variety of bioactive factors to the recipient cells via ligand-receptor interaction, direct membrane fusion, endocytosis, or phagocytosis. Ang1—angiopoietin 1, CXCR7 – chemokine (C-X-C motif) receptor 7, EGFr – epidermal growth factor receptor, IL-8 – interleukin 8, IL-1ra – IL-1 receptor antagonist, KGF – keratinocyte growth factor, mRNA – messenger RNA, miRNA – micro RNA, PS – phosphatidylserine, TGF-β – transforming growth factor beta, VEGF – vascular endothelial growth factor

Exosomes are formed by the inward budding of multi-vesicular bodies (MVBs), size ~ 40–100 nm, and rich in CD63, CD9, CD81, and tumor susceptibility gene 101 (Tsg 101). These vesicles are also enriched in annexins, ALG-2-interacting protein X (Alix), clathrin, heat shock proteins, and low amounts of phosphatidylserine (PS). Cytoskeleton activation is required for their release.

Microvesicles (shedding vesicles) are formed by budding from the plasma membrane, size ~ 80–1000 nm, and rich in integrins, selectins, and CD40 ligands. Their release is dependent on cytoskeleton activation as well as calcium influx. The lipid bilayer of microvesicles is enriched in cholesterol, sphingomyelin, ceramide, and PS.

Apoptotic bodies are derived from fragmentation of cells undergoing apoptosis, size ~ 1000–5000 nm, and rich in PS, nuclear fractions, and cellular organelles. While the role of cytoskeleton-associated molecules in the formation and the release of apoptotic bodies has been implicated, the mechanism responsible for relocation of fragmented DNA still remains unclear [18, 53, 62, 63].

It is now established that MSCs secrete all types of EVs [64]. The heterogeneous pool of MSC-EVs has been shown to express both EV- and MSC-specific surface markers, such as CD63, CD9, CD81, integrins, CD29, CD44, CD73, and α4-integrin [23, 65–67]. Similarly, both ubiquitous and MSC-specific proteins and nucleic acids are enveloped in these EVs (Fig. 1). Interestingly, certain proteins and nucleic acids are selectively enriched in EVs compared to their parental cells. For instance, Collino and colleagues [2010] identified that while microvesicles derived from bone marrow MSCs contain their parental cell-specific microRNAs (miR), the expression level of some was significantly higher in microvesicles compared to MSCs (miR-223, miR-451, and miR-564) [68]. It has also been shown that horizontal transfer of functional RNAs and proteins is involved in general cell functions, such as cell development, proliferation, survival, and differentiation, as well as regulation of the immune system [18], angiogenesis [69], and ATP generation [70]. Unequivocally, interest in exploring the therapeutic potential of MSC-EVs has evolved; however, at this stage, further investigation is warranted in regards to the unveiling of the composite profile of the contents of these vesicles and the elucidation of the potential therapeutic efficacy of these components.

Preparation of MSC-CM and MSC-EVs

MSC-CM is considered the least processed cell-free product from MSCs. Based on the source of MSCs, culture condition, culture duration, and collection method, different quantities of secreted factors may be detected in the CM [50]. Generally, MSCs are cultured in their growth media as monolayers or aggregates. Once cells reach approximately 80% confluence, serum-containing growth media are replaced with fresh media [36, 47, 49, 50, 71]. In order to decrease contamination of the CM by extrinsic sources, such as fetal bovine serum, serum-free media are commonly used at this step [57]. On the other hand, chemically defined media or EV-depleted serum containing media are suggested to reduce the effect of nutrition starvation on MSCs [72]. As previously mentioned, environmental signals influence the paracrine activity of MSCs; therefore, the cells can be exposed to different stimuli, including hypoxia or pro-inflammatory cytokines to promote the secretion of certain therapeutic molecules in vitro. At the end of the incubation period (commonly 24–48 h), the supernatant is collected from the MSC cultures. The cellular component is subsequently removed by density-gradient centrifugation or filtration. At this step, the cell-free product is considered MSC-CM. It is optional to concentrate MSC-CM before in vitro and in vivo applications. Following preparation, the CM can be stored at – 80 °C or subsequently processed for EV isolation.

There are several approaches to determine the yield of the MSC-CM. One of the most common approaches is based on the number of MSCs from which the CM was derived [47, 71, 73–76]. Other parameters, including total proteins and the concentration of certain soluble bioactive mediators, have also been considered for characterization and dosage determination of MSC-CM [46, 49, 50, 77]. A variety of techniques may be used to isolate and concentrate different fractions (e.g., exosomes or microvesicles) of EVs from CM; these include ultracentrifugation, filtration and chromatography, precipitation, and immuno-affinity [78]. Each method provides different degrees of purity and enrichment; however, none of the available methods can completely separate the different types of EVs from each other or from non-EV fractions (e.g. soluble proteins, cell-free nucleic acids, and membrane fractions). Combinations of two or more methods may be used to improve the purity of certain fractions of EVs. Assessment of isolated EVs is mainly done by determination of concentration and size distributions using different methods, such as nanoparticle tracking analysis (NTA), transmission electron microscopy, and flow cytometry. In addition, the amount of total proteins in EVs is commonly assessed and used to select EV dosage for in vitro and in vivo studies. Similar to CM, the concentration of EVs or their total protein can be normalized to the number of MSCs from which they are derived. The final product can further be concentrated and stored for short periods at 4 °C. For longer storage, EVs can be placed in ≤ – 20 °C without the need of cryopreservatives.

Therapeutic potential of MSC-CM in lung injury

So far, the ability of MSC-CM to significantly reduce the severity of lung injury, as effectively as MSCs, has been demonstrated in several in vitro and in vivo preclinical animal models (Table 2). To this end, Pati et al. showed

Table 2 Summary of therapeutic benefits of MSC-CM in preclinical animal models

CM Source	Route	Injury Model	Outcomes	Key Factor	Ref.
Mouse BM-MSC	IT	Mouse-ALI/LPS	↓ Neutrophils in BALF ↑ M2 in BALF	IGF-1	[74]
Human BM-MSC	IV	Rat-Pneumonia/*E. coli*	↑ Survival	LL-37	[81]
Rat BM-MSC	IT	Rat-Lung Injury/I/R	↓ Pro-inflammatory cytokines ↓ Neutrophils in BALF ↑ M2 & Treg in BALF		[82]
Mouse BMC	IN	Mouse-Asthma/OVA	↓ Airway inflammation ↓ Airway hyper-responsiveness ↓ Airway smooth muscle thickness ↑ IL-10 producing Treg & macrophages	APN	[83]
Mouse BM-MSC	IV	Neonatal Mouse-BPD/Hyperoxia	↓ Right ventricular hypertrophy ↓ Intrapulmonary arterioles muscularization ↓ Inflammatory cells & cytokines in BALF Preserve alveoli morphology ↑ Number of BASCs	Opn Csf1	[71, 84, 85]
Hyperoxia Preconditioned Rat BM-MSC	IP	Neonatal Rat- BPD/Hyperoxia	↓ PAH ↓ Right ventricular hypertrophy ↓ Pulmonary artery medial wall thickness Improved lung structure	STC-1	[87]
Rat BM-MSC	IT	Rat-Lung Fibrosis/ Bleomycin	↓ Lung fibrosis ↓ AEC apoptosis		[76]
Rat BM-MSC	IV	Rat-COPD/ cigarette smoke	↓ Lung emphysema ↓ Pulmonary artery medial wall thickness ↑ Number of small pulmonary vessels Protect lung fibroblasts		[91, 92]

AEC – alveolar epithelial cell, *ALI* – acute lung injury, *APN* – adiponectin, *BALF* – bronchoalveolar lavage fluid, *BASCs* – bronchoalveolar stem cells, *BM-MSC* – bone marrow-derived mesenchymal stem cells, *BPD* – bronchopulmonary dysplasia, *COPD* – chronic obstructive pulmonary disease, *Csf1* – macrophage colony stimulating factor 1 (M-CSF), E. coli – *Escherichia coli*, *IN* – intranasal, *IP* – intraperitoneally, *I/R* – ischemia reperfusion, *IT* – intratracheal, *IV* – intravenous, *LPS* – lipopolysaccharide, *M2* – macrophage type 2, *Opn* – osteopontin, *OVA* – ovalbumin, *PAH* – pulmonary artery hypertension, *STC-1* – stanniocalcin 1, *Treg* – regulatory T lymphocyte

that MSC-CM prevented endothelial cell permeability and restored the normal status of membrane adhesion molecules (β-catenin and VE-cadherin) in vitro. MSC-CM also reduced the adhesion of leukocytes to endothelial cells, thus suggesting that MSC-CM can moderate the inflammatory response of the injured endothelium by preserving vascular barrier integrity and preventing inflammatory cell binding to endothelial cells [79]. In another in vitro study, Ortiz et al. demonstrated the capability of MSC-CM to reduce the secretion of TNF-α by macrophages. Such anti-inflammatory effect of MSC-CM was suggested to be mediated by IL-1ra [10].

Lee and colleagues investigated alveolar fluid transport using whole human lungs in an ex vivo lung perfusion model. The idea of such experimental studies stemmed from the notion that impaired alveolar fluid clearance is associated with higher mortality in ARDS patients. In this study, the therapeutic benefits of MSCs and MSC-CM were evaluated by the extent of their ability to restore alveolar fluid clearance in ALI. The experimental design consisted of delivery of *Escherichia coli* (*E. coli*) endotoxin intra-bronchially to perfused lungs, followed by the administration of MSCs or MSC-CM one hour following induction of injury. Both treatments improved lung endothelial barrier integrity and the rate of alveolar fluid transport. This study also revealed the essential role of keratinocyte growth factor (KGF), a MSC component, in alveolar fluid transport. MSC pretreatment with KGF small-interference RNA (siRNA) decreased the effect of MSC-CM on alveolar fluid clearance. Conversely, this effect was restored by the addition of recombinant KGF protein to the CM [80].

Further studies to elucidate the anti-inflammatory potential of MSC-CM were extended to several small animal models of ALI. In this pursuit, Ionescu et al. showed that intratracheal (IT) administration of MSCs or MSC-CM reduced the total number of infiltrated neutrophils in bronchoalveolar lavage fluid (BALF) in mice with endotoxin-induced ALI. Of note, the administration of fibroblasts or fibroblast-CM did not reproduce the same effect thus demonstrating MSC specificity. Concurrently, the flow-cytometric analysis revealed that MSC and MSC-CM administration increased the percentage of inducible nitric oxide synthase (iNOS)-Ym1$^+$ alveolar macrophages in BALF, resembling the phenotype associated with alternatively activated macrophages (M2). Insulin-like growth factor 1 (IGF-1) was detected in MSC-CM, suggesting its role in polarization of alveolar macrophages to the M2 phenotype and protection of lungs from endotoxin-induced injury [74]. In another study, Devaney and colleagues reported that intravenous (IV) and IT administration of MSCs reduced the infiltration of neutrophils, IL-6, and the total amount of protein in BALF in a rat model of *E. coli*-induced pneumonia. MSCs also improved survival and bacterial clearance and preserved lung function. In contrast, MSC-CM improved animal survival without any significant mitigation of the severity of lung injury or inflammation [81]. Experimental evidence on the studies addressing the anti-inflammatory potential of MSC-CM revealed that MSC-CM pretreatment significantly reduced the amount of pro-inflammatory cytokines and the number of infiltrated neutrophils in BALF in a rat model of ischemia-reperfusion lung injury. In addition, the number of M2-like macrophages and T-regulatory lymphocytes in BALF fluid was increased in MSC-CM pretreated rats [82].

Likewise, in a mouse model of asthma, Ionescu et al. demonstrated that local delivery of CM derived from plastic-adherent bone marrow cells (BMC) is effective in reducing the number of pro-inflammatory cells in the lungs and airway hyper-responsiveness while increasing the percentage of IL-10 producing T-regulatory lymphocytes and macrophages. CM derived from lung fibroblasts did not produce the same effect as BMC-CM. Interestingly, adiponectin, an anti-inflammatory cytokine found in BMC-CM but not in fibroblast-CM, was shown to play a major role in conferring the protective effects of BMC-CM [83].

Additionally, the beneficial role of MSC-CM in protecting lung tissue from hyperoxia was studied in several small animal models of bronchopulmonary dysplasia (BPD). BPD and consequent pulmonary hypertension are serious complications in premature infants caused by mechanical ventilation and oxygen toxicity. As reported by Aslam and colleagues hyperoxia-induced BPD in neonatal mice can be prevented by IV administration of concentrated mouse MSC-CM similar to MSC treatment. This study also revealed that early administration of MSC-CM significantly decreased right ventricular hypertrophy and muscularization of intrapulmonary arterioles as well as preserved the number of alveoli with normal morphology in neonatal mice exposed to hyperoxia. In parallel, MSC-CM treatment was shown to dramatically reduce the number of inflammatory cells and cytokine levels in BALF of injured mice. Another important finding was reflected in the identification of two immunomodulatory molecules, osteopontin (Spp1 or Opn) and macrophage-colony-stimulating factor 1 (M-CSF or Csf1), exclusively present in higher extent in the MSC-CM. This suggests their plausible role in the therapeutic benefits of MSC-CM [71]. In a separate study from the same group, Hansmann observed that MSC-CM could also reverse the adverse effects of long-term exposure to hyperoxia on lung morphology and function [84]. With a view to identifying the mechanisms by which MSC-CM function, Tropea et al. observed that systemic administration of MSCs and their CM increased the number of bronchoalveolar stem cells (BASCs) in terminal bronchioles of lungs of neonatal mice 10 days post administration. Similarly, MSC-CM enhanced BASC colony growth in vitro; however, supplementation of BASC cultures with growth factors known to be present in MSC-CM (VEGF, HGF, KGF, or basic FGF) did not show a similar effect, thus ruling out the association of these MSC components in enhanced BASC colony growth [85]. It is noteworthy that the effect of daily administration of human MSC-CM, intraperitoneally, was observed to be comparable with a single administration of MSCs in protecting neonatal rats from BPD and pulmonary hypertension [86]. Since culture conditions can influence the secretion pattern of MSCs, Waszak and colleagues examined the effect of hyperoxia on the therapeutic potential of preconditioned MSC-CM in a rat model of BPD. Preconditioning MSCs under 95% O_2 improved therapeutic benefits of the CM compared with control MSC-CM or lung fibroblast-CM. Correlatively, the preconditioned MSC-CM was also shown to contain a higher amount of STC-1 [87], which is a pleiotropic protein with antioxidant, anti-apoptotic, and anti-inflammatory potential [37, 88–90].

Shen and colleagues examined the anti-apoptotic and anti-fibrotic benefits of MSC-CM in a chronic model of bleomycin-induced lung injury. Histological analysis of MSC-CM-treated rats revealed a significant reduction in lung fibrosis and apoptosis 28 days post-injury. Interestingly, the MSC-CM was able to promote proliferation and prevent apoptosis of human non-small cell lung cancer epithelial cells in vitro [76].

The therapeutic benefits of MSC-CM were also evaluated in a small animal model of cigarette-smoke-induced COPD. In addition to lung emphysema, cigarette smoke can cause apoptosis in lung fibroblasts. One of the roles of lung fibroblasts is to maintain the integrity of the alveolar structure; thus, their normal function is essential for the regeneration of the injured lung. Huh et al. showed that MSC and MSC-CM treatment significantly improved the histology of the emphysematous lungs and increased the number of small pulmonary vessels [91]. In a separate study, Kim et al. reported that MSC-CM reduced lung fibroblast apoptosis and increased their proliferation in vitro and in vivo. MSC-CM also restored the expression of extracellular matrix proteins and collagen gel contraction mediated at least in part by the PI3K/Akt pathway. Interestingly, the presence of both anti- and pro-fibrotic mediators was detected in MSC-CM [92].

Overall, these reports strongly suggest that administration of CM derived from MSCs can significantly attenuate cell death and inflammatory responses while improving tissue healing and endogenous regeneration in various lung injury models. However, the key mediators and the optimal conditions to produce them are still largely unknown.

Therapeutic potential of MSC-EVs in lung injury

Among the potential key mediators of MSCs, MSC-EVs are considered to bear therapeutic potential in lung injury. In order to establish a safe and effective alternative to live-cell transplantation, the therapeutic potential of different EV fractions was examined in a variety of preclinical animal models of lung injury as summarized in Table 3.

Gennai and colleagues used an ex vivo lung perfusion model to demonstrate the effect of MSC-EVs on alveolar fluid clearance rate in human lungs rejected for transplantation. MSC-EVs improved alveolar fluid clearance rate in a dose-dependent manner. Lung weight gain was also reduced by MSC-EV therapy compared to perfusion alone. Conversely, EVs derived from normal human lung fibroblasts had no beneficial effects. Further, MSC-EVs restored tracheal pressure, improved lung compliance, and reduced pulmonary artery pressure over six hours. The amount of lactate was also significantly lower in MSC-EV treated lungs compared to the control lungs. Since the anti-CD44 antibody attenuated the uptake of EVs by alveolar epithelial cells, the study suggested a key role of the CD44 receptor in internalizing EVs into recipient cells [93].

The studies on exploring therapeutic benefits of MSC-EVs have been examined in several ALI models. In this regard, an investigation by Zhu and colleagues recently showed that IT administration of MSC-EVs was associated with a reduction in pulmonary edema in *E. coli* endotoxin-induced ALI in mice. Additionally, MSC-EVs attenuated the influx of inflammatory cells and the presence of macrophage inflammatory protein 2 (MIP-2) in the alveoli. Both IT and IV administration of MSC-EVs were shown to dramatically increase the amount of KGF in BALF compared to injured untreated mice, maybe via transfer of KGF mRNA [22]. In another study, Li et al. preconditioned MSCs under anoxia for 60 min prior EV collection. Subsequently, EVs from both normal culture and preconditioned MSCs were observed to significantly reduce the total number of white blood cells, neutrophils, total proteins, and MIP-2 in BALF of endotoxin-injured mice; however, no significant differences were observed between the preconditioned MSC-EVs and control MSC-EVs [94].

Another report by Monsel and colleagues demonstrated that systemic administration of MSC-EVs improved survival and reduced lung inflammation and injury while promoting bacterial clearance in a murine model of *E. coli*-induced pneumonia. EVs harvested from MSCs preconditioned with a toll-like receptor (TLR)-3 agonist were shown to further increase KGF secretion and bacterial clearance. When examined in vitro, the MSC-EVs increased the phagocytic function of human macrophages and the ATP levels in alveolar epithelial type 2 cells. Preconditioned MSC-EVs were more effective in enhancing the anti-inflammatory and phagocytic activity of cultured macrophages, possibly by transferring cyclooxygenase-2 mRNA to activated monocytes resulting in an increase in production of PGE2 [95].

The direct effects of MSC-EVs on activated macrophages has also been studied by preconditioning alveolar macrophages (AMs) with MSC-EVs and administering them to mice with LPS-induced lung injury. Administration of pretreated AMs, but not control AMs, significantly reduced total proteins, TNF-α, and the total number of neutrophils in BALF. Mitochondrial transfer via MSC-EVs was shown to play an important role in carrying the anti-inflammatory and pro-phagocytic effects of MSCs on macrophages [96]. Phinney and colleagues demonstrated that under oxidative stress, MSCs donated mitochondria to macrophages via EVs. In addition, they revealed that IV administration of MSCs or their EVs in silica-exposed mice significantly reduced the infiltration of white blood cells and secretion of inflammatory mediators in BALF. MSCs and their EVs also reduced the size of the calcified nodules as well as the expression of pro-inflammatory [TNF, CCL2, and chemokine (C-X-C motif) ligand (CXCL) 1] and pro-fibrotic (TGF-β and IL-10) genes in the lung, 2 to 4 weeks post-injury. Interestingly, MSC-EVs, but not MSCs alone, reduced the accumulation of hydroxyproline in lung tissue [17]. Systemic administration of MSCs or EVs following silica exposure was shown to decrease collagen deposition in lung parenchyma and recruitment of neutrophils and lymphocytes into airways two weeks post-treatment. However, MSC-EV administration did not significantly reduce lung wet-to-dry ratio, as opposed to MSCs [97].

The therapeutic benefits of MSC-CM and MSC-EVs were compared in a mouse model of acute asthma. Systemic administration of both MSC-CM and EVs, but not lung fibroblast products, significantly abrogated the increase in airway hyper-responsiveness and lung inflammation. The amounts of T helper lymphocyte (Th)2- and Th17-associated cytokines were reduced in BALF while IL-10 levels were concomitantly increased. Blocking the release of secreted mediators in MSCs in vitro suppressed many protective effects of the cells [75].

In a murine model of hemorrhagic shock, MSCs and their EVs were shown to attenuate vascular permeability in injured lungs. Both treatments were able to suppress hemorrhagic-shock-induced RhoA GTPase activity in lungs. MSC-CM and recombinant angiopoietin 1 (Ang1),

Table 3 Summary of therapeutic benefits of MSC-EVs in preclinical animal models

EV Source	Route	Injury Model	Outcomes	Key Factor	Ref.
Human BM-MSC	IT, IV	Mouse-ALI/LPS	↓ Lung edema ↓ WBCs & neutrophils in BALF ↓ Total protein & MIP-2 in BALF ↑ KGF in BALF	KGF mRNA	[22]
Normoxia & Anoxia pretreated Human BM-MSC	IV	Mouse-ALI/LPS	↓ WBCs & neutrophils in BALF ↓ Total protein & MIP-2 in BALF		[94]
Untreated & Poly (I:C)–pretreated Human BM-MSC	IT, IV	Mouse-Pneumonia/*E. coli*	↓ Lung injury ↓ WBCs & neutrophils in BALF ↓ Total protein & MIP-2 in BALF ↓ E. coli count in BALF, lung, & blood ↑ Survival ↑ KGF in BALF	KGF mRNA & CD44	[95]
Human BM-MSC	EV-treated AM/ IN	Mouse-ALI/LPS	↓ Neutrophils in BALF ↓ Total protein & TNF-α in BALF	Mitochondria transfer	[96]
Human BM-MSC	IV	Mouse-Shock/Hemorrhage	↓ Vascular permeability ↓ RhoA GTPase activity in lung		[66]
Human WJ-MSC	IT	Mouse-Lung Injury/I/R	↓ Lung edema ↓ Airway resistance ↓ Pulmonary artery pressure ↓ Neutrophil in lung ↓ Inflammatroy cytokines in BALF ↑ KGF, PGE2, &IL-10 in BALF		[115]
Swine BM-MSC	IT	Swine-Influenza/SwIV	↓ Lung lesions ↓ WBCs in lung ↓ Inflammatory cytokines in lung ↓ Virus titer in nasal swap & lung	RNA	[101]
Mouse & Human BM-MSC	IV	Mouse-Asthma/AHE	↓ Airway hyper-responsiveness ↓ WBCs in BALF & lung ↓ Th2/Th17 related cytokines in BALF		[75]
Mouse BM-MSC	IV	Mouse-PAH/Hypoxia	↓ Right ventricular systolic pressure ↓ Vascular remodeling ↓ Macrophages & cytokines in lung ↓ STAT-3 in lung		[20]
Rat BM-MSC	IV	Rat-PAH/Monocrotaline	↓ Pulmonary artery pressure ↓ Pulmonary vascular remodeling ↓ Right ventricle pressure ↓ Right ventricular hypertrophy		[98]
Mouse & Human BM-MSC	IV	Mouse-PAH/ Monocrotaline	↓ Pulmonary vascular remodeling ↓ Right ventricle hypertrophy	miRNAs	[99]
Human WJ- & BM-MSC	IV	Neonatal Mouse-BPD/ Hyperoxia	↑ Alveolarization ↑ Lung funcion ↓ Lung fibrosis ↓ PAH ↓ Pulmonary vasular remodeling ↓ Pro-inflammatry genes in macrophages		[67]
Human UC-MSC	IT	Neonatal Rat-BPD/Hyperoxia	↑ Alveolarization & angiogenesis ↓ Alveolar epithelial cell death ↓ Macrophages & cytokines in lung	VEGF	[100]
Human BM-MSC	IV	Mouse-Lung Fibrosis/Silica	↓ Size of calcified nodules in lung ↓ Hydroxyproline in lung ↓ Inflammatory cells in BALF ↓ Cytokines in BALF	miRNAs & mitochondria transfer	[17]
Human BM-MSC	IV	Mouse-Lung Fibrosis/Silica	↓ Lung collagen ↓ WBCs in BALF		[97]
Human ASCs	IT	Mouse-COPD/ elastase	↓ Lung emphysema ↑ FGF2 in lung		[116]

AHE – *Aspergillus* hyphal extract, *ALI* – acute lung injury, *AM* – Alveolar macrophages, *ASCs* – adipose-derived mesenchymal stem cells, *BALF* – bronchoalveolar lavage fluid, *BM-MSC* – bone marrow-derived mesenchymal stem cells, *FGF2* – fibroblast growth factor 2, *IL-10* – interleukin 10, *IN* – intranasal, *I/R* – ischemia reperfusion, *IT* – intratracheal, *IV* – intravenous, *KGF* – keratinocyte growth factor, *LPS* – lipopolysaccharide, *MIP-2* – macrophage inflammatory protein 2, *miRNAs* – microRNAs, *OVA* – ovalbumin, *PAH* – pulmonary artery hypertension, *PGE2* – prostaglandin E2, *STAT-3* – signal transducer and activator of transcription 3, *SwIV* – swine influanza virus H1N1, *Th* – T helper lymphocyte, *UC-MSC* – umbilical cord blood-MSC, *VEGF* – vascular endothelial growth factor, *WBCs* – white blood cells, *WJ-MSC* – umbilical cord Wharton's jelly-MSC

but not EVs, significantly protected endothelial VE-cadherin junctions and reduced permeability in vitro. In vivo analysis of protein phosphorylation patterns also revealed some differences in signaling pathways activated by MSC-EVs compared to MSCs. Overall, these observations suggest that while MSC-EVs preserved pulmonary vasculature integrity similar to MSCs, their mechanism of action was not necessarily equivalent [66].

The effect of MSC-EVs on pulmonary vasculature was also demonstrated by Lee and colleagues. Studies by this group indicated that the administration of MSC-EVs, but not fibroblast-EVs, can protect against the elevation of right ventricular systolic pressure and pulmonary vascular remodeling in a murine model of hypoxia-induced pulmonary artery hypertension. The MSC-EVs mediated an anti-inflammatory effect by reducing the influx of lung macrophages and early inflammatory mediators. MSC-EV treatment also abrogated the hypoxia-induced phosphorylation of signal transducer and activator of transcription 3 (STAT-3), which plays a critical role in the response of pulmonary vasculature to hypoxia [20]. In a rat model of monocrotaline-induced pulmonary hypertension, IV administration of rat MSC-EVs decreased pulmonary artery pressure and remodeling as well as right ventricle pressure and hypertrophy. MSC-EVs were as effective as their parent cells in preventing pulmonary hypertension [98]. Similarly, IV administration of either mouse or human MSC-EVs was shown to reduce right ventricular hypertrophy and pulmonary vascular remodeling in monocrotaline-treated mice. Administration of the exosome fraction of MSC-EVs exerted higher therapeutic response compared to the microvesicle fraction. MicroRNA analysis revealed a significant increase in the levels of several anti-inflammatory and anti-proliferative microRNAs, including miRs-34a,-122,-124, and – 127 in MSC-exosomes compared to exosomes derived from plasma of healthy mice [99].

Similar to MSC-CM, MSC-EVs were shown to significantly reduce lung fibrosis, restore lung architecture, and improve alveolarization and lung function of neonatal mice exposed to 75% oxygen for 7 days. MSC-EV administration also reduced pulmonary arterial remodeling and hypertension associated with BPD. Additionally, MSC-EVs downregulated expression of genes associated with pro-inflammatory macrophages [67]. In a study conducted by Ahn and colleagues, EVs derived from UC-MSCs were as effective as their parental cells in preventing hypoxia-induced BPD in neonatal rats. Also, MSCs and their EVs reduced the inflammatory responses in the lungs in contrary to fibroblast-derived EVs that did not exhibit similar protective effects. Finally, the protective effect rendered by MSCs and EVs was partially abrogated by the knockdown of the VEGF gene in MSCs prior to EV isolation [100].

Recently, MSC-EVs were examined in a swine model of influenza virus-induced ALI. Local administration of MSC-EVs was able to significantly reduce the infiltration of inflammatory cells to the lungs, the thickening of alveolar walls, and the number of collapsed alveoli in infected swine. MSC-EVs were also able to reduce replication and shedding of influenza virus both in vivo and in vitro. It was suggested that the transfer of RNA to the infected cells might be an important factor in the observed anti-influenza activity by MSC-EVs [101].

Overall, cumulative studies described above suggest that in order to increase cell survival, preserve physiological function, and reduce immune/inflammatory responses, MSC-EVs can transfer bioactive mediators to injured cells and regulate their pathophysiologic responses. In most experiments, EVs appeared to be as potent as MSCs, possibly with lower health-associated risks.

MSC-EVs: From bench to bedside

In 2014, allogeneic MSC-EVs were administered to a patient with a steroid refractory graft-versus-host disease (GvHD). Not only the diarrhea volume of the patient was reduced after MSC-EV therapy, but also cutaneous and mucosal symptoms were improved within two weeks and the patient was in stable condition four months after EV treatments. Consequently, the dose of steroids given to the patient was reduced. Interestingly, the number of patient's peripheral blood mononuclear cells producing TNF-α, IL-1β, or IFN-γ was reduced more than 50% after the last EV administration [102].

In a separate study, forty patients with chronic kidney disease (CKD) were randomly divided into two groups to receive MSC-EVs or placebo treatment. Two doses of MSC-EVs were administered a week apart. The first dose was administered IV and the second intra-arterially. Of note, MSC-EV treatment, but not the placebo, was effective in improving estimated glomerular filtration rate and urinary albumin-to-creatinine ratio as well as reducing serum creatinine and blood urea. At twelve weeks after EV treatment, plasma levels of TNF-α were significantly reduced, whereas levels of IL-10 and TGF-β were increased [103]. In both studies, the MSC-EV administration was well-tolerated by patients without any side effects.

A phase II/III clinical trial is currently registered on clinicaltrials.gov evaluating the benefits of UC-MSC-EVs in type I diabetic patients [104]. In addition, recently, an Investigational New Drug clearance for allogeneic MSC-EVs was approved by the Food and Drug Administration for the treatment of severe second-degree burn patients. The company that received the approval is planning to conduct a multicenter phase I/IIa clinical trial in late 2018 [105].

Conclusions

Overall, current data suggest that MSC-derived products can effectively mimic the therapeutic effects of MSCs in preclinical models of lung injury. The use of CM or EVs may circumvent many of the safety concerns associated with the use of live cells, such as thrombogenicity. Also, unlike cells, CM and EVs are not able to proliferate or reprogram after administration, which decreases the risk of tumorigenicity [106–108]. From a therapeutic standpoint, MSC-EVs and other bioactive mediators are smaller than their parent cells, and thus might be distributed more efficiently into the lungs and other organs.

Another therapeutic advantage of EVs arises from their ability to protect their cargo from unfavorable environmental conditions, such as dramatic changes in pH or release of digestive (lytic) enzymes into the bloodstream and damaged tissue. Based on this concept, MSC-EVs are considered efficient vehicles for transporting delicate bioactive mediators to the distal airways. It is also thought that MSC-EVs can be used to deliver specific drugs to target organs. Such drugs can be delivered to EVs via MSCs that overexpress those factors, or can be loaded directly to the EVs after they have been released by the cells. Examples of different types of therapeutic cargo include siRNAs for silencing target genes and chemotherapeutic drugs, such as doxorubicin [109, 110].

In addition to their biological advantages, feasibility/logistical advantages set cell-free products apart. For instance, large-scale manufacturing of cell-free products is possible by repeated harvesting of CM from cultured MSCs. MSC-CM and EVs can be prepared and stored in small volumes, which could simplify dosing studies. Another great advantage is that CM and EVs can also be stored for several months at – 20 °C to – 80 °C without the need for cryopreservatives, unlike their parent cells [111]. Notably, cryopreservatives, such as dimethyl sulfoxide (DMSO), can be cytotoxic and have been reported to lyse EVs [112]. The potential capability to freeze-dry and lyophilize all or pertinent fractions of CM and EVs should be helpful in overcoming the logistical difficulties of storage and transport of these products in austere conditions.

There appear to be therapeutic advantages in using MSC-CM and EVs over live whole cells; yet, to develop safe and effective cell-free therapies, a significant knowledge gap needs to be addressed, including optimization of bioactive components, dosing regimens, and production methods. A growing number of studies have identified some of the key mediators in MSC-CM and EVs; however, there is a variability in the content of the secretome due to several factors. These include donor's condition (age, sex, and health status), the type of MSCs (e.g. bone marrow, adipose, or UC), the type of culture (flask or bioreactor), the type of media and supplements (e.g., fetal bovine serum, xeno-free, or chemically-defined media), and the microenvironment (e.g. oxygen tension and presence or absence of stress signals) [16, 104, 111]. Also, post-processing of CM and EVs (e.g. CM concentration and EV enrichment) as well as handling and storage can influence their quality [111]. Furthermore, various factors (e.g. methods of EV enrichment and storage) could influence the quantity of EVs present in the final product [104], making it difficult to estimate EV yield per MSC. In light of these limitations, it is essential to develop a series of potency assays for cell-free products in order to control their quality and quantity, and to predict their efficacy in vivo.

Based on currently available techniques, large numbers of MSCs are still required to produce an adequate amount of CM or EVs for clinical use, similar to the number of MSCs used for clinical trials (e.g. 10^6–10^7 cells/kg). In order to produce sufficient pools of MSCs, the cells need to be expanded in vitro for several population doublings. Although MSCs have been shown to be safe for up to 40 population doublings [16], it is important to frequently inspect them for cell senescence and chromosome instability, and eliminate defective cells. To overcome the low yield of MSCs and their products from primary cultures, genetic modification, such as immortalization, can be considered [113]. In addition, the technology to obtain CM and EVs from MSCs derived from induced pluripotent stem cells (iPSC-MSCs) might be beneficial [111, 114]. iPSC-MSCs have robust proliferation and differentiation capacities and can be generated either from allogeneic sources or patients [114]. These alternative approaches could also facilitate establishing universal donors to minimize donor-to-donor variability and produce large-scales of CM and EVs with consistent quality. The use of autologous MSCs and their products may be considered when allogeneic products are not available, especially in remote and austere conditions. However, since the effect of different disorders on endogenous stem cells and their products is not completely understood [16, 111], the application of autologous-based products needs to be carefully assessed.

To summarize, MSC-CM and EVs emerge as promising therapeutic tools for the treatment of acute and chronic lung diseases. However, there is a compelling need to gather additional knowledge. Furthermore, large-scale production of Good Manufacturing Practice (GMP)-graded MSC-CM and EVs needs to be developed so that cell-free therapy can be safely translated from the bench to the bedside.

Abbreviations

AEC: Alveolar Epithelial Cell; AHE: *Aspergillus* Hyphal Extract; ALI: Acute Lung Injury; Alix: Apoptosis-Linked Gene (ALG)-2-Interacting Protein X; AM: Alveolar Macrophages; Ang1: Angiopoietin 1; APN: Adiponectin; ARDS: Acute Respiratory Distress Syndrome; ASC: Adipose-derived Mesenchymal Stem/stromal Cell; BALF: Bronchoalveolar Lavage Fluid; BASCs: Bronchoalveolar Stem Cells; BMC: Bone Marrow Cells; BPD: Bronchopulmonary Dysplasia; CCL: Chemokine (C-C motif) ligand; CKD: Chronic kidney disease;

CM: Conditioned Media; COPD: Chronic Obstructive Pulmonary Disease; CXCL: Chemokine (C-X-C motif) ligand; CXCR: Chemokine (C-X-C motif) Receptor; DMSO: Dimethyl sulfoxide; E.coli: *Escherichia coli*; EGFr: Epidermal Growth Factor Receptor; EVs: Extracellular Vesicles; FGF: Fibroblast Growth Factor; G-CSF: Granulocyte Colony Stimulating Factor; GM-CSF: Granulocyte Monocyte Colony Stimulating Factor; GMP: Good Manufacturing Practice; GvHD: Graft-versus-Host Disease; HGF: Hepatocyte Growth Factor; HLA-DR: Human Leukocyte Antigen; HO-1: Hemeoxygenase 1; I/R: Ischemia Reperfusion; IDO: Indoleamine 2,3-Dioxygenase; IFN-γ: Interferon Gamma; IGF-1: Insulin-like Growth Factor 1; IL: Interleukin; IL-1ra: IL-1 Receptor Antagonist; iPSC-MSC: Induced Pluripotent Stem Cell-derived Mesenchymal Stem/stromal Cell; IN: Intranasal; iNOS: Inducible Nitric Oxide Synthase; IPF: Idiopathic Pulmonary Fibrosis; IT: Intratracheal; IV: Intravenous; KGF: keratinocyte Growth Factor; LIF: Leukemia Inhibitory Factor; LPS: Lipopolysaccharide; M2: Alternatively Activated Macrophages; MCP-1: Monocyte Chemotactic Protein 1; M-CSF (Csf1): Macrophage-Colony Stimulating Factor 1; MIP-2: Macrophage Inflammatory Protein 2; miRNA (miR): MicroRNA; MMP: Metalloproteinase; mRNA: Messenger RNA; MSCs: mesenchymal stem/stromal cells; MVBs: Multi-Vesicular Bodies; NTA: Nanoparticle Tracking Analysis.; Opn: (Spp1) Osteopontin.; OVA: Ovalbumin.; PAH: Pulmonary Artery Hypertension.; PDGF: Platelets Derived Growth Factor.; PGE2: Prostaglandin E2.; PS: Phosphatidylserine.; SDF-1: Stem Cell-Derived Factor 1.; siRNA: Small Interference RNA.; STAT-3: Signal transducer and activator of transcription 3.; STC-1: Stanniocalcin-1.; SwIV: Swine Influenza Virus H1N1.; TGF-β: Transforming Growth Factor beta.; Th: T Helper Lymphocyte.; TIMP-1: Tissue Inhibitor of Metalloproteinase 1.; TLR: Toll-like Receptor.; TNF-α: Tumor Necrosis Factor Alpha.; Treg: Regulatory T Lymphocyte.; Tsg 101: Tumor Susceptibility Gene 101.; TSG-6: TNF Stimulating Gene 6 Protein.; UC-MSC: Umbilical Cord Blood Mesenchymal Stem/stromal Cell.; VEGF: Vascular Endothelial Growth Factor.; WBC: White Blood Cell.; WJ-MSC: Umbilical Cord Warton's Jelly Mesenchymal Stem/stromal Cell.

Acknowledgements

The authors wish to thank the personnel of the Multi-Organ Support Technology (MOST) Task Area. Additionally, the authors would like to thank Dr. Subrata Haldar for reviewing and editing of the manuscript.

Funding

This work was supported by USAMRMC Combat Casualty Care RAD administered via the Multi-Organ Support Technology (MOST) Task Area, Grant number:
X_017_2018; PI: Arezoo Mohammadipoor.

Disclaimer

The opinions or assertions contained herein are the private views of the authors and are not to be construed as official or as reflecting the views of the Department of the Army or the Department of Defense.

Authors' contributions

A.M. contributed to the design and writing of the manuscript. B.A. contributed to the writing and critical revisions of the manuscript. A.B. contributed to the critical revisions. L.C. contributed to the funding and critical revisions. All authors read and approved the final manuscript.

Competing interests

The authors declare that they have no competing interests.

Author details

[1]Multi-Organ Support Technology (MOST) Task Area, US Army Institute of Surgical Research, Fort Sam Houston, TX, USA. [2]Oak Ridge Institute for Science and Education, Oak Ridge, TN, USA. [3]The Geneva Foundation, Tacoma, WA, USA.

References

1. Sueblinvong V, Weiss DJ. Stem cells and cell therapy approaches in lung biology and diseases. Transl Res. 2010;156(3):188–205.
2. Rubenfeld GD, Caldwell E, Peabody E, Weaver J, Martin DP, Neff M, Stern EJ, Hudson LD. Incidence and outcomes of acute lung injury. N Engl J Med. 2005;353(16):1685–93.
3. Matthay MA, Ware LB, Zimmerman GA. The acute respiratory distress syndrome. J Clin Invest. 2012;122(8):2731–40.
4. Przybysz TM, Heffner AC. Early treatment of severe acute respiratory distress syndrome. Emerg Med Clin North Am. 2016;34(1):1–14.
5. Batchinsky AI, Burkett SE, Zanders TB, Chung KK, Regn DD, Jordan BS, Necsoiu C, Nguyen R, Hanson MA, Morris MJ, et al. Comparison of airway pressure release ventilation to conventional mechanical ventilation in the early management of smoke inhalation injury in swine. Crit Care Med. 2011; 39(10):2314–21.
6. Batchinsky AI, Weiss WB, Jordan BS, Dick EJ Jr, Cancelada DA, Cancio LC. Ventilation-perfusion relationships following experimental pulmonary contusion. J Appl Physiol (1985). 2007;103(3):895–902.
7. The acute respiratory distress syndrome network. Ventilation with lower tidal volumes as compared with traditional tidal volumes for acute lung injury and the acute respiratory distress syndrome. N Engl J Med. 2000; 342(18):1301–8.
8. Ranieri VM, Rubenfeld GD, Thompson BT, Ferguson ND, Caldwell E, Fan E, Camporota L, Slutsky AS. Acute respiratory distress syndrome: the Berlin definition. Jama. 2012;307(23):2526–33.
9. Kreyer S, Scaravilli V, Linden K, Belenkiy SM, Necsoiu C, Li Y, Putensen C, Chung KK, Batchinsky AI, Cancio LC. Early utilization of extracorporeal CO2 removal for treatment of acute respiratory distress syndrome due to smoke inhalation and burns in sheep. Shock. 2016;45(1):65–72.
10. Ortiz LA, Dutreil M, Fattman C, Pandey AC, Torres G, Go K, Phinney DG. Interleukin 1 receptor antagonist mediates the antiinflammatory and antifibrotic effect of mesenchymal stem cells during lung injury. Proc Natl Acad Sci U S A. 2007;104(26):11002–7.
11. Xu J, Woods CR, Mora AL, Joodi R, Brigham KL, Iyer S, Rojas M. Prevention of endotoxin-induced systemic response by bone marrow-derived mesenchymal stem cells in mice. Am J Physiol Lung Cell Mol Physiol. 2007; 293(1):L131–41.
12. Gupta N, Su X, Popov B, Lee JW, Serikov V, Matthay MA. Intrapulmonary delivery of bone marrow-derived mesenchymal stem cells improves survival and attenuates endotoxin-induced acute lung injury in mice. J Immunol. 2007;179(3):1855–63.
13. Qin ZH, Xu JF, Qu JM, Zhang J, Sai Y, Chen CM, Wu L, Yu L. Intrapleural delivery of MSCs attenuates acute lung injury by paracrine/endocrine mechanism. J Cell Mol Med. 2012;16(11):2745–53.
14. Curley GF, Hayes M, Ansari B, Shaw G, Ryan A, Barry F, O'Brien T, O'Toole D, Laffey JG. Mesenchymal stem cells enhance recovery and repair following ventilator-induced lung injury in the rat. Thorax. 2012;67(6):496–501.
15. Antunes MA, Abreu SC, Cruz FF, Teixeira AC, Lopes-Pacheco M, Bandeira E, Olsen PC, Diaz BL, Takyia CM, Freitas IP, et al. Effects of different mesenchymal stromal cell sources and delivery routes in experimental emphysema. Respir Res. 2014;15:118.
16. Antebi B, Mohammadipoor A, Batchinsky AI, Cancio LC. The promise of mesenchymal stem cell therapy for acute respiratory distress syndrome. J Trauma Acute Care Surg. 2018;84(1):183–91.
17. Phinney DG, Di Giuseppe M, Njah J, Sala E, Shiva S, St Croix CM, Stolz DB, Watkins SC, Di YP, Leikauf GD, et al. Mesenchymal stem cells use extracellular vesicles to outsource mitophagy and shuttle microRNAs. Nat Commun. 2015;6:8472.
18. Lai RC, Yeo RW, Lim SK. Mesenchymal stem cell exosomes. Semin Cell Dev Biol. 2015;40:82–8.

19. Lai RC, Arslan F, Lee MM, Sze NS, Choo A, Chen TS, Salto-Tellez M, Timmers L, Lee CN, El Oakley RM, et al. Exosome secreted by MSC reduces myocardial ischemia/reperfusion injury. Stem Cell Res. 2010;4(3):214–22.
20. Lee C, Mitsialis SA, Aslam M, Vitali SH, Vergadi E, Konstantinou G, Sdrimas K, Fernandez-Gonzalez A, Kourembanas S. Exosomes mediate the cytoprotective action of mesenchymal stromal cells on hypoxia-induced pulmonary hypertension. Circulation. 2012;126(22):2601–11.
21. Li T, Yan Y, Wang B, Qian H, Zhang X, Shen L, Wang M, Zhou Y, Zhu W, Li W, et al. Exosomes derived from human umbilical cord mesenchymal stem cells alleviate liver fibrosis. Stem Cells Dev. 2013;22(6):845–54.
22. Zhu YG, Feng XM, Abbott J, Fang XH, Hao Q, Monsel A, Qu JM, Matthay MA, Lee JW. Human mesenchymal stem cell microvesicles for treatment of Escherichia coli endotoxin-induced acute lung injury in mice. Stem cells. 2014;32(1):116–25.
23. Wang Y, Lu X, He J, Zhao W. Influence of erythropoietin on microvesicles derived from mesenchymal stem cells protecting renal function of chronic kidney disease. Stem Cell Res Ther. 2015;6:100.
24. Friedenstein AJ, Chailakhjan RK, Lalykina KS. The development of fibroblast colonies in monolayer cultures of Guinea-pig bone marrow and spleen cells. Cell Tissue Kinet. 1970;3(4):393–403.
25. Zuk PA, Zhu M, Ashjian P, De Ugarte DA, Huang JI, Mizuno H, Alfonso ZC, Fraser JK, Benhaim P, Hedrick MH. Human adipose tissue is a source of multipotent stem cells. Mol Biol Cell. 2002;13(12):4279–95.
26. Miura M, Gronthos S, Zhao M, Lu B, Fisher LW, Robey PG, Shi S. SHED: stem cells from human exfoliated deciduous teeth. Proc Natl Acad Sci U S A. 2003;100(10):5807–12.
27. Lee MW, Choi J, Yang MS, Moon YJ, Park JS, Kim HC, Kim YJ. Mesenchymal stem cells from cryopreserved human umbilical cord blood. Biochem Biophys Res Commun. 2004;320(1):273–8.
28. In 't Anker PS, Scherjon SA, Kleijburg-van der Keur C, de Groot-swings GM, Claas FH, Fibbe WE, Kanhai HH. Isolation of mesenchymal stem cells of fetal or maternal origin from human placenta. Stem cells. 2004;22(7):1338–45.
29. Prockop DJ, Kota DJ, Bazhanov N, Reger RL. Evolving paradigms for repair of tissues by adult stem/progenitor cells (MSCs). J Cell Mol Med. 2010;14(9):2190–9.
30. Dominici M, Le Blanc K, Mueller I, Slaper-Cortenbach I, Marini F, Krause D, Deans R, Keating A, Prockop D, Horwitz E. Minimal criteria for defining multipotent mesenchymal stromal cells. The International Society for Cellular Therapy position statement. Cytotherapy. 2006;8(4):315–7.
31. Caplan AI, Dennis JE. Mesenchymal stem cells as trophic mediators. J Cell Biochem. 2006;98(5):1076–84.
32. Uccelli A, Moretta L, Pistoia V. Mesenchymal stem cells in health and disease. Nat Rev Immunol. 2008;8(9):726–36.
33. Matthay MA. Therapeutic potential of mesenchymal stromal cells for acute respiratory distress syndrome. Ann Am Thorac Soc. 2015;12(1):S54–7.
34. Konala VB, Mamidi MK, Bhonde R, Das AK, Pochampally R, Pal R. The current landscape of the mesenchymal stromal cell secretome: a new paradigm for cell-free regeneration. Cytotherapy. 2016;18(1):13–24.
35. Gunn WG, Conley A, Deininger L, Olson SD, Prockop DJ, Gregory CA. A crosstalk between myeloma cells and marrow stromal cells stimulates production of DKK1 and interleukin-6: a potential role in the development of lytic bone disease and tumor progression in multiple myeloma. Stem cells. 2006;24(4):986–91.
36. Hung SC, Pochampally RR, Chen SC, Hsu SC, Prockop DJ. Angiogenic effects of human multipotent stromal cell conditioned medium activate the PI3K-Akt pathway in hypoxic endothelial cells to inhibit apoptosis, increase survival, and stimulate angiogenesis. Stem cells. 2007;25(9):2363–70.
37. Block GJ, Ohkouchi S, Fung F, Frenkel J, Gregory C, Pochampally R, DiMattia G, Sullivan DE, Prockop DJ. Multipotent stromal cells are activated to reduce apoptosis in part by upregulation and secretion of stanniocalcin-1. Stem cells. 2009;27(3):670–81.
38. Ren G, Zhao X, Zhang L, Zhang J, L'Huillier A, Ling W, Roberts AI, Le AD, Shi S, Shao C, et al. Inflammatory cytokine-induced intercellular adhesion molecule-1 and vascular cell adhesion molecule-1 in mesenchymal stem cells are critical for immunosuppression. J Immunol. 2010;184(5):2321–8.
39. Choi H, Lee RH, Bazhanov N, Oh JY, Prockop DJ. Anti-inflammatory protein TSG-6 secreted by activated MSCs attenuates zymosan-induced mouse peritonitis by decreasing TLR2/NF-kappaB signaling in resident macrophages. Blood. 2011;118(2):330–8.
40. Zhang HC, Liu XB, Huang S, Bi XY, Wang HX, Xie LX, Wang YQ, Cao XF, Lv J, Xiao FJ, et al. Microvesicles derived from human umbilical cord mesenchymal stem cells stimulated by hypoxia promote angiogenesis both in vitro and in vivo. Stem Cells Dev. 2012;21(18):3289–97.
41. Lai RC, Tan SS, Yeo RW, Choo AB, Reiner AT, Su Y, Shen Y, Fu Z, Alexander L, Sze SK, et al. MSC secretes at least 3 EV types each with a unique permutation of membrane lipid, protein and RNA. J Extracell Vesicles. 2016;5:29828.
42. Nemeth K, Leelahavanichkul A, Yuen PS, Mayer B, Parmelee A, Doi K, Robey PG, Leelahavanichkul K, Koller BH, Brown JM, et al. Bone marrow stromal cells attenuate sepsis via prostaglandin E(2)-dependent reprogramming of host macrophages to increase their interleukin-10 production. Nat Med. 2009;15(1):42–9.
43. Bustos ML, Huleihel L, Meyer EM, Donnenberg AD, Donnenberg VS, Sciurba JD, Mroz L, McVerry BJ, Ellis BM, Kaminski N, et al. Activation of human mesenchymal stem cells impacts their therapeutic abilities in lung injury by increasing interleukin (IL)-10 and IL-1RN levels. Stem Cells Transl Med. 2013; 2(11):884–95.
44. Kim DS, Jang IK, Lee MW, Ko YJ, Lee DH, Lee JW, Sung KW, Koo HH, Yoo KH. Enhanced immunosuppressive properties of human mesenchymal stem cells primed by interferon-gamma. EBioMedicine. 2018;28:261–73.
45. van Poll D, Parekkadan B, Cho CH, Berthiaume F, Nahmias Y, Tilles AW, Yarmush ML. Mesenchymal stem cell-derived molecules directly modulate hepatocellular death and regeneration in vitro and in vivo. Hepatology. 2008;47(5):1634–43.
46. van Koppen A, Joles JA, van Balkom BW, Lim SK, de Kleijn D, Giles RH, Verhaar MC. Human embryonic mesenchymal stem cell-derived conditioned medium rescues kidney function in rats with established chronic kidney disease. PLoS One. 2012;7(6):e38746.
47. Chang CL, Leu S, Sung HC, Zhen YY, Cho CL, Chen A, Tsai TH, Chung SY, Chai HT, Sun CK, et al. Impact of apoptotic adipose-derived mesenchymal stem cells on attenuating organ damage and reducing mortality in rat sepsis syndrome induced by cecal puncture and ligation. J Transl Med. 2012;10:244.
48. Shrestha C, Zhao L, Chen K, He H, Mo Z. Enhanced healing of diabetic wounds by subcutaneous administration of human umbilical cord derived stem cells and their conditioned media. Int J Endocrinol. 2013;2013:592454.
49. Goolaerts A, Pellan-Randrianarison N, Larghero J, Vanneaux V, Uzunhan Y, Gille T, Dard N, Planes C, Matthay MA, Clerici C. Conditioned media from mesenchymal stromal cells restore sodium transport and preserve epithelial permeability in an in vitro model of acute alveolar injury. Am J Physiol Lung Cell Mol Physiol. 2014;306(11):L975–85.
50. Pawitan JA. Prospect of stem cell conditioned medium in regenerative medicine. Biomed Res Int. 2014;2014:965849.
51. Danieli P, Malpasso G, Ciuffreda MC, Cervio E, Calvillo L, Copes F, Pisano F, Mura M, Kleijn L, de Boer RA, et al. Conditioned medium from human amniotic mesenchymal stromal cells limits infarct size and enhances angiogenesis. Stem Cells Transl Med. 2015;4(5):448–58.
52. da Silva AF, Silva K, Reis LA, Teixeira VP, Schor N. Bone marrow-derived mesenchymal stem cells and their conditioned medium attenuate fibrosis in an irreversible model of unilateral ureteral obstruction. Cell Transplant. 2015;24(12):2657–66.
53. S ELA, Mager I, Breakefield XO, Wood MJ. Extracellular vesicles: biology and emerging therapeutic opportunities. Nat Rev Drug Discov. 2013;12(5):347–57.
54. McVey M, Tabuchi A, Kuebler WM. Microparticles and acute lung injury. Am J Physiol Lung Cell Mol Physiol. 2012;303(5):L364–81.
55. Quesenberry PJ, Goldberg LR, Aliotta JM, Dooner MS, Pereira MG, Wen S, Camussi G. Cellular phenotype and extracellular vesicles: basic and clinical considerations. Stem Cells Dev. 2014;23(13):1429–36.
56. Cocucci E, Racchetti G, Meldolesi J. Shedding microvesicles: artefacts no more. Trends Cell Biol. 2009;19(2):43–51.
57. Rani S, Ryan AE, Griffin MD, Ritter T. Mesenchymal stem cell-derived extracellular vesicles: toward cell-free therapeutic applications. Mol Ther. 2015;23(5):812–23.
58. Raposo G, Nijman HW, Stoorvogel W, Liejendekker R, Harding CV, Melief CJ, Geuze HJ. B lymphocytes secrete antigen-presenting vesicles. J Exp Med. 1996;183(3):1161–72.
59. Ratajczak J, Miekus K, Kucia M, Zhang J, Reca R, Dvorak P, Ratajczak MZ. Embryonic stem cell-derived microvesicles reprogram hematopoietic progenitors: evidence for horizontal transfer of mRNA and protein delivery. Leukemia. 2006;20(5):847–56.
60. Valadi H, Ekstrom K, Bossios A, Sjostrand M, Lee JJ, Lotvall JO. Exosome-mediated transfer of mRNAs and microRNAs is a novel mechanism of genetic exchange between cells. Nat Cell Biol. 2007;9(6):654–9.
61. Thery C. Exosomes: secreted vesicles and intercellular communications. F1000 Biol Rep. 2011;3:15.

62. Kourembanas S. Exosomes: vehicles of intercellular signaling, biomarkers, and vectors of cell therapy. Annu Rev Physiol. 2015;77:13–27.
63. Yu B, Zhang X, Li X. Exosomes derived from mesenchymal stem cells. Int J Mol Sci. 2014;15(3):4142–57.
64. Abreu SC, Weiss DJ, Rocco PR. Extracellular vesicles derived from mesenchymal stromal cells: a therapeutic option in respiratory diseases? Stem Cell Res Ther. 2016;7(1):53.
65. Bruno S, Grange C, Deregibus MC, Calogero RA, Saviozzi S, Collino F, Morando L, Busca A, Falda M, Bussolati B, et al. Mesenchymal stem cell-derived microvesicles protect against acute tubular injury. J Am Soc Nephrol. 2009;20(5):1053–67.
66. Potter DR, Miyazawa BY, Gibb SL, Deng X, Togaratti PP, Croze RH, Srivastava AK, Trivedi A, Matthay M, Holcomb JB, et al. Mesenchymal stem cell derived extracellular vesicles attenuate pulmonary vascular permeability and lung injury induced by hemorrhagic shock and trauma. J Trauma Acute Care Surg. 2017;84(2):245–56.
67. Willis GR, Fernandez-Gonzalez A, Anastas J, Vitali SH, Liu X, Ericsson M, Kwong A, Mitsialis SA, Kourembanas S. Mesenchymal stromal cell exosomes ameliorate experimental bronchopulmonary dysplasia and restore lung function through macrophage immunomodulation. Am J Respir Crit Care Med. 2017;197(1):104–16.
68. Collino F, Deregibus MC, Bruno S, Sterpone L, Aghemo G, Viltono L, Tetta C, Camussi G. Microvesicles derived from adult human bone marrow and tissue specific mesenchymal stem cells shuttle selected pattern of miRNAs. PLoS One. 2010;5(7):e11803.
69. Merino-Gonzalez C, Zuniga FA, Escudero C, Ormazabal V, Reyes C, Nova-Lamperti E, Salomon C, Aguayo C. Mesenchymal stem cell-derived extracellular vesicles promote angiogenesis: Potencial clinical application. Front Physiol. 2016;7:24.
70. Arslan F, Lai RC, Smeets MB, Akeroyd L, Choo A, Aguor EN, Timmers L, van Rijen HV, Doevendans PA, Pasterkamp G, et al. Mesenchymal stem cell-derived exosomes increase ATP levels, decrease oxidative stress and activate PI3K/Akt pathway to enhance myocardial viability and prevent adverse remodeling after myocardial ischemia/reperfusion injury. Stem Cell Res. 2013;10(3):301–12.
71. Aslam M, Baveja R, Liang OD, Fernandez-Gonzalez A, Lee C, Mitsialis SA, Kourembanas S. Bone marrow stromal cells attenuate lung injury in a murine model of neonatal chronic lung disease. Am J Respir Crit Care Med. 2009;180(11):1122–30.
72. Baglio SR, Rooijers K, Koppers-Lalic D, Verweij FJ, Perez Lanzon M, Zini N, Naaijkens B, Perut F, Niessen HW, Baldini N, et al. Human bone marrow- and adipose-mesenchymal stem cells secrete exosomes enriched in distinctive miRNA and tRNA species. Stem Cell Res Ther. 2015;6:127.
73. Dai W, Hale SL, Kloner RA. Role of a paracrine action of mesenchymal stem cells in the improvement of left ventricular function after coronary artery occlusion in rats. Regen Med. 2007;2(1):63–8.
74. Ionescu L, Byrne RN, van Haaften T, Vadivel A, Alphonse RS, Rey-Parra GJ, Weissmann G, Hall A, Eaton F, Thebaud B. Stem cell conditioned medium improves acute lung injury in mice: in vivo evidence for stem cell paracrine action. Am J Physiol Lung Cell Mol Physiol. 2012;303(11):L967–77.
75. Cruz FF, Borg ZD, Goodwin M, Sokocevic D, Wagner DE, Coffey A, Antunes M, Robinson KL, Mitsialis SA, Kourembanas S, et al. Systemic Administration of Human Bone Marrow-Derived Mesenchymal Stromal Cell Extracellular Vesicles Ameliorates Aspergillus Hyphal Extract-Induced Allergic Airway Inflammation in immunocompetent mice. Stem Cells Transl Med. 2015;4(11):1302–16.
76. Shen Q, Chen B, Xiao Z, Zhao L, Xu X, Wan X, Jin M, Dai J, Dai H. Paracrine factors from mesenchymal stem cells attenuate epithelial injury and lung fibrosis. Mol Med Rep. 2015;11(4):2831–7.
77. Timmers L, Lim SK, Hoefer IE, Arslan F, Lai RC, van Oorschot AA, Goumans MJ, Strijder C, Sze SK, Choo A, et al. Human mesenchymal stem cell-conditioned medium improves cardiac function following myocardial infarction. Stem Cell Res. 2011;6(3):206–14.
78. Witwer KW, Buzas EI, Bemis LT, Bora A, Lasser C, Lotvall J, Nolte-'t Hoen EN, Piper MG, Sivaraman S, Skog J, et al. Standardization of sample collection, isolation and analysis methods in extracellular vesicle research. J Extracell Vesicles. 2013;2:20360.
79. Pati S, Gerber MH, Menge TD, Wataha KA, Zhao Y, Baumgartner JA, Zhao J, Letourneau PA, Huby MP, Baer LA, et al. Bone marrow derived mesenchymal stem cells inhibit inflammation and preserve vascular endothelial integrity in the lungs after hemorrhagic shock. PLoS One. 2011; 6(9):e25171.
80. Lee JW, Fang X, Gupta N, Serikov V, Matthay MA. Allogeneic human mesenchymal stem cells for treatment of E. coli endotoxin-induced acute lung injury in the ex vivo perfused human lung. Proc Natl Acad Sci U S A. 2009;106(38):16357–62.
81. Devaney J, Horie S, Masterson C, Elliman S, Barry F, O'Brien T, Curley GF, O'Toole D, Laffey JG. Human mesenchymal stromal cells decrease the severity of acute lung injury induced by E. coli in the rat. Thorax. 2015;70(7): 625–35.
82. Hwang B, Liles WC, Waworuntu R, Mulligan MS. Pretreatment with bone marrow-derived mesenchymal stromal cell-conditioned media confers pulmonary ischemic tolerance. J Thorac Cardiovasc Surg. 2016;151(3):841–6.
83. Ionescu LI, Alphonse RS, Arizmendi N, Morgan B, Abel M, Eaton F, Duszyk M, Vliagoftis H, Aprahamian TR, Walsh K, et al. Airway delivery of soluble factors from plastic-adherent bone marrow cells prevents murine asthma. Am J Respir Cell Mol Biol. 2012;46(2):207–16.
84. Hansmann G, Fernandez-Gonzalez A, Aslam M, Vitali SH, Martin T, Mitsialis SA, Kourembanas S. Mesenchymal stem cell-mediated reversal of bronchopulmonary dysplasia and associated pulmonary hypertension. Pulmonary circulation. 2012;2(2):170–81.
85. Tropea KA, Leder E, Aslam M, Lau AN, Raiser DM, Lee JH, Balasubramaniam V, Fredenburgh LE, Alex Mitsialis S, Kourembanas S, et al. Bronchioalveolar stem cells increase after mesenchymal stromal cell treatment in a mouse model of bronchopulmonary dysplasia. Am J Physiol Lung Cell Mol Physiol. 2012;302(9):L829–37.
86. Pierro M, Ionescu L, Montemurro T, Vadivel A, Weissmann G, Oudit G, Emery D, Bodiga S, Eaton F, Peault B, et al. Short-term, long-term and paracrine effect of human umbilical cord-derived stem cells in lung injury prevention and repair in experimental bronchopulmonary dysplasia. Thorax. 2013;68(5): 475–84.
87. Waszak P, Alphonse R, Vadivel A, Ionescu L, Eaton F, Thebaud B. Preconditioning enhances the paracrine effect of mesenchymal stem cells in preventing oxygen-induced neonatal lung injury in rats. Stem Cells Dev. 2012;21(15):2789–97.
88. Wang Y, Huang L, Abdelrahim M, Cai Q, Truong A, Bick R, Poindexter B, Sheikh-Hamad D. Stanniocalcin-1 suppresses superoxide generation in macrophages through induction of mitochondrial UCP2. J Leukoc Biol. 2009;86(4):981–8.
89. Huang L, Garcia G, Lou Y, Zhou Q, Truong LD, DiMattia G, Lan XR, Lan HY, Wang Y, Sheikh-Hamad D. Anti-inflammatory and renal protective actions of stanniocalcin-1 in a model of anti-glomerular basement membrane glomerulonephritis. Am J Pathol. 2009;174(4):1368–78.
90. Mohammadipoor A, Lee RH, Prockop DJ, Bartosh TJ. Stanniocalcin-1 attenuates ischemic cardiac injury and response of differentiating monocytes/ macrophages to inflammatory stimuli. Transl Res. 2016;177:127–42.
91. Huh JW, Kim SY, Lee JH, Lee JS, Van Ta Q, Kim M, Oh YM, Lee YS, Lee SD. Bone marrow cells repair cigarette smoke-induced emphysema in rats. Am J Physiol Lung Cell Mol Physiol. 2011;301(3):L255–66.
92. Kim SY, Lee JH, Kim HJ, Park MK, Huh JW, Ro JY, Oh YM, Lee SD, Lee YS. Mesenchymal stem cell-conditioned media recovers lung fibroblasts from cigarette smoke-induced damage. Am J Physiol Lung Cell Mol Physiol. 2012; 302(9):L891–908.
93. Gennai S, Monsel A, Hao Q, Park J, Matthay MA, Lee JW. Microvesicles derived from human mesenchymal stem cells restore alveolar fluid clearance in human lungs rejected for transplantation. Am J Transplant Off J Am Soc Transplant Am Soc Transplant Surg. 2015;15(9):2404–12.
94. Li L, Jin S, Zhang Y. Ischemic preconditioning potentiates the protective effect of mesenchymal stem cells on endotoxin-induced acute lung injury in mice through secretion of exosome. Int J Clin Exp Med. 2015;8(3):3825–32.
95. Monsel A, Zhu YG, Gennai S, Hao Q, Hu S, Rouby JJ, Rosenzwajg M, Matthay MA, Lee JW. Therapeutic effects of human mesenchymal stem cell-derived microvesicles in severe pneumonia in mice. Am J Respir Crit Care Med. 2015;192(3):324–36.
96. Morrison TJ, Jackson MV, Cunningham EK, Kissenpfennig A, McAuley DF, O'Kane CM, Krasnodembskaya AD. Mesenchymal stromal cells modulate macrophages in clinically relevant lung injury models by extracellular vesicle mitochondrial transfer. Am J Respir Crit Care Med. 2017;196(10):1275–86.
97. Choi M, Ban T, Rhim T. Therapeutic use of stem cell transplantation for cell replacement or cytoprotective effect of microvesicle released from mesenchymal stem cell. Mol Cells. 2014;37(2):133–9.
98. Chen JY, An R, Liu ZJ, Wang JJ, Chen SZ, Hong MM, Liu JH, Xiao MY, Chen YF. Therapeutic effects of mesenchymal stem cell-derived microvesicles on

pulmonary arterial hypertension in rats. Acta Pharmacol Sin. 2014;35(9): 1121–8.
99. Aliotta JM, Pereira M, Wen S, Dooner MS, Del Tatto M, Papa E, Goldberg LR, Baird GL, Ventetuolo CE, Quesenberry PJ, et al. Exosomes induce and reverse monocrotaline-induced pulmonary hypertension in mice. Cardiovasc Res. 2016;110(3):319–30.
100. Ahn SY, Park WS, Kim YE, Sung DK, Sung SI, Ahn JY, Chang YS. Vascular endothelial growth factor mediates the therapeutic efficacy of mesenchymal stem cell-derived extracellular vesicles against neonatal hyperoxic lung injury. Exp Mol Med. 2018;50(4):26.
101. Khatri M, Richardson LA, Meulia T. Mesenchymal stem cell-derived extracellular vesicles attenuate influenza virus-induced acute lung injury in a pig model. Stem Cell Res Ther. 2018;9(1):17.
102. Kordelas L, Rebmann V, Ludwig AK, Radtke S, Ruesing J, Doeppner TR, Epple M, Horn PA, Beelen DW, Giebel B. MSC-derived exosomes: a novel tool to treat therapy-refractory graft-versus-host disease. Leukemia. 2014;28(4):970–3.
103. Nassar W, El-Ansary M, Sabry D, Mostafa MA, Fayad T, Kotb E, Temraz M, Saad AN, Essa W, Adel H. Umbilical cord mesenchymal stem cells derived extracellular vesicles can safely ameliorate the progression of chronic kidney diseases. Biomater Res. 2016;20:21.
104. Willis GR, Kourembanas S, Mitsialis SA. Toward exosome-based therapeutics: isolation, heterogeneity, and fit-for-purpose potency. Front Cardiovasc Med. 2017;4:63.
105. Exosome RNA Research and Industry News [https://www.exosome-rna.com/aegle-therapeutics-receives-ind-clearance-from-fda-for-stem-cell-derived-extracellular-vesicle-therapy/].
106. Monsel A, Zhu YG, Gudapati V, Lim H, Lee JW. Mesenchymal stem cell derived secretome and extracellular vesicles for acute lung injury and other inflammatory lung diseases. Expert Opin Biol Ther. 2016;16(7):859–71.
107. Lee JW, Fang X, Krasnodembskaya A, Howard JP, Matthay MA. Concise review: mesenchymal stem cells for acute lung injury: role of paracrine soluble factors. Stem cells. 2011;29(6):913–9.
108. Phinney DG, Pittenger MF. Concise review: MSC-derived exosomes for cell-free therapy. Stem cells. 2017;35(4):851–8.
109. Yeo RW, Lai RC, Zhang B, Tan SS, Yin Y, Teh BJ, Lim SK. Mesenchymal stem cell: an efficient mass producer of exosomes for drug delivery. Adv Drug Deliv Rev. 2013;65(3):336–41.
110. Batrakova EV, Kim MS. Development and regulation of exosome-based therapy products. Wiley Interdiscip Rev Nanomed Nanobiotechnol. 2016; 8(5):744–57.
111. Lener T, Gimona M, Aigner L, Borger V, Buzas E, Camussi G, Chaput N, Chatterjee D, Court FA, Del Portillo HA, et al. Applying extracellular vesicles based therapeutics in clinical trials - an ISEV position paper. J Extracell Vesicles. 2015;4:30087.
112. Lorincz AM, Timar CI, Marosvari KA, Veres DS, Otrokocsi L, Kittel A, Ligeti E. Effect of storage on physical and functional properties of extracellular vesicles derived from neutrophilic granulocytes. J Extracell Vesicles. 2014;3:25465.
113. Chen TS, Arslan F, Yin Y, Tan SS, Lai RC, Choo AB, Padmanabhan J, Lee CN, de Kleijn DP, Lim SK. Enabling a robust scalable manufacturing process for therapeutic exosomes through oncogenic immortalization of human ESC-derived MSCs. J Transl Med. 2011;9:47.
114. Hu GW, Li Q, Niu X, Hu B, Liu J, Zhou SM, Guo SC, Lang HL, Zhang CQ, Wang Y, et al. Exosomes secreted by human-induced pluripotent stem cell-derived mesenchymal stem cells attenuate limb ischemia by promoting angiogenesis in mice. Stem Cell Res Ther. 2015;6:10.
115. Stone ML, Zhao Y, Robert Smith J, Weiss ML, Kron IL, Laubach VE, Sharma AK. Mesenchymal stromal cell-derived extracellular vesicles attenuate lung ischemia-reperfusion injury and enhance reconditioning of donor lungs after circulatory death. Respir Res. 2017;18(1):212.
116. Kim YS, Kim JY, Cho R, Shin DM. Adipose stem cell-derived nanovesicles inhibit emphysema primarily via an FGF2-dependent pathway. Exp Mol Med. 2017;49(1):e284.

16

Heterogeneous burden of lung disease in smokers with borderline airflow obstruction

Cheryl S. Pirozzi[1*], Tian Gu[2], Pedro M. Quibrera[3], Elizabeth E. Carretta[3], MeiLan K. Han[4], Susan Murray[2], Christopher B. Cooper[5], Donald P. Tashkin[5], Eric C. Kleerup[5], Igor Barjaktarevic[5], Eric A. Hoffman[6], Carlos H. Martinez[2], Stephanie A. Christenson[7], Nadia N. Hansel[8], R. Graham Barr[9], Eugene R. Bleecker[10], Victor E. Ortega[11], Fernando J. Martinez[12], Richard E. Kanner[1], Robert Paine III[1,13] and for the NHLBI SubPopulations and InteRmediate Outcome Measures In COPD Study (SPIROMICS)

Abstract

Background: The identification of smoking-related lung disease in current and former smokers with normal FEV_1 is complex, leading to debate regarding using a ratio of forced expiratory volume in 1 s to forced vital capacity (FEV_1/FVC) of less than 0.70 versus the predicted lower limit of normal (LLN) for diagnosis of airflow obstruction. We hypothesized that the discordant group of ever-smokers with FEV_1/FVC between the LLN and 0.70 is heterogeneous, and aimed to characterize the burden of smoking-related lung disease in this group.

Methods: We compared spirometry, chest CT characteristics, and symptoms between 161 ever-smokers in the discordant group and 940 ever-smokers and 190 never-smokers with normal FEV_1 and $FEV_1/FVC > 0.70$ in the SPIROMICS cohort. We also estimated sensitivity and specificity for diagnosing objective radiographic evidence of chronic obstructive pulmonary disease (COPD) using different FEV_1/FVC criteria thresholds.

Results: The discordant group had more CT defined emphysema and non-emphysematous gas trapping, lower post-bronchodilator FEV_1 and FEF_{25-75}, and higher respiratory medication use compared with the other two groups. Within the discordant group, 44% had radiographic CT evidence of either emphysema or non-emphysematous gas trapping; an FEV_1/FVC threshold of 0.70 has greater sensitivity but lower specificity compared with LLN for identifying individuals with CT abnormality.

Conclusions: Ever-smokers with normal FEV_1 and $FEV_1/FVC < 0.70$ but > LLN are a heterogeneous group that includes significant numbers of individuals with and without radiographic evidence of smoking-related lung disease. These findings emphasize the limitations of diagnosing COPD based on spirometric criteria alone.

Keywords: Chronic obstructive pulmonary disease, Pulmonary function tests, Spirometry, Airway obstruction, Emphysema, Forced expiratory volume, Maximal Midexpiratory flow rate

Background

Airflow obstruction is a hallmark of chronic obstructive pulmonary disease (COPD), and by current recommendations [1] is confirmed by a reduced ratio of forced expiratory volume in 1 s (FEV_1) to forced vital capacity (FVC). To simplify the diagnosis of airflow obstruction, a fixed cut-off ratio of FEV_1/FVC ($FEV_1/FVC < 0.70$) is often used instead of predicted lower limit of normal (LLN) ($FEV_1/FVC < LLN$), defined as the lower fifth percentile of a reference population. [2, 3]

Because the predicted normal FEV_1/FVC declines with age, a fixed cut-off ratio of $FEV_1/FVC < 0.70$ has the potential for misclassification and over diagnosis in the elderly, [4–10] while using predicted LLN may better predict adverse clinical outcomes [11] and more accurately predict all-cause mortality. [4] Although there is a group of younger individuals for whom LLN is > 0.7, a particular challenge is presented by subjects who fall in a "discordant" group with FEV_1/FVC ratio > LLN but < 0.7. Compared to subjects with $FEV_1/FVC > 0.70$, the individuals in this

* Correspondence: Cheryl.pirozzi@hsc.utah.edu
[1]Division of Pulmonary and Critical Care Medicine, Department of Internal Medicine, University of Utah, 26 N 1900 E, Salt Lake City, UT 84132, USA
Full list of author information is available at the end of the article

discordant group have been found to have greater emphysema, airway wall thickening, and gas trapping, as well as greater risk for chronic obstructive pulmonary disease (COPD)-related hospitalization, emergency department visits, and mortality [12–16]. There has been recent interest in characterizing patients with mild smoking-related lung disease as evidenced by symptoms and radiographic abnormalities despite normal spirometry, [17, 18] highlighting the limitations of using spirometric criteria alone for diagnosis of COPD. We hypothesized that the discordant group of ever-smokers with FEV_1/FVC between the LLN and 0.70 is heterogeneous, containing some individuals with smoking-related lung disease and some with changes in lung function related to aging. We address this hypothesis by characterizing clinical, radiographic and physiologic features of ever-smokers in this discordant group and comparing them with the group of individuals with $FEV_1/FVC > 0.70$.[1]

Methods

SPIROMICS study methods

SPIROMICS is a multicenter prospective cohort study that has enrolled 2981 participants including never-smokers, smokers without airway obstruction and smokers with mild, moderate and severe COPD, with the goals of identifying new COPD subgroups and intermediate markers of disease progression [19]. Participants were 40–80 years old at baseline. "Smokers" were defined as current or former smokers with lifetime smoking history of greater than 20 pack-years. The study design and exclusion criteria have previously been described [19]. The research protocol was approved by the institutional review boards of all participating institutions and all participants gave written informed consent.

Subjects and measure of exposure

We analyzed data for three groups of subjects included in SPIROMICS: Group 1) current or former smokers (ever-smokers) with normal post-bronchodilator FEV_1 and $FEV_1/FVC >$ LLN but < 0.70 (**discordant group,** n = 161); Group 2) ever-smokers with normal FEV_1 and $FEV_1/FVC > 0.70$ ($n = 940$); and Group 3) never-smokers with normal FEV_1 and $FEV_1/FVC > 0.70$ ($n = 190$). In a supplementary analysis we also compared outcomes with a Group 4) patients with FEV_1/FVC in the 75% quartile of those less than LLN ($n = 379$).

Pulmonary function methods

Pulmonary function testing was performed and interpreted according to the 2005 ATS/ERS guidelines; post-bronchodilator spirometric measurements were used for analysis [20, 21]. NHANES III spirometric references values were used to calculate percent predicted values and LLN [22].

Outcomes

We compared respiratory symptoms, quality of life, medication use, CT metrics, FEV_1% predicted, forced expiratory flow rate between 25 and 75% of FVC or maximum mid-expiratory flow (FEF_{25-75}), 6 min walk distance (6MWD), and two prospective variables: annual FEV_1 change and exacerbation rate, between the three groups. Chronic bronchitis was defined as patient reported cough with sputum for at least 3 months for ≥2 years. Dyspnea was defined by the modified Medical Research Council (mMRC) dyspnea score, [23] stratified into two groups as mMRC ≥2 (moderate or severe dyspnea) vs mMRC 0–1 (mild or no dyspnea). Respiratory symptoms were also measured by the COPD Assessment Test (CAT) [24]. Quality of life was measured by the St. George's Respiratory Questionnaire (SGRQ) [25]. Medication use was defined as patient-reported regular use of inhaled bronchodilators and/or inhaled steroid. Annual FEV_1 change was defined using a regression model that incorporated the total number of study visits and spirometry measurements available for each participant. Each participant had a minimum of two spirometry measurements at least 200 days apart, with follow up ranging from 266 to 1749 days. Exacerbation rate was measured as the number of patient-reported events requiring health care utilization in the first year after study enrollment.

Multidetector-row computed tomography (MDCT) scans at full inspiration and full expiration were performed at the SPIROMICS baseline visit. Emphysema was defined using a threshold of <– 950 Hounsfield Units on full inspiration. Airway wall thickening was defined as the square root of the airway wall area for a standardized airway with an internal perimeter of 10 mm (Pi10) [26]. Parametric Response Mapping (PRM) was used to define functional small airways disease (fSAD), a measure of non-emphysematous gas trapping, as the percent of voxels with CT attenuation values > – 950 HU on the inspiratory exam and < – 856 HU on the expiratory scan, as previously described [27] using Imbio Lung Density software (Imbio, Minneapolis, MN).

Statistical analysis

Comparisons of categorical predictors across groups 1, 2 and 3 used chi-squared tests. For continuous variables, ANOVA was used to test for overall differences between the 3 groups; pairwise comparisons of continuous outcomes between any two groups were based on t-tests. [28] Multivariable linear regression was used to compare continuous measures (emphysema, fSAD, CT metrics, 6MWD, CAT score, quality of life, FEV_1, and FEF_{25-75}) between groups, adjusted for age, sex, race, smoking history (pack-years) and current smoking (yes/no). Multivariable logistic regression was used to compare binary clinical outcomes (emphysema present, fSAD present, chronic bronchitis, mMRC Dyspnea, and medication use) adjusted for the same patient characteristics described above.

Quantile regression models [29] applied to healthy never -smokers estimated the 95th percentile for PRM emphysema and, separately, the 95th percentile for PRM fSAD for a normal patient based on their age, sex, BMI and the scanner used. Hereafter, these estimated 95th percentiles will be used to define the upper limit of normal (ULN) for these PRM measures according to patient/scanner characteristics. Presence of emphysema or fSAD was defined when an individual's observed PRM emphysema percent or PRM fSAD percent was greater than the estimated ULN for a normal patient with similar patient/scanner characteristics. Sensitivity and specificity of each FEV_1/FVC cut-off for identifying individuals with radiographic CT evidence of smoking-related lung disease manifest as either emphysema and/or fSAD were estimated.

Results

We compared the discordant group (Group 1) with ever-smokers with normal spirometry (Group 2) and never-smokers (Group 3). The characteristics of the three groups are shown in Table 1. The discordant group had more male and white participants and was older than the other two groups.

Compared with ever-smokers with $FEV_1/FVC > 0.70$ (Group 2), the discordant individuals (Group 1) had lower post-bronchodilator FEV_1% predicted (92.1% vs 97.5%, $p < 0.001$) and reduced FEF_{25-75}% predicted (61.2% vs 102.3%, $p < 0.001$) (Table 2, Fig. 1). The two groups of ever-smokers did not differ significantly in 6MWD (437.5 vs 437.2 m, $p = 0.97$), SGRQ (22.5 vs 24.2, $p = 0.28$), or CAT score (10.7 vs 11.3, $p = 0.36$). More smokers in the discordant group reported regular use of either inhaled corticosteroids and/or bronchodilators than either ever-smokers with $FEV_1/FVC > 0.70$, Group 2, (34.4% vs. 25.1%, $p = 0.01$) or never-smokers, Group 3 (3.9%, $p < 0.001$). Groups 1 and 2 did not differ in the reported incidence of chronic bronchitis or moderate or severe dyspnea indicated by mMRC score ≥ 2. Nor did they differ with respect to FEV_1 decline per year, or exacerbations per year (Table 2).

The discordant group had a modest but significantly greater percentage of lung with CT scan-defined emphysema than Group 2 (2.1% vs 0.7%, $p < 0.001$) or Group 3 (0.3%, $p < 0.001$). Individuals in the discordant group also had significantly increased PRM fSAD as compared to Groups 2 and 3 (18.0% vs. 9.1% and 7.1%, respectively, $p < 0.001$), without detectable differences in airway thickness (Table 3, Fig. 1). Density plots illustrating the distribution of emphysema and small airways disease are presented in supplementary material (Additional file 1: Figure S1 and Additional file 2: Figure S2).

Using age-adjusted ULN for % emphysema, more individuals in the discordant group met CT criteria for the presence of emphysema compared with Groups 2 and 3 (38.7% vs. 17.4% ($p < 0.001$) and 8.2% ($p < 0.001$), respectively). Similarly, using age-adjusted ULN for PRM fSAD, more individuals in the discordant group also met CT criteria for the presence of fSAD compared with Groups 2 and 3 (15.3% vs. 7.8% ($p = 0.003$) and 2.9% ($p < 0.001$), respectively). In the discordant group, 44% of subjects had CT evidence of smoking-related lung disease, manifest as either emphysema or fSAD, compared with 20.7% ($p < 0.001$) of Group 2 and 9.4% ($p < 0.001$) of Group 3 subjects. Conversely, 56% of individuals in the discordant group had CT scans without radiographic evidence of smoking-related lung disease (Table 3, Fig. 2 , Additional file 3: Figure S3).

Within the discordant group, those with CT evidence of smoking-related lung disease did not have significantly greater respiratory symptoms, FEV_1 decline, exacerbations, or lower FEF_{25-75} compared with those without emphysema or fSAD (Table 4).

When compared to a fourth group of smokers with FEV_1/FVC in the 75% quartile of those less than LLN,

Table 1 Baseline characteristics for the three groups

Variable	Group 1 Ever-smokers, Normal FEV_1, $\frac{FEV1}{FVC}$ < 0.7 and > LLN (Discordant Group) ($n = 161$)	Group 2 Ever-smokers, Normal FEV_1, $\frac{FEV1}{FVC}$ > 0.7 ($n = 940$)	Group 3 Never-smokers, Normal FEV_1, $\frac{FEV1}{FVC}$ > 0.7 ($n = 190$)	P-value
Sex (% male)	70.8%	49.0%	37.9%	< 0.001*
Race (% white)	89.4%	68.2%	70.7%	< 0.001*
Current smoker (%)	32.5%	50.0%	0%	< 0.001*
Age (mean ± SD)	69.3 ± 6.4	60.4 ± 9.7	56.6 ± 10.2	< 0.001†
Smoking history in pack-years (mean ± SD)	48.3 ± 22.2	43.1 ± 27.3	Not Applicable	0.0‡

*Chi-Square test
†ANOVA
‡t-test

Table 2 Comparison of physiologic and clinical variables between ever-smokers with normal FEV_1 and FEV_1/FVC > LLN but < 0.70 ("discordant" group), ever-smokers with normal FEV_1 and $FEV_1/FVC > 0.70$, and never-smokers with normal FEV_1 and $FEV_1/FVC > 0.70$

Clinical Outcome	Group 1 Ever-smokers, Normal FEV_1, $\frac{FEV1}{FVC} < 0.7$ and > LLN (Discordant Group) ($n = 161$)	Group 2 Ever-smokers, Normal FEV_1, $\frac{FEV1}{FVC} > 0.7$ ($n = 940$)	Group 3 Never-smokers, Normal FEV_1, $\frac{FEV1}{FVC} > 0.7$ ($n = 190$)	Overall *p*-value* Unadjusted (Adjusted)	*P*-values for pairwise comparisons (Unadjusted) Group 1 vs. 2	Group 1 vs. 3	Group 2 vs. 3
FEV_1% predicted	92.1 ± 12.0	97.5 ± 12.8	102.0 ± 11.5	< 0.001 (< 0.001)	< 0.001	< 0.001	< 0.001**
$FEF_{25-75\%}$ % predicted	61.2 ± 11.0	102.3 ± 33.4	121.3 ± 32.5	< 0.001 (< 0.001)	< 0.001	< 0.001	< 0.001**
6MWD (m)	437.5 ± 109.6	437.2 ± 97.7	479.3 ± 103.4	< 0.001 (0.49)	0.97	< 0.001	< 0.001**
St George's Respiratory Questionnaire Total Score	22.5 ± 17.4	24.2 ± 19.1	8.8 ± 10.0	< 0.001 (< 0.001)	0.28	< 0.001	< 0.001**
COPD Assessment Test (CAT)	10.7 ± 7.4	11.3 ± 8.1	4.7 ± 6.0	< 0.001 (< 0.001)	0.36	< 0.001	< 0.001**
Use of either inhaled corticosteroid or bronchodilator	34.4%	25.1%	3.9%	< 0.001 (< 0.001)	0.01	< 0.001	< 0.001†
Chronic bronchitis	17.3%	17.8%	2.1%	< 0.001 (< 0.001)	0.88	< 0.001	< 0.001†
mMRC Dyspnea score ≥ 2	13.8%	13.6%	2.7%	< 0.001 (0.007)	0.95	< 0.001	< 0.001†
Change in FEV_1 (ml/year)	− 60.5 ± 120.5	−55.2 ± 127.5	−41.2 ± 99.7	0.32 (0.94)	0.64	0.17	0.19**
Exacerbation (#/year)	0.1 ± 0.4	0.1 ± 0.6	0.02 ± 0.1	0.02 (0.21)	0.50	0.13	0.006**

Emphysema = % of voxels with CT attenuation <− 950 Hounsfield Units (HU) on full inspiration. Functional small airways disease = % of voxels with CT attenuation > − 950 HU on the inspiratory exam and < − 856 HU on the expiratory scan, as determined via dynamic image registration (Parametric Response Mapping, PRM). Airway thickening = square root of the wall area for a standardized airway with an internal perimeter of 10 mm (Pi10)

*From likelihood ratio test comparing means of 3 groups from multivariable model with outcomes (rows) and group status as predictors adjusted for age, sex, race, smoking history (pack-years) and current smoking

***p*-values from 2 sample t-test

†Pairwise *p*-value form Wald test comparing means of 2 groups

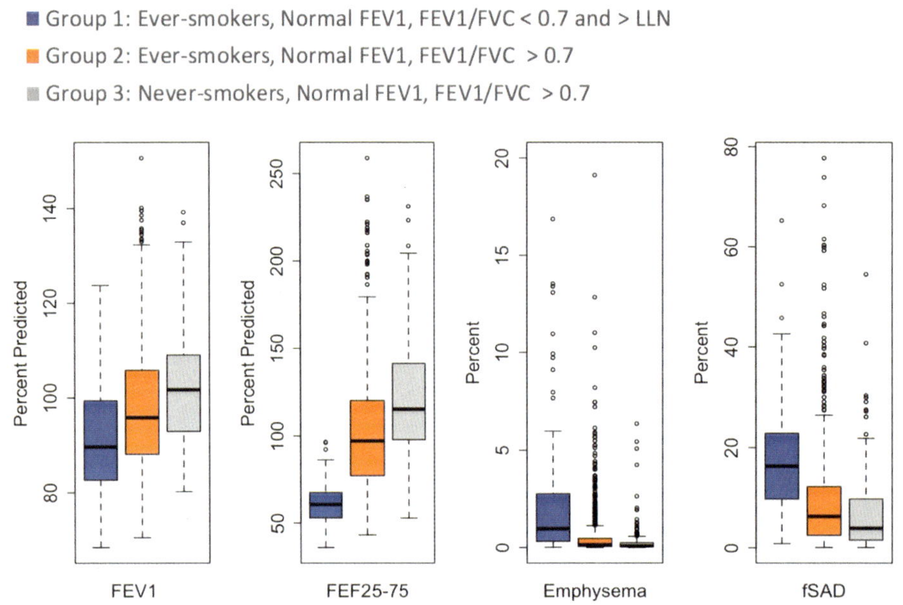

Fig. 1 Box plots demonstrating percent of predicted forced expiratory volume in 1 s (FEV_1%), forced expiratory flow rate between 25 and 75% of forced vital capacity ($FEF_{25-75\%}$), percent emphysema, and functional small airways disease by parametric response mapping (fSAD) in the three groups

Table 3 Comparison of CT variables between ever-smokers with normal FEV_1 and $FEV_1/FVC > LLN$ but < 0.70 ("discordant" group), ever-smokers with normal FEV_1 and $FEV_1/FVC > 0.70$, and never-smokers with normal FEV_1 and $FEV_1/FVC > 0.70$

Variable	Group 1 Ever-smokers, Normal FEV_1, $\frac{FEV1}{FVC} < 0.7$ and > LLN (Discordant Group) ($n = 161$)	Group 2 Ever-smokers, Normal FEV_1, $\frac{FEV1}{FVC} > 0.7$ ($n = 940$)	Group 3 Never-smokers, Normal FEV_1, $\frac{FEV1}{FVC} > 0.7$ ($n = 190$)	Overall *p*-value* from likelihood ratio test comparing association with group status Unadjusted (Adjusted)	P-values for pairwise comparisons (Unadjusted)		
					Group 1 vs. 2	Group 1 vs. 3	Group 2 vs. 3
Emphysema (%)	2.1 ± 2.9	0.7 ± 2.6	0.3 ± 0.9	< 0.001 (< 0.001)	< 0.001	< 0.001	< 0.001**
Functional small airways disease (%)	18.0 ± 10.6	9.1 ± 10.0	7.1 ± 8.3	< 0.001 (< 0.001)	< 0.001	< 0.001	< 0.001**
Airway wall thickening (Pi10)	3.70 ± 0.01	3.71 ± 0.00	3.69 ± 0.01	< 0.001 (0.17)	0.41	0.01	< 0.001**
Emphysema present > ULN	38.7%	17.4%	8.2%	< 0.001 (< 0.001)	< 0.001	< 0.001	0.004†
CT-defined functional small airway abnormality (fSAD) present > ULN	15.3%	7.8%	2.9%	< 0.001 (0.03)	0.003	< 0.001	0.03†
Either emphysema or fSAD present	44%	20.7%	9.4%	< 0.001 (< 0.001)	< 0.001	< 0.001	< 0.001†
Both emphysema and fSAD present	10%	4.5%	1.8%	0.002 (0.23)	0.007	0.005	0.11†

Presence of emphysema = ≥ upper limit of normal (ULN); Presence of fSAD = ≥ upper limit of normal (ULN). Emphysema = % of voxels with CT attenuation <– 950 Hounsfield Units (HU) on full inspiration. Functional small airways disease = % of voxels with CT attenuation > – 950 HU on the inspiratory exam and < – 856 HU on the expiratory scan, as determined via dynamic image registration (Parametric Response Mapping, PRM)
*From likelihood ratio test comparing means of 3 groups from multivariable model with outcomes (rows) and group status as predictors adjusted for age, sex, race, smoking history (pack-years) and current smoking
***P*-value from 2 sample t test
†Pairwise *p*-value form Wald test comparing means of 2 groups

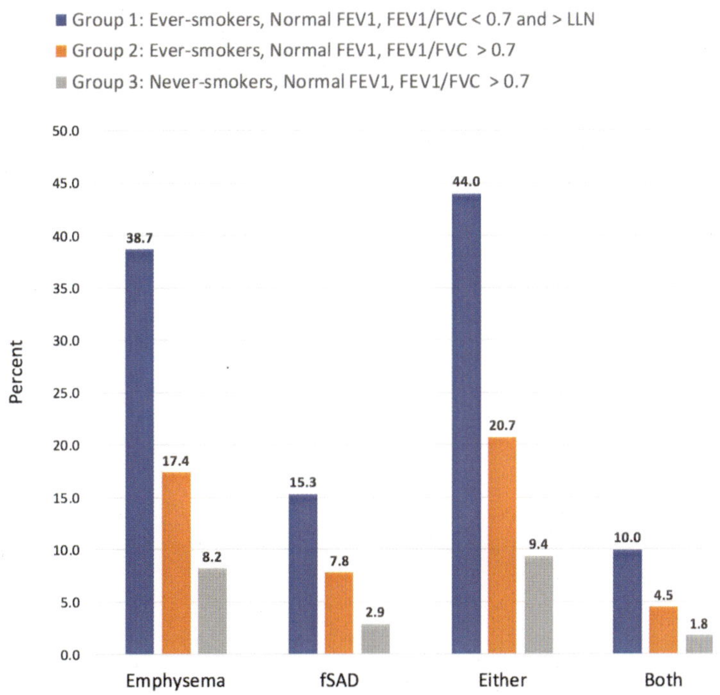

Fig. 2 Percent of patients in each group with emphysema and functional small airways disease (fSAD) present greater than the age-adjusted upper limit of normal (ULN) as measured by parametric response mapping (PRM) on chest CT

Table 4 Comparison of prospective FEV_1 decline, exacerbation rate and respiratory symptoms between those in the discordant group (Ever-smokers with normal FEV_1, $FEV_1/FVC < 0.70$ and > LLN) with CT findings of emphysema or functional small airways disease, and those without

	Ever-smokers with normal FEV_1, $FEV_1/FVC < 0.70$ and > LLN (discordant group, $n = 161$)			
	With fSAD or emphysema (44%)	Without fSAD or emphysema (56%)	*Adjusted *p*-value	Unadjusted *p*-value
Annual change in FEV_1 (ml/year)	−65.6 ± 113.0	−59.8 ± 130.6	0.26	0.79
Exacerbation (#/year)	0.13 ± 0.42	0.06 ± 0.24	0.90	0.25
COPD Assessment Test (CAT)	11.43 ± 7.44	9.88 ± 7.25	0.55	0.22
Chronic bronchitis (%)	14.3 ± 35.3	18.3 ± 38.9	0.58	0.52
$FEF_{25-75\%}$ % predicted	60.0 ± 11.6	62.2 ± 10.7	0.87	0.24

*Multivariate model adjusting for age, gender, race, pack year, and current smoking status

the discordant group had higher FEV_1 and $FEF_{25-75\%}$, fewer respiratory symptoms and exacerbations, less airway wall thickness and fewer % of people with fSAD, however did not differ in the amount of emphysema or FEV_1 decline (Additional file 4: Tables S1, S2 and S3).

A history of smoking had a significant association with symptoms in groups defined by either FEV_1/FVC threshold compared to never-smokers. When compared with never-smokers without airflow obstruction, both groups of ever-smokers had more chronic bronchitis, dyspnea, respiratory symptoms as measured by CAT, and lower quality of life by SGRQ (Table 2).

Finally, we evaluated the sensitivity and specificity of the two thresholds for FEV_1/FVC for identification of individuals with radiographic evidence of smoking-related lung disease (emphysema > age-adjusted ULN and/or PRM fSAD > age-adjusted ULN). A threshold of $FEV_1/FVC < 0.7$ had a sensitivity of 0.85 and specificity of 0.72 for identifying any radiographic abnormality. The FEV_1/FVC < LLN threshold had lower calculated sensitivity (0.78) and higher specificity (0.81) (Table 5). Thus the absolute ratio is more sensitive, while the LLN is more specific.

Discussion

In the SPIROMICS cohort, current or former smokers with normal FEV_1 who are diagnosed with COPD based on GOLD spirometric criteria, but who do not have airflow obstruction based on the LLN threshold, have more emphysema and functional small airways disease by CT, increased use of inhaled medications, and lower mid-expiratory flow compared with current or former smokers without airway obstruction, defined by $FEV_1/FVC > 0.70$. Almost half of individuals in this discordant group have CT evidence of smoking-related lung disease. Nevertheless, the discordant group did not have increased respiratory symptoms (chronic bronchitis, dyspnea, or CAT) or decreased exercise tolerance when compared with individuals with FEV_1/FVC ratio > 0.7.

Table 5 Calculated sensitivity and specificity for diagnosis of COPD defined by presence of radiographic CT evidence of smoking related lung disease, with emphysema > age adjusted upper limit of normal and/or functional small airways disease > ULN. $N = 2972$. LLN = lower limit of normal

Diagnostic criteria	Sensitivity	Specificity
$FEV_1/FVC < 0.7$	0.85	0.72
FEV_1/FVC < LLN	0.78	0.81

We have focused this analysis on individuals in this discordant group for three reasons. First, in reference populations the ratio of FEV_1/FVC decreases with advancing age, suggesting that use of a fixed threshold of 0.7 may inappropriately classify some individuals. Second, studies of this population may help elucidate the boundaries of normal aging in the setting of cigarette smoking. Finally, there has been recent interest in the clinical picture of smokers who may have smoking-related lung disease in the setting of little or no airflow obstruction [17, 18]. This study contributes to the discussion in each of these three areas.

Our findings support the presence of early/mild disease among individuals in this discordant group and thus provide potential pathophysiologic explanation for previous studies demonstrating increased risk for COPD-related health effects in this group, including increased adjusted risk of death, COPD-related emergency department visits and hospitalizations [13, 15]. These studies suggest that the LLN threshold lacks sensitivity, failing to identify a number of individuals with clinically significant disease.

However, because the predicted FEV_1/FVC may decline with normal age, using a fixed cut-off ratio of $FEV_1/FVC < 0.70$ increases diagnosis of obstruction in the elderly, and in very old adults has the potential to classify changes associated with aging as COPD [4–9]. In a cohort of adults 80 years and older, airflow obstruction defined by FEV_1/FVC < LLN, but not FEV_1/FVC between LLN and 0.70, was associated with increased mortality [4]. Similarly, small amounts of emphysema may occur due to aging-related changes rather than as a consequence of early smoking-related disease. In the multiethnic MESA cohort, full-lung CT scans of healthy nonsmokers revealed a small percent of emphysema (median 1.1%) that was increased in men and with age. [30] CT-defined functional small airway abnormality also increases with age [31]. Therefore, the predicted "normal" amount of emphysema and small airways disease increases with aging even in the absence of smoking exposure. An important question is how to distinguish between early/mild COPD and normal aging. In our study we used data from normal individuals to create age-adjusted upper limits of normal for both emphysema and PRM fSAD, suggesting that the CT abnormality we have identified in the discordant group is beyond that associated with normal aging. Our study extends previous findings by including innovative imaging parameters of small airways disease and comparisons with normal lung density [16].

We found significantly reduced $FEF_{25-75\%}$ and CT scan evidence of non-emphysematous air trapping in the discordant group. Reduction in mid-expiratory flow is generally assumed to be an indication of small airways disease [32–34]. We did not identify differences in airway wall thickness, manifest as path specific Pi10, associated with our discordant group. However, changes in lumen dimension may mask changes in wall thickening/thinning by this parameter [35]. CT air trapping is also thought to reflect small airways disease and has been associated with lower lung function and accelerated lung function decline [36, 37]. The functional small airways disease measurement using PRM helps to distinguish non-emphysematous air trapping from emphysema on CT [27]. Thus physiologic and CT scan data both point to subtle but potentially clinically important small airways abnormalities in this discordant group. Several studies have suggested that in the natural history of COPD, small airways may become narrowed or lost prior to the onset of emphysema [34, 38–40] and thus these abnormalities may be an earlier indication of smoking-related COPD. We evaluated two prospective variables: exacerbations in the first year after enrollment, and FEV_1 decline over a period of up to 4 years. Though we did not detect more FEV_1 decline or exacerbations in the discordant group or those with radiographic emphysema or fSAD, exacerbation rate was overall low in these patients with mild smoking-related lung disease. Longer follow up time will enhance our understanding of the significance of these mild radiographic and physiologic abnormalities as predictors of progression to COPD.

The choice of a threshold of FEV_1/FVC for diagnosing airflow obstruction may depend on the goals of testing and whether a more sensitive or specific test is preferred. In the SPIROMICS cohort, using a FEV_1/FVC threshold of 0.70 is more sensitive but less specific for identifying individuals with radiographic manifestations of COPD, while using LLN is more specific but less sensitive. As a screening test for early/mild disease in ever-smokers, a more sensitive test may be preferred. However, identifying airflow obstruction using either FEV_1/FVC threshold will incorrectly classify individuals.

There are several important features of this study. SPIROMICS is a large multi-center cohort whose subjects are extensively characterized for symptoms, physiology and radiology. MDCT scans performed at baseline allowed detailed assessment of emphysema, air trapping, and airway wall thickness and image analysis by PRM allowed differentiation of non-emphysematous air trapping from emphysema on CT. We recognize several limitations to our study. $FEF_{25-75\%}$ is an effort-dependent measurement like FEV_1 and we cannot exclude a confounding effect of limited effort or frailty. However, the subjects described in this report all had studies that met ATS criteria and had normal FVC. The specificity statistic is biased because the analysis data set is not a random sample. Additionally, never-smokers with $FEV_1/FVC < 0.7$ were not included in SPIROMICS and thus could not be compared in this analysis.

Conclusions

Ever-smokers who have normal FEV_1 and $FEV_1/FVC < 0.70$ but $>$ LLN (discordant group) have on average more emphysema and small airways disease, and increased respiratory medication use compared with those with $FEV_1/FVC > 0.70$. This is a heterogeneous group that includes a large number of individuals with CT evidence of either emphysema or non-emphysematous gas trapping, as well as many individuals without radiographic evidence of early smoking-related lung disease for whom it is likely that normal aging accounts for the apparent spirometric abnormality. The diagnosis of early/mild COPD requires a more sophisticated approach that goes beyond currently accepted spirometric criteria.

Endnotes

[1]Some of the results of these studies have been previously reported in the form of an abstract [41, 42].

Additional files

Additional file 1: Table S1. Baseline characteristics for the four groups. **Table S2.** Comparison of physiologic and clinical variables between ever-smokers with normal FEV_1 and $FEV_1/FVC >$ LLN but < 0.70 ("discordant" group, Group 1), ever-smokers with normal FEV_1 and $FEV_1/FVC > 0.70$ (Group 2), never-smokers with normal FEV_1 and $FEV_1/FVC > 0.70$ (Group 3) and ever-smokers with $FEV_1/FVC \leq$ LLN and > 75th quartile (Group 4). **Table S3.** Comparison of CT variables between ever-smokers with normal FEV_1 and $FEV_1/FVC >$ LLN but < 0.70 ("discordant" group, Group 1), ever-smokers with normal FEV_1 and $FEV_1/FVC > 0.70$ (Group 2), never-smokers with normal FEV_1 and $FEV_1/FVC > 0.70$ (Group 3) and ever-smokers with $FEV_1/FVC \leq$ LLN and > 75th quartile (Group 4). (DOCX 100 kb)

Additional file 2: Figure S1. Density plot of the distribution of emphysema. (PNG 58 kb)

Additional file 3: Figure S2. Density plot of the distribution of functional small airways disease. (PNG 55 kb)

Additional file 4: Figure S3. Venn diagram illustrating patients within the discordant group (ever-smokers with normal FEV_1 and $FEV_1/FVC >$ LLN but < 0.70) who have emphysema, functional small airways disease (fSAD), and both on chest CT imaging. (PDF 34 kb)

Additional file 5: Heterogeneous Burden of Lung Disease in Smokers with Borderline Airflow Obstruction. (DOCX 73 kb)

Abbreviations

6MWD: 6 min walk distance; CAT: COPD Assessment Test; COPD: Chronic obstructive pulmonary disease; CT: Computed tomography; FEF_{25-75}: Forced expiratory flow rate between 25 and 75% of FVC; FEV_1: Forced expiratory volume in 1 s; fSAD: Functional small airways disease; FVC: Forced vital capacity; LLN: Lower limit of normal; mMRC: Modified Medical Research Council; Pi10: Square root of the airway wall area for a standardized airway with an internal perimeter of 10 mm; PRM: Parametric Response Mapping; SGRQ: St. George's Respiratory Questionnaire; ULN: Upper limit of normal

Acknowledgements

The authors thank the SPIROMICS participants and participating physicians, investigators and staff for making this research possible. More information about the study and how to access SPIROMICS data is at www.spiromics.org. We would like to acknowledge the following current and former investigators of the SPIROMICS sites and reading centers: Neil E Alexis, PhD; Wayne H Anderson, PhD; R Graham Barr, MD, DrPH; Eugene R Bleecker, MD; Richard C Boucher, MD; Russell P Bowler, MD, PhD; Elizabeth E Carretta, MPH; Stephanie A Christenson, MD; Alejandro P Comellas, MD; Christopher B Cooper, MD, PhD; David J Couper, PhD; Gerard J Criner, MD; Ronald G Crystal, MD; Jeffrey L Curtis, MD; Claire M Doerschuk, MD; Mark T Dransfield, MD; Christine M Freeman, PhD; MeiLan K Han, MD, MS; Nadia N Hansel, MD, MPH; Annette T Hastie, PhD; Eric A Hoffman, PhD; Robert J Kaner, MD; Richard E Kanner, MD; Eric C Kleerup, MD; Jerry A Krishnan, MD, PhD; Lisa M LaVange, PhD; Stephen C Lazarus, MD; Fernando J Martinez, MD, MS; Deborah A Meyers, PhD; John D Newell Jr., MD; Elizabeth C Oelsner, MD, MPH; Wanda K O'Neal, PhD; Robert Paine, III, MD; Nirupama Putcha, MD, MHS; Stephen I. Rennard, MD; Donald P Tashkin, MD; Mary Beth Scholand, MD; J Michael Wells, MD; Robert A Wise, MD; and Prescott G Woodruff, MD, MPH. The project officers from the Lung Division of the National Heart, Lung, and Blood Institute were Lisa Postow, PhD, and Thomas Croxton, PhD, MD.

Notation of prior abstract publication/presentation

Evidence of Clinical COPD in Smokers with Airway Obstruction Diagnosed with FEV_1/FVC Ratio of Less than 0.70 but Not Less than Predicted Lower Limit of Normal. Presented at the American Thoracic Society International Conference, May 19, 2015, Denver, CO, USA.

Funding

SPIROMICS was supported by contracts from the NIH/NHLBI (HHSN268200900013C, HHSN268200900014C, HHSN268200900015C, HHSN268200900016C, HHSN268200900017C, HHSN268200900018C HHSN268200900019C, HHSN268200900020C), which were supplemented by contributions made through the Foundation for the NIH from AstraZeneca; Bellerophon Therapeutics; Boehringer-Ingelheim Pharmaceuticals, Inc.; Chiesi Farmaceutici SpA; Forest Research Institute, Inc.; GSK; Grifols Therapeutics, Inc.; Ikaria, Inc.; Nycomed GmbH; Takeda Pharmaceutical Company; Novartis Pharmaceuticals Corporation; Regeneron Pharmaceuticals, Inc.; and Sanofi. This analysis was also supported by R01 HL122438 and K24 HL138188.

Authors' contributions

CP, RP, and RK conceived and supervised the overall study. TG, PQ, EC, MKH, and SM participated in the statistical analysis. CP wrote the first draft of the manuscript. RK, MKH, CC, DT, EK, IB, EH, CM, SC, NH, GB, EB, VO, FM, TG, SM, PQ, EC, and RP participated in writing of the manuscript, provided important intellectual content, and read, edited, and approved the final manuscript.

Competing interests

Dr. Tashkin reports personal fees from Boehringer-Ingelheim, personal fees from AstraZeneca, personal fees from Sunovion, personal fees from Theravance/Innoviva, personal fees from Mylan, outside the submitted work. Dr. Kleerup reports grants from NIH, grants from Foundation for the NIH, during the conduct of the study; grants from Boehringer Ingelheim, grants from Novartis, grants from Pearl/AstraZeneca, grants from Sunovion/Sepracor, outside the submitted work. Boehringer Ingelheim and GlaxoSmithKline supplied inhalers for pulmonary function testing in this study. Dr. Han reports personal fees from GSK, personal fees from BI, personal fees from AZ, non-financial support from Sunovion, non-financial support from Novartis, outside the submitted work. Dr. Cooper reports grants from Equinox Health Clubs, personal fees from Equinox Health Clubs, grants from Amgen, personal fees from PulmonX, GlaxoSmithKline, outside the submitted work; and works with scientific engagement for the GlaxoSmithKline Global Respiratory Franchise. Dr. Barjaktarevic reports grants from NIH, during the conduct of the study; personal fees from Astra Zeneca, from Grifols, from CSL Behring, outside the submitted work. Dr. Hoffman is a founder and shareholder of VIDA Diagnostics, a company commercializing lung image analysis software developed, in part, at the University of Iowa. Dr. Christenson reports personal fees from AstraZeneca, non-financial support from Genentech, grants from MedImmune, outside the submitted work. Dr. Hansel reports grants and personal fees from AstraZeneca, grants and personal fees from GSK, grants from Boehringer Ingelheim, grants from NIH, grants from COPD Foundation, outside the submitted work. Dr. Bleecker has undertaken clinical trials through his employer, Wake Forest School of Medicine and University of Arizona, for AstraZeneca, MedImmune, Boehringer Ingelheim, Cephalon/Teva, Genentech, Johnson and Johnson (Janssen), Novartis, Regeneron, and Sanofi Genzyme, personal fees from ERB, has also served as a paid consultant for AztraZeneca, MedImmune, Boehringer Ingelheim, Glaxo Smith Kline, Novartis, Regeneron, and Sanofi Genzyme, outside the submitted work. Dr. Martinez reports grants from NHLBI, during the conduct of the study; grants from National Institutes of Health, personal fees from Continuing Education, personal fees from Forest Laboratories, other from Janssen, personal fees from GlaxoSmithKline, personal fees from Nycomed/Takeda, personal fees from AstraZeneca, personal fees from Boehringer Ingelheim, personal fees from Bellerophon (formerly Ikaria), personal fees from Genentech, personal fees from Novartis, personal fees from Pearl, personal fees from Roche, personal fees from Sunovion, personal fees from Theravance, personal fees from CME Incite, personal fees from Annenberg Center for Health Sciences at Eisenhower, personal fees from Integritas, personal fees from InThought, personal fees from National Association for Continuing Education, personal fees from Paradigm Medical Communications, LLC, personal fees from PeerVoice, personal fees from UpToDate, personal fees from Haymarket Communications, personal fees from Western Society of Allergy and Immunology, from Proterixbio (formerly Bioscale), personal fees from Unity Biotechnology, personal fees from ConCert Pharmaceuticals, personal fees from Lucid, personal fees from Methodist Hospital, personal fees from Columbia University, personal fees from Prime Healthcare Ltd., personal fees from WebMD, personal fees from PeerView Network, personal fees from California Society of Allergy and Immunology, personal fees from Chiesi, personal fees from Puerto Rico Thoracic Society, outside the submitted work. Ms. Carretta reports funding from the National Heart, Lung, and Blood Institute, the Foundation for the NIH, Genentech, and the COPD Foundation during the conduct of the study. Dr. Paine reports grants from National Heart Lung and Blood Institute, grants from COPD Foundation, during the conduct of the study; grants from Department of Veterans Affairs, outside the submitted work.

Author details

[1]Division of Pulmonary and Critical Care Medicine, Department of Internal Medicine, University of Utah, 26 N 1900 E, Salt Lake City, UT 84132, USA. [2]Department of Biostatistics, University of Michigan, Ann Arbor, MI, USA. [3]Department of Biostatistics, Collaborative Studies Coordinating Center, University of North Carolina at Chapel Hill, Chapel Hill, NC, USA. [4]Department of Internal Medicine, University of Michigan, Ann, MI, USA. [5]Department of Medicine, UCLA David Geffen School of Medicine, Los Angeles, CA, USA. [6]Department of Radiology, University of Iowa, Iowa City, IA, USA. [7]Department of Medicine, University of California, San Francisco, CA, USA. [8]Department of Medicine, Johns Hopkins University, Baltimore, MD, USA. [9]Department of Medicine, Columbia University, New York, NY, USA.

[10]Department of Medicine, University of Arizona, Tucson, AZ, USA.
[11]Department of Medicine, Wake Forest University, Winston-Salem, NC, USA.
[12]Department of Medicine, Weill Cornell Medical College, New York, NY, USA.
[13]Department of Veterans Affairs Medical Center, Salt Lake City, UT, USA.

References

1. Vestbo J, Hurd SS, Agustí AG, Jones PW, Vogelmeier C, Anzueto A, Barnes PJ, Fabbri LM, Martinez FJ, Nishimura M, Stockley RA, Sin DD, Rodriguez-Roisin R. Global strategy for the diagnosis, management, and prevention of chronic obstructive pulmonary disease: GOLD executive summary. Am J Respir Crit Care Med. 2013;187:347–65.
2. Crapo RO, Morris AH, Gardner RM. Reference spirometric values using techniques and equipment that meet ATS recommendations. Am Rev Respir Dis. 1981;123:659–64.
3. Pellegrino R, Viegi G, Brusasco V, Crapo RO, Burgos F, Casaburi R, Coates A, van der Grinten CPM, Gustafsson P, Hankinson J, Jensen R, Johnson DC, MacIntyre N, McKay R, Miller MR, Navajas D, Pedersen OF, Wanger J. Interpretative strategies for lung function tests. Eur Respir J. 2005:948–68.
4. Turkeshi E, Vaes B, Andreeva E, Matheï C, Adriaensen W, Van Pottelbergh G, Degryse J-M. Airflow limitation by the global lungs initiative equations in a cohort of very old adults. Eur Respir J. 2015;46(1):123–32.
5. Vollmer WM, Gíslason T, Burney P, Enright PL, Gulsvik A, Kocabas A, Buist AS. Comparison of spirometry criteria for the diagnosis of COPD: results from the BOLD study. Eur Respir J. 2009;34:588–97.
6. Swanney MP, Ruppel G, Enright PL, Pedersen OF, Crapo RO, Miller MR, Jensen RL, Falaschetti E, Schouten JP, Hankinson JL, Stocks J, Quanjer PH. Using the lower limit of normal for the FEV_1/FVC ratio reduces the misclassification of airway obstruction. Thorax. 2008;63:1046–51.
7. Vaz Fragoso CA, Concato J, McAvay G. Chronic obstructive pulmonary disease in older persons: a comparison of two spirometric definitions. Respiratory. 2010;104(8):1189–96.
8. Hansen JE, Sun X-G, Wasserman K. Spirometric criteria for airway obstruction: use percentage of FEV_1/FVC ratio below the fifth percentile, not. CHEST. 2007;131:349–55.
9. Quanjer PH. Correctly defining criteria for diagnosing chronic obstructive pulmonary disease matters. Am J Respir Crit Care Med. 2014;189:230.
10. Vaz Fragoso CA, McAvay G, Van Ness PH, Casaburi R, Jensen RL, MacIntyre N, Gill TM, Yaggi HK, Concato J. Phenotype of Normal spirometry in an aging population. Am J Respir Crit Care Med. 2015;192:817–25.
11. van Dijk W, Tan W, Li P, Guo B, Li S, Benedetti A, Bourbeau J, CanCOLD study group. Clinical relevance of fixed ratio vs lower limit of normal of FEV_1/FVC in COPD: patient-reported outcomes from the CanCOLD cohort. Ann Fam Med. 2015;13:41–8.
12. Bhatt SP, Sieren JC, Dransfield MT, Washko GR, Newell JD, Stinson DS, Zamba GKD, Hoffman EA, COPDGene Investigators. Comparison of spirometric thresholds in diagnosing smoking-related airflow obstruction. Thorax. 2014;69:409–14.
13. Mannino DM, Sonia Buist A, Vollmer WM. Chronic obstructive pulmonary disease in the older adult: what defines abnormal lung function? Thorax. 2007;62:237–41.
14. Mohamed Hoesein FAA, Zanen P, Lammers J-WJ. Lower limit of normal or FEV_1/FVC. Respir Med. 2011;105:907–15.
15. Izquierdo Alonso JL, De Lucas Ramos P, Rodríguez Glez-Moro JM. The use of the lower limit of Normal as a criterion for COPD excludes patients with increased morbidity and high consumption of health-care resources. Archivos de Bronconeumología (English Edition). 2012;48:223–8.
16. Hoesein FAAM, de Jong PA, Lammers J-WJ, Mali WP, Schmidt M, de Koning HJ, van der Aalst C, Oudkerk M, Vliegenthart R, van Ginneken B, van Rikxoort EM, Zanen P. Computed tomography structural lung changes in discordant airflow limitation. PLoS One. 2013;8:e65177.
17. Woodruff PG, Barr RG, Bleecker E, Christenson SA, Couper D, Curtis JL, Gouskova NA, Hansel NN, Hoffman EA, Kanner RE, Kleerup E, Lazarus SC, Martinez FJ, Paine R, Rennard S, Tashkin DP, Han MK, SPIROMICS research group. Clinical significance of symptoms in smokers with preserved pulmonary function. N Engl J Med. 2016;374:1811–21.
18. Regan EA, Lynch DA, Curran-Everett D, Curtis JL, Austin JHM, Grenier PA, Kauczor H-U, Bailey WC, DeMeo DL, Casaburi RH, Friedman P, Van Beek EJR, Hokanson JE, Bowler RP, Beaty TH, Washko GR, Han MK, Kim V, Kim SS, Yagihashi K, Washington L, McEvoy CE, Tanner C, Mannino DM, Make BJ, Silverman EK, Crapo JD. Clinical and radiologic disease in smokers with Normal spirometry. JAMA Intern Med. 2015;175:1539.
19. Couper D, LaVange LM, Han M, Barr RG, Bleecker E, Hoffman EA, Kanner R, Kleerup E, Martinez FJ, Woodruff PG, Rennard S, SPIROMICS research group. Design of the Subpopulations and Intermediate Outcomes in COPD study (SPIROMICS). Thorax. 2014;69:491–4.
20. Miller MR, Hankinson J, Brusasco V, Burgos F, Casaburi R, Coates A, Crapo R, Enright P, van der Grinten CPM, Gustafsson P, Jensen R, Johnson DC, MacIntyre N, McKay R, Navajas D, Pedersen OF, Pellegrino R, Viegi G, Wanger J. ATS/ERS task force: standardisation of spirometry. Eur Respir J. 2005;26(2):319–38.
21. Miller MR, Crapo R, Hankinson J, Brusasco V, Burgos F, Casaburi R, Coates A, Enright P, van der Grinten CPM, Gustafsson P, Jensen R, Johnson DC, MacIntyre N, McKay R, Navajas D, Pedersen OF, Pellegrino R, Viegi G, Wanger J. ATS/ERS task force: general considerations for lung function testing. Eur Respir J. 2005;26:153–61.
22. Hankinson JL, Odencrantz JR, Fedan KB. Spirometric reference values from a sample of the general U.S. population. Am J Respir Crit Care Med. 1999;159:179–87.
23. Bestall JC, Paul EA, Garrod R, Garnham R, Jones PW, Wedzicha JA. Usefulness of the Medical Research Council (MRC) dyspnoea scale as a measure of disability in patients with chronic obstructive pulmonary disease. Thorax. 1999;54:581–6.
24. Jones PW, Harding G, Berry P, Wiklund I, Chen W-H, Kline Leidy N. Development and first validation of the COPD assessment test. Eur Respir J. 2009;34:648–54.
25. Jones PW, Quirk FH, Baveystock CM, Littlejohns P. A self-complete measure of health status for chronic airflow limitation. The St. George's respiratory questionnaire. Am Rev Respir Dis. 1992;145:1321–7.
26. Nakano Y, Wong JC, de Jong PA, Buzatu L, Nagao T, Coxson HO, Elliott WM, Hogg JC, Paré PD. The prediction of small airway dimensions using computed tomography. Am J Respir Crit Care Med. 2005;171:142–6.
27. Galbán CJ, Han MK, Boes JL, Chughtai KA, Meyer CR, Johnson TD, Galbán S, Rehemtulla A, Kazerooni EA, Martinez FJ, Ross BD. Computed tomography-based biomarker provides unique signature for diagnosis of COPD phenotypes and disease progression. Nat Med. 2012;18:1711–5.
28. Welch BL. The generalization of `student"s" problem when several different population variances are involved. Biometrika. 1947;34:28.
29. Koenker R (2012). Package 'quantreg'. http://cran.r-project.org/web/packages/quantreg/quantreg.pdf, accessed 15 Aug 2018.
30. Hoffman EA, Ahmed FS, Baumhauer H, Budoff M, Carr JJ, Kronmal R, Reddy S, Barr RG. Variation in the percent of emphysema-like lung in a healthy, nonsmoking multiethnic sample. The MESA lung study. Ann Am Thorac Soc. 2014;11:898–907.
31. Martinez CH, Diaz AA, Meldrum C, Curtis JL, Cooper CB, Pirozzi C, Kanner RE, Paine R, Woodruff PG, Bleecker ER, Hansel NN, Barr RG, Marchetti N, Criner GJ, Kazerooni EA, Hoffman EA, Ross BD, Galbán CJ, Cigolle CT, Martinez FJ, Han MK, SPIROMICS Investigators. Age and small airway imaging abnormalities in subjects with and without airflow obstruction in SPIROMICS. Am J Respir Crit Care Med. 2017;195:464–72.
32. McFadden ER Jr, Linden DA. A reduction in maximum mid-expiratory flow rate. A spirographic manifestation of small airway disease. Am J Med. 1972; 52(6):725–37.
33. Gelb AF, Zamel N. Simplified diagnosis of small-airway obstruction. N Engl J Med. 1973;288:395–8.
34. van den Berge M, ten NHT H, Cohen J, Douma WR, Postma DS. Small airway disease in asthma and COPD: clinical implications. CHEST. 2011;139:412–23.
35. Smith BM, Hoffman EA, Rabinowitz D, Bleecker E, Christenson S, Couper D, Donohue KM, Han MK, Hansel NN, Kanner RE, Kleerup E, Rennard S, Barr RG. Comparison of spatially matched airways reveals thinner airway walls in COPD. The multi-ethnic study of atherosclerosis (MESA) COPD study and the Subpopulations and intermediate outcomes in COPD study (SPIROMICS). Thorax. 2014;69:987–96.
36. Mets OM, de Jong PA, van Ginneken B, Kruitwagen CLJJ, Prokop M, Oudkerk M, Lammers J-WJ, Zanen P. CT air trapping is independently associated with lung function reduction over time. PLoS One. 2013;8:e61783.
37. Bommart S, Marin G, Bourdin A, Molinari N, Klein F, Hayot M, Vachier I, Chanez P, Mercier J, Vernhet-Kovacsik H. Relationship between CT air trapping criteria and lung function in small airway impairment quantification. BMC Pulm Med. 2014;14:29.

38. McDonough JE, Yuan R, Suzuki M, Seyednejad N, Elliott WM, Sanchez PG, Wright AC, Gefter WB, Litzky L, Coxson HO, Paré PD, Sin DD, Pierce RA, Woods JC, McWilliams AM, Mayo JR, Lam SC, Cooper JD, Hogg JC. Small-airway obstruction and emphysema in chronic obstructive pulmonary disease. N Engl J Med. 2011;365:1567–75.
39. Hogg JC, Chu F, Utokaparch S, Woods R, Elliott WM, Buzatu L, Cherniack RM, Rogers RM, Sciurba FC, Coxson HO, Paré PD. The nature of small-airway obstruction in chronic obstructive pulmonary disease. N Engl J Med. 2004; 350:2645–53.
40. Verbanck S, Schuermans D, Meysman M, Paiva M, Vincken W. Noninvasive assessment of airway alterations in smokers. Am J Respir Crit Care Med. 2004;170:414–9.
41. Pirozzi CS, Paine R, Tashkin DP, Kleerup EC, Woodruff PG, Han MK, Quibrera PM, Carretta E, Kanner R: Evidence of Clinical COPD in Smokers with Airway Obstruction Diagnosed with FEV_1/FVC Ratio of Less than 0.70 but Not Less than Predicted Lower Limit of Normal. In *American Thoracic Society International Conference Abstracts*. American Thoracic Society; 2015:A4473–A4473.
42. Pirozzi CS, Gu T, Quibrera P, Carretta E, Han MK, Murray S, Cooper CB, Tashkin DP, Kleerup EC, Hoffman EA, Martinez C, Christenson S, Hansel NN, Barr RG, Bleecker ER, Ortega VE, Martinez FJ, Kanner RE, Paine R: Heterogeneous Burden of Emphysema and Functional Small Airway Abnormalities in Smokers with FEV_1/FVC Ratio Above Lower Limit of Normal but Below 0.7. In American Thoracic Society International Conference Abstracts. Am J Respir Crit Care Med 2018;197:A6397

Association of lung function with cardiovascular risk: a cohort study

Bin Wang[1,2], Yun Zhou[1,2], Lili Xiao[1,2], Yanjun Guo[1,2], Jixuan Ma[1,2], Min Zhou[1,2], Tingming Shi[3], Aijun Tan[4], Jing Yuan[1,2] and Weihong Chen[1,2*]

Abstract

Background: The potential effects of pulmonary dysfunction on cardiovascular diseases (CVD) are receiving attention. We aimed to investigate and quantify the cross-sectional and longitudinal associations between lung function and overall cardiovascular risk among Chinese general population.

Methods: We studied 4019 participants from the Wuhan-Zhuhai cohort, with a follow-up of 3 years. A multivariable risk algorithm generated from the Framingham study was used to calculate individuals' overall cardiovascular risk i.e. 10-Year CVD Risk, which was further classified into 2 categories: low (< 10%) and high (≥10%) CVD risk. General linear model and logistic regression model were separately used to assess the associations of lung function with continuous and dichotomous 10-Year CVD Risk.

Results: Cross-sectionally, each 5% decrease in FEV_1/FVC was associated with a 0.47% increase in 10-Year CVD Risk ($P < 0.001$). The adjusted odds ratio (OR) (95% confidence interval [CI]) for the prevalence of high CVD risk (10-Year CVD Risk≥10%) was 1.12 (1.07, 1.17) corresponding to each 5% decrease in FEV_1/FVC. The OR (95% CI) for high CVD risk in the lowest group of FEV_1/FVC (< 70% i.e. chronic obstructive pulmonary disease [COPD]) was 2. 37 (1.43, 3.91) when compared with the highest group. Longitudinally, the adjusted risk ratio (RR) (95% CI) for the incidence of high CVD risk was 1.14 (1.03, 1.25) with each 5% decrease in baseline FEV_1/FVC. Compared with the highest group of FEV_1/FVC, the RR (95% CI) for high CVD risk in the lowest group (COPD) was 4.06 (1.46, 11.26). Analyses of 10-Year CVD Risk with FVC or FEV_1 showed similar trends and significant associations (all $P < 0.05$).

Conclusion: Reduced lung function was cross-sectionally and longitudinally associated with increased cardiovascular risk in Chinese general population.

Keywords: Lung function, Chronic obstructive pulmonary disease, Cardiovascular disease, Cohort study

Background

Cardiovascular diseases (CVD), including coronary disease, cerebrovascular disease, peripheral vascular disease and cardiac failure, are leading causes of morbidity and mortality in China and worldwide [1, 2]. To better prevent and control CVD, a global multivariable risk algorithm based on traditional CVD risk factors including sex, age, total and high density lipoprotein (HDL) cholesterol, systolic blood pressure and treatment for hypertension, smoking and diabetes status, was generated from the Framingham study [3]. The model has been demonstrated to have good discrimination power and be able to estimate overall CVD risk in the next ten years (10-Year CVD Risk) for individuals without CVD [3]. The 10-Year CVD Risk provides useful and elegant composite measures of the classical risk factors for CVD and reflects overall cardiovascular risk of individuals, thus it has been well recognized and widely used in fields of clinic and public health [3–5].

It is well known that cardiovascular and respiratory systems are closely linked with each other in physiology and pathophysiology. Cardiovascular dysfunction could

* Correspondence: wchen@mails.tjmu.edu.cn
[1]Department of Occupational & Environmental Health, School of Public Health, Tongji Medical College, Huazhong University of Science and Technology, Wuhan 430030, Hubei, China
[2]Key Laboratory of Environment and Health, Ministry of Education & Ministry of Environmental Protection, and State Key Laboratory of Environmental Health (Incubating), School of Public Health, Tongji Medical College, Huazhong University of Science and Technology, Wuhan 430030, Hubei, China
Full list of author information is available at the end of the article

affect lung function, in turn, pulmonary dysfunction may cause adverse cardiovascular outcomes [6, 7]. Pulmonary function, a noninvasive clinical diagnostic parameter, is often used to evaluate the conditions of the respiratory system and identify the severity of pulmonary impairments such as asthma and chronic obstructive pulmonary disease (COPD) [8]. Accumulating evidence suggested that pulmonary dysfunction was positively and independently associated with CVD morbidity [9–15] and mortality [16–20]. A cross-sectional study conducted among 9688 Korean general population without obstructive lung disease found that forced vital capacity (FVC) was inversely related to 10-Year CVD Risk [21]. However, it is still largely unknown whether the reduction of lung function parameters like forced expiratory volume in 1 s (FEV_1) and the ratio of FEV_1 to FVC (FEV_1/FVC) are related to current and future CVD risk such as 10-Year CVD Risk. Further analysis on their associations in both cross-sectional and longitudinal ways will help better clarify and understand the potential effect of lung function decline on CVD.

Therefore, in present study, we investigated and quantified the cross-sectional and longitudinal associations between lung function (including parameters of FEV_1, FVC and FEV_1/FVC) and the 10-Year CVD Risk in a Chinese general population.

Methods

Study population

The study participants were from the Wuhan-Zhuhai cohort, a Chinese community-based prospective cohort, which has been described previously [22]. Briefly, the cohort was established between 2011 and 2012, comprising 4812 participants aged 18 to 80 years who lived in Wuhan or Zhuhai city in China for more than 5 years. Standardized questionnaires and extensive physical examinations were carried out at baseline and 3 years later. For cross-sectional analysis, participants less than 30 years old (n = 260) or previously diagnosed with CVD (n = 317) were excluded, as 10-Year CVD Risk estimation was inapplicable for this population [3]. We also excluded 216 subjects with missing data or outliers (>mean ± 3SD) on indexes of blood test, anthropometry, blood pressure or pulmonary function. Finally, a total of 4019 participants were included in our cross-sectional study. For longitudinal analysis, we further excluded 2196 individuals who did not attend physical examinations, or had missing data or outliers on indexes of blood test, anthropometry or blood pressure at 3-year follow-up. After further excluding 752 participants with 10-Year CVD Risk ≥10% at baseline, 1071 subjects were included in our longitudinal study. Individuals included and excluded in our study showed no differences with respect to basic demographic characteristics such as sex, body mass index, smoking status, drinking status, education levels, abdominal obesity, etc. ($P > 0.05$).

Lung function test

Lung function test was performed in accordance with the recommendation of American Thoracic Society [23]. In brief, spirometry was conducted by specialists using digital spirometers (Chestgraph HI-101, CHEST Ltd., Tokyo, Japan), which were calibrated each day before testing, according to the manufacturer's instruction. All individuals were suggested not to smoke for at least 1 h and not to have a big meal for 2 h before the test. Each participant was informed to keep a sitting position, wear a nose clip, and then breathe through the mouth-piece after at least 5 min of normal breathing during the testing procedure. Three acceptable volume-time curves of pulmonary function parameters were obtained after three satisfactory blows of each participant performed. Lung function parameters including FVC, FEV_1 and FEV_1/FVC were mainly used in our study. COPD was defined as FEV_1/FVC < 70%, which was further classified into four stages according to Global Initiative for Chronic Obstructive Lung Disease (GOLD) [24]: GOLD 1 (mild: FEV_1/FVC < 70% and $FEV_1 \geq 80\%$ predicted), GOLD 2 (moderate: FEV_1/FVC < 70% and $50\% \leq FEV_1 < 80\%$ predicted), GOLD 3 (severe: FEV_1/FVC < 70% and $30\% \leq FEV_1 < 50\%$ predicted) and GOLD 4 (very severe: FEV_1/FVC < 70% and $FEV_1 < 30\%$ predicted).

Ten-year CVD risk calculation and classification

Sex-specific 10-Year CVD Risk was calculated by a multivariable risk factor algorithm that incorporated age, total cholesterol, HDL cholesterol, systolic blood pressure and treatment for hypertension, current smoking, and diabetes status, as described previously [3]. According to the Framingham study [3] and Framingham database derived practice guideline [25], 10-Year CVD Risk was further classified into 2 categories: low (< 10%) and high (≥10%) CVD risk.

Ascertainment of covariates and CVD risk factors

Body mass index (BMI) was calculated by dividing weight (kg) by the squared value of height (m). Active physical activity was defined as regular exercise ≥2 times per week and each time ≥ 20 min within the last 6 months. Education degree was classified into 3 levels: middle school or below, high school, and university or above. Smokers comprised both current and former smokers, and smoking amount (pack-years) for each smoker was computed as packs of cigarettes per day multiplied by years of smoking. Participants were divided into drinkers (including current and former drinkers) and nondrinkers. Abdominal obesity was defined as waist circumference ≥ 90 cm for men or ≥ 80 cm for women. Blood lipids and fasting glucose levels were determined in the clinical laboratory of hospitals. Blood pressure was measured on the right arm of the seated participant with a validated automatic oscillometric device. Diabetes was defined as fasting plasma glucose ≥7.0 mmol/L, or taking oral hypoglycemic medication or insulin, or self-reported physician-diagnosed diabetes.

Statistical analyses

Subjects were divided into four groups based on quartiles (Q) of FVC or FEV_1 or clinical thresholds of FEV_1/FVC level (L1 < 70%; L2 70% ~ < 80%; L3 80% ~ < 90%; L4 ≥ 90%), for which 70% is a clinical threshold of COPD diagnosis and 80% is a critical value of normal lung function. Baseline characteristics across groups of FEV_1/FVC were compared by variance analysis for continuous variables and Cochran-Armitage trend test for dichotomous variables. Analysis of covariance was used to compare 10-Year CVD Risk by groups of lung function parameters, with adjusting for gender, height, weight, abdominal obesity, smoking amount, drinking status, low density lipoprotein (LDL), physical activity, city and education levels. Age was not included in the statistic models for adjustment again, because as a dependent variable, 10-Year CVD Risk was estimated by a multivariable risk factor algorithm where age has been included, further adjustment for age in the statistic models again will lead to overcorrection and conservative association between lung function and CVD risk.

Association of lung function with continuous 10-Year CVD Risk was assessed using general linear model, with adjustment for potential confounders as mentioned above. The association was quantified by using estimated changes and 95% confidence intervals (CIs) of 10-Year CVD Risk with each 5% decrease of FEV_1/FVC or each 50-mL decrease of FVC or FEV_1 in continuous analyses. We also estimated changes (95% CI) of 10-Year CVD Risk across groups of lung function parameters in categorical analyses with the highest group (L4 or Q4) as the reference.

Logistic regression model was used to calculate the odds ratios (ORs), risk ratios (RRs) and 95% CI for dichotomous 10-Year CVD Risk (individuals with 10-Year CVD Risk ≥10% were regarded as cases) according to the decreasing of baseline lung function level, with adjusting for potential covariates as mentioned above. All statistical analyses were performed with SAS version 9.4 (SAS Institute, Cary, NC), and all *p*-values were two sided with a significant level at 0.05.

Results

Baseline characteristics

The baseline characteristics of the participants based on groups of FEV_1/FVC are presented in Table 1. The mean age of 4019 participants (1304 men; 32.45%) was 53.98 years. Without adjustment for any confounder, the number of smokers, drinkers and participants with high 10-Year CVD Risk (≥10%), as well as age, smoking amount, low density lipoprotein and 10-Year CVD Risk significantly increased across decreasing FEV_1/FVC groups ($P < 0.001$). In further analysis with COPD patients (group L1: FEV_1/FVC < 70%), we found an upward trend of 10-Year CVD Risk as the progresses of COPD (from GOLD 1 to GOLD 4, $P_{trend} = 0.041$) (Table S1). And COPD patients with older age, male sex, smoking or drinking habits achieved higher CVD risk ($P < 0.05$) (Additional file 1: Table S1).

Association of pulmonary function with 10-year CVD risk

With adjustment for potential covariates, leastsquares means of 10-Year CVD Risk by groups of lung function parameters at baseline are shown in Fig. 1. The highest 10-Year CVD Risk was observed in the lowest group of lung function parameters (L1 [COPD group] or Q1) when compared with those in other groups. Upward trend of 10-Year CVD Risk was significantly associated with decreased lung function groups.

Table 2 presents an inverse relationship between lung function and continuous 10-Year CVD Risk at baseline. After adjusting for potential confounders, each 5% decrease in FEV_1/FVC was associated with a 0.47% increase in 10-Year CVD Risk ($P < 0.001$). Remarkably monotonic increase of 10-Year CVD Risk was shown when FEV_1/FVC gradually decreased ($P_{trend} < 0.001$). Similar trends and significant associations were also observed between FVC and FEV_1 and 10-Year CVD Risk (Table 2).

Table 3 shows a negative association between lung function and dichotomous10-Year CVD Risk at baseline. After adjusting for potential confounders, the OR (95%CI) for the prevalence of high CVD risk (10-Year CVD Risk ≥10%) was 1.12 (1.07, 1.17) with each 5% decrease in FEV_1/FVC. Compared with the highest FEV_1/FVC group, multi-variate adjusted ORs (95%CI) gradually increased when lung function decreased. From the second highest to the lowest FEV_1/FVC group (COPD), they were 1.11 (0.94, 1.31), 1.63 (1.31, 2.03), 2.37 (1.43, 3.91) for high CVD risk. Similar trends and significant relationships were also shown between FVC and FEV_1 and 10-Year CVD Risk (Table 3).

After 3 years of follow-up, we recalculated the 10-Year CVD Risk for the 1071 participants included in our longitudinal study, and 214 incident cases of high CVD risk (10-Year CVD Risk ≥10%) were identified. RRs for the incidence of high CVD risk are shown in Table 4. A negative association between baseline lung function and incidence of high CVD risk was observed. The RR (95%CI) was 1.14 (1.03, 1.25) corresponding to each 5% decline in FEV1/FVC. The categorical analysis also showed a significant monotonic RR increase of high CVD risk as the decreasing

Table 1 Baseline characteristics of study participants by groups of FEV_1/FVC and in all participants ($N = 4019$)

Variables		FEV_1/FVC (%)				
	All participants	L4 (≥90)	L3 (80 ~ < 90)	L2 (70 ~ < 80)	L1 (< 70)	P_{trend}
No. subjects	4019	1606	1664	648	101	
No. subjects in Wuhan city	2536 (63.10)	855 (53.24)	1085 (65.2)	511 (78.86)	85 (84.16)	< 0.001
Age, years	53.98 ± 11.21	52.14 ± 11.02	54.23 ± 11.02	56.69 ± 11.16	61.51 ± 10.58	< 0.001
male sex	1304 (32.45)	485 (30.20)	509 (30.59)	261 (40.28)	49 (48.51)	< 0.001
Body mass index, kg/m^2	24.05 ± 3.36	24.08 ± 3.45	24.12 ± 3.31	23.93 ± 3.27	23.30 ± 3.23	0.105
Education levels						
Middle school or below	2505 (62.33)	958 (59.65)	1042 (62.62)	428 (66.05)	77 (76.24)	< 0.001
High school	1100 (27.37)	457 (28.46)	458 (27.52)	167 (25.77)	18 (17.82)	0.035
University or above	414 (10.30)	191 (11.89)	164 (9.86)	53 (8.18)	6 (5.94)	0.002
Physical activity	1967 (48.94)	791 (49.25)	836 (50.24)	298 (45.99)	42 (41.58)	0.120
Smokers[a]	886 (22.05)	307 (19.12)	351 (21.09)	192 (29.63)	36 (35.64)	< 0.001
Smoking amount, pack-years[b]	5.29 ± 14.09	4.26 ± 12.79	4.71 ± 13.12	8.38 ± 17.37	11.45 ± 20.29	< 0.001
Drinkers[a]	714 (17.77)	257 (16.00)	276 (16.59)	154 (23.77)	27 (26.73)	< 0.001
Abdominal obesity	1795 (44.66)	707 (44.02)	774 (46.51)	280 (43.21)	34 (33.66)	0.392
LDL, mmol/L	3.10 ± 1.02	2.98 ± 1.02	3.15 ± 1.02	3.23 ± 1.02	3.19 ± 0.89	< 0.001
10-Year CVD Risk, %	10.24 ± 9.11	9.16 ± 8.50	10.21 ± 9.10	12.25 ± 9.81	15.11 ± 10.25	< 0.001
10-Year CVD Risk						
Low (< 10%)	2452 (61.01)	1050 (65.38) ()(65.38)	1033 (62.08)	329 (50.77)	40 (39.60)	< 0.001
High (≥10%)	1567 (38.99)	556 (34.62)	631 (37.92)	319 (49.23)	61 (60.40)	< 0.001

Abbreviations: *FEV_1/FVC* the ratio of forced expiratory volume in the 1 s to forced vital capacity, *LDL* low density lipoprotein
Values are n (%) or mean ± SD
[a]Smokers/drinkers included both current and former smokers/drinkers
[b]Smoking amount was calculated among both current and former smokers

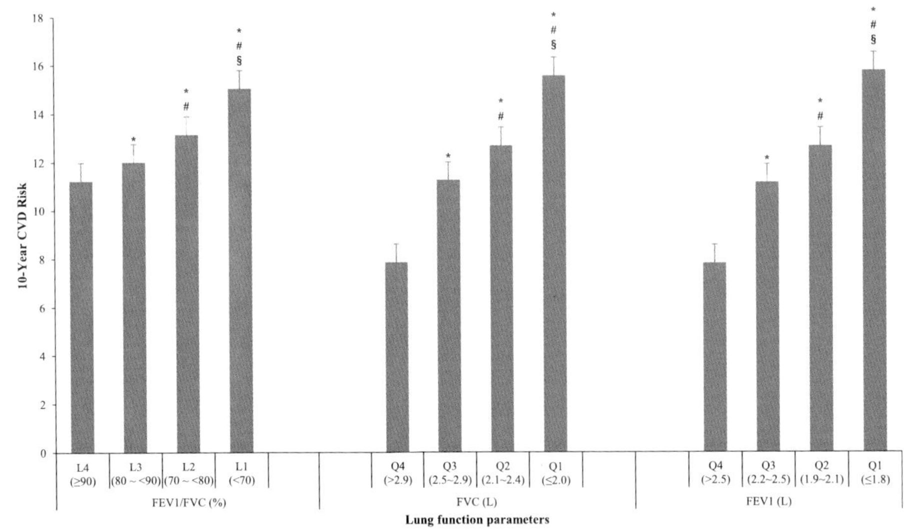

Fig. 1 The 10-Year CVD Risk in all participants by groups of lung function parameters using analysis of covariance. Abbreviations: FEV_1, forced expiratory volume in 1 s; FVC, forced vital capacity; FEV_1/FVC, the ratio of FEV_1 to FVC. * Significant differences between L4/Q4 and any other lung function group at $P < 0.05$; # significant differences between L3/Q3 and any other lung function group at $P < 0.05$; § significant differences between L2/Q2 and any other lung function group at $P < 0.05$. Adjusted for gender (male/female), height (continuous, m), weight (continuous, kg), abdominal obesity (yes/no), smoking amount (continuous, pack-year), drinking status (drinker/nondrinker), low density lipoprotein (continuous, mmol/L), physical activity (active/inactive), city (Wuhan/Zhuhai) and education levels (middle school or below, high school, university or above)

Table 2 Association between lung function and 10-Year CVD Risk ($N = 4019$)

Lung function parameters	Estimated changes (95% CI) by continuous lung function parameters[a]	Estimated changes (95% CI) by groups of lung function parameters				P_{trend}
FEV_1/FVC (%)		L4 (≥90)	L3 (80 ~ < 90)	L2 (70 ~ < 80)	L1 (< 70)	
	0.47 (0.34, 0.60)	0.00 (ref.)	0.78 (0.28, 1.28)	1.91 (1.24, 2.59)	3.82 (2.34, 5.30)	< 0.001
FVC (L)		Q4 (> 2.9)	Q3 (2.5~ 2.9)	Q2 (2.1~ 2.4)	Q1 (≤2.0)	
	0.24 (0.22, 0.26)	0.00 (ref.)	3.40 (2.71, 4.08)	4.83 (4.08, 5.58)	7.72 (6.92, 8.51)	< 0.001
FEV_1 (L)		Q4 (> 2.5)	Q3 (2.2~ 2.5)	Q2 (1.9~ 2.1)	Q1 (≤1.8)	
	0.28 (0.25, 0.30)	0.00 (ref.)	3.33 (2.65, 4.01)	4.85 (4.10, 5.60)	7.96 (7.21, 8.71)	< 0.001

Abbreviations: *FEV_1* forced expiratory volume in 1 s; *FVC* forced vital capacity, *FEV_1/FVC* the ratio of FEV_1 to FVC, *CI* confidence interval
Adjusted for gender (male/female), height (continuous, m), weight (continuous, kg), abdominal obesity (yes/no), smoking amount (continuous, pack-year), drinking status (drinker/nondrinker), low density lipoprotein (continuous, mmol/L), physical activity (active/inactive), city (Wuhan/Zhuhai) and education levels (middle school or below, high school, university or above)
[a]Estimated changes of 10-Year CVD Risk were calculated by each 5% decrease of FEV_1/FVC or each 50-mL decrease of FVC or FEV_1 in continuous analyses

of FEV_1/FVC groups ($P_{trend} = 0.021$). Compared with the highest FEV_1/FVC group, the RRs (95%CI) for high CVD risk were 1.15 (0.80, 1.65), 1.41 (0.85, 2.34), 4.06 (1.46, 11.26) from the second highest to the lowest FEV_1/FVC group (COPD). Similarly, significant negative associations of FVC and FEV_1 with 10-Year CVD Risk were observed with all P and $P_{trend} < 0.001$ (Table 4).

Discussion

In the present study, negative cross-sectional and longitudinal associations were identified between lung function and 10-Year CVD Risk. After adjusting for potential confounders, increased prevalence and incidence of high CVD risk (10-Year CVD Risk ≥10%) were observed with the decline of lung function level. Additionally, when 10-Year CVD Risk was further classified into ≥6%/< 6% or > 20%/≤ 20% as also proposed by the Framingham study [3] and practice guideline derived from Framingham database [25], similar trends and significant associations with lung function were also found (data not shown). Our findings help to understand the correlation between lung function and current and future CVD risk. They also have significant implications for public health. Lung function test is a noninvasive clinical diagnostic method and is easy taken after routing training. The significant relationship between reduced lung function and increased CVD risk in ten years indicated that improving lung function or preventing lung function decline may help to prevent CVD.

Lung function has been linked to CVD risk in previous studies [21, 26, 27]. The 4th Korea National Health and Nutrition Examination Survey found that FVC decline was cross-sectionally associated with increased 10-Year CVD Risk [21]. Similarly, a study by Arcari et al. on Italian general population showed that FVC or FEV_1 reduction was cross-sectionally associated with elevated 10-Year CVD Risk [27]. However, they did not find the association between FEV_1/FVC, a mainly clinical diagnostic indicator for obstructive lung diseases such as COPD, and 10-Year CVD Risk, which is inconsistent with our findings. In our study, we found that not only FVC and FEV_1 but also

Table 3 Odds ratios for 10-Year CVD Risk according to lung function parameters ($N = 4019$)

Variables	ORs (95% CI) by Continuous lung function[a]	ORs (95% CI) by groups of lung function parameters				P_{trend}
FEV_1/FVC (%)		L4 (≥90)	L3 (80 ~ < 90)	L2 (70 ~ < 80)	L1 (< 70)	
N (≥10% / < 10%)	1567/2452	556/1050	631/1033	319/329	61/40	
Adjusted OR (95% CI)	1.12 (1.07, 1.17)	1.00 (ref.)	1.11 (0.94, 1.31)	1.63 (1.31, 2.03)	2.37 (1.43, 3.91)	< 0.001
FVC (L)		Q4 (> 2.9)	Q3 (2.5~ 2.9)	Q2 (2.1~ 2.4)	Q1 (≤2.0)	
N (≥10% / < 10%)	1567/2452	358/526	347/683	343/715	519/528	
Adjusted OR (95% CI)	1.07 (1.06, 1.08)	1.00 (ref.)	2.34 (1.79, 3.06)	4.33 (3.18, 5.90)	9.82 (7.11, 13.56)	< 0.001
FEV_1 (L)		Q4 (> 2.5)	Q3 (2.2~ 2.5)	Q2 (1.9~ 2.1)	Q1 (≤1.8)	
N (≥10% / < 10%)	1567/2452	363/554	311/690	284/608	609/600	
Adjusted OR (95% CI)	1.09 (1.08, 1.10)	1.00 (ref.)	2.33 (1.77, 3.07)	4.10 (3.00, 5.60)	10.37 (7.58, 14.19)	< 0.001

Abbreviations: *FEV_1* forced expiratory volume in 1 s, *FVC* forced vital capacity, *FEV_1/FVC* the ratio of FEV_1 to FVC *OR* odds ratio; *CI* confidence interval
Adjusted for gender (male/female), height (continuous, m), weight (continuous, kg), abdominal obesity (yes/no), smoking amount (continuous, pack-year), drinking status (drinker/nondrinker), low density lipoprotein (continuous, mmol/L), physical activity (active/inactive), city (Wuhan/Zhuhai) and education levels (middle school or below, high school, university or above)
[a]Odds ratios were estimated by each 5% decrease of FEV_1/FVC or each 50-mL decrease of FVC or FEV_1 in continuous analyses

Table 4 Risk ratios for 10-Year CVD Risk according to lung function parameters ($N = 1071$)

Variables	RRs (95% CI) by Continuous lung function[a]	RRs (95% CI) by groups of lung function parameters				p_{trend}
FEV_1/FVC (%)		L4 (≥90)	L3 (80 ~ < 90)	L2 (70 ~ < 80)	L1 (< 70)	
N (≥10% / < 10%)	214/857	82/377	90/361	33/110	9/9	
Adjusted RR (95% CI)	1.14 (1.03, 1.25)	1.00 (ref.)	1.15 (0.80, 1.65)	1.41 (0.85, 2.34)	4.06 (1.46, 11.26)	0.021
FVC (L)		Q4 (> 2.8)	Q3 (2.5~ 2.8)	Q2 (2.1~ 2.4)	Q1 (≤2.0)	
N (≥10% / < 10%)	214/857	60/197	29/211	61/266	64/183	
Adjusted RR (95% CI)	1.04 (1.02, 1.06)	1.00 (ref.)	1.10 (0.58, 2.10)	2.07 (1.11, 3.85)	3.19 (1.68, 6.06)	< 0.001
FEV_1 (L)		Q4 (> 2.5)	Q3 (2.2~ 2.5)	Q2 (1.9~ 2.1)	Q1 (≤1.8)	
N (≥10% / < 10%)	214/857	46/180	43/235	49/243	76/199	
Adjusted RR (95% CI)	1.07 (1.05, 1.09)	1.00 (ref.)	2.46 (1.28, 4.76)	3.33 (1.63, 6.81)	6.49 (3.19, 13.18)	< 0.001

Abbreviations: FEV_1, forced expiratory volume in 1 s; FVC, forced vital capacity; FEV_1/FVC, the ratio of FEV_1 to FVC; RR, risk ratio; CI, confidence interval
Adjusted for gender (male/female), height (continuous, m), weight (continuous, kg), abdominal obesity (yes/no), smoking amount (continuous, pack-year), drinking status (drinker/nondrinker), low density lipoprotein (continuous, mmol/L), physical activity (active/inactive), city (Wuhan/Zhuhai) and education levels (middle school or below, high school, university or above)
[a]Risk ratios were estimated by each 5% decrease of FEV_1/FVC or each 50-mL decrease of FVC or FEV_1 in continuous analyses

FEV_1/FVC reduction was cross-sectionally and longitudinally associated with increased10-Year CVD Risk. Such discrepancy between our study and the published data may be partly due to the differences in race, genetics and lifestyles of the study population. For example, as a common risk factor for CVD, cigarette smoking rate was 22.05% in our study, lower than the mean smoking rate (28.10%) for adults in China [28]. Physical activity rate, a protective factor of CVD, was 48.94% in our study, much higher than the average level (11.90%) of Chinese adults [29]. These factors may lead to more obvious effect of lung function decline on CVD. Additionally, compared with the participants in our study (average BMI: 24.05 kg/m^2), the subjects included in Arcari's study had higher BMI with a mean value of 27.6 kg/m^2, which was considered as overweight and on the brink of obesity [30]. As risk factors for CVD [25, 31], overweight and obesity may partly conceal the effects of FEV_1/FVC on the risk of CVD in Arcari's study.

Furtherly, we noted that participants with COPD ($FEV_1/FVC < 70\%$) achieved the highest 10-Year CVD Risk in our present study. This result is consistent with those reported by Ford and colleagues. They found that aged adults with obstructive or restrictive impairment had an increased 10-Year CVD Risk compared with those with normal lung function [26]. Besides, accumulating evidence suggested that COPD patients have an elevated risk of CVD and cardiovascular death, and nearly two fifths of COPD patients die of CVD [17, 18, 32].

The underlying mechanisms between pulmonary dysfunction and CVD remain incompletely understood. Generally, pulmonary and cardiovascular functions are closely related in both physiological and pathological conditions. At the circumstance of lung function decline, cardiac pumping function has to increase compensatorily to ensure the body's oxygen need, which may result in cardiac and vascular overloads, and even cardiovascular injuries [33, 34]. If these situations were not improved timely, cardiovascular events might occur in the near future [33]. Additionally, shared risk factors may partly explain the association between poor lung function and elevated CVD risk [7]. It is well documented that several risk factors for lung function reduction, such as aging and smoking, are also well-established risk factors for CVD [3]. And traditional cardiovascular risk factors such as hypertension, dyslipidemia and diabetes mellitus are common in subjects with lung function impairment including COPD [35]. Air pollutants like particulate matters and polycyclic aromatic hydrocarbons are notable risk factors for both poor lung function and cardiovascular events [36–38]. However, the still observed association between lung function and CVD after adjusting for shared risk factors suggested the involvement of additional explanations [20].

Further explanations could be inflammation and oxidative stress, which were reported to have important contributions to both lung function decline and CVD risk increase [7]. Evidence has shown that inflammation markers such as C-reactive protein, fibrinogen and inflammation-sensitive plasma proteins were involved in the inverse relationship between lung function and CVD risk [20, 21, 39]. As a major driving mechanism in the pathophysiology of lung function impairment, elevated oxidative stress in local pulmonary microenvironment may directly affect cardiovascular system [7]. Previous studies suggested that oxidative stress may cause vascular dysfunction through inactivating the endothelial-derived nitric oxide by superoxide anion

[40]. Generation of reactive oxygen species (ROS) could promote inflammation in the vascular wall by inducing the production of pro-inflammatory genes and cytokines via the activation of NF-κB [41], whereas in turn, inflammatory cytokines (TNF-α, IL-6, etc.) could increase ROS production by NADPH oxidases [42, 43], causing a vicious circle that exacerbates vascular dysfunction [44]. Moreover, oxidative stress and inflammation could also alter the vascular structure by promoting vascular remodeling, stiffness and atherosclerosis [44–46]. Therefore, the inflammation and increased oxidative stress in pulmonary dysfunction may independently increase CVD risk by altering vascular structure and promoting vascular dysfunction and insufficiency [7]. Besides, evidence has shown that pulmonary dysfunction specific inflammation and oxidative stress may elevate cardiovascular risk also through increasing susceptibility to thrombotic or embolic events [47–49].

The strengths of our study include a relative large study population and a 3-year follow-up. Based on that, we could investigate the cross-sectional relationship between lung function and CVD risk and longitudinally evaluate the changes after 3 years. And to our knowledge, it is the first prospective study to investigate the relationship between lung function and 10-Year CVD Risk. However, there are still several limitations. First, rather than clinically diagnosed CVD, we evaluated the risk of CVD using a global multivariable risk algorithm, which was clinically used to estimate the 10-Year CVD Risk of individuals. Nevertheless, as an available endpoint, 10-Year CVD Risk do provide useful and elegant composite measures of the classical risk factors for CVD and represent individuals' overall cardiovascular risk. Moreover, we are not unique in using 10-Year CVD Risk as a composite measure of CVD risk (endpoint), and a similar method was also taken by studies draw from Cardiovascular Risk Factor Multiple Evaluation in Latin America Study [50], Louisville Healthy Heart Study [51], Lifestyle Interventions and Independence for Elders Study [52], International Mobility in Aging Study [53], etc. Second, the CVD risk was merely estimated at baseline and at 3 years of follow-up, and the follow-up time may be relatively short. Further long-time longitudinal study may help to accurately evaluate such relationship.

Conclusions

Our study clearly demonstrated that reduced lung function was cross-sectionally and longitudinally associated with increased CVD risk in a general Chinese population. It suggests that improve lung function or prevent lung function decline may help to prevent CVD. Further studies with long-time follow-up are needed to validate our findings and illuminate the potential mechanisms.

Abbreviations

BMI: body mass index; CI: confidence interval; COPD: chronic obstructive pulmonary disease; CVD: cardiovascular diseases; FEV_1: forced expiratory volume in 1 s; FEV_1/ FVC: the ratio of FEV_1 to FVC; FVC: forced vital capacity; GOLD: global initiative for chronic obstructive lung disease; HDL: high density lipoprotein; IL-6: Interleukin-6; LDL: low density lipoprotein; NADPH: Nicotinamide adenine dinucleotide phosphate; NF-κB: nuclear factor kappa B; OR: odds ratio; ROS: reactive oxygen species; RR: risk ratio; TNF-α: tumour necrosis factor alpha

Acknowledgments

All volunteers who participated in this study and all members of the study team are greatly acknowledged.

Funding

This study was supported by National Key Research and Development Program (2016YFC1303903 and 2016YFC0901101); Key Program of the National Natural Science Foundation of China (91543207); Fundamental Research Funds for the Central Universities, HUST (2016YXZD044 and 2016JCTD116).

Authors' contributions

WC was responsible for the design of the Wuhan-Zhuhai cohort study and funding obtaining. BW, YZ and WC conceived and designed this study. BW and YZ performed statistical analyses. BW interpreted the data and drafted the manuscript. All authors contributed to the data collection, manuscript revision, important intellectual content and final version approval. WC has full access to all the data in the study and takes responsibility for the integrity of the data and the accuracy of the data analysis.

Competing interests

The authors declare that they have no competing interests.

Author details

[1]Department of Occupational & Environmental Health, School of Public Health, Tongji Medical College, Huazhong University of Science and Technology, Wuhan 430030, Hubei, China. [2]Key Laboratory of Environment and Health, Ministry of Education & Ministry of Environmental Protection, and State Key Laboratory of Environmental Health (Incubating), School of Public Health, Tongji Medical College, Huazhong University of Science and Technology, Wuhan 430030, Hubei, China. [3]Hubei Provincial Key Laboratory for Applied Toxicology, Hubei Provincial Center for Disease Control and Prevention, Wuhan 430079, Hubei, China. [4]Zhuhai Center for Disease Control and Prevention, Zhuhai 519060, Guangdong, China.

References

1. He J, Gu D, Wu X, Reynolds K, Duan X, Yao C, Wang J, Chen CS, Chen J, Wildman RP, et al. Major causes of death among men and women in China. N Engl J Med. 2005;353:1124–34.
2. Lopez AD, Mathers CD, Ezzati M, Jamison DT, Murray CJ. Global and regional burden of disease and risk factors, 2001: systematic analysis of population health data. Lancet. 2006;367:1747–57.
3. D'Agostino RB Sr, Vasan RS, Pencina MJ, Wolf PA, Cobain M, Massaro JM, Kannel WB. General cardiovascular risk profile for use in primary care: the Framingham heart study. Circulation. 2008;117:743–53.
4. Grundy SM, Pasternak R, Greenland P, Smith S Jr, Fuster V. Assessment of cardiovascular risk by use of multiple-risk-factor assessment equations: a statement for healthcare professionals from the American Heart Association and the American College of Cardiology. Circulation. 1999;100:1481–92.
5. Park KH, Kim MK, Kim HS, Park WJ, Cho GY, Choi YJ. Clinical significance of Framingham risk score, flow-mediated dilation and pulse wave velocity in patients with stable angina. Circ J. 2011;75:1177–83.

6. Burroughs Pena MS, Dunning A, Schulte PJ, Durheim MT, Kussin P, Checkley W, Velazquez EJ. Pulmonary function and adverse cardiovascular outcomes: can cardiac function explain the link? Respir Med. 2016;121:4–12.
7. Austin V, Crack PJ, Bozinovski S, Miller AA, Vlahos R. COPD and stroke: are systemic inflammation and oxidative stress the missing links? Clin Sci (Lond). 2016;130:1039–50.
8. Vogelmeier CF, Criner GJ, Martinez FJ, Anzueto A, Barnes PJ, Bourbeau J, Celli BR, Chen R, Decramer M, Fabbri LM, et al. Global strategy for the diagnosis, management, and prevention of chronic obstructive lung disease 2017 report. GOLD executive summary. Am J Respir Crit Care Med. 2017;195:557–82.
9. Iribarren C, Tolstykh IV, Eisner MD. Are patients with asthma at increased risk of coronary heart disease? Int J Epidemiol. 2004;33:743–8.
10. Engstrom G, Melander O, Hedblad B. Population-based study of lung function and incidence of heart failure hospitalisations. Thorax. 2010; 65:633–8.
11. Georgiopoulou VV, Kalogeropoulos AP, Psaty BM, Rodondi N, Bauer DC, Butler AB, Koster A, Smith AL, Harris TB, Newman AB, et al. Lung function and risk for heart failure among older adults: the health ABC study. Am J Med. 2011;124:334–41.
12. Agarwal SK, Heiss G, Barr RG, Chang PP, Loehr LR, Chambless LE, Shahar E, Kitzman DW, Rosamond WD. Airflow obstruction, lung function, and risk of incident heart failure: the atherosclerosis risk in communities (ARIC) study. Eur J Heart Fail. 2012;14:414–22.
13. Soderholm M, Zia E, Hedblad B, Engstrom G. Lung function as a risk factor for subarachnoid hemorrhage: a prospective cohort study. Stroke. 2012; 43:2598–603.
14. Johnston AK, Mannino DM, Hagan GW, Davis KJ, Kiri VA. Relationship between lung function impairment and incidence or recurrence of cardiovascular events in a middle-aged cohort. Thorax. 2008;63:599–605.
15. Lee HM, Liu MA, Barrett-Connor E, Wong ND. Association of lung function with coronary heart disease and cardiovascular disease outcomes in elderly: the rancho Bernardo study. Respir Med. 2014;108:1779–85.
16. Schunemann HJ, Dorn J, Grant BJ, Winkelstein W Jr, Trevisan M. Pulmonary function is a long-term predictor of mortality in the general population: 29-year follow-up of the Buffalo health study. Chest. 2000;118:656–64.
17. Sin DD, Man SF. Chronic obstructive pulmonary disease as a risk factor for cardiovascular morbidity and mortality. Proc Am Thorac Soc. 2005;2:8–11.
18. Sin DD, Wu L, Man SF. The relationship between reduced lung function and cardiovascular mortality: a population-based study and a systematic review of the literature. Chest. 2005;127:1952–9.
19. Engstrom G, Hedblad B, Janzon L. Reduced lung function predicts increased fatality in future cardiac events. A population-based study. J Intern Med. 2006;260:560–7.
20. Min KB, Min JY. Reduced lung function, C-reactive protein, and increased risk of cardiovascular mortality. Circ J. 2014;78:2309–16.
21. Kang HK, Park HY, Jeong BH, Koh WJ, Lim SY. Relationship between forced vital capacity and Framingham cardiovascular risk score beyond the presence of metabolic syndrome: the fourth Korea National Health and nutrition examination survey. Medicine (Baltimore). 2015;94:e2089.
22. Song Y, Hou J, Huang X, Zhang X, Tan A, Rong Y, Sun H, Zhou Y, Cui X, Yang Y, et al. The Wuhan-Zhuhai (WHZH) cohort study of environmental air particulate matter and the pathogenesis of cardiopulmonary diseases: study design, methods and baseline characteristics of the cohort. BMC Public Health. 2014;14:994.
23. Standardization of Spirometry, Update. American Thoracic Society. Am J Respir Crit Care Med. 1995(152):1107–36.
24. Tan WC, Bourbeau J, Aaron SD, Zhou G, Maltais F, Hernandez P, Fitzgerald JM, Marciniuk DD, Walker BL, Sin DD. Global initiative for chronic obstructive lung disease 2017 classification and lung function decline in chronic obstructive pulmonary disease. Am J Respir Crit Care Med. 2018;197:670–3.
25. National Cholesterol Education Program Expert Panel on Detection E, treatment of high blood cholesterol in a. third report of the National Cholesterol Education Program (NCEP) expert panel on detection, evaluation, and treatment of high blood cholesterol in adults (adult treatment panel III) final report. Circulation. 2002;106:3143–421.
26. Ford ES, Wheaton AG, Mannino DM, Presley-Cantrell L, Li C, Croft JB. Elevated cardiovascular risk among adults with obstructive and restrictive airway functioning in the United States: a cross-sectional study of the National Health and nutrition examination survey from 2007-2010. Respir Res. 2012;13:115.
27. Arcari A, Magnacca S, Bracone F, Costanzo S, Persichillo M, Di Castelnuovo A, de Curtis A, Zito F, Schunemann HJ, Donati MB, et al. Relation between pulmonary function and 10-year risk for cardiovascular disease among healthy men and women in Italy: the Moli-sani project. Eur J Prev Cardiol. 2013;20:862–71.
28. Li Q, Hsia J, Yang G. Prevalence of smoking in China in 2010. N Engl J Med. 2011;364:2469–70.
29. Zhang N, Du SM, Ma GS. Current lifestyle factors that increase risk of T2DM in China. Eur J Clin Nutr. 2017;71:832–8.
30. Loinard C, Ginouvès A, Vilar J, Cochain C, Zouggari Y, Recalde A, Duriez M, Lévy BI, Pouysségur J, Berra E. Clinical guidelines: identification, evaluation, and treatment of overweight and obesity in adults - statistical data included. Circulation. 2009;120:50–9.
31. Hubert HB, Feinleib M, McNamara PM, Castelli WP. Obesity as an independent risk factor for cardiovascular disease: a 26-year follow-up of participants in the Framingham heart study. Circulation. 1983;67:968–77.
32. Barnes PJ, Celli BR. Systemic manifestations and comorbidities of COPD. Eur Respir J. 2009;33:1165–85.
33. Wilkins MR, Ghofrani HA, Weissmann N, Aldashev A, Zhao L. Pathophysiology and treatment of high-altitude pulmonary vascular disease. Circulation. 2015;131:582–90.
34. Mcphee SJ, Hammer GD. Pathophysiology of disease an introduction to clinical medicine, sixth edition. Maidenhead: Open University Press; 2010.
35. Mannino DM, Thorn D, Swensen A, Holguin F. Prevalence and outcomes of diabetes, hypertension and cardiovascular disease in COPD. Eur Respir J. 2008;32:962–9.
36. Zhou Y, Sun H, Xie J, Song Y, Liu Y, Huang X, Zhou T, Rong Y, Wu T, Yuan J, Chen W. Urinary polycyclic aromatic hydrocarbon metabolites and altered lung function in Wuhan, China. Am J Respir Crit Care Med. 2016;193:835–46.
37. Hu C, Hou J, Zhou Y, Sun H, Yin W, Zhang Y, Wang X, Wang G, Chen W, Yuan J. Association of polycyclic aromatic hydrocarbons exposure with atherosclerotic cardiovascular disease risk: a role of mean platelet volume or club cell secretory protein. Environ Pollut. 2017;233:45–53.
38. Pinault LL, Weichenthal S, Crouse DL, Brauer M, Erickson A, Donkelaar AV, Martin RV, Hystad P, Chen H, Fines P, et al. Associations between fine particulate matter and mortality in the 2001 Canadian census health and environment cohort. Environ Res. 2017;159:406–15.
39. Engstrom G, Lind P, Hedblad B, Wollmer P, Stavenow L, Janzon L, Lindgarde F. Lung function and cardiovascular risk: relationship with inflammation-sensitive plasma proteins. Circulation. 2002;106:2555–60.
40. Miller AA, Budzyn K, Sobey CG. Vascular dysfunction in cerebrovascular disease: mechanisms and therapeutic intervention. Clin Sci (Lond). 2010;119:1–17.
41. Marchesi C, Paradis P, Schiffrin EL. Role of the renin-angiotensin system in vascular inflammation. Trends Pharmacol Sci. 2008;29:367–74.
42. Basuroy S, Bhattacharya S, Leffler CW, Parfenova H. Nox4 NADPH oxidase mediates oxidative stress and apoptosis caused by TNF-alpha in cerebral vascular endothelial cells. Am J Physiol Cell Physiol. 2009;296:C422–32.
43. Schrader LI, Kinzenbaw DA, Johnson AW, Faraci FM, Didion SP. IL-6 deficiency protects against angiotensin II induced endothelial dysfunction and hypertrophy. Arterioscler Thromb Vasc Biol. 2007;27:2576–81.
44. Moskowitz MA, Lo EH, Iadecola C. The science of stroke: mechanisms in search of treatments. Neuron. 2010;67:181–98.
45. Husain K, Hernandez W, Ansari RA, Ferder L. Inflammation, oxidative stress and renin angiotensin system in atherosclerosis. World J Biol Chem. 2015;6:209–17.
46. Faraci FM. Protecting against vascular disease in brain. Am J Physiol Heart Circ Physiol. 2011;300:H1566–82.
47. Maclay JD, McAllister DA, Johnston S, Raftis J, McGuinnes C, Deans A, Newby DE, Mills NL, MacNee W. Increased platelet activation in patients with stable and acute exacerbation of COPD. Thorax. 2011;66:769–74.
48. Tohgi H, Konno S, Takahashi S, Koizumi D, Kondo R, Takahashi H. Activated coagulation/fibrinolysis system and platelet function in acute thrombotic stroke patients with increased C-reactive protein levels. Thromb Res. 2000; 100:373–9.
49. Dayal S, Wilson KM, Motto DG, Miller FJ Jr, Chauhan AK, Lentz SR. Hydrogen peroxide promotes aging-related platelet hyperactivation and thrombosis. Circulation. 2013;127:1308–16.
50. Schargrodsky H, Hernandez-Hernandez R, Champagne BM, Silva H, Vinueza R, Silva Aycaguer LC, Touboul PJ, Boissonnet CP, Escobedo J, Pellegrini F, et al. CARMELA: assessment of cardiovascular risk in seven Latin American cities. Am J Med. 2008;121:58–65.

18

Serum AGE/RAGEs as potential biomarker in idiopathic pulmonary fibrosis

Carlos Machahua[1,2], Ana Montes-Worboys[1,2,3], Lurdes Planas-Cerezales[1,3], Raquel Buendia-Flores[1], Maria Molina-Molina[1,2,3*†] and Vanesa Vicens-Zygmunt[1,3†]

Abstract

Background: The soluble receptor for advanced glycation end-products (sRAGE) has been suggested that it acts as a decoy for capturing advanced glycation end-products (AGEs) and inhibits the activation of the oxidative stress and apoptotic pathways. Lung AGEs/sRAGE is increased in idiopathic pulmonary fibrosis (IPF). The objective of the study was to evaluate the AGEs and sRAGE levels in serum as a potential biomarker in IPF.

Methods: Serum samples were collected from adult patients: 62 IPF, 22 chronic hypersensitivity pneumonitis (cHP), 20 fibrotic non-specific interstitial pneumonia (fNSIP); and 12 healthy controls. In addition, 23 IPF patients were re-evaluated after 3-year follow-up period. Epidemiological and clinical features were recorded: age, sex, smoking habits, and lung function. AGEs and sRAGE were evaluated by ELISA, and the results were correlated with pulmonary functional test values.

Results: IPF and cHP groups presented a significant increase of AGE/sRAGE serum concentration compared with fNSIP patients. Moreover, an inverse correlation between AGEs and sRAGE levels were found in IPF, and serum sRAGE at diagnosis correlated with FVC and DLCO values. Additionally, changes in serum AGEs and sRAGE correlated with % change of FVC, DLCO and TLC during the follow-up. sRAGE levels below 428.25 pg/ml evolved poor survival rates.

Conclusions: These findings demonstrate that the increase of AGE/sRAGE ratio is higher in IPF, although the levels were close to cHP. AGE/sRAGE increase correlates with respiratory functional progression. Furthermore, the concentration of sRAGE in blood stream at diagnosis and follow-up could be considered as a potential prognostic biomarker.

Keywords: AGEs, RAGEs, IPF, Biomarker

Background

Idiopathic pulmonary fibrosis (IPF) is the most frequent form of fibrotic interstitial lung diseases (ILDs), which presents a variable outcome and is generally fatal within 2–4 years from diagnosis [1]. Histologically, IPF is characterized by an usual interstitial pneumonia (UIP) pattern; where honeycombing areas with collagen deposition and fibroblast foci are situated next to structurally preserved areas [2]. Advances in the knowledge of the pathogenesis have been focused in integrating the different factors involved in IPF with the purpose of improving the diagnosis, management and treatment [3].

In clinical practice, some fibrosing lung entities such as chronic hypersensitivity pneumonitis (cHP) and fibrotic nonspecific interstitial pneumonia (fNSIP) represent a challenge in the differential diagnosis for IPF as there are clinical and radiological similarities [4–8]. Even after an invasive procedure such as lung biopsy, it occasionally remains difficult to differentiate IPF from cHP [9, 10]. Though some features may be similar to IPF [11], the prognosis is better for fNSIP and cHP, and the treatment differs [12]. The proteomic analysis could be a useful tool to differentiate between these entities and to reach an accurate diagnosis, attempting to avoid invasive diagnostic procedures [13]. In the last decades, serum and broncoalveolar biological markers have been

* Correspondence: mariamolinamolina@hotmail.com
†Maria Molina-Molina and Vanesa Vicens-Zygmunt contributed equally to this work.
1Pneumology Research Group, IDIBELL, L'Hospitalet de Llobregat, Barcelona, Spain
2Biomedical Research Network Centers in Respiratory Diseases (CIBERES), Barcelona, Spain
Full list of author information is available at the end of the article

extensively studied in IPF for diagnosis and prognosis [14–17]. However, despite the progress in identifying new biomolecules involved in IPF pathogenesis, none improve the differential diagnosis and monitoring of the clinical course [18].

Recent studies have reported the implication of advanced glycation end-products (AGEs) and their receptor (RAGE) with IPF and other fibrotic ILDs [19]. In fact, a previous study within our group reported an AGE-RAGE imbalance in lung tissue from IPF patients compared to controls [20]. The RAGE is an immunoglobulin superfamily protein [21] implicated in the maintenance of alveolar structures in lung tissue [22] and the development and differentiation of Type I pneumocytes [23]. Its soluble form (sRAGE) is secreted directly to the extracellular matrix (ECM) through loss of its transmembrane region by cleavage [24, 25]. This is of particular interest because sRAGE has been proposed as an AGE decoy [26]. Some groups have suggested that sRAGE bind AGEs, blocking the cell signaling pathway of AGEs or attenuating their effects [27–29]. AGEs are the result of non-enzymatic reactions between a reducing sugar monosaccharides with a free amino group of proteins [30], widely studied in oxidative stress, inflammation and aging [31, 32]. AGEs also contribute to abnormal wound healing by acting on signaling pathway in cells [33] and ECM protein cross-links [34]; these changes may alter the physicochemical properties of collagen fibers modifying the tissue stiffness [35]. Given that RAGE is highly expressed in lung tissue [36], sRAGE could be a possible serum or plasma biomarker to study the pulmonary disorder.

Some studies of blood [37] and bronchoalveolar lavage [38] indicate a correlation between lung injury and the levels of sRAGE [39–41]. Nevertheless, there is scarce information about the specificity of AGE-RAGE imbalance in IPF [42, 43]. Therefore, our study aims to evaluate the potential utility of serological AGEs and sRAGE levels in IPF.

Methods

Ethical statement and patient recruitment

Patients were recruited in the outpatient Unit of ILDs from University Hospital of Bellvitge: 62 IPF, 22 cHP, and 20 fNSIP. The patient's diagnosis was discussed in the multidisciplinary committee and was established in accordance with the American Thoracic Society/European Respiratory Society criteria [5, 12, 44]. Twelve healthy subjects age-matched were recruited as control. The inclusion criteria of healthy volunteers were the absence of chronic illness and pulmonary functional test abnormalities. We collected serum samples after 3 years from 23 IPF patients in order to analyze the changes of AGEs-sRAGE levels and the progression of the disease. Lung transplantation and mortality were reported. These patients and those that return to their original care centers were excluded for the second serological evaluation.

This observational prospective study was approved by the Ethics Committee of University Hospital of Bellvitge (CEIC, ref. PR082/15) and all patients signed the written informed consent before their inclusion.

Pulmonary function test (PFT)

Spirometry, lung volume, and Diffusing Capacity of Lung for Carbon Monoxide (DLCO) were measured in the Medisoft® bodybox Plethysmograph at the PFT laboratory. Three reproducible spirometry measurements were performed (with a difference of less than 150 ml between each one) to obtain the Forced Vital Capacity (FVC) and Total Lung Capacity (TLC). Two maneuvers were recorded to register the best value by DLCO single-breath technique.

Sample collection, processing and measurement

Peripheral blood samples were collected from participants in a BD Vacutainer® SST™ tubes (Becton, Dickinson and Company, USA), and serum faction were obtained using standardized procedures. AGE and sRAGE were measured by specific commercial ELISA kit; Human RAGE

Table 1 Group features

Patient characteristics	Control	IPF	cHP	fNSIP
Subjects (n)	12	62	22	20
Gender (Male/Female)	9 / 3	53 / 9	10 / 12	5 / 15
Age (yr.)	69.11 ± 5.97	68.43 ± 8.57	64.74 ± 11.36	63.33 ± 11.62
Smoking (Former/Never)	5 / 7	43 / 19	12 / 10	5 / 15
Pack-years	20.23 ± 26.07	31.28 ± 20.74	19.25 ± 27.39	20.70 ± 11.67
Smoking cessation (yr.)	7.67 ± 9.07	15.17 ± 8.69	18.56 ± 10.38	9.00 ± 4.58
% FVC	116.20 ± 14.23**	78.71 ± 20.33	82.59 ± 15.98	81.40 ± 25.93
% DLCO	103.10 ± 2.62**	50.41 ± 20.75	56.98 ± 19.40	59.11 ± 27.67
% TLC	112.75 ± 18.31**	79.79 ± 18.69	80.88 ± 17.82	83.61 ± 19.90

Data represent the mean ± SD, *cHP* chronic hypersensitivity pneumonitis, *DLCO* diffusing capacity for carbon monoxide, *fNSIP* fibrotic non-specific interstitial pneumonia, *FVC* forced vital capacity, *IPF* idiopathic pulmonary fibrosis, *TLC* Total lung capacity. (**) p-value < 0.01

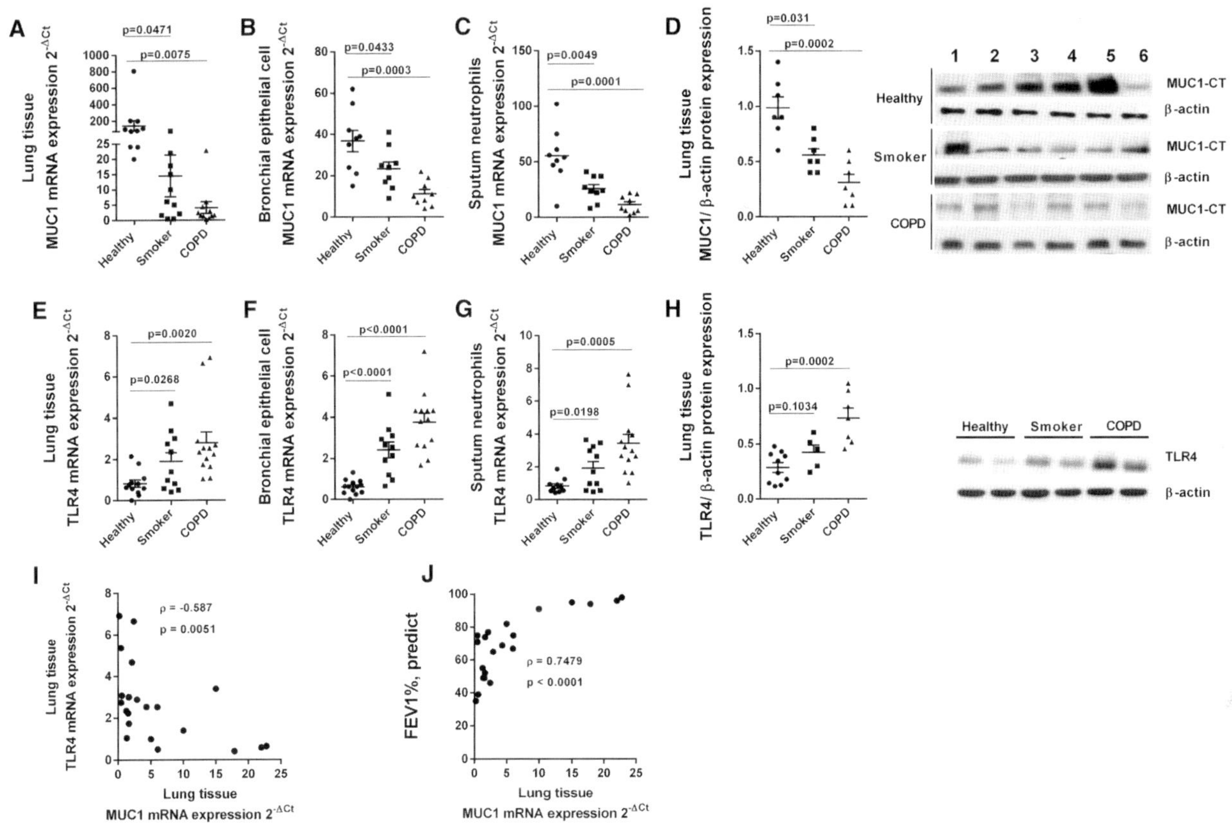

Fig. 1 MUC1 downregulation and TLR4 overexpression in lung tissue from heavy smokers and COPD patients. Lung tissue from healthy (*n* = 10), smokers (*n* = 11) and COPD patients (*n* = 13) were analysed. MUC1 mRNA gene expression in lung tissue homogenates (**a**), bronchial epithelial cells (**b**) and sputum neutrophils (**c**). **d** MUC1-CT protein expression in lung homogenates.TLR4 mRNA gene expression in lung tissue homogenates (**e**), bronchial epithelial cells (**f**) and sputum neutrophils (**g**). **h** MUC1-CT protein expression in lung homogenates. **i** Correlation of TL4 and MUC1 gene expression in lung tissue from smokers and COPD patients. **j** Correlation of FEV1% and MUC1 gene expression in lung tissue from smokers and COPD patients. Gene expression was analyzed by real time PCR using the $2^{-\Delta Ct}$ as described in methods. Protein expression was analyzed by western blot. Representative western blot are showed. Data are presented as median with interquartile range. "P" exact values were obtained following Kruskal Wallis test. FEV1%: forced expiratory volume in 1 s

TLR4 protein expression only reach significant differences in COPD patients (Fig. 1h). The expression of MUC1 and TLR4 in lung tissue from smokers and COPD patients was inversely correlated ($\rho = -0.587$; $P = 0.0051$; Fig. 1i). The FEV1% of smokers and COPD patients was directly correlated with MUC1 lung tissue expression ($\rho = -0.7479$; $P < 0.0001$; Fig. 1j).

Corticosteroid anti-inflammatory effects are impaired in cells from smokers and COPD patients stimulated with cigarette smoke

Cigarette smoke extract (CSE) dose-dependently decreased MUC1 expression in primary bronchial epithelial cells (HBECs) from healthy subjects reaching 73% inhibition at 10% CSE concentration (Fig. 2a). Dexamethasone 1 μM inhibited the LPS-induced IL-8, GM-CSF and MIP3α to 98, 82 and 48% of inhibition respectively (Fig. 2b-d). Similar findings were observed when CSE 5% was used as stimulus (Fig. 2b-c). In contrast, HBECs stimulated with the LPS and CSE combination were resistant to the anti-inflammatory effects of dexamethasone on the IL-8, GM-CSF and MIP3α release (Fig. 2b-e). HBECs from COPD showed higher IL-8 levels than cells from smokers and healthy subjects in response to LPS and CSE (Fig. 2f). Dexamethasone showed more %maximum inhibitory effect (%Emax) on IL-8 release in HBECs from healthy subjects (%Emax 60%) compared with cells from smokers (%Emax 24.5%) and COPD patients (%Emax 21.2%) (Fig. 2g).

CSE dose-dependently decreased MUC1 expression in sputum neutrophils, reaching 96% of inhibition after CSE 10% exposure (Fig. 3a). Similar results were observed in neutrophils from peripheral blood (data not shown). LPS and CSE increased IL-8 and MMP9 release in cultured peripheral blood neutrophils which was significantly higher in neutrophils from COPD patients (Fig. 3b-d). Dexamethasone showed impaired anti-inflammatory effects on the LPS and CSE-induced

Quantikine ELISA Kit (DRG00; R&D Systems, USA) and Human AGEs ELISA Kit (CSB-E09412h; Cusabio Biotech Co., China), following the manufacturer's recommendations.

Statistical analysis

The results were expressed as mean [SD] or median [interquartile range] and were compared using one-way ANOVA or Student's t test, followed by the appropriate post hoc analysis.

To evaluate the power of AGEs/sRAGE to discriminate between the fibrotic ILDs, receiver operating characteristic (ROC) analyses were performed: the levels of AGE and sRAGE in blood serum were considered as a continuous variable and the diagnostic classification was accepted as a dichotomous variable. Cutoff points were calculated by the ROC curves with the highest possible sensitivity and specificity, and their discriminative potential was quantified following 3 different diagnostic accuracy measures: Diagnostic effectiveness (Accuracy), Likelihood ratio for positive test results (LR+), and Youden's index (J). To determine the serum levels that predict 3-year survival rates in the whole IPF cohort, ROC curve analysis was also performed, and the rate was estimated by Kaplan–Meier analysis using log-rank test as statistic contrast. In addition, Pearson's correlations were performed to test the relation among PFT, sRAGE and AGE serum levels at the beginning of the study and at the end of the 3-year follow-up. Statistical software SPSS statistic 24 (IBM, USA) was used for statistical analyses. Significant differences were accepted when the p value was < 0.05 (*) or < 0.01 (**).

Results

Clinical characteristics

Clinical features of IPF, cHP, fNSIP and control groups are included in Table 1. IPF patients were predominantly males and former smokers. No statistical differences among the studied groups were found in age, pack-years, nor smoking cessation. Regarding PFTs, control subjects showed better results in the percentage of predicted FVC, DLCO and TLC than fibrotic ILDs, as expected ($p < 0.01$).

AGEs and sRAGEs serum concentration in pulmonary fibrosis

AGEs levels were significantly higher in serum samples from IPF and cHP compared with control and fNSIP patients ($p < 0.01$). There were no statistical differences in AGEs serum levels between IPF and cHP groups, and no differences were observed when fNSIP was compared to control (Fig. 1a).

On the other hand, a significant decrease in sRAGE concentration was observed in serum samples from IPF and cHP patients compared to fNSIP and control donors

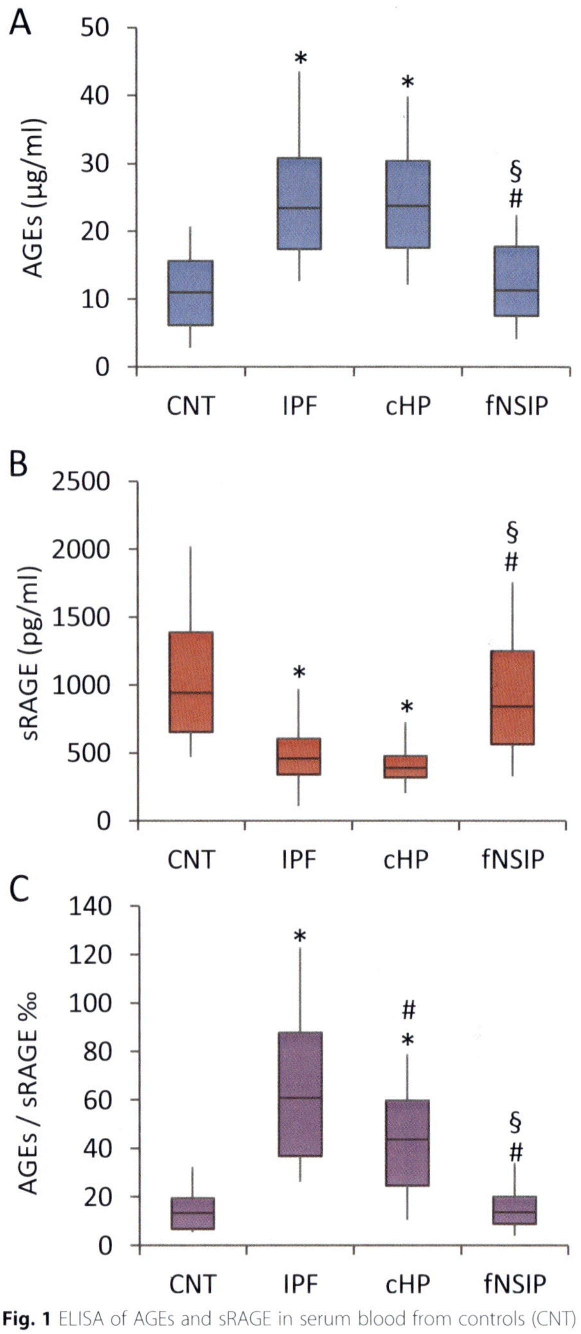

Fig. 1 ELISA of AGEs and sRAGE in serum blood from controls (CNT) and fibrosing ILDs. **a** and **b** ELISA for total AGEs and sRAGE showed significant differences between control group with IPF and cHP (*$p < 0.01$), and differences between fNSIP patients with IPF (#$p < 0.01$) and cHP (§$p < 0.01$) groups. However, there were no significant differences between IPF with cHP and control with fNSIP. **c** AGEs/sRAGE ratio estimated by ELISA was greater in IPF and cHP groups compared with control (*$p < 0.01$). The ratio also allowed to distinguish between IPF patients with cHP and fNSIP (#$p < 0.05$), and cHP with fNSIP group (§$p < 0.01$), whereas this did not distinguish between control and fNSIP patients. Data were analyzed by one-way ANOVA following by the appropriate post-hoc analysis

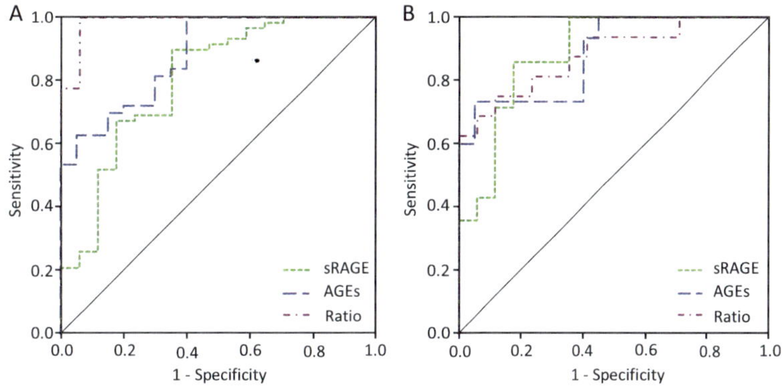

Fig. 2 ROC curve for total AGEs, sRAGE levels and Ages/sRAGE ratio. **a** AGEs and sRAGE showed a good capability to differentiate between IPF patients and fNSIP group (AUC = 0.879 and 0.801, respectively), whereas the AGEs/sRAGE ratio had higher predictable capability (AUC 0.987, CI = 0.959–1.000) to discriminate between both. **b** Comparing cHP and fNSIP, all the three indicators (AGEs, sRAGE levels and AGE/sRAGE ratio) showed AUC values quite good to be considered diagnostic tests (AGEs = 0.883, sRAGE = 0.887, Ratio = 0.882). Data were evaluated by ROC analyses; blood serum levels of AGE and sRAGE were considered as a continuous variable, and the diagnostic classification was accepted as a dichotomous variable

($p < 0.01$). There were no significant differences comparing IPF and cHP (Fig. 1b).

The serum AGE/sRAGE ratio of each patient was analyzed from the ELISA results. An increase of 4.20 and 4.48-fold was observed in IPF patients compared with fNSIP and control subjects, respectively ($p < 0.01$). Furthermore, the ratio was statistically significant higher in IPF patients than cHP patients ($p < 0.05$). In addition, the AGE/sRAGE ratio was 2.84-fold higher in cHP as compared to fNSIP ($p < 0.01$). AGE/sRAGE ratio in fNSIP was similar to the control group (Fig. 1c).

AGE and sRAGE as a discriminative factor between IPF and fNSIP

We performed a ROC curve analysis to evaluate the potential IPF specificity of AGEs and sRAGE levels in blood serum (Additional file 1). The results showed that serum sRAGE and AGEs levels present a high capacity to differentiate IPF patients from fNSIP (AUC = 0.801 and 0.879, respectively), and between cHP and fNSIP patients (AUC = 0.887 and 0.883, respectively) (Fig. 2a, b). Furthermore, the AGE/sRAGE ratio also distinguished between fNSIP and IPF (AUC = 0.987, CI = 0.959–1.000), and between cHP and fNSIP (AUC = 0.882, CI = 0.766–0.998).

On the other hand, AGEs and sRAGE levels did not demonstrate capability to differentiate IPF and cHP (AUC = 0.383 and 0.507, respectively), while ratio showed very low differential power (AUC = 0.713, CI = 0.569–0.856).

To evaluate the discriminative potential of AGEs, sRAGE and AGE/sRAGE, optimal cut-off points were obtained from the ROC curve. Table 2 showed that AGEs/sRAGE ratio had a higher diagnostic effectiveness (accuracy = 98.28%, LR+ = 17.00, J = 0.94) than serum levels of AGEs and sRAGE separate values to distinguish between IPF and fNSIP patients. Moreover, although the diagnostic accuracy and the Youden's index of the three parameters were quite similar, serum levels of AGEs were more appropriate than sRAGE and the AGEs/sRAGE ratio to differentiate between cHP and fNSIP (LR+ = 14.67, 4.86, and 6.38; respectively).

AGE and sRAGE correlation with PFTs

Pearson's test showed that increased levels of AGEs correlated with lower sRAGE in IPF patients ($r = -0.541$,

Table 2 Cut-off values and diagnostic accuracy measures of AGEs, sRAGE and AGEs/sRAGE ratio

	IPF – fNSIP			cHP – fNSIP		
Indicators	AGE	sRAGE	Ratio	AGE	sRAGE	Ratio
Cut-off value	19.25 μg/ml	782.59 pg/ml	25.65 ‰	20.92 μg/ml	529.57 pg/ml	24.87 ‰
Sensitivity (%)	69.77	89.66	100.00	73.33	85.71	75.00
Specificity (%)	85.00	64.71	94.12	95.00	82.35	88.24
Accuracy (%)	74.60	84.00	98.28	85.71	83.87	81.82
LR+	4.65	2.54	17.00	14.67	4.86	6.38
J	0.55	0.54	0.94	0.68	0.68	0.63

AGE advanced glycation end-product, *cHP* chronic hypersensitivity pneumonitis, *fNSIP* fibrotic non-specific interstitial pneumonia, *J* Youden's index, *LR+* Likelihood ratio for positive test results, *IPF* idiopathic pulmonary fibrosis, *sRAGE* soluble receptor for advanced glycation end-products

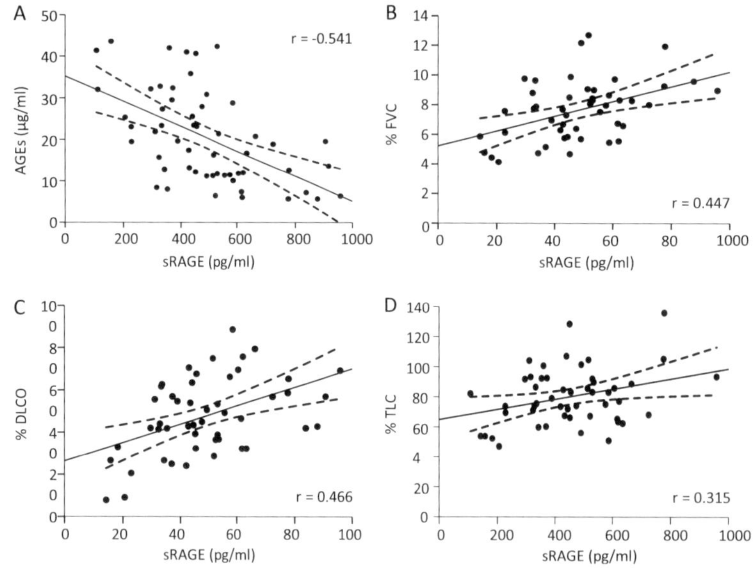

Fig. 3 Pearson's correlation between sRAGE, AGEs and PFT in IPF patients. **a** Results showed a negative relationship between sRAGE and AGEs in serum samples from IPF patients. **b, c, d** There was a positive correlation between sRAGE serum levels and percentages values of FVC, DLCO and TLC in IPF samples. The lineal relationship between the variables was analyzed by Pearson's correlations coefficient

$p < 0.01$) (Fig. 3a). Meanwhile, cHP patients also showed a negative correlation ($r = -0.496$, $p < 0.05$), fNSIP patients did not show any significant correlation (Additional file 2).

Pearson's test also showed that lower levels of sRAGE in serum samples from IPF patients correlated with worse lung functionalism: % predicted of FVC ($r = 0.447$, $p < 0.01$), DLCO ($r = 0.466$, $p < 0.01$) and TLC ($r = 0.315$; $p < 0.05$) (Fig. 3b, c, d). However, the concentration of AGEs did not show any correlation with PFTs in IPF (data not shown). Regarding cHP and fNSIP samples, there was also a positive correlation between sRAGE and PFTs, whereas AGEs levels did not show any correlation in either entity (cHP and fNSIP).

AGEs-sRAGE concentration in the follow-up of IPF patients

Twenty-three IPF patients were re-evaluated 3-years after their inclusion. Table 3 show a decrease in the lung

Table 3 ELISA measurements and lung function from IPF patients at 3-year interval

Patient characteristics	Initial	3 yrs.	*p*-value
sRAGE (pg/ml)	461.53 ± 191.77	375.78 ± 143.25	0.029*
AGEs (µg/ml)	19.07 ± 8.63	17.19 ± 8.45	0.340
Ratio (‰)	52.58 ± 34.58	41.13 ± 14.91	0.079
% FVC	89.21 ± 19.50	79.14 ± 20.63	0.001**
% DLCO	57.84 ± 11.54	48.68 ± 12.73	0.000**
% TLC	87.22 ± 16.89	76.47 ± 15.57	0.000**

Data represent the mean ± SD, *AGE* advanced glycation end-product, *DLCO* diffusing capacity for carbon monoxide, *FVC* forced vital capacity, *sRAGE* soluble receptor for advanced glycation end-products, *TLC* Total lung capacity. (*) *p*-value < 0.05, (**) *p*-value < 0.01

functional values, with a significant decrease in the mean FVC. Regarding ELISA analyses, only sRAGE serum levels showed a significant decrease between the basal level and 3-years after ($p < 0.05$) (Fig. 4a).

In addition, the ROC analysis of the whole IPF group showed sRAGE levels as a reliable predictor of the 3-year follow-up (AUC = 0.724, 95% CI = 0.586–0.863, $p < 0.01$). Survival estimation by Kaplan–Meier was lower in IPF patients with serum concentrations of sRAGE under 428.25 pg/mL at the basal level ($p = 0.014$) (Fig. 4b).

Furthermore, we correlated the changes in serum sRAGE and AGEs from IPF patients adjusted over time (Δ ELISA in a month = [ELISA final − ELISA initial]/month) with the percentage of change of lung function in the same interval (change of % predicted PFT = [PFT final − PFTs initial]/month). The results show a relationship between variations in sRAGE, AGEs and their ratio levels with the lung functional values (% predicted) of FVC, TLC and DLCO (Table 4). IPF patients with a decrease in sRAGE serum levels during the follow-up usually showed a significant decline in % predicted DLCO as well (Fig. 5a). On the other hand, an increase of AGEs serum levels was highly associated with a DLCO decline, while no changes in DLCO associated no changes in AGEs serum levels (Fig. 5b).

With regards to the AGEs/sRAGE ratio, a negative correlation with % predicted DLCO was observed as well. Therefore, IPF patients with an increase of the AGEs/sRAGE ratio had a more rapid decline in DLCO (Fig. 5c). Furthermore, an increment of AGEs in serum was correlated with a loss of their receptor in IPF

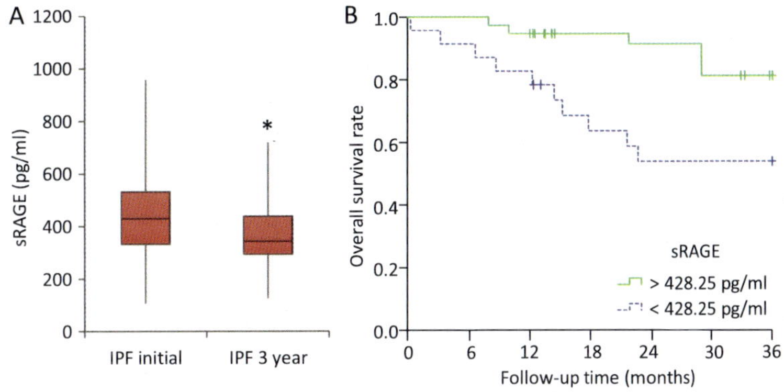

Fig. 4 Serum levels and predictive capability of sRAGE for 3-year survival rates. **a** Results showed a significant decrease of sRAGE in IPF patients beyond 3-years. **b** Kaplan–Meier analysis showed IPF patients with sRAGE levels in serum under 428.25 pg/ml had lower survival rate ($p = 0.014$) at 3-yr follow-up. Comparison of AGEs/sRAGE levels in follow-up were analyzed by Paired sample t-test, the threshold of sRAGE levels in blood were calculated by ROC analysis and survival rate was estimated by Kaplan–Meier analysis using log-rank test as statistic contrast

patients, maintaining a negative correlation over time (Additional file 3).

Discussion

Some reports have shown an association between the blood sRAGE levels and the state of alveolar epithelium and lung injury [40, 45, 46]. Furthermore, previous results from our group found AGEs increased in IPF lungs [20]. The present results suggest that serum AGEs and sRAGE are different in IPF than in fNSIP, and their ratio is even higher than in cHP, which could be a useful information for the differential diagnosis of these fibrotic ILDs. Moreover, low levels of sRAGE at diagnosis predict poor survival in IPF. Finally, the AGE and RAGE changes correlate with lung functional changes over time.

While the radiological fNSIP pattern may be similar to IPF, the histological pattern is completely different. Therefore, lung biopsy is required in some cases to differentiate both entities. In this case, finding biological lung markers that could be measured in blood samples to differentiate both entities would be of interest for the clinical practice. Serum AGEs and sRAGE show a completely different pattern in IPF and fNSIP, probably due to the lack of fibroblastic foci and honeycombing in fNSIP lungs and the pathogenic differences [11]. Lung RAGEs are expressed in alveolar epithelial cells and lungs with usual interstitial pneumonia pattern show lower RAGEs expression than NSIP lungs [20]. Manichaiku et al. showed lower plasma levels in IPF and HP patients than control subjects [47]. The decrease of RAGEs is not present in all fibrotic ILDs; fNSIP presents serum RAGEs and AGEs similar to normal subjects.

Table 4 Correlation between changes in ELISA measurements and lung function

Correlations	Change of PFT	r	R^2	*P*-value
Δ sRAGE	FVC	0.437	0.191	0.042*
	DLCO	0.586	0.343	0.005**
	TLC	0.412	0.170	0.057
Δ AGEs	FVC	−0.452	0.204	0.027*
	DLCO	−0.747	0.557	0.000**
	TLC	−0.486	0.237	0.022*
Δ Ratio	FVC	−0.479	0,230	0.018*
	DLCO	−0.704	0.495	0.000**
	TLC	−0.352	0.124	0.100

AGE advanced glycation end-product, *DLCO* diffusing capacity for carbon monoxide, *FVC* forced vital capacity, *PFT* pulmonary function test, *r* correlation coefficient, R^2 coefficient of determination, *sRAGE* soluble receptor for advanced glycation end-products, *TLC* Total lung capacity. (*) *p*-value < 0.05, (**) *p*-value < 0.01

Lungs are the main source of RAGEs in healthy conditions [36]. Several studies concluded that cleaving full length RAGE (FL-RAGE), the transmembrane form, is the main way to produce the soluble form of alveolar epithelial cells (AECs) from healthy human lungs [48]. This might suggest that decrease in sRAGE found in IPF patients could be interpreted as a lack of RAGE synthesis or the loss of AECs. Thus, variations in the serum sRAGE levels would reflect the possible changes in lung function. The association between serum sRAGE and PFTs, as well as the changes over time would support this hypothesis. Longitudinal changes in FVC and DLCO have been found to have important prognostic value in IPF [49]. However, predicting prognosis at diagnosis remains a challenge. In our IPF cohort, patients with lower levels of sRAGE at the beginning of this study (under 428.25 pg/mL) showed worse lung-transplant progression free survival rate at 3 years, in accordance with previous observations from Yamaguchi and colleagues [37].

The decrease of sRAGE might be related to the progressive loss of alveolar structures in lung fibrosis lung. Chronic lung diseases that cause a progressive destruction of the alveolar structures such as chronic obstructive pulmonary disease (COPD) showed low levels of

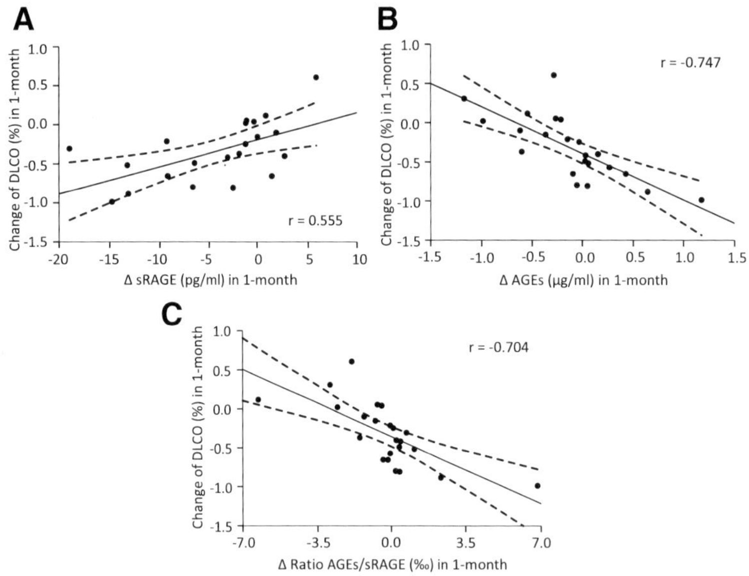

Fig. 5 Correlation between changes in DLCO and differences in sRAGE-AGEs levels in IPF patients. **a** In IPF patients, a decline of DLCO was related with a decrease of sRAGE in serum ($r = 0.555$, $p < 0.01$). **b and c** On the contrary, AGEs levels and the AGEs/sRAGE ratio were negatively correlated with the percentage of changes in DLCO in IPF patients ($r = -0.747$ and -0704, respectively, $p < 0.01$), meaning poor lung function in patients with an increase of AGEs-sRAGE imbalance over time. The changes in serum sRAGE and AGEs and lung function from IPF patients was calculated, adjusting over time: **Δ** ELISA in a month = [ELISA final − ELISA initial]/month; change of % predicted PFT = [PFT final − PFTs initial]/month. Pearson's correlation coefficients were performed to analyze the lineal relationship between the variables

sRAGE compared with controls [39, 50]. Those results have been correlated with a deterioration in lung function over time. Similarly, mechanical damage of lung showed low levels of sRAGE [41, 51]. On the other hand, the downregulation of RAGE has also been related to several pro-fibrotic pathways [52, 53]. There are some reports that showed a predisposition to develop a spontaneous pulmonary fibrosis in RAGE null mice [54]. All these findings suggest that the destruction of alveolar structures by fibrotic changes might favor the loss of RAGEs in IPF patients, and this downregulation of sRAGE, at the same time, could favor the fibrosis progression.

Regarding AGEs levels in serum, although a significant increase has been found in IPF and cHP compared to fNSIP, the measurement in the IPF group at the beginning of the study was not associated with pulmonary functional values. However, changes in AGEs levels over time were associated with FVC, TLC and DLCO decline. AGEs are increased in IPF lungs and have been associated with myofibroblast formation and ECM stiffness in vitro [55]. In addition, if sRAGE decreases, the pro-fibrotic effect of AGEs could increase due to the decreased decoy effect [56]. Our results also showed that those IPF patients with higher AGEs/sRAGE ratio showed a faster decline in DLCO. These findings indicate that an increase of AGEs or the AGEs/sRAGE ratio might indicate the degree of remodeling changes due to pulmonary fibrosis.

Some limitations of the study are the small number of the included cases in each group and the lack of validating cohort. Furthermore, no other possible biomarkers have been measured in our cohort in order to compare the differences or supplementary value for diagnostic and prognostic purposes. However, the results are useful for inclusion of this biomarker in longitudinal multicenter studies to evaluate potential biomarkers in fibrotic ILDs.

In the last few years, extensive reviews had been done to evaluate the multiple potential serum markers proposed, some of them implied in ECM remodeling or AEC dysfunction, suggesting a much better diagnostic accuracy and practicality when they were evaluated together [57–59]. Our model base on AGEs-sRAGE estimation and ratio also emphasizes the need to mix biomarkers for improving predictive power.

Conclusions

In conclusion, these results demonstrate that the ratio AGEs/sRAGE could be considered as a new potential serum biomarker for aiding in the differential diagnosis between the most common fibrosing ILDs, although a prospective multicenter study for validating this pivotal results would be required. Furthermore, serum sRAGE level is a prognostic biomarker in IPF.

Additional files

Additional file 1: ROC statistics for sRAGE and AGE serum levels. AGE: advanced glycation end-product, AUC: area under the curve, cHP: chronic hypersensitivity pneumonitis, fNSIP: fibrotic non-specific interstitial

pneumonia, CI: confidence interval, IPF: idiopathic pulmonary fibrosis, sRAGE: soluble receptor for advanced glycation end-products, ROC: Receiver operating characteristic. (*) *p*-value < 0.05, (**) *p*-value < 0.01. (XLSX 9 kb)

Additional file 2: Correlation between RAGE, AGE and PFT. AGE: advanced glycation end-product, cHP: chronic hypersensitivity pneumonitis, DLCO: diffusing capacity for carbon monoxide, fNSIP: fibrotic non-specific interstitial pneumonia, FVC: forced vital capacity, IPF: idiopathic pulmonary fibrosis, r: correlation coefficient, R^2: coefficient of determination, sRAGE: soluble receptor for advanced glycation end-products, TLC: Total lung capacity. (*) *p*-value < 0.05, (**) *p*-value < 0.01. (XLSX 9 kb)

Additional file 3: AGEs-sRAGE correlation in IPF patients during follow-up. IPF patients with a decline of AGEs in serum showed an increase of soluble fragment of the receptor in blood. (PDF 109 kb)

Abbreviations
AECs: Alveolar Epithelial Cells; AGEs: Advanced glycation end-products; AUC: Area Under the Curve; cHP: Chronic Hypersensitivity Pneumonitis; COPD: chronic obstructive pulmonary disease; DLCO: Diffusing Capacity for Carbon Monoxide; ECM: Extracellular Matrix; FL-RAGE: Full-length RAGE; fNSIP: Fibrotic non-specific interstitial pneumonia; FVC: Forced Vital Capacity; ILDs: Interstitial Lung Diseases; IPF: Idiopathic Pulmonary Fibrosis; J: Youden's index; LR+: Likelihood ratio for positive test results; PFT: Pulmonary Function Test; RAGE: Receptor for AGEs; ROC: Receiver Operating Characteristic; sRAGE: Soluble RAGE; TLC: Total Lung Capacity; UIP: Usual Interstitial Pneumonia

Acknowledgments
The author wants to thank Jose Palma from Hospital of Bellvitge for helping in the management of PFTs, and Jessica Germaine Schull for correcting the spelling.

Funding
This research was supported by the Spanish Pneumology and Thoracic Surgeon Society (SEPAR, 010/2017), the Catalan Pneumology Society (SOCAP), the Catalan Foundation of Pulmonology (FUCAP), and the Institute of Health Carlos III (ISCIII, PI15/00710), co-funded by FEDER funds/European Regional Development Fund (ERDF) – "a Way to Build Europe". We thank CERCA Programme / Generalitat de Catalunya for institutional support.

Authors' contributions
CM set up and performed the several assessments, interpreted the data, and drafted the manuscript. AMW oversaw the experimental assays and revised the draft of the manuscript. LPC prepared the samples, accomplished the database of the patients. RB handled and prepared the samples. MMM conceived, designed and oversaw the experiments, and helped to draft the manuscript. WZ conceived the study, and participated in its design and coordination and helped to draft the manuscript. All authors read and approved the final manuscript.

Competing interests
The authors declare that they have any competing interests (both financial and non-financial) related to this manuscript.

Author details
[1]Pneumology Research Group, IDIBELL, L'Hospitalet de Llobregat, Barcelona, Spain. [2]Biomedical Research Network Centers in Respiratory Diseases (CIBERES), Barcelona, Spain. [3]Unit of Interstitial Lung Diseases, Department of Pneumology, University Hospital of Bellvitge, C. Feixa Llarga sn., 08907 L'Hospitalet de Llobregat, Barcelona, Spain.

References

1. Buendía-Roldán I, Mejía M, Navarro C, Selman M. Idiopathic pulmonary fibrosis: clinical behavior and aging associated comorbidities. Respir Med. 2017;129:46–52.
2. Lynch JP, Huynh RH, Fishbein MC, Saggar R, Belperio JA, Weigt SS. Idiopathic pulmonary fibrosis: epidemiology, clinical features, prognosis, and management. Semin Respir Crit Care Med. 2016;37:331–57.
3. Daccord C, Maher TM. Recent advances in understanding idiopathic pulmonary fibrosis. F1000Research. 2016;5:1046.
4. Vourlekis JS, Schwarz MI, Cool CD, Tuder RM, King TE, Brown KK. Nonspecific interstitial pneumonitis as the sole histologic expression of hypersensitivity pneumonitis. Am J Med. 2002;112:490–3.
5. Travis WD, Costabel U, Hansell DM, King TE, Lynch DA, Nicholson AG, et al. An official American Thoracic Society/European Respiratory Society statement: update of the international multidisciplinary classification of the idiopathic interstitial pneumonias. Am J Respir Crit Care Med. 2013;188:733–48.
6. Grunes D, Beasley MB. Hypersensitivity pneumonitis: a review and update of histologic findings. J Clin Pathol. 2013;66:888–95.
7. Spagnolo P, Rossi G, Cavazza A, Bonifazi M, Paladini I, Bonella F, et al. Hypersensitivity pneumonitis: a comprehensive review. J Investig Allergol Clin Immunol. 2015;25:237–50.
8. Nathan SD, Brown AW, King CS. Diseases that mimic idiopathic pulmonary fibrosis. In: Guide to clinical Management of Idiopathic Pulmonary Fibrosis. Cham: Springer International Publishing; 2016. p. 33–41.
9. Takemura T, Akashi T, Kamiya H, Ikushima S, Ando T, Oritsu M, et al. Pathological differentiation of chronic hypersensitivity pneumonitis from idiopathic pulmonary fibrosis/usual interstitial pneumonia. Histopathology. 2012;61:1026–35.
10. Morell F, Villar A, Montero MÁ, Muñoz X, Colby TV, Pipvath S, et al. Chronic hypersensitivity pneumonitis in patients diagnosed with idiopathic pulmonary fibrosis: a prospective case-cohort study. Lancet Respir Med. 2013;1:685–94.
11. Glaspole I, Goh NSL. Differentiating between IPF and NSIP. Chron Respir Dis. 2010;7:187–95.
12. Vasakova M, Morell F, Walsh S, Leslie K, Raghu G. Hypersensitivity pneumonitis: perspectives in diagnosis and management. Am J Respir Crit Care Med. 2017;196:680–9.
13. Vasakova M, Poletti V. Fibrosing interstitial lung diseases involve different pathogenic pathways with similar outcomes. Sarcoidosis Vasc Diffus Lung Dis. 2015;32:246 50.
14. van den Blink B, Wijsenbeek MS, Hoogsteden HC. Serum biomarkers in idiopathic pulmonary fibrosis. Pulm Pharmacol Ther. 2010;23:515–20.
15. Ley B, Brown KK, Collard HR. Molecular biomarkers in idiopathic pulmonary fibrosis. AJP Lung Cell Mol Physiol. 2014;307:L681–91.
16. Guiot J, Moermans C, Henket M, Corhay J-L, Louis R. Blood biomarkers in idiopathic pulmonary fibrosis. Lung. 2017;195:273–80.
17. Drakopanagiotakis F, Wujak L, Wygrecka M, Markart P. Biomarkers in idiopathic pulmonary fibrosis. Matrix Biol. 2018;69:404–21.
18. Maher TM. PROFILEing idiopathic pulmonary fibrosis: rethinking biomarker discovery. Eur Respir Rev. 2013;22:148–52.
19. Oczypok EA, Perkins TN, Oury TD. All the "RAGE" in lung disease: the receptor for advanced glycation endproducts (RAGE) is a major mediator of pulmonary inflammatory responses. Paediatr Respir Rev. 2017;23:40–9.
20. Machahua C, Montes-Worboys A, Llatjos R, Escobar I, Dorca J, Molina-Molina M, et al. Increased AGE-RAGE ratio in idiopathic pulmonary fibrosis. Respir Res. 2016;17:144.
21. Hudson BI, Lippman ME. Targeting RAGE signaling in inflammatory disease. Annu Rev Med. 2018;69:349–64.
22. Uchida T, Shirasawa M, Ware LB, Kojima K, Hata Y, Makita K, et al. Receptor for advanced glycation end-products is a marker of type I cell injury in acute lung injury. Am J Respir Crit Care Med. 2006;173:1008–15.
23. Katsuoka F, Kawakami Y, Arai T, Imuta H, Fujiwara M, Kanma H, et al. Type II alveolar epithelial cells in lung express receptor for advanced glycation end products (RAGE) gene. Biochem Biophys Res Commun. 1997;238:512–6.
24. Hudson BI, Carter AM, Harja E, Kalea AZ, Arriero M, Yang H, et al. Identification, classification, and expression of RAGE gene splice variants. FASEB J. 2008;22:1572–80.
25. Raucci A, Cugusi S, Antonelli A, Barabino SM, Monti L, Bierhaus A, et al. A soluble form of the receptor for advanced glycation endproducts (RAGE) is produced by proteolytic cleavage of the membrane-bound form by the sheddase a disintegrin and metalloprotease 10 (ADAM10). FASEB J. 2008;22:3716–27.

26. Yan SF, Ramasamy R, Schmidt AM. Soluble RAGE: therapy and biomarker in unraveling the RAGE axis in chronic disease and aging. Biochem Pharmacol. 2010;79:1379–86.
27. Tae HJ, Kim JM, Park S, Tomiya N, Li G, Wei W, et al. The N-glycoform of sRAGE is the key determinant for its therapeutic efficacy to attenuate injury-elicited arterial inflammation and neointimal growth. J Mol Med. 2013;91:1369–81.
28. Izushi Y, Teshigawara K, Liu K, Wang D, Wake H, Takata K, et al. Soluble form of the receptor for advanced glycation end-products attenuates inflammatory pathogenesis in a rat model of lipopolysaccharide-induced lung injury. J Pharmacol Sci. 2016;130:226–34.
29. Blondonnet R, Audard J, Belville C, Clairefond G, Lutz J, Bouvier D, et al. RAGE inhibition reduces acute lung injury in mice. Sci Rep. 2017;7:7208.
30. Ott C, Jacobs K, Haucke E, Navarrete Santos A, Grune T, Simm A. Role of advanced glycation end products in cellular signaling. Redox Biol. 2014;2: 411–29.
31. Byun K, Yoo YC, Son M, Lee J, Jeong GB, Park YM, et al. Advanced glycation end-products produced systemically and by macrophages: a common contributor to inflammation and degenerative diseases. Pharmacol Ther. 2017;177:44–55.
32. Chaudhuri J, Bains Y, Guha S, Kahn A, Hall D, Bose N, et al. The role of advanced glycation end products in aging and metabolic diseases: bridging association and causality. Cell Metab. 2018;28:337–52.
33. Sukkar MB, Ullah MA, Gan WJ, Wark PAB, Chung KF, Hughes JM, et al. RAGE: a new frontier in chronic airways disease. Br J Pharmacol. 2012;167:1161–76.
34. Avery NCC, Bailey AJJ. The effects of the Maillard reaction on the physical properties and cell interactions of collagen. Pathol Biol. 2006;54:387–95.
35. Gautieri A, Passini FS, Silván U, Guizar-Sicairos M, Carimati G, Volpi P, et al. Advanced glycation end-products: mechanics of aged collagen from molecule to tissue. Matrix Biol. 2017;59:95–108.
36. Mukherjee TK, Mukhopadhyay S, Hoidal JR. Implication of receptor for advanced glycation end product (RAGE) in pulmonary health and pathophysiology. Respir Physiol Neurobiol. 2008;162:210–5.
37. Yamaguchi K, Iwamoto H, Horimasu Y, Ohshimo S, Fujitaka K, Hamada H, et al. AGER gene polymorphisms and soluble receptor for advanced glycation end product in patients with idiopathic pulmonary fibrosis. Respirology. 2017;22:965–71.
38. Willems S, Verleden SE, Vanaudenaerde BM, Wynants M, Dooms C, Yserbyt J, et al. Multiplex protein profiling of bronchoalveolar lavage in idiopathic pulmonary fibrosis and hypersensitivity pneumonitis. Ann Thorac Med. 2013;8:38.
39. Iwamoto H, Gao J, Pulkkinen V, Toljamo T, Nieminen P, Mazur W. Soluble receptor for advanced glycation end-products and progression of airway disease. BMC Pulm Med. 2014;14:68.
40. Yonchuk JG, Silverman EK, Bowler RP, Agustí A, Lomas DA, Miller BE, et al. Circulating soluble receptor for advanced glycation end products (sRAGE) as a biomarker of emphysema and the RAGE axis in the lung. Am J Respir Crit Care Med. 2015;192:785–92.
41. Negrin LL, Halat G, Prosch H, Hüpfl M, Hajdu S, Heinz T. Soluble receptor for advanced glycation end products quantifies lung injury in Polytraumatized patients. Ann Thorac Surg. 2017;103:1587–93.
42. Inghilleri S, Morbini P, Campo I, Zorzetto M, Oggionni T, Pozzi E, et al. Factors influencing oxidative imbalance in pulmonary fibrosis: an immunohistochemical study. Pulm Med. 2011;2011:421409.
43. Kyung SY, Byun KH, Yoon JY, Kim YJ, Lee SP, Park JW, et al. Advanced glycation end-products and receptor for advanced glycation end-products expression in patients with idiopathic pulmonary fibrosis and NSIP. Int J Clin Exp Pathol. 2013;7:221–8.
44. Raghu G, Collard HR, Egan JJ, Martinez FJ, Behr J, Brown KK, et al. An official ATS/ERS/JRS/ALAT statement: idiopathic pulmonary fibrosis: evidence-based guidelines for diagnosis and management. Am J Respir Crit Care Med. 2011; 183:788–824.
45. Jabaudon M, Blondonnet R, Roszyk L, Pereira B, Guérin R, Perbet S, et al. Soluble forms and ligands of the receptor for advanced glycation end-products in patients with acute respiratory distress syndrome: an observational prospective study. PLoS One. 2015;10(8):e0135857.
46. Hoonhorst SJM, Lo Tam Loi AT, Pouwels SD, Faiz A, Telenga ED, van den Berge M, et al. Advanced glycation endproducts and their receptor in different body compartments in COPD. Respir Res. 2016;17:46.
47. Manichaikul A, Sun L, Borczuk AC, Onengut-Gumuscu S, Farber EA, Mathai SK, et al. Plasma soluble receptor for advanced glycation end products in idiopathic pulmonary fibrosis. Ann Am Thorac Soc. 2017;14:628–35.
48. Ohlmeier S, Mazur W, Salmenkivi K, Myllärniemi M, Bergmann U, Kinnula VL. Proteomic studies on receptor for advanced glycation end product variants in idiopathic pulmonary fibrosis and chronic obstructive pulmonary disease. Proteomics Clin Appl. 2010;4:97–105.
49. Cottin V, Hansell DM, Sverzellati N, Weycker D, Antoniou KM, Atwood M, et al. Effect of emphysema extent on serial lung function in patients with idiopathic pulmonary fibrosis. Am J Respir Crit Care Med. 2017;196:1162–71.
50. Wu L, Ma L, Nicholson LFB, Black PN. Advanced glycation end products and its receptor (RAGE) are increased in patients with COPD. Respir Med. 2011; 105:329–36.
51. Benjamin JT, Van der Meer R, Slaughter JC, Steele SRN, Plosa EJ, Sucre JM, et al. Inverse relationship between soluble RAGE and risk for bronchopulmonary dysplasia. Am J Respir Crit Care Med. 2018;197:1083–6.
52. Ding H, Ji XH, Chen R, Ma T, Tang Z, Fen Y, et al. Antifibrotic properties of receptor for advanced glycation end products in idiopathic pulmonary fibrosis. Pulm Pharmacol Ther. 2015;35:34–41.
53. Song JS, Kang CM, Park CK, Yoon HK, Lee SY, Ahn JH, et al. Inhibitory effect of receptor for advanced glycation end products (RAGE) on the TGF-β-induced alveolar epithelial to mesenchymal transition. Exp Mol Med. 2011; 43:517–24.
54. Englert JM, Hanford LE, Kaminski N, Tobolewski JM, Tan RJ, Fattman CL, et al. A role for the receptor for advanced glycation end products in idiopathic pulmonary fibrosis. Am J Pathol. 2008;172:583–91.
55. Vicens-Zygmunt V, Estany S, Colom A, Montes-Worboys A, Machahua C, Sanabria AAJ, et al. Fibroblast viability and phenotypic changes within glycated stiffened three-dimensional collagen matrices. Respir Res. 2015;16:82.
56. Prasad K. Low levels of serum soluble receptors for advanced glycation end products, biomarkers for disease state: myth or reality. Int J Angiol. 2014;23: 11–6.
57. Rosas IO, Richards TJ, Konishi K, Zhang Y, Gibson K, Lokshin AE, et al. MMP1 and MMP7 as potential peripheral blood biomarkers in idiopathic pulmonary fibrosis. PLoS Med. 2008;5:e93.
58. Hamai K, Iwamoto H, Ishikawa N, Horimasu Y, Masuda T, Miyamoto S, et al. Comparative study of circulating MMP-7, CCL18, KL-6, SP-A, and SP-D as disease markers of idiopathic pulmonary fibrosis. Dis Markers. 2016;2016:1–8.
59. Jenkins RG, Simpson JK, Saini G, Bentley JH, Russell AM, Braybrooke R, et al. Longitudinal change in collagen degradation biomarkers in idiopathic pulmonary fibrosis: an analysis from the prospective, multicentre PROFILE study. Lancet Respir Med. 2015;3:462–72.

19

MUC1 deficiency mediates corticosteroid resistance in chronic obstructive pulmonary disease

Javier Milara[1,2,3,9*†], Lucía Díaz-Platas[4†], Sonia Contreras[5], Pilar Ribera[5], Inés Roger[3], Beatriz Ballester[5], Paula Montero[5], Ángel Cogolludo[3,6], Esteban Morcillo[3,5,7] and Julio Cortijo[3,5,8]

Abstract

Background: Lung inflammation in COPD is poorly controlled by inhaled corticosteroids (ICS). Strategies to improve ICS efficacy or the search of biomarkers who may select those patients candidates to receive ICS in COPD are needed. Recent data indicate that MUC1 cytoplasmic tail (CT) membrane mucin can mediate corticosteroid efficacy in chronic rhinosinusitis. The objective of this work was to analyze the previously unexplored role of MUC1 on corticosteroid efficacy in COPD in vitro and in vivo models.

Methods: MUC1-CT expression was measured by real time PCR, western blot, immunohistochemistry and immunofluorescence. The inflammatory mediators IL-8, MMP9, GM-CSF and MIP3α were measured by ELISA. The effect of MUC1 on inflammation and corticosteroid anti-inflammatory effects was measured using cell siRNA in vitro and Muc1-KO in vivo animal models.

Results: MUC1-CT expression was downregulated in lung tissue, bronchial epithelial cells and lung neutrophils from smokers ($n = 11$) and COPD ($n = 11$) patients compared with healthy subjects ($n = 10$). MUC1 was correlated with FEV1% ($\rho = 0.7479$; $p < 0.0001$) in smokers and COPD patients. Cigarette smoke extract (CSE) decreased the expression of MUC1 and induced corticosteroid resistance in human primary bronchial epithelial cells and human neutrophils. MUC1 Gene silencing using siRNA-MUC1 impaired the anti-inflammatory effects of dexamethasone and reduced glucocorticoid response element activation. Dexamethasone promoted glucocorticoid receptor alpha (GRα) and MUC1-CT nuclear translocation and co-localization that was inhibited by CSE. Lung function decline and inflammation induced by lipopolysaccharide and cigarette smoke in Muc1 KO mice was resistant to dexamethasone.

Conclusions: These results confirm a role for MUC1-CT mediating corticosteroid efficacy in COPD.

Keywords: Chronic obstructive pulmonary disease, MUC1, Corticosteroid resistance

Background

Chronic obstructive pulmonary disease (COPD) is a chronic inflammatory, progressive and debilitating lung disease. It is a major cause of chronic morbidity, the fourth leading cause of death worldwide and is projected to be the third leading cause of death by 2020 [1]. The primary cause of COPD is chronic exposure to cigarette smoke, which leads to airway inflammation and remodeling, thus increasing airflow limitation. In contrast with the magnitude of COPD, therapeutic options remains limited, and none of the available drugs have demonstrated to reduce lung function decline and mortality. The current first-line maintenance treatment for COPD involves the use of bronchodilators, including long-acting muscarinic antagonists (LAMAs) and long-acting beta 2 agonists (LABAs). Combination treatment with LAMA and LABA improves respiratory function, reduces symptoms and exacerbations compared to monotherapy or inhaled corticosteroids (ICS)/LABA combinations. Anti-inflammatory options for COPD are limited to corticosteroids and phosphodiesterase 4 inhibitors. While inhaled corticosteroids (ICS) have

* Correspondence: xmilara@hotmail.com
† Javier Milara and Lucía Díaz-Platas contributed equally to this work.
1 Department of Pharmacology, Faculty of Medicine, Jaume I University, Castellón de la Plana, Spain
2 Pharmacy Unit, University General Hospital Consortium, Valencia, Spain
Full list of author information is available at the end of the article

shown good activity in asthma, they are much less effective in improving lung function and have little or no effect on controlling the underlying chronic inflammation in COPD patients [2]. Triple therapy based on ICS in combination with LABAs and LAMAs is indicated in severe COPD at risk of exacerbations [3], however the use of ICS is under debate and needs more evidence to adequately select the COPD phenotype that takes advantage of this combination.

The loss of corticosteroid anti-inflammatory efficacy is a characteristic feature in COPD patients. Several molecular mechanisms of corticosteroid resistance have now been identified involving phosphorylation and modifications of glucocorticoid receptor (GR), and loss of histone deacetylase-2 (HDAC2) activity/ expression between others [4]. In patients with corticosteroid resistance, alternative anti-inflammatory treatments are being investigated as well as drugs that may reverse the molecular mechanisms of glucocorticoid resistance. Therefore, the understanding of corticosteroid resistant mechanisms, as biomarkers of therapeutic response, could be of potential value to individualize COPD therapy.

Mucin 1 (MUC1) is a member of membrane-bound mucins that has been associated with airway epithelial anti-inflammatory effects through the inhibition of bacteria and virus activation of toll-like receptors (TLR)-2–9 [5–8]. The MUC1 protein acts as a membrane receptor comprising two polypeptide subunits: an N-terminal extracellular subunit and a C-terminal subunit. A highly conserved cytoplasmic tail (CT) in the C-terminal subunit modulates multiple intracellular signals [9] implicated in different cellular processes such as cellular adherent junction maintenance and morphogenesis [10]. In COPD, MUC1-CT dysregulation promotes the loss of bronchial epithelial barrier integrity [11]. There are several intracellular mediators that can interact with MUC1-CT. Recent data published by our group indicate that MUC1-CT is downregulated in patients with chronic rhinosinusitis with nasal polyps who did not respond to systemic corticosteroids [12]. In vitro studies demonstrated that MUC1-CT forms a complex with GR in response to corticosteroids, mediating the nuclear complex translocation and the induction of anti-inflammatory gene expression. Although MUC1 could be a potential biomarker of corticosteroid response, currently there is no evidence on the association of the lack of MUC1-CT expression and corticosteroid resistance in COPD. The present work analyzes the association of MUC1-CT with corticosteroid efficacy using multiple approaches, including translational, cellular in vitro and animal in vivo models.

Materials and methods

Unless stated otherwise, all reagents used were obtained from Sigma Chemical Co. (Madrid, Spain).

Patients

Sputum neutrophils, peripheral blood neutrophils and bronchial epithelial cells were obtained from COPD patients, healthy smokers and healthy non-smoker subjects. Clinical characteristics of patients are defined in Table 1. Twenty-two patients with COPD, defined according to Global Initiative for Chronic Obstructive Lung Disease (GOLD) 2013 guidelines, were enrolled in this study. Patients were aged 67.5 ± 8 years, had forced expiratory volume in 1 s (FEV_1) of 48.6 ± 8% predicted, and all were prescribed an inhaled corticosteroid, long-acting anticholinergic and long-acting beta 2 agonists. All COPD patients were current smokers and bronchitic. The minimum washout period in stable COPD patients for sampling sputum or blood was 4 days, which avoided effects of chronic medication on the results.COPD patients in this study were classified as GOLD 2 (moderate disease; $n = 3$) and GOLD 3 (severe disease; $n = 19$). There were no exacerbations of the disease within 2 weeks prior to taking blood samples. Fifteen age-matched non-smoking control healthy subjects with normal lung function (age 66 ± 4 years old, FEV1 98 ± 3% predicted) and fifteen healthy smokers (age 65 ± 9 years old, FEV1 89 ± 6% predicted) were also recruited. Routine lung function tests were performed to evaluate forced vital capacity (FVC), FEV1 and FEV1/FVC ratio using a Vitalograph® alpha III spirometer (Vitalograph, Maids Moreton, UK).

Peripheral human lung tissue was obtained from 3 types of subjects (Thoracic Surgery and Pathology Services of the University General Consortium Hospital and University and Polytechnic Hospital La Fe, Spain): A) Patients with COPD who were underwent surgery for organ transplantation program ($n = 15$). B) Lung explants of non-smoker healthy donor subjects from the transplant program (were used as controls), without any lung disease ($n = 11$). C) Smoker donor subjects with normal lung function and lung cancer who were undergoing lung surgery for treatment purposes (lung tissue used in this work was as far as possible of the solitary cancer lesion; $n = 12$). Inclusion criteria comprised either non-smokers or current smokers with or without COPD who were free of symptoms of upper respiratory tract infection. After selection based on lung function, all lung tissue samples chosen for the study were checked histologically using the following exclusion criteria: (1) presence of tumor, (2) presence of post stenotic pneumonia, and (3) fibrosis of lung parenchyma. This project was approved by the local ethics committee of General University Hospital, Valencia, Spain, and written informed consent was taken from each patient or volunteer before starting blood sampling and lung function testing.

Isolation and culture of primary bronchial epithelial cells

Human bronchial epithelial cells (HBECs) from small bronchi were isolated as previously outlined [13]. Small

Table 1 Clinical features

	Healthy ($n = 15$)	Smokers ($n = 15$)	COPD ($n = 22$)
Age, yr. (mean (SD)	66 ± 4	65 ± 9	67.5 ± 8
Sex (M/F)	11/4	12/3	17/5
Tobacco consumption, pack-yr	0	24.1 ± 6	30.5 ± 8
FEV1, % pred	98 ± 3	89 ± 6	48.6 ± 8*
FVC, % pred	91 ± 2	90 ± 4	91.5 ± 6
FEV1/FVC %	94 ± 5	88 ± 1	61.2 ± 10*
GOLD 1 (mild) patients, no.	0	0	0
GOLD 2 (moderate) patients, no.	0	0	3
GOLD 3 (severe) patients, no.	0	0	19
GOLD 4 (very severe) patients, no.	0	0	0
Receiving inhaled steroids, no.	0	0	22
Receiving theophyllines, no.	0	0	0
Receiving long-acting b2-agonist, no.	0	0	22
Receiving anticholinergics, no.	0	0	22
Total peripheral blood neutrophils	$4.2 \pm 0.6 \times 10^9$/L	$6.5 \pm 0.9 \times 10^9$/L*	$9.5 \pm 2.1 \times 10^9$/L*

COPD Chronic obstructive pulmonary disease, *FEV1* Forced expiratory volume in 1 s, *FVC* Forced vital capacity; Pack-yr = 1 year smoking 20 cigarettes-day. % pred, % predicted. Data are mean ± SDs. * $P < 0.05$ related to Healthy subjects

pieces of human bronchi (0.5–1 mm internal diameter) were excised from microscopically normal lung areas, carefully dissected from lung parenchyma and plated on collagen-coated culture dishes (10 μg/cm^2 rat type I collagen; Sigma) in bronchial epithelial growth medium (BEGM), comprising bronchial epithelial basal medium (BEBM) supplemented with bovine pituitary extract (52 μg/ml, hydrocortisone 0.5 μg/ml), human recombinant epidermal growth factor ([EGF] 25 ng/ml), epinephrine (0.5 μg/ml), transferrin (10 μg/ml), insulin (5 μg/ml), retinoic acid (50 nM), triiodo-L-thyronine (6.5 ng/ml), gentamycin (40 μg/ml), amphotericin B (50 ng/ml), and bovine serum albumin (1.5 μg/ml). Small bronchi were oriented with the epithelial layer in contact with the culture plate. After a period of ~ 1–2 weeks, bronchial epithelial cells were observed around the bronchi. After trypsinization (passage 2–4), cells were cultured accordingly for different experiments. All the experiments performed in this study with primary HBEC were done on monolayer cultures. The identity of the monolayer as bronchial epithelial cells was confirmed using morphological criteria and immunofluorescence for cytokeratin 5 (KRT5) as well as later use of in vitro differentiation in air-liquid interface as pseudo-stratified bronchial epithelium with basal cells, ciliated cells, columnar, and goblet cells (data not shown). Cell viability was assessed by vital trypan blue exclusion analysis using the Countness® automated cell counter (Life Technologies, Madrid, Spain). Cell viability was > 98% in all cell cultures.

The bronchial epithelial BEAS2B cell line was obtained from American Type Culture Collection and cultured in BEGM media with supplements (Lonza, Madrid, Spain) on collagen-coated culture dishes (10 μg cm^{-2}; rat type I collagen) at 37 °C with 5% CO_2 in humidified air. The culture medium was replaced every 48 h.

Human neutrophil isolation from sputum and peripheral blood

Neutrophils were isolated from peripheral venous blood and cultured as previously outlined [14]. using 3% dextran 500 (in 0.9% saline) together with Ficoll-Paque Histopaque 1077 (Amersham Pharmacia Biotech, Barcelona, Spain) at a ratio of 2:1. The neutrophil preparations were > 97% pure as assessed by Giemsa staining and had viability of > 99% as measured by trypan blue exclusion. Neutrophils from spontaneous sputum (~ 2 ml) were collected and processed with dithiothreitol using established methods [15]. Sputum cell pellets were resuspended in RPMI 1640 supplemented with 10% foetal calf serum, 1% penicillin–streptomycin and 1 mmol L-glutamine/L at a concentration of 1×10^6 cells/ml. An aliquot containing 4×10^5 cells was incubated on a 24-well plate for 1 h at 37 °C in humidified 5% CO_2. Preparations containing < 95% neutrophils were discarded. Neither the purity nor the viability of the cell preparations was affected by the different experimental conditions of the study.

Preparation of cigarette smoke extract solutions

Cigarette smoke extract (CSE) was prepared as previously outlined [16]. Briefly, the smoke of a research cigarette (2R4F; Tobacco Health Research, University of Kentucky, KY, USA) was generated by a respiratory

pump (Apparatus Rodent Respirator 680; Harvard, Germany) through a puffing mechanism similar to the human smoking pattern (3 puffs/min; 1 puff volume of 35 ml; each puff duration lasting 2 s with 0.5 cm above the filter) and was bubbled into a flask containing 25 ml of pre-warmed (37 °C) Roswell Park Memorial Institute (RPMI)-1640 culture medium. The CSE solution was sterilized by filtration through a 0.22 μm cellulose acetate sterilizing system (Corning, USA). The resulting CSE solution was considered 100% CSE and was used within 30 min of preparation. CSE 10% approximately corresponds to the exposure associated with smoking of two packs per day [17]. The quality of the prepared CSE solution was assessed based on the absorbance at 320 nm, which is the specific light absorption wavelength of peroxynitrite. Stock solutions with an absorbance value of 3.0 ± 0.1 were used. To test for cytotoxicity and apoptosis due to CSE, bronchial epithelial cells were treated with CSE concentrations of up to 10% for 24 h. No significant differences in the lactate dehydrogenase supernatant level (lactate dehydrogenase cytotoxicity assay; Cayman, Spain) or in the number of apoptotic cells (annexin V-FITC) were observed in comparison with the control group [18].

Histology and immunofluorescence analysis

Lung histology was conducted as previously reported in the smoking animal model [19]. Tissue blocks (4 μm thickness) were stained with haematoxylin-eosin for assessment of the inflammatory lung infiltration. Immunofluorescence of MUC1-CT and GRα were analyzed in bronchial epithelial cell cultures and in bronchial epithelium from animals.

The in vitro cell culture of human bronchial epithelial cells was fixed (4% paraformaldehyde, 30 min, at room temperature) after appropriate treatments. Cells were permeabilized (20 mM HEPES at pH 7.6, 300 mM sucrose, 50 mM NaCl, 3 mM $MgCl_2$, 0.5% Triton X-100), blocked (10% goat serum in PBS), and incubated with the primary antibodies MUC1-CT (rabbit anti-human polyclonal MUC1-CT antibody (Novus Biologicals (NBP1–60046)) and GRα (mouse anti-human monoclonal glucocorticoid receptor α antibody (GRα; BD Biosciences (611227)) overnight at 4 °C, followed by secondary antibody anti-rabbit/ mouse rhodamine/FITC- (1:100, Molecular Probes). Cell nuclei were marked with 49–6-diaidino-2-phenylindole dihydrochloride (1:10,000; DAPI).

Mouse lung tissue was fixed in paraformaldehyde (4%) for 48 h and embedded in Tissue-Tek® OCT™ cryosectioning compound (Sakura Finetek Europe BV, Leiden). Blocks were cut into 10 μm thick sections, permeabilized in Triton X 100 (0.1% in PBS) for 5 min, blocked in 10% goat serum in PBS and co-immunostained with MUC1-CT and GRα antibodies for 24 h at 4 °C followed by a secondary FITC or rhodamine conjugated anti-mouse/rabbit IgG antibody and finally DAPI (2 μg/ml) to mark nuclei (Molecular Probes, Leiden, The Netherlands).

Colocalization of MUC1-CT and GRα was performed using a confocal spectral Leica TCS SP2 microscope with × 1000 magnification and 3× zoom. Red (HeNe 543 nm), green (HeNe 488 nm), and blue (Ar 351 nm, 364 nm) lasers were used. Colocalization studies were performed using the Leica confocal software v2.61.

Cell stimulations and IL-8, GM-CSF, MIP3a and MMP-9 assays

Primary HBECs or isolated human neutrophils from non-smoker, smoker, and smokers with COPD were adjusted to 500 × 10^6 cells per well in 6-well plates and incubated in BEGM culture medium at 37 °C with 5% CO_2. Cells were then treated in the presence or absence of dexamethasone (0.1 nM-1 μM; Sigma Aldrich, Madrid, Spain), for 1 h. After drug incubation, HBECs or neutrophils were stimulated with the TLR4 agonist lipopolysaccharide (LPS) (Invivogene, Toulouse, France) at 1 μg/ml final concentration alone or in combination with CSE at the indicated times as previously outlined [12, 20].

In additional experiments, scrambled siRNA control or MUC1 gene-targeted siRNA were transfected to Beas2B cells for 48 h. Cells were then incubated with dexamethasone 1 μM for 1 h and stimulated with/ without CSE.

Supernatants were collected and centrifuged at 120 g for 5 min. IL-8, GM-CSF, MIP3α or MMP9 were measured in cell-free supernatants using commercially available enzyme-linked immunosorbent assay kits (R&D Systems, Nottingham, UK).

Real-time RT-PCR and siRNA experiments

Total RNA was isolated from HBECs, human neutrophils, human and animal lung tissue using TriPure® Isolation Reagent (Roche, Indianapolis, USA). The integrity of the extracted RNA was confirmed with Bioanalyzer (Agilent, Palo Alto, CA, USA). Reverse transcription was performed in 300 ng of total RNA with a TaqMan reverse transcription reagents kit (Applied Biosystems, Perkin-Elmer Corporation, CA, USA). cDNA was amplified with specific primers and probes predesigned by Applied Biosystems for TLR4 (Hs00152939_m1), MUC1 (Hs00159357_m1) and MKP1 (Hs00610256_g1) for human samples, and MUC1 (Mm0 0449604_m1), GRα (Mm00449604_m1), MKP1 (Mm004 57274_g1), CD200 (Mm00487740_m1), RGS2 (Mm00 501385_m1), TSC22D3 (Mm00726417_m1), IL-8 (Mm042 08136_m1), IL-13 (Mm99999190_m1) and CRISPLD (Mm01240812_m1) for mouse samples in a 7900HT Fast Real-Time PCR System (Applied Biosystems) using Universal Master Mix (Applied Biosystems).

MKP1 is a mitogen-activated protein kinase phosphatase whose expression is increased by corticosteroids and induces the degradation/ de-phosphorylation of several

kinases such as ERK1/2 and p38, thus increasing the anti-inflammatory properties of corticosteroids [21].

RGS2 is a GTPase-activating protein that switches off signaling from Gq-linked G protein-coupled receptors (GPCRs). In airway smooth muscle, RGS2 is upregulated in a positive cooperative manner by glucocorticoid and LABA, and exerts a bronchoprotective effect; in epithelial and other cells RGS2 expression may attenuate pro-inflammatory mediator release [22].

TSC22D3 is a glucocorticoid-inducible gene that inhibits the transcriptional activity of both NF-kB and AP-1. Glucocorticoid-induced TSC22D3 expression may also be modestly enhanced by LABAs. It is reported that induction of this gene suppresses various indices of inflammation [23].

Previously known to mediate several other functions, CRISPLD2 was recently found to encode as a novel, secreted, mammalian LPS binding protein in both humans and mice. Enhancement of fluticasone propionate induced CRISPLD2 expression could contribute to the reduction in exacerbations in COPD produced by infections with gram-negative bacteria by downregulating TLR4-mediated proinflammatory responses [24].

CD200 is a glucocorticoid-inducible gene. Pulmonary alveolar macrophages have high constitutive expression of CD200R. Signaling through this receptor involves the interaction of CD200R-bearing cells with other cells (e.g., airway epithelia) that express CD200. Studies in mice have shown that the CD200/CD200R interaction blunts macrophage activation measured as proinflammatory cytokine generation. Acute exacerbations of COPD are triggered, primarily, by prolonged bouts of excessive inflammation in response to bacterial and viral infections. Pharmacological upregulation of CD200 on epithelial and other airway cells in COPD could attenuate inflammation and reduce exacerbation frequency [25].

Expression of the target gene was expressed as the fold increase or decrease relative to the expression of human GAPDH (4310884E) or mouse GAPDH (4352339E) as an endogenous control (Applied Biosystems). The mean value of the replicates for each sample was calculated and expressed as the cycle threshold (Ct). The level of gene expression was then calculated as the difference (ΔCt) between the Ct value of the target gene and the Ct value of GAPDH. The fold changes in the target gene mRNA levels were designated $2^{-\Delta Ct}$.

Small interfering RNA (siRNA), including the scrambled siRNA control, was purchased from Ambion (Huntingdon, Cambridge, UK). MUC1 gene-targeted siRNA (identification no. 4392420) was designed by Ambion. Beas2b cells were transfected with siRNA (50 nM) in serum and antibiotic-free medium. After 6 h, the medium was aspirated and replaced with medium containing serum for a further 42 h before cell stimulation. The transfection reagent used was lipofectamine-2000 (Invitrogen, Paisley, UK) at a final concentration of 2 μg/ml.

Western blotting analysis

Western blotting analysis was used to detect changes in lung tissue expression of MUC1-CT, TLR-4, phospho-ERK1/2, MKP1, GRα and phospho-GR-Ser226, phos pho-p38. Lung tissue from human and mouse were homogenized and lysed on ice with a lysis buffer comprising a complete inhibitor cocktail plus 1 mM ethylen ediaminetetraacectic acid (Roche Diagnostics Ltd., West Sussex, UK) with 20 mM Tris base, 0.9% NaCl, 0.1% Triton X-100, 1 mM dithiothreitol, and 1 mg/mL pepstatin A. The Bio-Rad assay (Bio-Rad Laboratories Ltd., Herts, UK) was used according to the manufacturer's instructions to quantify the level of protein in each sample to ensure equal protein loading. Sodium dodecyl sulfate polyacrylamide gel electrophoresis was used to separate the proteins according to their molecular weight. Briefly, 15 μg of proteins (denatured) along with a molecular weight protein marker (Bio-Rad Kaleidoscope marker; Bio-Rad Laboratories) were loaded onto an acrylamide gel consisting of a 5% acrylamide stacking gel stacked on top of a 10% acrylamide resolving gel and run through the gel by application of 100 V for 1 h. Proteins were transferred from the gel to a polyvinylidene difluoride membrane using a wet-blotting method. The membrane was blocked with 5% Marvel in PBS containing 0.1% Tween20 (PBS-T), probed with polyclonal MUC1-CT antibody (Novus Biologicals (NBP1–60046)), monoclonal phospho-ERK1/2 (Sigma-Aldrich (M9692)), monoclonal TLR4 antibody (Novus Biologicals (H00007099-M02)), monoclonal glucocorticoid receptor α antibody (GRα; BD Biosciences (611227)), monoclonal phospho-GR-Ser226 antibody (Novus Biologicals (NB100–92540)), polyclonal Mitogen Activated Protein Kinase Phosphatase 1 antibody (MKP1) (Assay Biotech (B1099), and monoclonal phospho-p38 antibody (Cell Signaling (4511)), and normalized to total mouse anti-human β-actin antibody (monoclonal antibody, catalog no. A1978; Sigma). The enhanced chemiluminescence method of protein detection using enhanced chemiluminescence reagents (ECL Plus; Amersham GE Healthcare, Buckinghamshire, UK) was used to detect labeled proteins. Densitometry of films was performed using the Image J 1.42q software (available at http://rsb.info.nih.gov/ij/, USA). Results of target protein expression are expressed as the percentage of the densitometry of the endogenous controls β-actin.

Immunoprecipitation

Equal amounts of protein (200 μg) were incubated with 2 μg of anti-GRα or anti-MUC1-CT antibodies and the IgG isotype control. The immune complexes were precipitated with protein G on Sepharose 4B fast flow beads

(Sigma (P-3296)) overnight at 4 °C. After washing three times with NET buffer containing 50 mM Tris-HCl at pH 8.0, 150 mM NaCl, and 0.1% Nonidet P-40, the bound materials were eluted from the immunoprecipitates in reducing SDS-PAGE loading buffer containing 10% SDS, 1 M Tris-HCl at pH 6.8, 50% glycerol, 10% 2-mercaptoethanol, and 2% bromophenol blue at 100 °C for 10 min. Immunoprecipitated protein complexes were assayed by western blotting as described above and probed using anti-GRα or anti-MUC1-CT antibodies, as appropriate.

Glucocorticoid response element transfection assay

Beas2B epithelial cells were seeded (40.000 cells/well) and cultured for 24 h under a 5% CO_2/air atmosphere at 37 °C in 96-well plates containing Dulbecco's modified Eagle's Medium (DMEM). The Cignal GRE Reporter Assay Kit (QIAGEN, Cat no. 336841) was used to monitor the activity of glucocorticoid receptor-induced signal transductions pathways in cultured cells, following the manufacturer's indications. First, cells were transfected with MUC1 gene-targeted siRNA or scrambled siRNA control as described above. 24 h later, cells were transfected with Cignal Reporter (100 ng), Cignal negative control (100 ng) and Cignal positive control (100 ng) in Opti-MEM serum-free culture medium using Lipofectamine 2000 Reagent (Invitrogen) as transfection reagent. Subsequently, cells were incubated with the transfection reagents at 37 °C in a 5% CO2 incubator for 16 h. After this incubation period, cells were pre-incubated during 6 h with different dexamethasone concentrations (0.1 nM-1 μM) in DMEM.

After this 6 h period, the luciferase assay was developed by using Dual-Luciferase Reporter Assay System (Promega, Cat N° 1910) following the manufacturer's protocol for developing the assay. In brief, growth medium was removed from the cultured cells and the surface of the cultured cells was washed gently with phosphate buffered saline (PBS). After removing completely the rinse solution, Passive Lysis Buffer 1X was added. The culture plate was then placed on an orbital shaker, with gentle shaking at room temperature for 15 min. In the meantime, Luciferase Assay Reagent II (LAR II) was prepared by resuspending the provided lyophilized Luciferase Assay Substrate in 10 mL of the supplied Luciferase Assay Buffer II. A volume of 100 μl of LAR II was predispensed in the appropriate number of wells of a white 96-well plate. Then, a volume of 20 μl of cell lysate was added into the wells containing LAR II, and mixed by pipetting 2 or 3 times. The white plate was placed in the luminometer (Victor), reading was initiated and the Firefly luciferase activity was measured. In the meantime, the Stop & Glo Reagent was prepared, just before use, by diluting 1 volume of the Stop & Glo Substrate to 50 volumes of Stop & Glo Buffer. Following the first measure, 100 μl of Stop & Glo Reagent was dispensed in the corresponding wells. The plate was replaced in the luminometer and a second reading was initiated and the Renilla Luciferase activity was recorded. Data are expressed as 2xGRE fold induction of luciferase relative to unstimulated cells.

Inflammatory cigarette smoke animal model

Experimentation and handling were performance in accordance with the guidelines of the Committee of Animal Ethics and Well-being of the University of Valencia (Valencia, Spain). The animal studies followed the ARRIVE guidelines [26]. Mice studies used pathogen-free female C57BL/6 of 12 weeks years old (Harlan Iberica®, Barcelona, Spain). Muc1-KO mice C57BL/6 animals were originally generate by Sandra Gendler (Mayo Clinic, NY, USA) [27] and donated by the animalerie Institut de Médecine Prédictive et de Recherche Thérapeutique, (Lille Cedex, France). Mice were housed with free access to water and food under standard conditions: relative humidity 55 ± 10%; temperature 22 ± 3 °C; 15 air cycles/ per hour; 12/12 h Light/Dark cycle.

The experimental procedure started at day 0 with the basal measure of micro-computed tomography (CT) coupled to positron emission tomography (PET) lung image analysis (micro-CT-PET Albira Imaging System (Oncovision®, Spain) and measure of lung function by plethysmography of whole body (Miami, Florida, USA). At day 1 intranasal lipopolysaccharide (LPS from Salmonella Typhimurium, Sigma Aldrich, Madrid, Spain) or vehicle (sterile deionized water) was administered at 75 μg in 25 μl as previously outlined to induce an inflammatory response [28]. Between days 2 to day 3, mice were exposed to cigarette smoke of 6 cigarettes (2R4F; Tobacco Health Research, University of Kentucky, KY, USA). Between day 4 and day 5 mice were exposed to cigarette smoke of 8 cigarettes. The last day of procedure (day 6), mice were exposed to cigarette smoke of 10 cigarettes, and anlaysis of micro-CT-PET and lung function were assessed. Each cigarette exposure was programed to be consumed in 5 min followed by 8 min of airway exposure using a flux of 5 L/min [29]. A nose only system (TSE systems, Bad Homburg, Germany) was employed for cigarette smoking. Each drag had 1.9 s, and the period of time between drags was 20 s. Control animals received same conditions inhaling air instead of cigarette smoke. Dexamethasone was given at 10 mg/kg/day and 3 mg/kg/day in methocel 10% suspensions, once daily, p.o. by gavage in a volume of 10 mL/kg, starting at day 1 until day 6 of the experimental procedure. Dexamethasone was administer 1 h before cigarette smoke exposure. The account for experimental groups was estimated in a number of 8 mice ($n = 8$) based in previous findings [29]. The primary outcome was the

50% reduction of the lung inflammation (SUV) by dexamethasone 3 mg/kg/day. The sample size was calculated for an effect size f of 1.8, α error of 0.05 and power of 0.96, using one tailed analysis of variance (ANOVA).

Different experimental groups were assigned as follow: 1) Intranasal sterile deionized water + airway nose only system exposure (n = 8); 2) Intranasal sterile deionized water + airway nose only system exposure + dexamethasone 10 mg/kg/day (n = 8); 3) Intranasal LPS + airway nose only system exposure (n = 8); 4) Intranasal LPS + cigarette smoke nose only system exposure (n = 8); 5) Intranasal LPS + cigarette smoke nose only system exposure + dexamethasone 10 mg/kg/day (n = 8); 6) Intranasal LPS + cigarette smoke nose only system exposure + dexamethasone 3 mg/kg/day (n = 8); 7) Intranasal LPS + airway nose only system exposure + 10 mg/kg/day (n = 8); 8) Intranasal LPS + airway nose only system exposure + 3 mg/kg/day.

Micro-CT-PET analysis

The animal images were acquired at day 0 and 6 using the multimodal micro-PET-CT system (micro-CT-PET Albira Imaging System (Oncovision®, Spain). Animals were anesthesized with intraperitoneal mixture of ketamin (70 mg/Kg) and medetomidin (0.25 mg/kg). After 10 min of stabilization animals were injected intraperitoneally with 300 μCi.

fludeoxyglucose ^{18}F (^{18}F-FDG). After 30 min, the animals were allocated in supine position in a cradle made of plexiglas to acquire micro-CT and PET images.

Acquisitions of both PET and CT were made with an offset of 10 mm in length to visualize the lung region. Acquisition by CT (Carestream Molecular Imaging, Woodbridge, CT) was performed with good acquisition quality, high dose (400 μA) and high voltage (45Kv) with the Step & Shoot acquisition mode and FBP reconstruction algorithm (Filtered Back Projection). In the PET mode, the studies were programmed with a field of vision (Field Of View (FOV)) of 80 mm, an acquisition time of 90 s per projection during 15 min. The images were reconstructed using the OSEM Cross algorithm with a number of iterations of 3 using the standard reconstruction parameters of the Albira Suite 5.0 Reconstructor software. The images were analyzed and quantified using the PMOD analysis software version 3.2 (PMOD Technologies LTD, Zurich, Switzerland). Once acquired, the PET / CT images were reconstructed and merged.

Volumes of interest (VOI) of the lung region were determined for the CT images. The VOI was analyzed for each subject for their different days of acquisition. For PET images, the VOI obtained in the CT image of each subject was taken as a template and it was extrapolated to the PET image and subsequently quantified. The quantification of images provided the number of accounts acquired per pixel unit. This value was relativized by the dose injected and by subject weight, resulting in the standard uptake value (SUV).

Statistical analysis

Statistical analysis of results was carried out by parametric (animal and cellular studies) or non-parametric (human tissue studies) analysis as appropriate. $P < 0.05$ was considered statistically significant. Non-parametric tests were used to compare results from human samples of control patients, smoker and COPD patients. In this case, data were displayed as medians and interquartile range values. When the comparisons concerned more than two groups, analysis of variance (Kruskal-Wallis test) was first performed. In the case of a global significant difference, between-group comparisons were assessed by the Dunn's post-hoc test, which generalizes the Bonferroni adjustment procedure. When the comparisons concerned only 2 groups, between-group differences were analyzed by the Mann Whitney test. Results from animal and cellular in vitro mechanistic cell experiments were expressed as mean ± SE of n experiments since normal distribution for each data set was confirmed by histogram analyses and Kolmogorov–Smirnov test. In this case, statistical analysis was carried out by parametric analysis. Two-group comparisons were analysed using the two-tailed Student's paired t-test for dependent samples, or unpaired t-test for independent samples. Multiple comparisons were analysed by one-way or two-way analysis of variance followed by Bonferroni post hoc test. Variable correlations were implemented using spearman ρ analysis.

Results

MUC1 expression is decreased in lung tissue from smokers and COPD patients

Lung tissue, bronchial epithelial cells and neutrophils were isolated from healthy, current smokers and COPD patients based in the clinic characteristic described in Table 1. The gene mRNA expression of MUC1 decreased from 143 ($2^{-\Delta Ct}$) in healthy lung tissue to 15 ($2^{-\Delta Ct}$) and 4 ($2^{-\Delta Ct}$) in lug tissue from smokers and COPD patients respectively (Fig.1a). Similar results were observed in bronchial epithelial cells and sputum neutrophils from smokers and COPD patients (Fig. 1b, c). In the same way, MUC1-CT protein expression was down-regulated in lung tissue from smokers and COPD patients to a 65 and 30% of control respectively (Fig. 1d). The MUC1-CT expression showed the same pattern of MUC1-CT distribution in lung tissue from healthy, smoker and COPD patients (data not shown), mainly located in bronchial epithelial cells and alveolar type II cells as previously described [30]. TLR4 mRNA expression was significantly upregulated in lung tissue, bronchial epithelial cells and sputum neutrophils from smokers and COPD patients (Fig. 1e-g), while

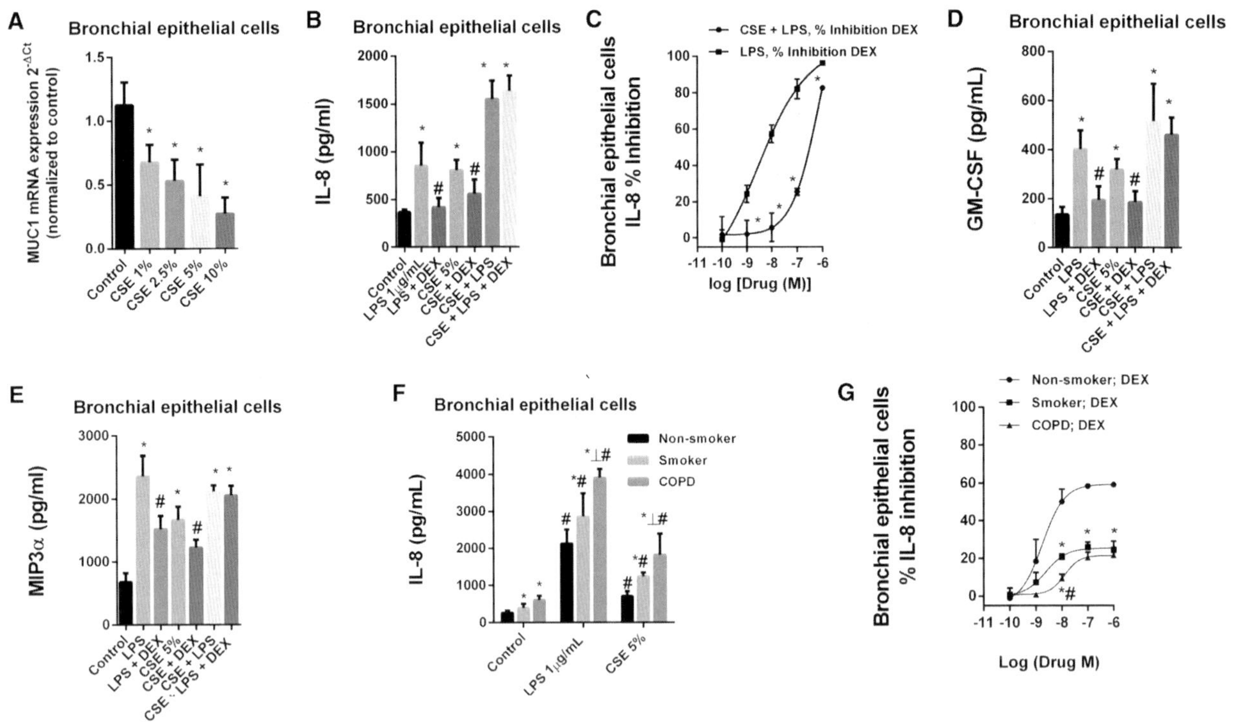

Fig. 2 Cigarette smoke mediates corticosteroid resistance and decreases MUC1 expression in human bronchial epithelial cells (HBEC). **a** Cigarette smoke extract (CSE) decreased the mRNA gene expression of MUC1 in HBEC from healthy subjects. **b**-**e** HBECs stimulated with lipopolysaccharide (LPS) and CSE 5% were resistant to the anti-inflammatory effects of dexamethasone on IL-8, GM-CSF and MIP3α release. **f** Both LPS and CSE induce higher IL-8 release in HBECs from smokers and COPD patients than in cells from healthy subjects. **g** Dexamethasone shows lesser inhibitory effect on LPS-induced IL-8 release in cells from smokers and COPD patients than in cells from healthy subjects. The results are shown as mean ± SE of $n = 4$ cell populations from healthy subjects (**a**-**g**), smokers (**f**, **g**) and COPD (**f**, **g**) patients. Gene expression was analyzed by real time PCR using the $2^{-\Delta Ct}$ as described in methods. Two-way ANOVA followed by Bonferroni post-hoc tests. **a**, **b**, **d** and **e** $*P < 0.05$ compared with control; #P < 0.05 compared with stimulus. (**c**) *P < 0.05 compared with CSE+ LPS group. **f** *P < 0.05 compared with non-smoker group; #P < 0.05 compared with control group; ⊥ P < 0.05 compared with smoker group. **g** *P < 0.05 compared with non-smoker group; #P < 0.05 compared with smoker group

IL-8 and MMP9 release, in neutrophils from smokers and COPD patients (Fig. 3f-i).

MUC1 mediates corticosteroid anti-inflammatory effects in vitro

Beas2b bronchial epithelial cells transiently transfected with siRNA-MUC1 were resistant to the effects of dexamethasone which did not increase the anti-inflammatory MKP1 and MUC1 expression (Fig. 4a, b). In the same way, in transiently transfected Beas2b cells with siRNA-MUC1, dexamethasone did not reduce IL-8 and GM-CSF release in response to CSE (Fig. 4c, d). Corticosteroids mediate part of its anti-inflammatory effects through transactivation of genes that encode proteins with anti-inflammatory properties, such as MKP1, via direct interaction of the agonist-bound GR to glucocorticoid response elements (GREs). In this work, cells were transfected with GRE reporter construct in siRNA-MUC1 cells and siRNA(−) cells and incubated with dexamethasone 1 μM during 4 h. Treatment of 2xGRE Beas2B reporter cells with dexamethasone (0.1 nM to 1 μM) for 4 h induced GRE dependent transcription in a concentration-dependent manner that was significantly lower in siRNA-MUC1 than in siRNA(−) control cells (Fig. 4e).

Confocal immunofluorescence for GRα and MUC1-CT revealed that both proteins are co-expressed in the cytoplasm of primary HBECs around the nucleus. After dexamethasone addition the GRα-MUC1-CT complex was translocated to the cell nucleus. However, pre-treated cells with CSE 5% for 24 h decreased MUC1-CT expression and blocked GRα-MUC1-CT nucleus translocation (Fig. 4f). HBECs incubated with CSE5% for 24 h showed a decreased expression of MUC1-CT, and an increased expression of GR phosphorylated at serine 226 (GR-Ser226), p-ERK1/2 and p-P38 expression (Fig. 4g). The proteasomal inhibitor MG-132 5 μM inhibited the loss of expression of MUC1-CT induced by CSE5% and reversed the increase of GR-Ser226 (Fig. 4h). Immunoprecipitation experiments revealed that MUCI-CT forms a complex with GRα that is dissociated by CSE in a concentration-dependent manner (Fig. 4i). The incubation of HBECs

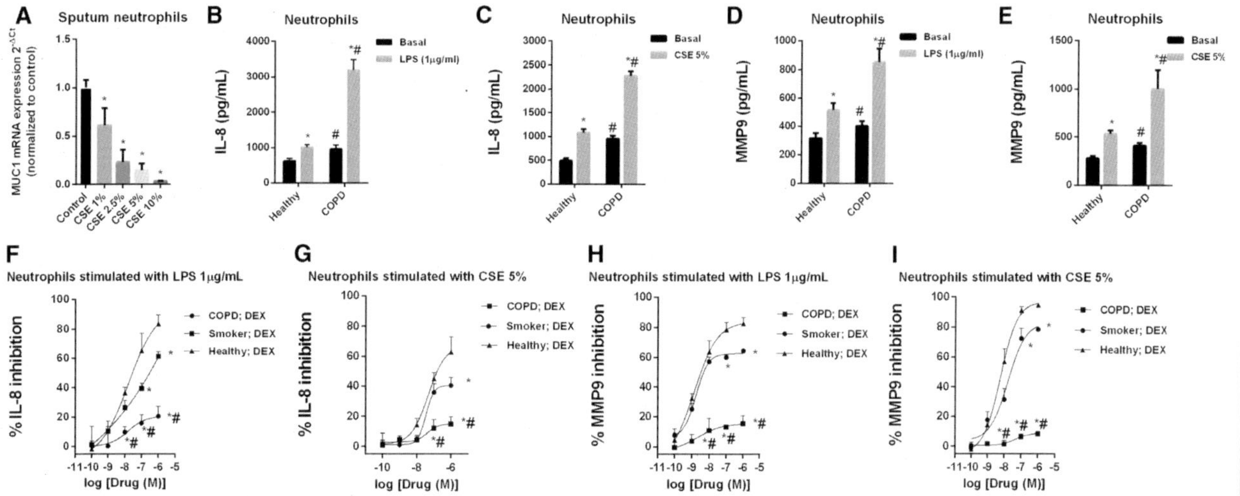

Fig. 3 Cigarette smoke mediates corticosteroid resistance and decreases MUC1 expression in human neutrophils. **a** Cigarette smoke extract (CSE) decreased the mRNA gene expression of MUC1 in sputum neutrophils from smokers. **b-e** Peripheral blood neutrophils from healthy and COPD patients were stimulated with (**b**, **d**) lipopolysaccharide (LPS) or (**c**, **e**) with cigarette smoke extract (CSE) during 6 h, and IL-8 and MMP9 levels were measured by ELISA. **f-i** Peripheral blood neutrophils form healthy, smokers and COPD patients were incubated with dexamethasone for 1 h and stimulated with LPS or CSE for 6 h. The results are shown as mean ± SE of $n = 4$ cell populations from healthy subjects, smokers and COPD patients. Gene expression was analyzed by real time PCR using the $2^{-\Delta Ct}$ as described in methods. Two-way ANOVA followed by Bonferroni post-hoc tests. **a-e** *$P < 0.05$ compared with control/basal; #$P < 0.05$ compared with healthy group. **f-i** *$P < 0.05$ compared with healthy group; #$P <$ 0.05 compared with smoker group

with CSE 5% during 24 h prevented the formation of GRα-MUC1-CT complex induced by dexamethasone (Fig. 4j).

MUC1 mediates corticosteroid anti-inflammatory effects in vivo

Dexamethasone administered at 3–10 mg/kg/day orally improved respiratory resistance (enhanced pause (Penh)), decreased inflammatory cells (Additional file 1: Data S1A-D), and IL-8/IL-13 (Additional file 1: Data S2A and S2B) in bronchoalveolar lavage (BAL) fluid of WT control animals treated with LPS and in a lesser extent in LPS + CS treated animals. In Mucl KO animals, dexamethasone did not improve Penh neither number of inflammatory cells nor IL8/IL13 cytokines in BAL fluid (Additional file 1: Data S1 and S2). Mucl KO mice showed predominant neutrophil inflammation after LPS or LPS + CS exposure (Additional file 1: Figure S1). Lung hematoxylin & eosin histology showed lesser lung inflammatory cell infiltrates in lung sections from WT animals treated with dexamethasone in both groups: animals exposed to LPS and LPS + CS (Additional file 1: Figure S3). In contrast, dexamethasone did not reduced inflammatory cell infiltrates in Mucl KO animals (Additional file 1: Figure S3).

In lung tissue, LPS and LPS + CS administration increased IL-8 and IL-13 mRNA expression (Fig. 5a, b). Dexamethasone inhibited IL-8 and IL-13 expression only in WT animals stimulated with LPS ($P < 0.05$) but not in animals stimulated with LPS + CS (Fig. 5a, b). In Mucl KO mice dexamethasone did not inhibited IL-8 and IL-13 expression (Fig. 5a, b). Lung tissue from WT control mice increased Mucl expression in response to dexamethasone (Fig. 5c). Furthermore, LPS stimulus increased the expression of Mucl in WT animals (Fig. 5c). MUC1-KO mice did not show Mucl expression in lung tissue confirming the KO nature (Fig. 5c). GRα expression was not affected by experimental conditions (Fig. 5d).

Corticosteroids can enhance genes that encode proteins with anti-inflammatory properties. In this work, dexamethasone elevated the expression of corticosteroid-inducible anti-inflammatory genes MKP1, CRISPLD, CD200, RGS2 and TSC22D3 in lung tissue of WT control animals stimulated with LPS, but not in animals stimulated with LPS + CS (Fig 6a-e). Furthermore, dexamethasone did not increase the expression of the anti-inflammatory genes in Mucl KO mice (Fig. 6a-e).

Micro-CT-PET image analysis detected an increase of fludeoxyglucose ^{18}F (^{18}F-FDG) signal expressed as standard uptake value (SUV) in animals treated with LPS and LPS + CS (Fig. 7). Dexamethasone decrease SUV values at 3 mg and 10 mg/kg/day in WT animals stimulated with LPS, while only dexamethasone 10 mg/kg/day was effective inhibiting SUV in animals treated with LPS + CS. In Mucl-KO animals, dexamethasone did not reduce SUV values (Fig. 7).

We observed that both LPS and LPS + CS can enhance the GR phosphorylation at ser^{226}, while dexamethasone

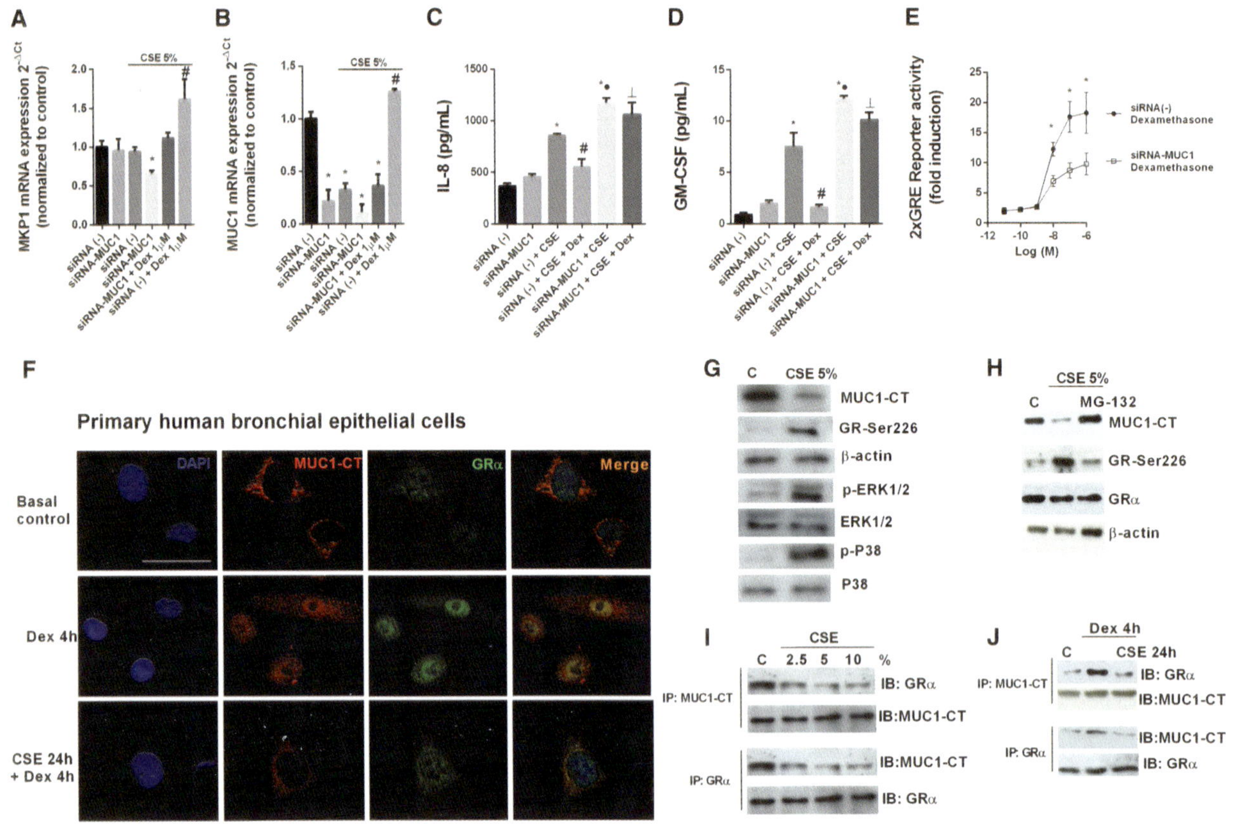

Fig. 4 MUC1 mediates dexamethasone anti-inflammatory effects. **a-e** Bronchial epithelial Beas2b cells were transiently transfected with siRNA-MUC1 or with control siRNA(−) for 48 h, incubated with dexamethasone (Dex) for 1 h and (**a-d**) stimulated with cigarette smoke extract (CSE) during 24 h. **a**, **b** MKP1 and MUC1 mRNA gene expression was analyzed by real time PCR. **c**, **d** IL-8 and GM-CSF release was measured by ELISA. **e** Glucocorticoid response element (GRE) activation was measured after 4 h of dexamethasone incubation at different concentrations in Beas2b cells transfected with Cignal GRE Reporter Assay. **f** Confocal co-immunofluorescence analysis of glucocorticoid alpha (GRα) and MUC1-CT co-localization in primary human bronchial epithelial cells (HBECs) treated with dexamethasone during 4 h, and in cells incubated with CSE for 24 h followed by the incubation with dexamethasone for 4 h. DAPI was used to mark cell nuclei. Scale bar: 5 μm. **g** Protein expression measured by western blot in HBEC stimulated with CSE during 24 h. **h** HBECs were incubated with MG132 5 μM during 1 h followed by CSE stimulation during 24 h. Western blot of different proteins was analysed. **i** Immunoprecipitation of MUC1-CT and GRα in HBECs stimulated with different concentrations of CSE. **j** Immunoprecipitation of MUC1-CT and GRα in HBECs incubated with CSE during 24 h followed by the stimulation with dexamethasone during 4 h. Representative western blot are showed. The results are shown as mean ± SE of n = 4 independent experiments. Gene expression was analyzed by real time PCR using the $2^{-\Delta Ct}$ as described in methods. One-way ANOVA followed by Bonferroni post-hoc tests. **a**, **b** **P* < 0.05 compared with siRNA(−) transfected cells; #*P* < 0.05 compared with siRNA-MUC1 + Dex group. **c**, **d**) **P* < 0.05 compared with siRNA(−) transfected cells; # and •*P* < 0.05 compared with siRNA(−) + CSE group; ⊥*P* < 0.05 compared with siRNA(−) + CSE + Dex group. **e** **P* < 0.05 compared with siRNA-MUC1 + Dex group

reduces GR-ser[226] expression in lung tissue of WT control mice (Fig. 8a, b). However, dexamethasone showed impaired effects reducing GR-ser[226] expression in Muc1 KO animals. LPS inflammation, but not LPS + CS, increased the expression of Muc1-CT in lung tissue from WT control animals (Fig. 8c). Neither LPS nor LPS + CS modified the Muc1-CT distribution (data not shown). Furthermore, dexamethasone at the highest dose, increased the Muc1-CT expression (Fig. 8c). The anti-inflammatory effects of corticosteroids are partially mediated by the inhibition of the phosphorylation of different intracellular pathways. Thus, for example, p38 and ERK1/2 phosphorylations are typically enhanced by LPS and in cells from COPD patients. In this work, dexamethasone reduced the phosphorylation of p38 and ERK1/2 at 3 mg and 10 mg/kg/day in WT controls stimulated with LPS, but only at 10 mg/kg/day when it was stimulated with LPS + CS. In Muc1 KO animals, dexamethasone showed lesser effect inhibiting p38 and ERK1/2 phosphorylation (Fig. 8d-f).

Confocal immunofluorescence showed a Muc1-CT-GRα co-localization in the bronchial epithelial cell cytoplasm of WT mice. The treatment with dexamethasone induced the bronchial epithelial cell nuclear translocation of the Muc1-CT-GRα complex (Fig. 9). In Muc1 KO animals GRα was expressed in

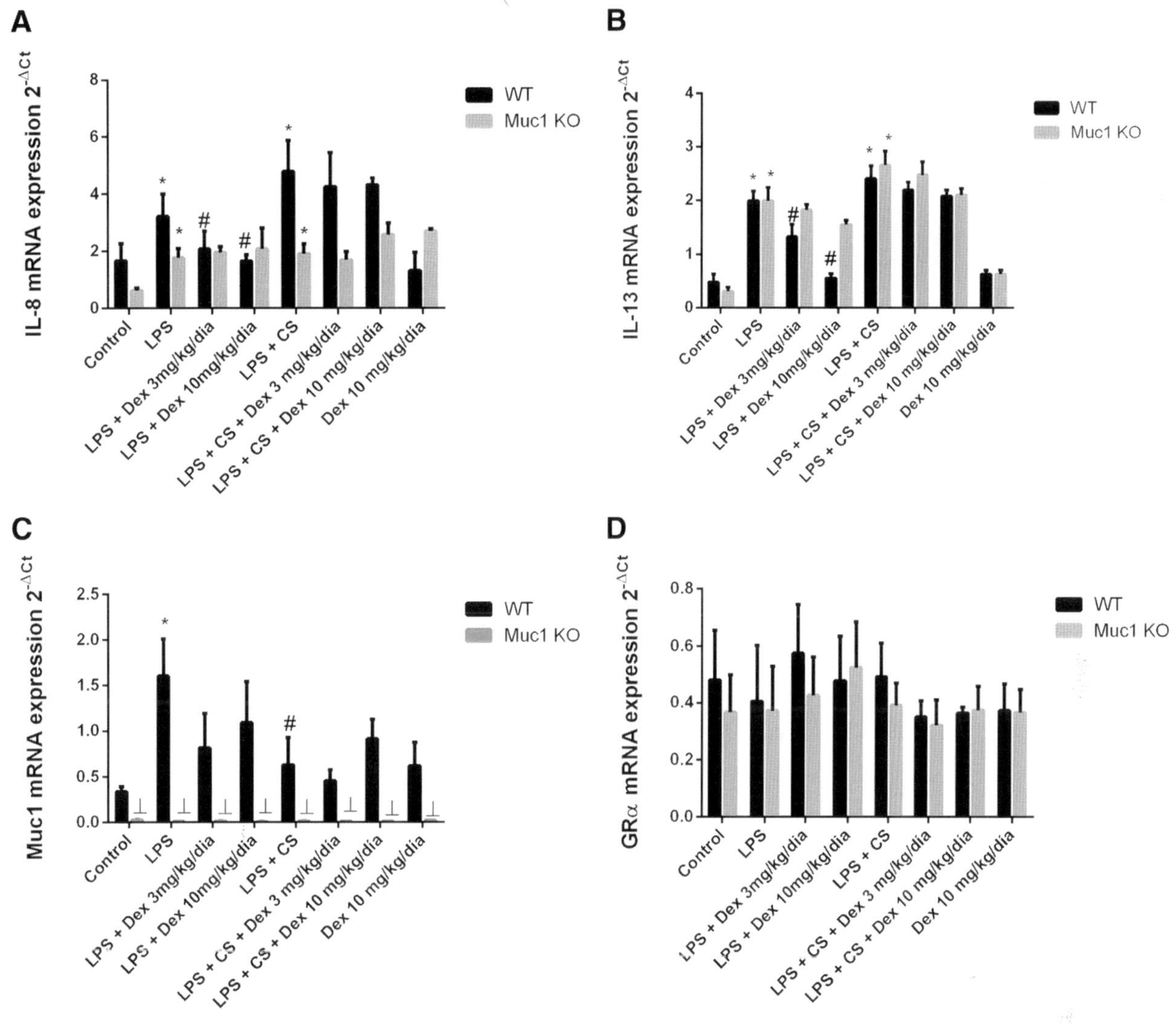

Fig. 5 Muc1 KO mice is resistant to the anti-inflammatory effects of dexamethasone in a model of acute cigarette smoke inflammation. C57BL/6 Muc1 KO mice and WT mice were undergoing intranasal instillation of 75 μg of lipopolysaccharide (LPS) at day 1. Between days 2 and 3, animals were exposed to cigarette smoke (or control air) of 6 cigarettes followed by 8 cigarettes (or control air) at days 4 and 5, and 10 cigarettes (or control air) at day 6. Vehicle or dexamethasone at 3 mg/kg/day and 10 mg/kg/day was administered orally once a day between day 1 and 6. Animals were sacrificed at day 6 and lungs were homogenized to analyze the gene mRNA expression of (**a**) IL-8, (**b**) IL-13, (**c**) Muc1 and (**d**) GRα. Gene expression was analyzed by real time PCR using the $2^{\Delta Ct}$ as described in methods. Results are the mean ± SE of $n = 8$ animals per experimental group. One-way ANOVA followed by Bonferroni post-hoc tests. *$P < 0.05$ compared with control. #$P < 0.05$ compared with LPS. ⊥$P < 0.05$ compared with WT. KO: knock out; WT: wild type; CS: cigarette smoke; LPS: lipopolysaccharide

bronchial epithelial cell cytoplasm, but nuclear translocation in response to dexamethasone was not observed (Fig. 9).

Discussion

The present work shows that the loss of MUC1-CT expression mediates corticosteroid resistance in in vitro and in vivo models relevant to the COPD pathology. MUC1-CT was downregulated in lung tissue, isolated bronchial epithelial cells and neutrophils from heavy smokers and COPD patients resistant to corticosteroids. Furthermore, cigarette smoke extract decreased MUC1-CT expression. In vitro cell MUC1 gene silencing and animal in vivo MUC1 KO model of COPD inflammation demonstrated that corticosteroids mediate part of their anti-inflammatory effects by forming MUC1-CT-GRα complexes that translocate to the cell nucleus to increase the expression of anti-inflammatory genes. These results support previous findings in corticosteroid resistant chronic rhinosinusitis with nasal polyps (CRSwNP) [12] which may be of potential value to explain, almost in part, the loss of corticosteroid efficacy in COPD.

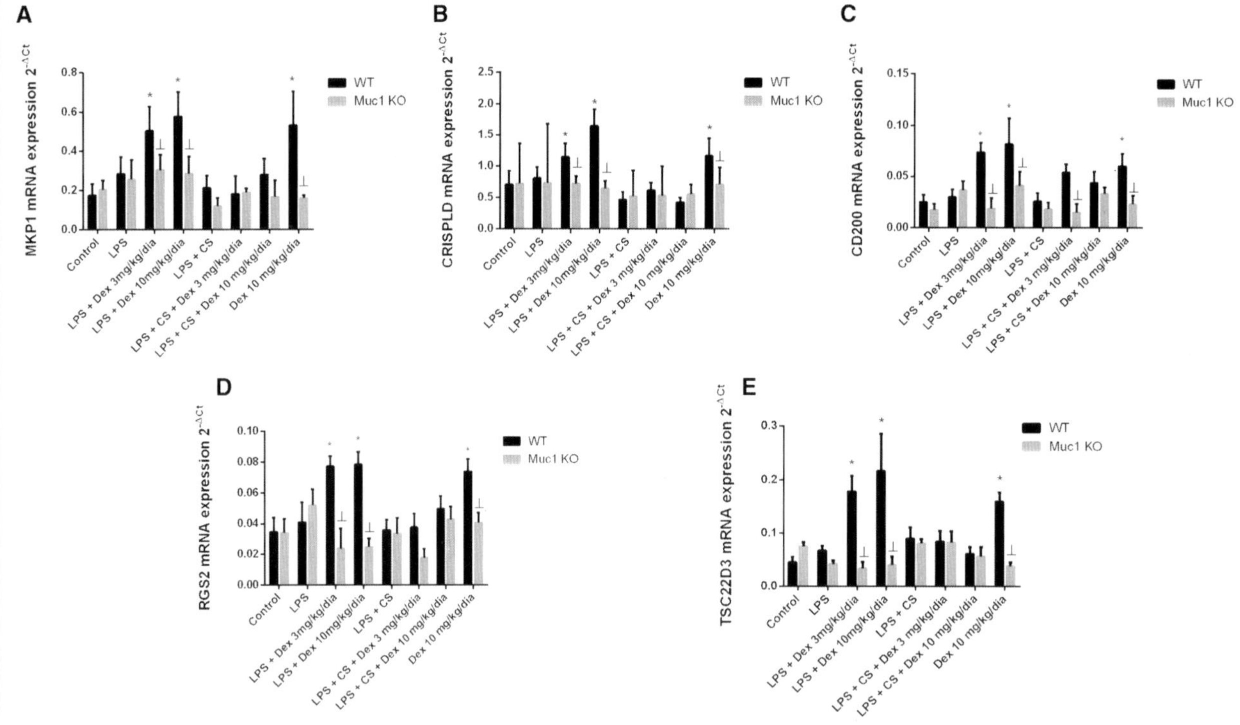

Fig. 6 Corticosteroid anti-inflammatory inducible genes expression is resistant to dexamethasone in Muc1 KO mice. C57BL/6 Muc1 KO mice and WT mice were undergoing intranasal instillation of 75 µg of lipopolysaccharide (LPS) at day 1. Between days 2 and 3, animals were exposed to cigarette smoke (or control air) of 6 cigarettes followed by 8 cigarettes (or control air) at days 4 and 5, and 10 cigarettes (or control air) at day 6. Vehicle or dexamethasone at 3 mg/kg/day and 10 mg/kg/day was administered orally once a day between day 1 and 6. Animals were sacrificed at day 6 and lungs were homogenized to analyze the gene mRNA expression of different corticosteroid-inducible genes such as (**a**) MKP1, (**b**) CRISPLD, (**c**) CD200, (**d**) RGS2 and (**e**) TSC22D3. Gene expression was analyzed by real time PCR using the $2^{\Delta Ct}$ as described in methods. Results are the mean ± SE of n = 8 animals per experimental group. One-way ANOVA followed by Bonferroni post-hoc tests. **P* < 0.05 compared with control. ┴*P* < 0.05 compared with WT. KO: knock out; WT: wild type; CS: cigarette smoke; LPS: lipopolysaccharide

The use of ICS in COPD is currently under debate. Recent clinical trials using fixed-dose combinations of LAMA/LABA have demonstrated more effectiveness than the LAMA or LABA alone in terms of improvement in trough FEV1, transitional dyspnea index (TDI) and St. George's Respiratory Questionnaire (SGRQ) scores [31]. The recent study FLAME showed that the combination of indacaterol (110 µg) plus glycopyrronium (50 µg) was superior to salmeterol (50 µg) plus fluticasone (500 µg) improving FEV_1 and preventing acute exacerbations of COPD in both moderate and severe COPD patients [32, 33]. However the LABA/ICS combination or the triple therapy LABA/LAMA/ICS seems superior in the cases of very severe airflow limitation [32]. The evidence that dual bronchodilation can prevent or at least delay the onset of acute exacerbations of COPD raises the fundamental questions whether it makes sense to switch all patients from a LABA/ICS regimen to a LABA/LAMA regimen on the basis of the improvement in lung function and the lower exacerbation rates [34] or there is a subgroup of patients with COPD who may benefit the most from this therapy. Perhaps the nature of COPD exacerbations (viral or bacterial) or the inflammatory phenotype (eosinophils vs neutrophils) could help us to appropriately select the correct regimen therapy. In this regard, the role of elevated blood eosinophils as a biomarker for the identification of candidates for ICS treatment is currently debated, although recent pooled analysis have ruled out the association of blood eosinophils as predictor of ICS good response [35].

Therefore, there is a need to understand the different cellular and molecular mechanisms implicated in the loss of corticosteroid efficacy in COPD. A good understanding of corticosteroid resistance could be of potential value to design new strategies such as the addition of novel drugs to reverse corticosteroid resistance [36] or the analysis of corticosteroid resistance biomarkers to avoid ICS therapy. Between the different molecular processes associated to the loss of corticosteroid efficacy, the most analyzed process involves the activation of phosphatidylinositide 3-kinase (PI3K) δ that switch off histone deacetylase 2 (HDAC2) to avoid the correct GRα-corticosteroid inhibition of NF-kB–dependent inflammatory gene expression

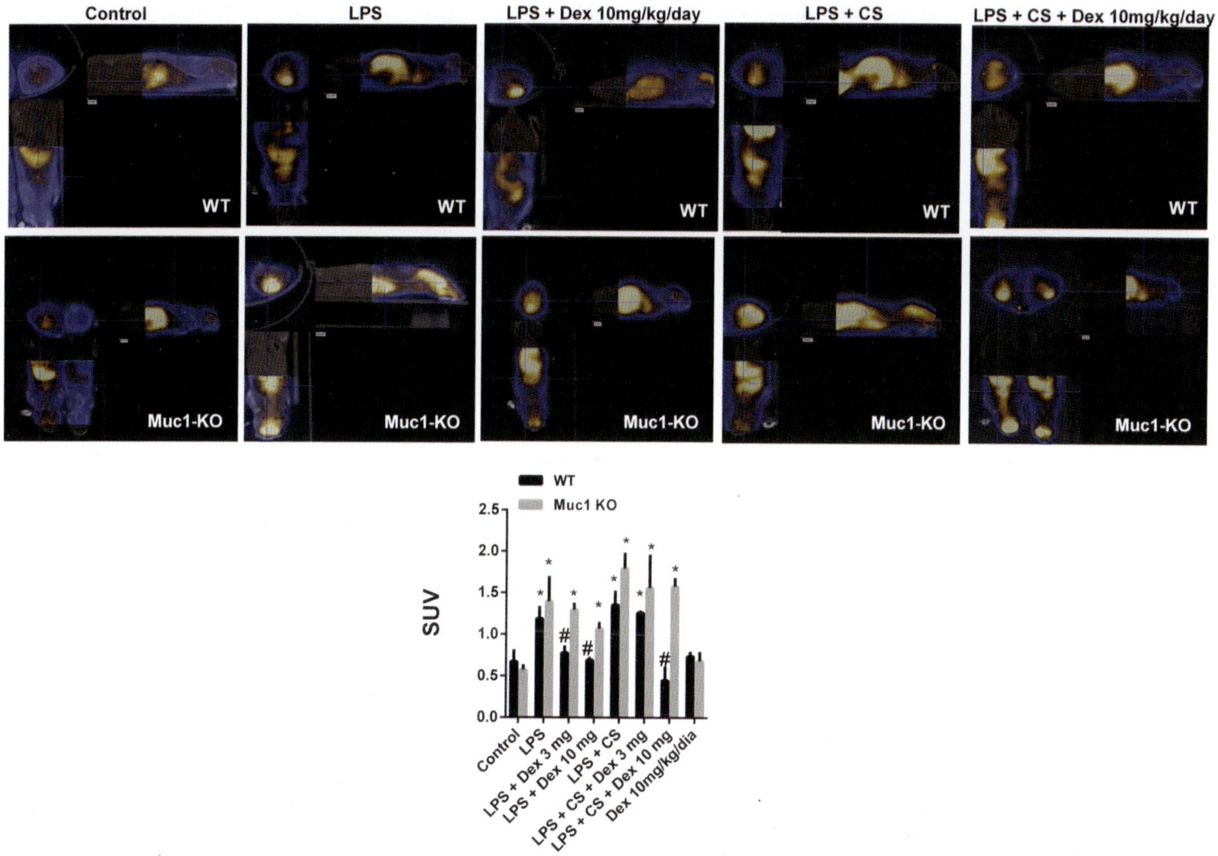

Fig. 7 Muc1 KO mice is resistant to the anti-inflammatory effects of dexamethasone in a model of acute cigarette smoke inflammation analysed by micro-CT-PET. C57BL/6 Muc1 KO mice and WT mice were undergoing intranasal instillation of 75 μg of lipopolysaccharide (LPS) at day 1. Between days 2 and 3, animals were exposed to cigarette smoke (or control air) of 6 cigarettes followed by 8 cigarettes (or control air) at days 4 and 5, and 10 cigarettes (or control air) at day 6. Vehicle or dexamethasone at 3 mg/kg/day and 10 mg/kg/day was administered orally once a day between day 1 and 6. Computed tomography (CT) followed by positron emission tomography (PET) of fludeoxyglucose ^{18}F (^{18}F-FDG) was measured as standard uptake value (SUV). Representative images are showed. Results are the mean ± SE of n = 8 animals per experimental group. One-way ANOVA followed by Bonferroni post-hoc tests. *$P < 0.05$ compared with control. #$P < 0.05$ compared with LPS/ LPS + CS. KO: knock out; WT: wild type; CS: cigarette smoke; LPS: lipopolysaccharide

[37]. Also, GRα modifications such as the phosphorylation at specific serine residues of GRα, such as ser^{226}, impedes nuclear translocation, leading to steroid resistance [38]. The sustained inflammation in COPD is believed to increase and perpetuate the GR-ser^{226} status [38]. In this regard, the innate immune system through the chronic stimulation of TLRs activates intracellular p38, ERK1/2 and JNK1 intracellular pathways that can phosphorylate GRα at ser^{226} [39, 40]. TLR4 is activated by lipopolysaccharide (LPS) of gram negative bacteria and cigarette smoke, and its expression appears to be chronically elevated in bronchial epithelial cells from stable severe and very severe COPD patients, contributing to airway chronic inflammation [41]. In this work we confirmed this observations, showing an increase of TLR4 expression in bronchial epithelial cells and neutrophils from heavy smokers and COPD patients. Unlike TLR4, the expression of MUC1-CT was decreased in lung tissue, bronchial epithelial cells and neutrophils from heavy smokers and COPD patients. Cytoplasmic MUC1-CT mediates anti-inflammatory effects through the interaction with TLR signal components [8, 42]. Therefore, the higher expression of TLR4 and low expression of MUC1-CT implicates a greater inflammatory response. In this work, both, LPS and CSE promoted a higher inflammatory response in bronchial epithelial cells and neutrophils from heavy smokers and COPD patients. Furthermore, bronchial epithelial cells transiently transfected with siRNA-MUC1 showed higher amounts of IL-8 and GM-CSF than siRNA controls in response to CSE. In this line, Muc1-KO animals showed higher amount of BAL inflammatory cells and inflammation, thus confirming the anti-inflammatory role of MUC1-CT.

In contrast to our findings, recent data indicate that sputum MUC1 is increased in the acute phase of COPD exacerbation and also in the BALF of mice

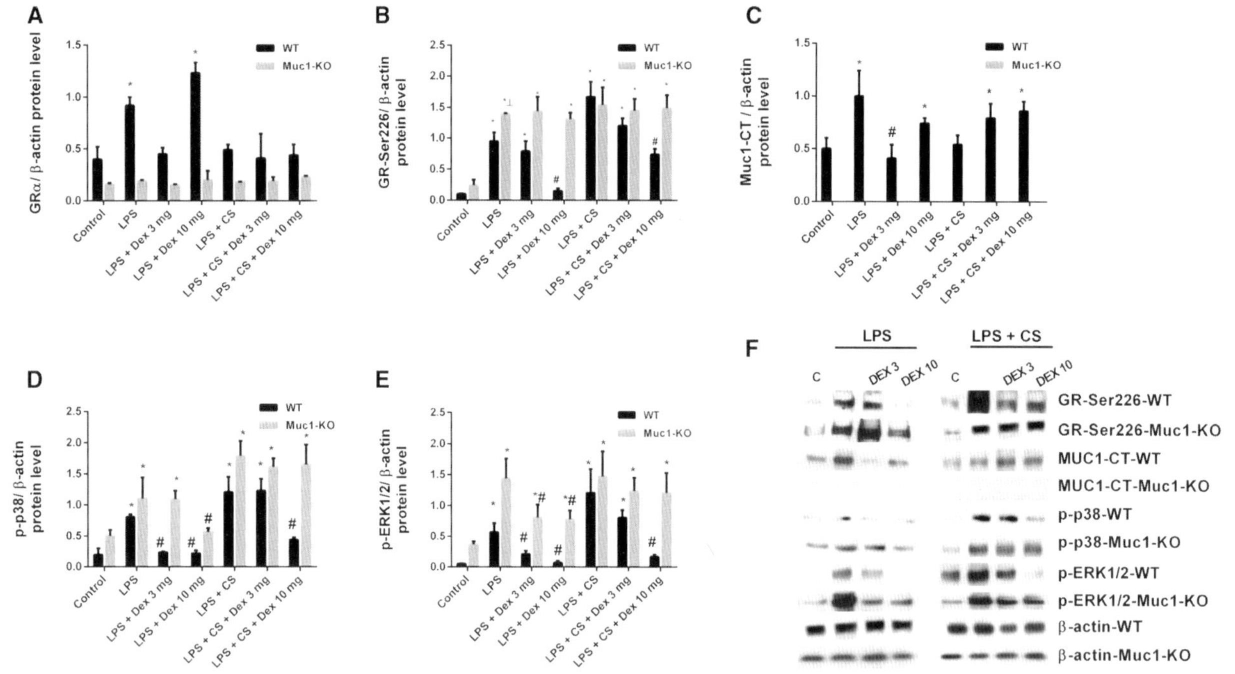

Fig. 8 Mechanistic pathways involved in corticosteroid resistance of Muc1 KO mice. C57BL/6 Muc1 KO mice and WT mice were undergoing intranasal instillation of 75 μg of lipopolysaccharide (LPS) at day 1. Between days 2 and 3, animals were exposed to cigarette smoke (or control air) of 6 cigarettes followed by 8 cigarettes (or control air) at days 4 and 5, and 10 cigarettes (or control air) at day 6. Vehicle or dexamethasone at 3 mg/kg/day and 10 mg/kg/day was administered orally once a day between day 1 and 6. Animals were sacrificed at day 6 and lungs were homogenized to analyze protein expression of (**a**) glucocorticoid receptor alpha (GRα), (**b**) GR phosphorylated at ser226 (GR-ser^{226}), (**c**) Muc1 cytoplasmic tail (CT), (**d**) phospho-p38 and (**e**) phopho-ERK1/2. Protein expression was normalized to β-actin. **f** Representative western blots are showed. Results are the mean ± SE of n = 8 animals per experimental group. One-way ANOVA followed by Bonferroni post-hoc tests. *$P < 0.05$ compared with control. #$P < 0.05$ compared with LPS/ LPS + CS. KO: knock out; WT: wild type; CS: cigarette smoke; LPS: lipopolysaccharide

instilled with intranasal LPS [43]. In this work, intranasal instillation of LPS also increased MUC1 expression in lung tissue that was abrogated with the combination of CS. Difference observed could be explained by the nature of COPD patients studied, since we analyzed samples from stable COPD and not from exacerbations that can trigger MUC1 transiently as anti-inflammatory endogenous control to limit excessive inflammation [43].

The lack of MUC1-CT not only promoted a higher inflammation but reduced the anti-inflammatory effect of corticosteroids. As commented above, the over-activation of TLR4 in absence of MUC1-CT could increase the chronic phosphorylation of p38 and ERK1/2 to promote GR-ser^{226} and consequently inducing corticosteroid resistance. In this work, dexamethasone was unable to inhibit p38 and ERK1/2 phosphorylations in lungs from Muc1 KO mice, thus allowing sustained and elevated levels of GR-ser^{226} which has been related with the lack of GRα cell nuclear translocation [12]. These data was corroborated in confocal microscope and immunoprecipitation in vitro studies using bronchial epithelial cells, showing nuclear translocation of MUC1-CT-GRα complex after dexamethasone stimulation that was inhibited by cigarette smoke pre-incubation. Similar results were observed in vivo in mice Muc1 KO bronchial epithelial cells. The interaction of MUC1-CT forming a complex with GRα has been observed previously in beas2b bronchial epithelial cells and nasal polyp tissue confirming the results of this study [12]. However, MUC1-CT can interact with other proteins. This is the case of the estrogen receptor (ER)-α and β-catenin that can form complexes with MUC1-CT to stabilize and protect ERα and β-catenin from their ubiquitination and degradation allowing nuclear translocation of both proteins [11, 44]. These findings are in line with a possible protective role of MUC1-CT on GRα. In this work, the proteasomal inhibitor MG-132 prevented the CSE-induced MUC1-CT decrease, suggesting that CSE mediates MUC1-CT downregulation via proteasomal degradation. In the same way, proteasomal inhibition reduced the GR-ser^{226} expression, suggesting that MUC1-CT could protect GRα against phosphorylation at serine 226.

Corticosteroids mediates part of their anti-inflammatory effects through the activation of GRE gene regions, thus

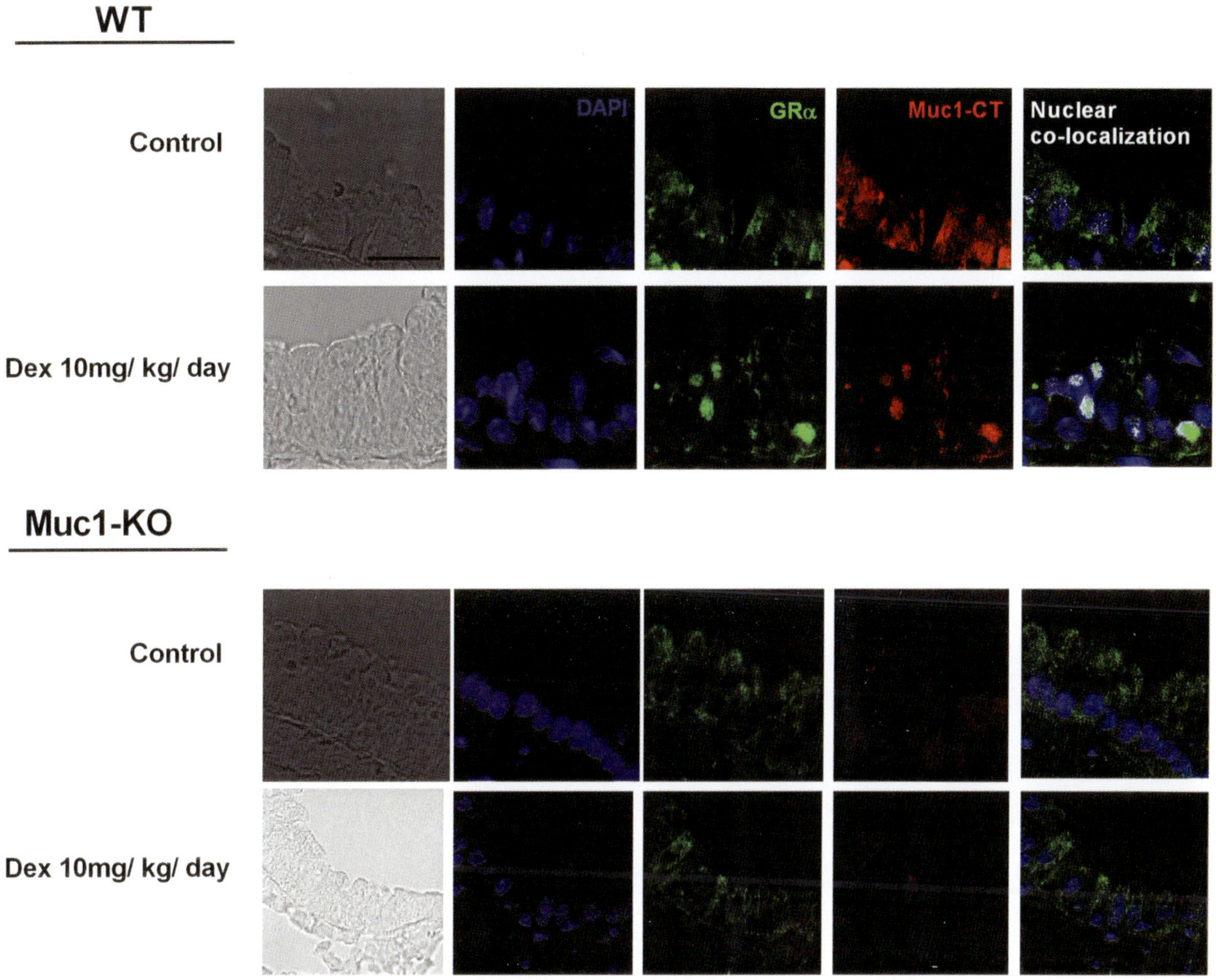

Fig. 9 Dexamethasone induces Muc1-CT nuclear translocation and co-localization with GRα in bronchial epithelium of WT mice but not in MUC1 KO mice. C57BL/6 Muc1 KO mice and WT mice were undergoing dexamethasone 10 mg/kg/day (orally) for 6 days. Animals were sacrificed at day 6 and lungs were fixed in paraformaldehyde (4%) for 48 h and embedded in Tissue-Tek® OCT™ cryosectioning compound. Lung slices were immunostained with MUC1-cytoplasmic tail (CT) and glucocorticoid receptor alpha (GRα) antibodies with rhodamine/fluorescein secondary antibodies. DAPI was used to mark cell nucleus. Representative con-focal images are showed. Scale bar: 5 μm

increasing the expression of corticosteroid dependent anti-inflammatory genes. In this work, bronchial epithelial cells transfected with siRNA-MUC1 showed an impaired GRE activation in response to growing concentrations of dexamethasone that was translated in a lack of expression of corticosteroid inducible anti-inflammatory MKP1 gene. Similar findings were observed in Muc1 KO mice, in which corticosteroid-inducible anti-inflammatory genes MKP1, CRISPLD, CD200, RGS2 and TSC22D3 were resistant to dexamethasone. Interestingly, WT control animals stimulated with LPS and CS were also resistant to the effect of dexamethasone increasing anti-inflammatory genes and inhibiting inflammatory cytokines such as IL8 and IL13 which related CS with resistance to corticosteroids as previously outlined [4].

However, although the findings of this study provide a rational explanation for the lack of efficacy of corticosteroids in patients with COPD, other mechanisms may also be implicated [37], thus sharing different mechanisms that can contribute to the final COPD phenotype.

Conclusions

We have demonstrated a new role for MUC1-CT in the modulation of the anti-inflammatory effects of corticosteroids in COPD. Our findings suggest a possible explanation for why corticosteroids cannot repress inflammation in COPD, thus contributing to the amount of knowledge of corticosteroid resistance processes in COPD which may be of potential value to develop new strategies to the COPD treatment.

Abbreviations

COPD: Chronic obstructive pulmonary disease; CSE: Cigarette smoke extract; ERK1/2: Extracellular signal–regulated kinases; GM-CSF: Granulocyte-macrophage colony-stimulating factor; GRE: Glucocorticoid response element; GRα: Glucocorticoid receptor alpha; HBEC: Human bronchial epithelial cells; HDAC2: Histone deacetylase; ICS: Inhaled corticosteroids; LABA: Long-acting beta 2 agonists; LAMA: Long-acting muscarinic antagonist; LPS: Lipopolysaccharide; MIP3α: Macrophage Inflammatory Protein-3; MKP1: Mitogen-activated protein kinase phosphatase 1; MMP9: Matrix metallopeptidase 9; MUC1-CT: Mucin 1 cytoplasmic tail; PET: Positron emission tomography; SUV: Standard uptake value; TLR: Toll like receptor

Acknowledgments

We thank the personnel of the Dept. of Pathology at the General University Hospital of Valencia and the animal housing facilities of the University of Valencia, Spain.

Funding

This work was supported by the grants SAF2017–82913-R (JC), SAF2014–55399-R (AC), FIS PI14/01733 (JM), FIS PI17/02158 (JM), SAF2015–65368-R (EM), CIBERES (CB06/06/0027), TRACE (TRA2009–0311; Spanish Government), and by research grants from the Regional Government Prometeo 2017/023/UV (JC, EM), ACIF/2016/341 (BB), ACIF/2017/A/370 (PR) from "Generalitat Valenciana". Funding entities did not contribute to the study design or data collection, analysis and interpretation nor to the writing of the manuscript.

Authors' contributions

Conception and design: JM, LDP, EM and JC. Data acquisition: JM, LDP, SC, PR, IR, BB, PM and AC. Analysis and interpretation: JM, LDP, SC, PR, IR, BB, PM, AC, EM and JC. All authors read and approved the final manuscript.

Competing interests

The authors declare that they have no competing interests.

Author details

[1]Department of Pharmacology, Faculty of Medicine, Jaume I University, Castellón de la Plana, Spain. [2]Pharmacy Unit, University General Hospital Consortium, Valencia, Spain. [3]CIBERES, Health Institute Carlos III, Valencia, Spain. [4]Unidade Radiofármacos PET, GALARIA, Santiago de Compostela, A Coruña, Spain. [5]Department of Pharmacology, Faculty of Medicine, University of Valencia, Valencia, Spain. [6]Department of Pharmacology, School of Medicine, Universidad Complutense de Madrid, Madrid, Spain. [7]Health Research Institute INCLIVA, Valencia, Spain. [8]Research and teaching Unit, University General Hospital Consortium, Valencia, Spain. [9]Unidad de Investigación Clínica, Consorcio Hospital General Universitario, Avenida tres cruces s/n, E-46014 Valencia, Spain.

References

1. Mathers CD, Loncar D. Projections of global mortality and burden of disease from 2002 to 2030. PLoS Med. 2006;3:e442.
2. Roche N, Marthan R, Berger P, Chambellan A, Chanez P, Aguilaniu B, Brillet PY, Burgel PR, Chaouat A, Devillier P, et al. Beyond corticosteroids: future prospects in the management of inflammation in COPD. Eur Respir Rev. 2011;20:175–82.
3. Welte T, Miravitlles M, Hernandez P, Eriksson G, Peterson S, Polanowski T, Kessler R. Efficacy and tolerability of budesonide/formoterol added to tiotropium in patients with chronic obstructive pulmonary disease. Am J Respir Crit Care Med. 2009;180:741–50.
4. Barnes PJ. Glucocorticosteroids. Handb Exp Pharmacol. 2017;237:93–115.
5. Kim KC, Lillehoj EP. MUC1 mucin: a peacemaker in the lung. Am J Respir Cell Mol Biol. 2008;39:644–7.
6. Kyo Y, Kato K, Park YS, Gajghate S, Umehara T, Lillehoj EP, Suzaki H, Kim KC. Antiinflammatory role of MUC1 mucin during infection with nontypeable Haemophilus influenzae. Am J Respir Cell Mol Biol. 2012;46:149–56.
7. Li Y, Dinwiddie DL, Harrod KS, Jiang Y, Kim KC. Anti-inflammatory effect of MUC1 during respiratory syncytial virus infection of lung epithelial cells in vitro. Am J Physiol Lung Cell Mol Physiol. 2010;298:L558–63.
8. Ueno K, Koga T, Kato K, Golenbock DT, Gendler SJ, Kai H, Kim KC. MUC1 mucin is a negative regulator of toll-like receptor signaling. Am J Respir Cell Mol Biol. 2008;38:263–8.
9. Hattrup CL, Gendler SJ. Structure and function of the cell surface (tethered) mucins. Annu Rev Physiol. 2008;70:431–57.
10. Bafna S, Kaur S, Batra SK. Membrane-bound mucins: the mechanistic basis for alterations in the growth and survival of cancer cells. Oncogene. 2010; 29:2893–904.
11. Chen YT, Gallup M, Nikulina K, Lazarev S, Zlock L, Finkbeiner W, McNamara N. Cigarette smoke induces epidermal growth factor receptor-dependent redistribution of apical MUC1 and junctional beta-catenin in polarized human airway epithelial cells. Am J Pathol. 2010;177:1255–64.
12. Milara J, Peiro T, Armengot M, Frias S, Morell A, Serrano A, Cortijo J. Mucin 1 downregulation associates with corticosteroid resistance in chronic rhinosinusitis with nasal polyps. J Allergy Clin Immunol. 2015;135:470–6.
13. Milara J, Armengot M, Banuls P, Tenor H, Beume R, Artigues E, Cortijo J. Roflumilast N-oxide, a PDE4 inhibitor, improves cilia motility and ciliated human bronchial epithelial cells compromised by cigarette smoke in vitro. Br J Pharmacol. 2012;166:2243–62.
14. Milara J, Juan G, Peiro T, Serrano A, Cortijo J. Neutrophil activation in severe, early-onset COPD patients versus healthy non-smoker subjects in vitro: effects of antioxidant therapy. Respiration. 2012;83:147–58.
15. Pizzichini E, Pizzichini MM, Efthimiadis A, Evans S, Morris MM, Squillace D, Gleich GJ, Dolovich J, Hargreave FE. Indices of airway inflammation in induced sputum: reproducibility and validity of cell and fluid-phase measurements. Am J Respir Crit Care Med. 1996;154:308–17.
16. Milara J, Ortiz JL, Juan G, Guijarro R, Almudever P, Martorell M, Morcillo EJ, Cortijo J. Cigarette smoke exposure up-regulates endothelin receptor B in human pulmonary artery endothelial cells: molecular and functional consequences. Br J Pharmacol. 2010;161:1599–615.
17. Su Y, Han W, Giraldo C, De Li Y, Block ER. Effect of cigarette smoke extract on nitric oxide synthase in pulmonary artery endothelial cells. Am J Respir Cell Mol Biol. 1998;19:819–25.
18. Milara J, Peiro T, Serrano A, Cortijo J. Epithelial to mesenchymal transition is increased in patients with COPD and induced by cigarette smoke. Thorax. 2013;68:410–20.
19. Cortijo J, Iranzo A, Milara X, Mata M, Cerda-Nicolas M, Ruiz-Sauri A, Tenor H, Hatzelmann A, Morcillo EJ. Roflumilast, a phosphodiesterase 4 inhibitor, alleviates bleomycin-induced lung injury. Br J Pharmacol. 2009;156:534–44.
20. Milara J, Lluch J, Almudever P, Freire J, Xiaozhong Q, Cortijo J. Roflumilast N-oxide reverses corticosteroid resistance in neutrophils from patients with chronic obstructive pulmonary disease. J Allergy Clin Immunol. 2014;134:314–22.
21. Ralph JA, Ahmed AU, Santos LL, Clark AR, McMorrow J, Murphy EP, Morand EF. Identification of NURR1 as a mediator of MIF signaling during chronic arthritis: effects on glucocorticoid-induced MKP1. Am J Pathol. 2010;177:2366–78.
22. Holden NS, Bell MJ, Rider CF, King EM, Gaunt DD, Leigh R, Johnson M, Siderovski DP, Heximer SP, Giembycz MA, Newton R. beta2-adrenoceptor agonist-induced RGS2 expression is a genomic mechanism of bronchoprotection that is enhanced by glucocorticoids. Proc Natl Acad Sci U S A. 2011;108:19713–8.
23. Mittelstadt PR, Ashwell JD. Inhibition of AP-1 by the glucocorticoid-inducible protein GILZ. J Biol Chem. 2001;276:29603–10.
24. Wang ZQ, Xing WM, Fan HH, Wang KS, Zhang HK, Wang QW, Qi J, Yang HM, Yang J, Ren YN, et al. The novel lipopolysaccharide-binding protein CRISPLD2 is a critical serum protein to regulate endotoxin function. J Immunol. 2009;183:6646–56.
25. Snelgrove RJ, Goulding J, Didierlaurent AM, Lyonga D, Vekaria S, Edwards L, Gwyer E, Sedgwick JD, Barclay AN, Hussell T. A critical function for CD200 in lung immune homeostasis and the severity of influenza infection. Nat Immunol. 2008;9:1074–83.

26. Kilkenny C, Browne WJ, Cuthill IC, Emerson M, Altman DG. Improving bioscience research reporting: the ARRIVE guidelines for reporting animal research. PLoS Biol. 2010;8:e1000412.
27. Spicer AP, Rowse GJ, Lidner TK, Gendler SJ. Delayed mammary tumor progression in Muc-1 null mice. J Biol Chem. 1995;270:30093–101.
28. Al Faraj A, Sultana Shaik A, Pureza MA, Alnafea M, Halwani R. Preferential macrophage recruitment and polarization in LPS-induced animal model for COPD: noninvasive tracking using MRI. PLoS One. 2014;9:e90829.
29. Wollin L, Pieper MP. Tiotropium bromide exerts anti-inflammatory activity in a cigarette smoke mouse model of COPD. Pulm Pharmacol Ther. 2010;23:345–54.
30. Ishikawa N, Hattori N, Yokoyama A, Kohno N. Utility of KL-6/MUC1 in the clinical management of interstitial lung diseases. Respir Investig. 2012;50:3–13.
31. Calzetta L, Rogliani P, Matera MG, Cazzola M, Systematic Review A. With meta-analysis of dual bronchodilation with LAMA/LABA for the treatment of stable COPD. Chest. 2016;149:1181–96.
32. Wedzicha JA, Banerji D, Chapman KR, Vestbo J, Roche N, Ayers RT, Thach C, Fogel R, Patalano F, Vogelmeier CF, Investigators F. Indacaterol-Glycopyrronium versus salmeterol-fluticasone for COPD. N Engl J Med. 2016; 374:2222–34.
33. Vogelmeier C, Zhong N, Humphries MJ, Mezzi K, Fogel R, Bader G, Patalano F, Banerji D. Indacaterol/glycopyrronium in symptomatic patients with COPD (GOLD B and GOLD D) versus salmeterol/fluticasone: ILLUMINATE/LANTERN pooled analysis. Int J Chron Obstruct Pulmon Dis. 2016;11:3189–97.
34. Donohue JF. Another choice for prevention of COPD exacerbations. N Engl J Med. 2016;374:2284–6.
35. Roche N, Chapman KR, Vogelmeier CF, Herth FJF, Thach C, Fogel R, Olsson P, Patalano F, Banerji D, Wedzicha JA. Blood eosinophils and response to maintenance chronic obstructive pulmonary disease treatment. Data from the FLAME Trial. Am J Respir Crit Care Med. 2017;195:1189–97.
36. Koenderman L, Chilvers ER. Future treatment in patients with chronic obstructive pulmonary disease: to reverse or not to reverse steroid resistance-that is the question. J Allergy Clin Immunol. 2014;134:323–4.
37. Barnes PJ. Corticosteroid resistance in patients with asthma and chronic obstructive pulmonary disease. J Allergy Clin Immunol. 2013;131:636–45.
38. Kobayashi Y, Ito K, Kanda A, Tomoda K, Mercado N, Barnes PJ. Impaired dual-specificity protein phosphatase DUSP4 reduces corticosteroid sensitivity. Mol Pharmacol. 2017;91:475–81.
39. Li LB, Goleva E, Hall CF, Ou LS, Leung DY. Superantigen-induced corticosteroid resistance of human T cells occurs through activation of the mitogen-activated protein kinase kinase/extracellular signal-regulated kinase (MEK-ERK) pathway. J Allergy Clin Immunol. 2004;114:1059–69.
40. Mercado N, Hakim A, Kobayashi Y, Meah S, Usmani OS, Chung KF, Barnes PJ, Ito K. Restoration of corticosteroid sensitivity by p38 mitogen activated protein kinase inhibition in peripheral blood mononuclear cells from severe asthma. PLoS One. 2012;7:e41582.
41. Di Stefano A, Ricciardolo FLM, Caramori G, Adcock IM, Chung KF, Barnes PJ, Brun P, Leonardi A, Ando F, Vallese D, et al. Bronchial inflammation and bacterial load in stable COPD is associated with TLR4 overexpression. Eur Respir J. 2017;5:23–49.
42. Kato K, Lillehoj EP, Park YS, Umehara T, Hoffman NE, Madesh M, Kim KC. Membrane-tethered MUC1 mucin is phosphorylated by epidermal growth factor receptor in airway epithelial cells and associates with TLR5 to inhibit recruitment of MyD88. J Immunol. 2012;188:2014–22.
43. Zheng Z, Qi Y, Xu X, Jiang H, Li Z, Yang Q, Zhang C, Zhang K, Chen R, Wang J, Lu W. Sputum mucin 1 is increased during the acute phase of chronic obstructive pulmonary disease exacerbation. J Thorac Dis. 2017;9: 1873–82.
44. Wei X, Xu H, Kufe D. MUC1 oncoprotein stabilizes and activates estrogen receptor alpha. Mol Cell. 2006;21:295–305.

20

Primary immunodeficiency diseases in lung disease: warning signs, diagnosis and management

Pere Soler-Palacín[1*], Javier de Gracia[1,6], Luis Ignacio González-Granado[2], Carlos Martín[3], Carlos Rodríguez-Gallego[4], Silvia Sánchez-Ramón[5] and Lung ID-Signal Group

Abstract

Background: Pulmonary complications are common in primary immunodeficiency diseases (PID) and contribute to morbidity and mortality in these patients. However, their varied presentation and a general lack of awareness of PID in this setting make early diagnosis and treatment difficult. The aim of this study was to define the warning signs of PID in patients with respiratory manifestations, the necessary diagnostic tests, and the therapeutic management of both children and adults.

Methods: A review of the literature was performed, and 43 PID interdisciplinary specialists were consulted.

Results: This document identifies the pulmonary and extrapulmonary manifestations that should prompt a suspicion of PID, the immunological and respiratory tests that should be included in the diagnostic process according to the level of care, recommendations regarding the use of immunoglobulin replacement therapy according to the specific immunodeficiency, and the minimum recommended immunological and pulmonary monitoring in these patients.

Conclusions: This document is the first to combine scientific evidence with the opinion of a broad panel of experts specializing in the treatment of patients with immunodeficiencies. It aims to provide a useful tool for all practitioners who are regularly involved in the management of these patients.

Keywords: "Immunoglobulins/deficiency"[mesh], "Antibodies/deficiency"[mesh], "Immunoglobulins/administration and dosage"[mesh], "Respiratory Tract Infections"[mesh], "Immunologic Deficiency Syndromes"[mesh]

Background

Immunodeficiency diseases (ID) are disorders involving a quantitative and/or functional disorder in the immune response [1] that may lead to a greater risk of infections, immune dysregulation, autoimmune phenomena, inflammation, and cancer. These IDs are classified as primary immunodeficiency diseases (PIDs) if their origin is genetic, and secondary (SID) if acquired.

PIDs comprise a heterogeneous group of more than 300 diseases. The Primary Immunodeficiencies Classification Committee of the International Union of Immunological Societies (IUIS) divides PIDs into 8 groups (9, if we include PID phenocopies), depending on their clinical and immunological phenotype [2]. The various congenital or acquired defects can affect both the innate and the acquired immune system [3]. The most common PIDs are predominantly antibody disorders (56.66%), other well defined PIDs (13.91%), phagocytic disorders (8.73%), predominantly T cell deficiencies (7.47%), and complement deficiencies (4.89%) [4].

The prevalence of PID in Europe and the United States ranges from 41 to 83 per 100,000 inhabitants, depending on the study [5, 6]. The diagnosis of PID often emerges from a picture of recurrent or unusual infections, autoimmune diseases, inflammatory processes or cancers. A careful approach must be taken in the early detection of these signs, in order to avoid unnecessary testing, but without delaying diagnosis. However, since their clinical presentation varies widely and understanding of this area is often limited, underdiagnosis and

* Correspondence: psoler@vhebron.net
[1]Hospital U. Vall d'Hebron, P. de la Vall d'Hebron, 119-129, 08035 Barcelona, Spain
Full list of author information is available at the end of the article

delayed diagnosis are common, generating significant morbidity and mortality [7] and a major social and economic impact [8]. Generally, the early clinical manifestations of PID occur during childhood, but they also are frequently encountered in the second or third decade of life, or even in older patients [9]. Moreover, there are different clinical presentations across various age categories and these presentations in children could widely differ from adult patients with PID [10].

New warning signs alerting to a suspicion of PID are being increasingly described, based on clinical presentations - mainly infectious diseases - and, in some cases, family history. Fifteen years ago, the Jeffrey Modell Foundation (JMF) defined the warning signs of suspected PID in children and adults [8, 11]. This document is a useful basis, but one that needs to be updated, as it does not refer to the autoimmune, inflammatory or malignant manifestations of PIDs, which can be the main clinical presentation in some of these diseases [12]. In addition, a follow-up study by Subbarayan *et at* highlighted the low sensitivity and specificity of these warning signs, recommending that PID awareness initiatives should be mainly targeted at hospital pediatricians and families with a history of PID although these initiatives should also include the general public [13].

Pulmonary complications in PID are common and significantly contribute to the morbidity and mortality of patients. Recurrent respiratory tract infections often constitute the first warning sign in some PIDs and are often the main cause of death in adults with PID [14, 15].

The aim of this study was to define which warning signs should alert to the suspicion of PID in patients with respiratory manifestations, and to develop proposals for intervention in these cases. This document is aimed at primary care (PC) professionals and specialists who see both adult and pediatric patients with respiratory diseases. This study is part of the ID-Signal Project, which aims to generate a series of documents based on the clinical manifestations of IDs dedicated to non-immunologists who may take care of patients with PID or SID in their clinical practice.

Methods

Initially, an interdisciplinary expert group formed of 2 pulmonologists, 2 immunologists and 2 pediatricians specializing in immunodeficiencies identified items to be addressed in the areas of clinical and laboratory testing, diagnostic imaging, functional tests, and therapeutic approach, and prepared a series of recommendations. A review of the literature was then performed, which acted as a basis for a discussion of the contents of the document in an in-person meeting. The main conclusions and recommendations were forwarded to an external panel of experts for their individual evaluation, depending on their specialty. Although we could have done a Delphi process involving at least two rounds, we preferred a single consultation to have a general view of the opinion of a larger group of experts and to make the process easier. The external panel consisted of 43 experts from all over Spain, with experience in the diagnosis and treatment of PID, working in Spanish National Health System centers. In total, 19 immunologists specializing in adults (adult immunologists, AI), 15 pediatric specialists in immunodeficiencies (pediatric immunologists, PI), 5 pulmonologists taking care of adults (adult pulmonologists, AP), and 4 pediatric specialists in pulmonology (pediatric pulmonologists, PP) participated.

This panel indicated their level of agreement on a scale of 1 to 4, with 1 reflecting "strongly disagree" and 4 "strongly agree", and they could also add comments when necessary. The results were pooled and the percentages of votes in the categories 1 and 2 (disagree) and in the categories 3 and 4 (agreement) were calculated. Unanimity was determined when 100% of the experts agreed with recommendation/conclusion; consensus, when at least 80% of the experts agreed without unanimity; majority, when more than 65% and less than 80% of the experts agreed with the recommendation/conclusion; and disagreement, when the percentage of agreement was 65% or less.

Results and discussion

Lung diseases that should prompt a suspicion of PID

In general, lung complications caused by PID include respiratory tract infections, interstitial lung disease (ILD), and cancers [14]. Recurrent lung infections are often the first warning sign in both adult and pediatric PID patients. These recurrent infections often cause permanent lung damage if appropriate treatment is not promptly initiated. Usually, there are also frequent upper respiratory infections previous to the lower ones, so an optimal pulmonary management should encompass the upper airway [16]. Airway damage can manifest as air trapping, thickening of the bronchial walls, atelectasis and/or bronchiectasis [14, 17]. The pathogens most commonly associated with pneumonia in patients with ID will depend on the type of immunodeficiency presented by the patient but generally include *Streptococcus pneumoniae* and *Haemophilus influenzae*, followed by *Mycoplasma* spp., *Staphylococcus* spp., *Moraxella* spp., *Pseudomonas aeruginosa*, and other viral pathogens, and more rarely *Pneumocystis jirovecii* and various fungi [18].

However, since mortality due to infectious complications has declined, non-infectious complications have begun to account for a large number of the poor clinical outcomes observed in some of these patients [19]. Thus, several histological patterns of ILD have been identified in patients with PID, especially in those with a diagnosis of common variable immunodeficiency disease (CVID), including granulomatous lung disease, lymphoid interstitial pneumonia (LIP), non-specific interstitial pneumonia (NSIP), and organizing pneumonia, and more than one may co-exist in the same patient [14].

The patient profile (adult or pediatric) and pulmonary manifestations (infectious or non-infectious) that lead to a consultation in PC or with a respiratory medicine specialist may be different. Manifestations that should prompt a suspicion of PID are included in Table 1. A respiratory medicine specialist must ensure that pneumonia is confirmed on radiology: this will be suggestive of PID, particularly if disease appears in different sites. Cases of slow-progressing disease must be investigated, and pneumonias that do not resolve with multiple course of antibiotics and require hospital admission, intravenous antibiotics or intensive care assistance, should be noted, along with a high frequency of pneumonias across time (one pneumonia per year for more than one year). Slow-progressing pneumonitis or bronchitis in an infant that requires admission, particularly in the intensive care unit, should be considered as potential

Table 1 Respiratory manifestations indicating a suspicion of PID in primary care and pulmonology clinics

Respiratory Manifestions with suspicion of PID in PC	N (Composition of panel)	Votes in agreement (%)	Degree of agreement
Adult patient			
Recurrent bronchial infections (≥ 2/year), with cough and purulent expectoration	23* (AI, AP)	87.0	**Consensus**
Idiopathic bronchiectasis	23* (AI, AP)	100.0	**Unanimity**
Recurrent pneumonias**	23* (AI, AP)	100.0	**Unanimity**
Chronic bronchial infection	23* (AI, AP)	91.3	**Consensus**
Need for prolonged antibiotic treatment for respiratory infections	23* (AI, AP)	95.7	**Consensus**
Pediatric patient			
Recurrent pneumonias**	19 (PI, PP)	100.0	**Unanimity**
Idiopathic bronchiectasis	19 (PI, PP)	100.0	**Unanimity**
Respiratory manifestations with suspicion of PID in pulmonolgy unit	**N (Composition panel)**	**Votes in agreement (%)**	**Degree of agreement**
Infections			
Adult and pediatric patients			
Recurrent bronchial infections (≥ 2/year), with cough and purulent expectoration	43 (AI, AP, PI, PP)	86.0	**Consensus**
Idiopathic bronchiectasis	43 (AI, AP, PI, PP)	100.0	**Unanimity**
Recurrent pneumonias**	43 (AI, AP, PI, PP)	97.7	**Consensus**
Chronic bronchial infection	43 (AI, AP, PI, PP)	90.7	**Consensus**
Need for prolonged antibiotic treatment for respiratory infections	43 (AI, AP, PI, PP)	93.0	**Consensus**
Pulmonary abscess and pneumatocele	43 (AI, AP, PI, PP)	90.7	**Consensus**
Infections caused by rare or opportunistic microorganisms	43 (AI, AP, PI, PP)	100.0	**Unanimity**
Infants			
Severe infantile bronchiolitis or pneumonia	43 (AI, AP, PI, PP)	93.0	**Consensus**
NON-INFECTIOUS			
Adult and pediatric patients			
Granulomatous-lymphocytic interstitial lung disease	43 (AI, AP, PI, PP)	100.0	**Unanimity**
Bronchiolitis obliterans	43 (AI, AP, PI, PP)	72.1	Majority
Lymphoproliferative syndrome	43 (AI, AP, PI, PP)	90.7	**Consensus**
Alveolar proteinosis	43 (AI, AP, PI, PP)	86.0	**Consensus**
Recurrent serositis	43 (AI, AP, PI, PP)	76.7	Majority
Thymic disorders: thymoma (adult), thymic aplasia (infant)	43 (AI, AP, PI, PP)	100.0	**Unanimity**

AI: adult immunologists; AP: adult pulmonologists; PC: primary care; PI: pediatric immunologists; PID: primary immunodeficiency disease; PP: pediatric pulmonologists
*One value is missing. ** One pneumonia per year for more than one year

manifestations of PID, although severe bronchiolitis may be relatively common in healthy infants.

Classification of respiratory diseases by PID type

PIDs have been divided into several categories, according to their clinical characteristics and immune system involvement. In any case, we must remember that inclusion in one category or another involves an important academic component, and in routine practice, the clinical context of the patient will help guide their classification. There are some lung manifestations that should lead to the suspicion of a specific PID. This is the case of pneumatocele and AD-hyperIgE syndrome, bronchiectasis and antibody deficiencies, severe bronchiolitis and severe combined immunodeficiencies or pulmonary fungal infections and phagocyte disorders, among others. However, most lung diseases can occur in a wide range of PID, in which a wide but phased diagnostic protocol is recommended.

Table 2 identifies the respiratory pathogens that are most commonly associated with each type of PID; several manifestations only achieved a majority agreement but not consensus, possibly due to the limited experience available in certain types of manifestations. Discrepancies were found for other manifestations ("abscess and pneumatocele" and "bronchiolitis obliterans", with agreements of 55.8 and 60.5%, respectively).

Table 2.

EXTRAPULMONARY manifestations that should suggest PID

It is very important that the specialist who evaluates a patient with suspected PID due to lung problems also takes in account the presence of extrapulmonary manifestations that might support the clinical suspicion of PID, since one of the main characteristics of PID is its ability to affect multiple organs or systems simultaneously or sequentially. PID may present with skin [20–22], gastrointestinal [23], or autoimmune [24–26] manifestations, among others. Table 3 (adapted from JC Aldave [27]) lists the main extrapulmonary clinical manifestations, with their degrees of agreement. Two common extrapulmonary manifestations did not reach consensus.

On the other hand, there are some histopatological findings which would prompt the clinician to consider a diagnosis of PID before having the suspicious of it. This is the case of granulomas or the absence of plasma cells in a gastrointestinal biopsy.

Diagnostic tests to be performed in patients with suspected PID

A large number of PIDs can be diagnosed from a detailed clinical history that includes a family history of PID, consanguinity, or family members who died at a young age, a comprehensive physical examination, blood tests, and a determination of serum immunoglobulin (Ig) levels. These tests are available in the vast majority of laboratories, even in PC. The physical examination should be detailed and ordered by body system, and it is important to assess the patient's nutritional status, with particular attention to height and weight and sequelae from previous infections. The presence of lymphadenopathies or the absence of nodal chains, tonsils, hepatosplenomegaly, etc. must be determined, since in some cases these parameters may orient the professional towards a specific PID. A complete blood count (CBC) with a differential count provides important information on suspected cytopenias (neutropenia, monocytopenia, lymphopenia, or thrombocytopenia) and qualitative cellular changes [9]. The determination of serum Igs (IgG, IgM, IgA, and IgE) is the first step in the evaluation of humoral immunity, and will help diagnose or at least point to a suspicion of quantitative Ig deficiencies, such as congenital agammaglobulinemia, CVID, or selective IgA deficiency, and humoral changes associated with other defects, such as hyper-IgE or hyper-IgM syndrome [9]. On the other side, quantification of calculated globulin (CG, total protein minus albumin [28]), T-cell recombination excision circles (TREC) and kappa-deleting element recombination circles (KREC) may help identify PIDs early in PC. Recently, a study by Pecoraro et al showed that a screening calculated globulin test could be used as a tool to reduce diagnostic delays, improve long-term prognosis and reduce the healthcare costs of antibody deficiency [29].

There are obvious differences between diagnosis in children and adults since, usually, most severe PID are diagnosed in childhood while recurrent respiratory infections, which can be caused by many other non-immunological entities and are the clue for the diagnosis during adulthood. Adolescents are a special population with mixed manifestations. Therefore, first line diagnostic tests in adults are almost specifically based on ruling primary antibody deficiency out (immunoglobulin levels and antibody production assessment), while clinical manifestations will orient the initial tests in childhood (e.g. burst oxidation tests in invasive fungal infections, complement pathway assessment if recurrent bacteremia...).

It is important to assess the results according to the reference values for each age, since there are significant differences which, if not taken into account, can cause PID to be overlooked [30]. In addition, it is always important that the suspected diagnosis is oriented to avoiding unnecessary studies that result in a waste of time and resources. However, when the diagnosis is uncertain and suspicion is high, additional tests, such as functional or molecular studies, are needed, and these must be conducted in reference centers. In fact, some of the

Table 2 Common respiratory manifestations by PID type

Common respiratory manifestations by PID type	N (Composition of panel)	Votes in agreement (%)	Degree of agreement
Predominantly T cell deficiency (combined and PID-related syndromes)			
Recurrent bronchitis	43 (AI, AP, PI, PP)	72.1	Majority
Idiopathic bronchiectasis	43 (AI, AP, PI, PP)	76.7	Majority
Recurrent pneumonias*	43 (AI, AP, PI, PP)	88.4	**Consensus**
Repeated pneumonia in child	43 (AI, AP, PI, PP)	88.4	**Consensus**
Chronic bronchial infection	43 (AI, AP, PI, PP)	79.1	Majority
Prolonged antibiotic treatment with poor response	43 (AI, AP, PI, PP)	86.0	**Consensus**
Abscess and pneumatocele	43 (AI, AP, PI, PP)	55.8	Discrepancy
Infections caused by rare microorganisms	43 (AI, AP, PI, PP)	100.0	**Unanimity**
Pneumonitis or bronchitis with hospitalization in infants	43 (AI, AP, PI, PP)	86.0	**Consensus**
Interstitial lung disease	43 (AI, AP, PI, PP)	93.0	**Consensus**
Bronchiolitis obliterans	43 (AI, AP, PI, PP)	67.4	Majority
Alveolar proteinosis	43 (AI, AP, PI, PP)	76.7	Majority
Absent thymus or aplasia	43 (AI, AP, PI, PP)	95.3	**Consensus**
Antibody deficiencies			
Recurrent bronchitis	43 (AI, AP, PI, PP)	90.7	**Consensus**
Idiopathic bronchiectasis	43 (AI, AP, PI, PP)	97.7	**Consensus**
Recurrent pneumonias*	43 (AI, AP, PI, PP)	97.7	**Consensus**
Repeated pneumonia in child	43 (AI, AP, PI, PP)	97.7	**Consensus**
Chronic bronchial infection	43 (AI, AP, PI, PP)	90.7	**Consensus**
Prolonged antibiotic treatment with poor response	43 (AI, AP, PI, PP)	97.7	**Consensus**
Pneumonia due to encapsulated bacteria	43 (AI, AP, PI, PP)	97.7	**Consensus**
Interstitial lung disease	43 (AI, AP, PI, PP)	79.1	Majority
Bronchiolitis obliterans	43 (AI, AP, PI, PP)	60.5	Discrepancy
Pulmonary lymphoma	43 (AI, AP, PI, PP)	69.8	Majority
Thymoma	43 (AI, AP, PI, PP)	88.4	**Consensus**
Immune deregulation			
Recurrent bronchitis	43 (AI, AP, PI, PP)	69.8	Majority
Idiopathic bronchiectasis	43 (AI, AP, PI, PP)	74.4	Majority
Chronic bronchial infection	43 (AI, AP, PI, PP)	65.1	Majority
Pneumonia due to encapsulated bacteria	43 (AI, AP, PI, PP)	67.4	Majority
Interstitial lung disease	43 (AI, AP, PI, PP)	81.4	**Consensus**
Phagocyte disorders			
Recurrent pneumonias*	43 (AI, AP, PI, PP)	90.7	**Consensus**
Prolonged antibiotic treatment with poor response	43 (AI, AP, PI, PP)	88.4	**Consensus**
Abscess and pneumatocele	43 (AI, AP, PI, PP)	97.7	**Consensus**
Infections caused by rare microorganisms	43 (AI, AP, PI, PP)	97.7	**Consensus**
Alveolar proteinosis	43 (AI, AP, PI, PP)	69.8	Majority
Innate immunity disorder			
Recurrent pneumonias*	43 (AI, AP, PI, PP)	97.7	**Consensus**
Pneumonia due to encapsulated bacteria	43 (AI, AP, PI, PP)	95.3	**Consensus**
Abscess and pneumatocele	43 (AI, AP, PI, PP)	83.7	**Consensus**
Infections caused by rare microorganisms	43 (AI, AP, PI, PP)	90.7	**Consensus**
Complement deficiency			

Table 2 Common respiratory manifestations by PID type *(Continued)*

Common respiratory manifestations by PID type	N (Composition of panel)	Votes in agreement (%)	Degree of agreement
Recurrent bronchitis	43 (AI, AP, PI, PP)	65.1	Majority
Idiopathic bronchiectasis	43 (AI, AP, PI, PP)	72.1	Majority
Recurrent pneumonias*	43 (AI, AP, PI, PP)	83.7	**Consensus**
Repeated pneumonia in child	43 (AI, AP, PI, PP)	83.7	**Consensus**
Chronic bronchial infection	43 (AI, AP, PI, PP)	67.4	Majority
Autoinflammatory disease			
Recurrent serositis	43 (AI, AP, PI, PP)	100.0	**Unanimity**

AI: adult immunologists; AP: adult pulmonologists; PI: pediatric immunologists; PID: primary immunodeficiency disease; PP: pediatric pulmonologists
* One pneumonia per year for more than one year

warning signs alone (signature signs) as opportunistic infections, or high burden of infection should lead to the referral of the patient to a higher level of care, so that the appropriate tests could be performed.

With regard to tests that are specifically "pulmonary" in a patient with suspected PID, tests adapted to the disease and based on the clinical history are recommended: this is the case for lung function tests and high-resolution computed tomography (HRCT) to evaluate the lung structure, sputum cultures to detect respiratory infections, and sputum cell counts (neutrophils and eosinophils), among others [31]. Chest X-rays may be valuable in acute processes but they are of little use for demonstrating the presence of bronchiectasis or non-infectious pulmonary complications [32, 33]. The sensitivity of lung function tests for the early detection of complications, such as bronchiectasis, is low, and they should always include, if possible, the evaluation of diffusing capacity of the lung for carbon monoxide (DLCO). HRCT, on the other hand, is highly sensitive and specific, and has an important role in the multidisciplinary approach to these conditions, and in the detection, characterization, and quantification of the degree of lung damage, the treatment plan, and follow-up of patients. It is currently the gold standard for the detection and characterization of bronchiectasis [14, 16].

Tables 4 and 5 include immunological and pulmonary tests, respectively, that must be performed when PID is suspected, divided into levels of care. Even though, in the last years the use of next-generation sequencing has become an essential route for diagnosing PID and it is usually performed earlier in the diagnostic algorithm of a patient with suspected PID. Meanwhile, protein and functional testing remain to be tested in reference centers if available. Although all the immunological tests (Table 4) reached consensus, some interesting proposals that the authors agreed to include outside of the table are provided. These include protein expression and genetic studies in the third level for phagocyte deficiencies; determination of IgD levels, C-reactive protein (CRP), erythrocyte sedimentation rate (ESR) in the baseline level for autoinflammatory diseases; serial determination of mevalonate in urine during the acute episode in the second level for autoinflammatory diseases; and replacement of tetanus serologies with tetanus/diphtheria. Pulmonary tests (Table 5) were divided into

Table 3 Most common extrapulmonary manifestations of PID (adapted from JC Aldave, JFM) [27]

MOST COMMON EXTRAPULMONARY MANIFESTATIONS OF PID	N (Composition of panel)	Votes in agreement (%)	Degree of agreement
Recurrent or complicated sinusitis	43 (AI, AP, PI, PP)	100.0	**Unanimity**
Recurrent or complicated otitis	43 (AI, AP, PI, PP)	93.0	**Consensus**
Other extrapulmonary infections requiring admission	43 (AI, AP, PI, PP)	88.4	**Consensus**
Ectodermal dysplasia	43 (AI, AP, PI, PP)	72.1	Majority
Chronic diarrhea or malabsorption	43 (AI, AP, PI, PP)	93.0	**Consensus**
Difficult-to-treat giardiasis	43 (AI, AP, PI, PP)	93.0	**Consensus**
Autoimmune cytopenias or other autoimmunity	43 (AI, AP, PI, PP)	93.0	**Consensus**
Lymphadenopathies and hepatosplenomegaly	43 (AI, AP, PI, PP)	97.7	**Consensus**
Related cancers, especially associated with viruses	43 (AI, AP, PI, PP)	83.7	**Consensus**
Family history of ID or consistent manifestations	43 (AI, AP, PI, PP)	88.4	**Consensus**
Post-vaccinal infections	43 (AI, AP, PI, PP)	79.1	Majority

AI: adult immunologists; AP: adult pulmonologists; ID: immunodeficiency; PI: pediatric immunologists; PID: primary immunodeficiency disease; PP: pediatric pulmonologists

Table 4 Immunological tests additional to baseline tests in patients with suspected PID

Baseline level	First level[a]	Second level[b]	Third level[b]	N (Composition of panel)	Votes in agreement (%)	Degree of agreement
Combined						
Complete blood count IgA, IgG, IgM and IgE levels Biochemical analysis[e]	Lymphocyte populations	Extended phenotype, lymphocyte function	Protein expression Functional and genetic studies	34 (AI, AP)	91.2	**Consensus**
PID-associated syndromes						
Complete blood count IgA, IgG, IgM and IgE levels Biochemical analysis[e]	Karyotype ± CGH Array	Studies according to specific suspicion	Protein expression Functional and genetic studies	33* (AI, AP)	87.9	**Consensus**
Antibody production deficiency[c]						
Complete blood count IgA, IgG, IgM and IgE levels Biochemical analysis[e]	Basic antibody production study (ASLO, hemaglutinins and tetanus)	IgG subclasses Response to *Salmonella typhi* or pneumococcus Response to tetanus toxoid[d] and *H. influenzae* (optional) Lymphocyte populations with extended phenotype B	Protein expression Functional and genetic studies	34 (AI, AP)	91.2	**Consensus**
Immune deregulation						
Complete blood count IgA, IgG, IgM and IgE levels Biochemical analysis[e]	Autoantibody panel (ANA and NOSAB, anti-neutrophils) Targeted hormone study Coombs test Vitamin B12 with neural tube defects Soluble FAS ligand Ferritin Triglycerides Fibrinogen Calcium and phosphorus	Treg Soluble CD25 FoxP3	Protein expression Functional and genetic studies	33* (AI, AP)	97.0	**Consensus**
Phagocyte deficiencies[d]						
Complete blood count IgA, IgG, IgM and IgE levels Biochemical analysis[e]	Oxidation test (DHR) Basic lymphocyte subpopulations	CD18/11b	–	34 (AI, AP)	91.2	**Consensus**
Innate immunity disorder						
Complete blood count IgA, IgG, IgM and IgE levels Biochemical analysis[e]	Studies according to clinical suspicion	–	Protein expression Functional and genetic studies	34 (AI, AP)	97.1	**Consensus**
Complement deficiency						
Complete blood count IgA, IgG, IgM and IgE levels Biochemical analysis[e]	CH50, C3, C4, autoimmunity studies	AP50 Factor quantification	Protein expression Functional and genetic studies	34 (AI, AP)	94.1	**Consensus**

Table 4 Immunological tests additional to baseline tests in patients with suspected PID *(Continued)*

Autoinflammatory diseases[d]						
Complete blood count IgA, IgG, IgM and IgE levels Biochemical analysis[e]	Inflammatory markers CRP ESR	SAA	Genetic studies	33* (AI, AP)	84.8	**Consensus**

AI: adult immunologists; ANA: antinuclear antibodies, ASLO: antistreptolysin O; Coombs: antiglobulin test; CRP: C-reactive protein; DHR: dihydrorhodamine 123; DNT: double negative alpha/beta T cells; ESR: erythrocyte sedimentation rate; NOSAB: non-specific autoantibodies; PI: pediatric immunologists; SAA: serum amyloid A; Treg: regulatory T cells

[a]First-level tests will be carried out in primary care or hospital centers which have laboratories with the necessary resources

[b]Second and third-level tests will be carried out in reference centers

[c] These tests will also be performed in any PID that includes antibody production deficiencies as part of the entity

[d] Proposals for changes are included throughout the text

[e] Biochemical analysis includes, at least: blood urea nitrogen, creatinine, liver enzymes, C-reactive protein and albumin

*One value is missing

Table 5 Respiratory tests to be conducted in adult (consensus) and pediatric (no consensus) patients with suspected PID

First level[a]	Second level[b]	Third level[c]	N (Composition of panel)	Votes in agreement (%)	Degree of agreement
Adults					
Refer to pulmonologist when warning signs detected	Spirometry* Plethysmography DLCO HRCT +/– abdominal ultrasound Sputum culture (bacteria, mycobacteria, and fungi), if expectoration	Exercise stress tests. Bronchoscopy with bronchoalveolar lavage and transbronchial cryobiopsy. Open lung biopsy or by video-assisted thoracoscopy in case of interstitial lung disease.	5 (AP)	100.0	**Unanimity**
Children					
Spirometry, if possible according to patient age and availability Chest X-ray	Spirometry (technically possible ≥3 years) Plethysmography (≥ 6–7 years, if available) DLCO (≥ 6–7 years) Lung HRCT +/– abdominal ultrasound Sputum culture, if expectoration (induced sputum, if no expectoration)	Lung function studies by age: • In infants: plethysmography; tidal volume determination; tidal or raised volume rapid thoracoabdominal compression technique. • In preschoolers: oscillometry; oscillatory resistance. Bronchoscopy with bronchoalveolar lavage, in the case of localized or diffuse bronchiectasis or interstitial lung disease, even if patient is expectorating. Open lung biopsy or video-assisted thoracoscopy in case of interstitial lung disease Transbronchial cryobiopsy in children > 7 years as alternative to lung biopsy	4 (PP)	50.0	Discrepancy

AP: adult pulmonologists; DLCO: diffusing capacity of the lung for carbon monoxide; HRCT: high-resolution computed tomography; PP: pediatric pulmonologists
[a]First-level tests will be carried out in PC centers
[b] First-level tests will be carried out by respiratory specialists
[c] Third-level tests will be carried out immunologists or in reference center
* Spirometry may be performed as part of level 1 when available at the primary care setting

Table 6 Minimum tests to be performed during monitoring of the patient with PID and respiratory symptoms

TESTS	N (Composition of panel)	Votes in agreement (%)	Degree of agreement
Patient visit every 6–12 months.	34 (AI, AP)	91.2	**Consensus**
Immunological studies (complete blood count, biochemistry with LDH and Igs) every 6–12 months.	34 (AI, AP)	91.2	**Consensus**
In the event of RT with gammaglobulins, IgG trough values must be measured more frequently, at least during dose adjustment.	34 (AI, AP)	100.0	**Unanimity**
Respiratory tests: • Annual lung function tests are recommended every year. • Spirometry must be performed every 4–6 months in the absence of lung disease. • The sputum culture must be performed at each visit if patient is expectorating and in case of any exacerbation.	9 (AP, PP)	100.0	**Unanimity**
Lung CT every 2–3 years if the patient has pulmonary involvement and every 5 years otherwise. Radiation must be minimized in case of radiosensitive ID.	9 (AP, PP)	100.0	**Unanimity**
Extrapulmonary tests should be performed according to the patient's symptoms or manifestations.	43 (AI, PI, AP, PP)	97.7	**Consensus**

AI: adult immunologists; AP: adult pulmonologists; ID: immunodeficiency; Ig: immunoglobulins; LDH: lactate dehydrogenase; PI: pediatric immunologists; PID: primary immunodeficiency disease; PP: pediatric pulmonologists; RT: replacement therapy

adults and children. Discrepancies emerged regarding the use of these tests in children, so they could not be validated.

Immunoglobulin replacement therapy in PID

Immunoglobulin replacement therapy (IGRT) is essential in patients with PIDs that directly affect B cell function and antibody production, primarily in severe cases, but also in patients in whom involvement is not obvious from routine testing [34]. IGRT has brought about a significant change in the prognosis of patients with PID. The mortality of CVID has fallen from 29% in 1971 (before the introduction of intravenous Ig) to 19.6% in 2012 [35]. In pulmonary complications of PID, IGRT has halved the number of bacterial pneumonias [36]; however, this treatment does not appear to improve other recurrent respiratory infections [36].

There are currently 6 PID phenotypes for which IGRT is indicated or may be indicated [37]: agammaglobulinemia due to the absence of B cells; hypogammaglobulinemia with impaired specific antibody production; selective antibody deficiencies (IGRT use must be individually evaluated); hypogammaglobulinemia with normal-quality antibody response; isolated deficiency of an IgG subclass with recurrent infections; and recurrent infections due to an unknown immune mechanism.

Since IGRT was introduced in the 1980s, the administered dose of Ig has been gradually increased to achieve higher IgG plasma concentrations [38]. For example, in the case of patients with CVID, IgG plasma concentrations to prevent bacterial infections may range between 5 and 17 g/L, although trough concentrations of IgG of around 8–10 g/L are often recommended. These levels can be achieved with a dose range of 0.2–1.2 g/kg/month. Doses must be individualized, and higher doses are required in patients with bronchiectasis and those with certain phenotypes [38].

IGRT can be administered by 2 routes: subcutaneous (SCIG) and intravenous (IVIG); the muscular route has fallen into disuse. There is also a facilitated SCIG which improves its bioavailability and allows infusions every 3–4 weeks [39]. Adequate doses administered by both routes provide physiological IgG concentrations [40, 41], although the kinetics are different: intravenous administration produces a rapid increase in IgG plasma concentrations, while subcutaneous administration produces more gradual increases in plasma levels [41, 42] and more stable serum concentrations [40, 43]. SCIG can be particularly beneficial in patients with low IgG concentrations despite intravenous treatment, since higher mean serum values can be achieved with lower doses of immunoglobulin [44–46]. Both routes of administration have shown equivalence in terms of efficacy and safety [37, 45, 47], although the incidence of serious systemic adverse effects is higher with IVIG and more mild local effects are observed with SCIG [42, 45, 48].

Different factors must be considered when selecting the route of administration, as not all patients benefit equally from both [49]. Firstly, SCIG is associated with a better quality of life for both patients and their caregivers [46, 50, 51]. A review of 25 studies showed improved health-related quality of life in patients who switched IVIG administration in the hospital for home-administered SCIG [45]. This same review also concluded that SCIG therapy was more cost-effective, mainly due to the reduction in days missed from school or work [45]. The subcutaneous route is also more appropriate for patients with difficulties for venous access, and does not appear to adversely affect renal function [37, 41]. However, the patient must be trained, and the equipment and infrastructure required for correct administration may not be easily achieved for all patients. Finally, patient preferences are fundamental when decisions are being made. Multidisciplinary long-term monitoring programs must be implemented that are flexible regarding the alternate use of both routes, depending on the life circumstances of each patient [52, 53]. Despite all, the decision of which route and location of therapy is best may change with age and personal circumstances and requires ongoing re-evaluation; however patients who are stable and managing well with a specific route should not be swapped onto different products for non-clinical reasons.

Monitoring PID patients with pulmonary involvement

Survival and quality of life of patients with certain PIDs has improved significantly in recent years, particularly as a result of better diagnosis and treatment of infections and other comorbidities, the development of highly potent antimicrobial agents, and the development of specific therapeutic alternatives, such as IgG and others [54]. However, we must not allow the reduction in the number of infections and hospitalizations to generate a lower perception of severity that might lead to a relaxation in the regular clinical monitoring of the disease [9].

The decision on the frequency of evaluations of PID patients depends on several factors, including the type of PID, clinical conditions, and age. There is currently no internationally agreed consensus on the follow-up of patients with PID and lung involvement, but it has been suggested that patients should be evaluated at least once every 6–12 months with a full clinical history and physical examination [9]. Whenever possible, this evaluation should be performed by an expert in PID [55].

The literature reviewed proposes that the follow-up of patients with pulmonary complications should include serial lung function tests and imaging studies, along with regular sputum cultures [9, 56]. Chest X-ray will only be indicated if acute pulmonary involvement is suspected. It is recommended that HRCTs are performed every 3–5 years in patients under treatment, depending on their clinical stability [57].

Table 6 sets out the recommendations on the minimum tests to be performed during the clinical monitoring of the PID patient with pulmonary symptoms.

Conclusions

This study is the first to focus on PID from a pulmonary point of view, addressing the diagnosis, treatment and follow-up of both adult and pediatric patients, while simultaneously including the opinion and clinical experience of more than 40 experts from different fields and specialties who regularly treat these deficiencies. This document is intended to be a useful tool for both primary care professionals and specialists who are treating patients with lung disease, helping them to identify the warning signs of PID in order to make an early diagnosis or else to refer the patient to a specialized unit, thus avoiding unnecessary complications. Other approaches that may help an early identification of PIDs should include education and awareness for specialists. Finally, future possible shortcomings of the study will involve other medical specialties and other clinical manifestations of IDs.

Abbreviations

AI: Adult immunologists; ANA: Antinuclear antibodies; AP: Adult pulmonologists; ASLO: Antistreptolysin O; CG: Calculated globulin; COOMBS: Antiglobulin test; CRP: C-reactive protein; CVID: Common variable immunodeficiency; DHR: Dihydrorhodamine 123; DLCO: Diffusing capacity of the lung; DNT: Double negative alpha/beta T cells; ESR: Erythrocyte sedimentation rate; HRCT: High-resolution computed tomography; ID: Immunodeficiency; Ig: Immunoglobulins; IGRT: Immunoglobulin replacement therapy; ILD: Interstitial lung disease; IUIS: International Union of Immunological Societies; IVIG: Intravenous Ig; JMF: Jeffrey Modell Foundation; KREC: Kappa-deleting element recombination circles; LDH: Lactate dehydrogenase; NOSAB: Non-organ-specific autoantibodies; NSIP: Non-specific interstitial pneumonia; PC: Primary care; PI: Pediatric immunologists; PID: Primary immunodeficiency disease; PP: Pediatric pulmonologists; RT: Replacement therapy; SAA: Serum amyloid A; SCIG: Subcutaneous Ig; SID: Secondary immunodeficiency diseases; TREC: T-cell recombination excision circles; Treg: Regulatory T cells

Acknowledgements

The authors of this work would like to thank CSL Behring for the financial support provided for the conduct of this study, the ID-Signal Group for their participation as members of the external panel, and Cristina Valiente and Verónica Albert of GOC Networking, for their methodological support throughout the course of the study.
The Lung ID-Signal Group consists of the following members: Óscar Asensio, Luis Allende, Laia Alsina, Ana María Bielsa, Luis Borderías, Sara Calleja-Antolín, Carmen Cámara, Javier Carbone, Carmen Carreras, Francisco Casas, Ana De Andrés, Angela Deyá, Romina Dieli, Amparo Escribano, Luis Fernández-Pereira, José Mª García Ruiz de Morales, Juana Gil-Herrera, Manel Juan, Pilar Llobet, Marcos López-Hoyos, M. Carmen Luna-Paredes, Andrea Martín-Nalda, Mónica Martínez, Josefa Melero, Ana Méndez-Echevarría, Pedro Moral, Antonio Moreno, Olaf Neth, María Núñez, Gonzalo Ocejo-Vinyals, Juliana Ochoa-Grullón, Peter Olbrich, Ricardo Pujol, Daniel Pleguezuelo, Eva Polverino, Jaime Pons, Esther Quintana-Gallego, José Tomás Ramos, Carmen Rodríguez, Juan Luis Santos-Pérez, M. Elena Seoane, Montserrat Vendrell and Alexandru Vlagea.

Funding

This study was funded by CSL Behring.

Authors' contributions

PSP made substantial contributions to the conception and design of the document, to the first draft of the document (before the evaluation of the external panel of experts), and also to the analysis and interpretation of data from the external panel of experts; he has also been involved in drafting and revising the manuscript critically for important intellectual content and has given final approval of the version to be published. JG made contributions the first draft of the document (before the evaluation of the external panel of experts) and to the interpretation of data from the external panel of experts; he also has been involved in revising the manuscript and has given final approval of the version to be published. LIG made contributions the first draft of the document (before the evaluation of the external panel of experts) and to interpretation of data from the external panel of experts; he also has been involved in revising the manuscript and has given final approval of the version to be published. CM made contributions the first draft of the document (before the evaluation of the external panel of experts) and to interpretation of data from the external panel of experts; he also has been involved in revising the manuscript and has given final approval of the version to be published. CR made contributions to the first draft of the document (before the evaluation of the external panel of experts) and to the interpretation of data from the external panel of experts; he also has been involved in revising the manuscript and has given final approval of the version to be published. SSR made substantial contributions to the conception and design of the document, to the first draft of the document (before the evaluation of the external panel of experts), and also to the analysis and interpretation of data from the external panel of experts; he also has been involved in drafting and revising the manuscript critically for important intellectual content and has given final approval of the version to be published.

Competing interests

- PSP reports receiving personal fees from CSL Behring and grants from the Jeffrey Modell Foundation during the conduct of the study; and personal fees from Shire SL, and from Grifols, outside the context of the submitted work.
- JG reports receiving personal fees from CLS Berhing, from the Fundación Victor Griffols, and from Shire SL, outside the context of the submitted work.
- LIG reports receiving grants from Fondo de Investigación Sanitaria Carlos III and from Shire SL, and grants and personal fees from CSL Behring, during the conduct of the study.
- CM reports receiving personal fees from CSL Behring, outside the context of the submitted work.
- CR reports receiving personal fees from CSL Behring, during the conduct of the study.
- SSR has served as speaker, consultant and advisory member for or has received research funding from CSL Behring, Grifols, Shire and Octapharma.

Author details

[1]Hospital U. Vall d'Hebron, P. de la Vall d'Hebron, 119-129, 08035 Barcelona, Spain. [2]Hospital U. 12 Octubre, Av. Cordoba, s/n, 28041 Madrid, Spain. [3]Hospital U. Miguel Servet, P. Isabel la Católica, 1-3, 50009 Zaragoza, Spain. [4]H. Son Espases, C. de Valldemossa, 79, 07120 Palma, Balearic Islands, Spain. [5]Hospital Clínico San Carlos, C. del Prof Martín Lagos, s/n, 28040 Madrid, Spain. [6]Hospital Universitari Vall d'Hebron - Institut de Recerca, Barcelona, Spain.

References

1. de Vries E. European Society for Immunodeficiencies m. patient-centred screening for primary immunodeficiency, a multi-stage diagnostic protocol designed for non-immunologists: 2011 update. Clin Exp Immunol. 2012;167: 108–19.
2. Picard C, Bobby Gaspar H, Al-Herz W, et al. International Union of Immunological Societies: 2017 primary immunodeficiency diseases committee report on inborn errors of immunity. J Clin Immunol. 2018;38: 96–128.
3. Costa-Carvalho BT, Grumach AS, Franco JL, et al. Attending to warning signs of primary immunodeficiency diseases across the range of clinical practice. J Clin Immunol. 2014;34:10–22.
4. Mahlaoui N, Gathmann B, Kindle G, Ehl S. ESID registry working party steering committee, ESID society. The European Society for Immunodeficiencies (ESID) registry: recent advancements in the epidemiology of primary Immunodeficiencies and how does that translate in clinical care. Int J Public Health. 2014;1:25–7.
5. Bousfiha AA, Jeddane L, Ailal F, et al. Primary immunodeficiency diseases worldwide: more common than generally thought. J Clin Immunol. 2013;33:1–7.
6. Kobrynski L, Powell RW, Bowen S. Prevalence and morbidity of primary immunodeficiency diseases, United States 2001-2007. J Clin Immunol. 2014; 34:954–61.
7. Plebani A, Soresina A, Rondelli R, et al. Clinical, immunological, and molecular analysis in a large cohort of patients with X-linked agammaglobulinemia: an Italian multicenter study. Clin Immunol. 2002;104: 221–30.
8. Modell V, Gee B, Lewis DB, et al. Global study of primary immunodeficiency diseases (PI)--diagnosis, treatment, and economic impact: an updated report from the Jeffrey Modell Foundation. Immunol Res. 2011;51:61–70.
9. Roxo Junior P. Primary immunodeficiency diseases: relevant aspects for pulmonologists. Jornal brasileiro de pneumologia : publicacao oficial da Sociedade Brasileira de Pneumologia e Tisilogia. 2009;35:1008–17.
10. Jesenak M, Banovcin P, Jesenakova B, Babusikova E. Pulmonary manifestations of primary immunodeficiency disorders in children. Front Pediatr. 2014;2:77.
11. Jeffrey Modell Foundation. 10 Warning Signs of Primary Immunodeficiency for Adults. Disponible en: http://www.info4pi.org/aboutPI/pdf/Adult10WarningSigns-FINAL.pdf.
12. Arkwright PD, Gennery AR. Ten warning signs of primary immunodeficiency: a new paradigm is needed for the 21st century. Ann N Y Acad Sci. 2011; 1238:7–14.
13. Subbarayan A, Colarusso G, Hughes SM, et al. Clinical features that identify children with primary immunodeficiency diseases. Pediatrics. 2011;127:810–6.
14. Hampson FA, Chandra A, Screaton NJ, et al. Respiratory disease in common variable immunodeficiency and other primary immunodeficiency disorders. Clin Radiol. 2012;67:587–95.
15. Verma N, Grimbacher B, Hurst JR. Lung disease in primary antibody deficiency. Lancet Respir Med. 2015;3:651–60.
16. Baumann U, Routes JM, Soler-Palacín P, Jolles S. The lung in primary Immunodeficiencies: new concepts in infection and inflammation. Front Immunol. 2018;9:1837.
17. Serra G, Milito C, Mitrevski M, et al. Lung MRI as a possible alternative to CT scan for patients with primary immune deficiencies and increased radiosensitivity. Chest. 2011;140:1581–9.
18. Fried AJ, Bonilla FA. Pathogenesis, diagnosis, and management of primary antibody deficiencies and infections. Clin Microbiol Rev. 2009;22:396–414.
19. Nonas S. Pulmonary manifestations of primary immunodeficiency disorders. Immunol Allergy Clin N Am. 2015;35:753–66.
20. Chu EY, Freeman AF, Jing H, et al. Cutaneous manifestations of DOCK8 deficiency syndrome. Arch Dermatol. 2012;148:79–84.
21. Zhang Q, Davis JC, Lamborn IT, et al. Combined immunodeficiency associated with DOCK8 mutations. N Engl J Med. 2009;361:2046–55.
22. Al-Herz W, Nanda A. Skin manifestations in primary immunodeficient children. Pediatr Dermatol. 2011;28:494–501.
23. Kobrynski LJ, Mayer L. Diagnosis and treatment of primary immunodeficiency disease in patients with gastrointestinal symptoms. Clin Immunol. 2011;139:238–48.
24. Cunningham-Rundles C. Autoimmunity in primary immune deficiency: taking lessons from our patients. Clin Exp Immunol 2011;164 Suppl 2:6–11.
25. Moraes-Vasconcelos D, Costa-Carvalho BT, Torgerson TR, Ochs HD. Primary immune deficiency disorders presenting as autoimmune diseases: IPEX and APECED. J Clin Immunol. 2008;28(Suppl 1):S11–9.
26. Arason GJ, Jorgensen GH, Ludviksson BR. Primary immunodeficiency and autoimmunity: lessons from human diseases. Scand J Immunol. 2010;71: 317–28.
27. Warning signs of Primary Immunodeficiency for specialty care physicians. (Accessed Sept.-19-2018, at http://downloads.info4pi.org/pdfs/Diagnostic-Algorithm-for-Specialty-Care-Physicians.pdf.)
28. Jolles S, Borrell R, Zouwail S, et al. Calculated globulin (CG) as a screening test for antibody deficiency. Clin Exp Immunol. 2014;177:671–8.
29. Pecoraro A, Jolles S, Crescenzi L, et al. Validation of calculated globulin (CG) as a screening test for antibody deficiency in an Italian University hospital. Curr Pharm Biotechnol. 2018.

30. Garcia-Prat M, Vila-Pijoan G, Martos Gutierrez S, et al. Age-specific pediatric reference ranges for immunoglobulins and complement proteins on the Optilite. J Clin Lab Anal. 2018:e22420.
31. Ozerovitch L. Primary immune deficiency in bronchiectasis. Nurs Times. 2016;112:16–9.
32. Thickett KM, Kumararatne DS, Banerjee AK, Dudley R, Stableforth DE. Common variable immune deficiency: respiratory manifestations, pulmonary function and high-resolution CT scan findings. QJM. 2002;95: 655–62.
33. Sala Cunill A, Soler-Palacín P, Martín De Vicente C, Labrador Horrillo M, Luengo Sánchez O, Figueras Nadal C. Common variable immunodeficiency. Prognostic factors for lung damage Med Clin (Barc). 2010;134:64–7.
34. Perez EE, Orange JS, Bonilla F, et al. Update on the use of immunoglobulin in human disease: a review of evidence. J Allergy Clin Immunol. 2017;139: S1–s46.
35. Resnick ES, Moshier EL, Godbold JH, Cunningham-Rundles C. Morbidity and mortality in common variable immune deficiency over 4 decades. Blood. 2012;119:1650–7.
36. Jolles S. Subclinical infection and dosing in primary immunodeficiencies. Clin Exp Immunol. 2014;178(Suppl 1):67–9.
37. Stiehm ER, Orange JS, Ballow M, Lehman H. Therapeutic use of immunoglobulins. Adv Pediatr Infect Dis. 2010;57:185–218.
38. Lucas M, Lee M, Lortan J, Lopez-Granados E, Misbah S, Chapel H. Infection outcomes in patients with common variable immunodeficiency disorders: relationship to immunoglobulin therapy over 22 years. J Allergy Clin Immunol 2010;125:1354–1360 e4.
39. Wasserman RL. Overview of recombinant human hyaluronidase-facilitated subcutaneous infusion of IgG in primary immunodeficiencies. Immunotherapy. 2014;6:553–67.
40. Berger M. Subcutaneous administration of IgG. Immunol Allergy Clin N Am. 2008;28:779–802 viii.
41. Gardulf A. Immunoglobulin treatment for primary antibody deficiencies: advantages of the subcutaneous route. BioDrugs. 2007;21:105–16.
42. Haddad É, Barnes D, Kafal A. Home therapy with subcutaneous immunoglobulins for patients with primary immunodeficiency diseases. Transfus Apher Sci. 2012;46:315–21.
43. Gaspar J, Gerritsen B, Jones A. Immunoglobulin replacement treatment by rapid subcutaneous infusion. Arch Dis Child. 1998;79:48–51.
44. Thépot S, Malphettes M, Gardeur A, et al. Immunoglobulin dosage and switch from intravenous to subcutaneous immunoglobulin replacement therapy in patients with primary hypogammaglobulinemia: decreasing dosage does not alter serum IgG levels. J Clin Immunol. 2010;30:602–6.
45. Lingman-Framme J, Fasth A. Subcutaneous immunoglobulin for primary and secondary immunodeficiencies: an evidence-based review. Drugs. 2013; 73:1307–19.
46. Berger M, Murphy E, Riley P, Bergman GE, Investigators VT. Improved quality of life, immunoglobulin G levels, and infection rates in patients with primary immunodeficiency diseases during self-treatment with subcutaneous immunoglobulin G. South Med J. 2010;103:856–63.
47. Gardulf A, Nicolay U, Asensio O, et al. Rapid subcutaneous IgG replacement therapy is effective and safe in children and adults with primary immunodeficiencies--a prospective, multi-national study. J Clin Immunol. 2006;26:177–85.
48. Jiang F, Torgerson TR, Ayars AG. Health-related quality of life in patients with primary immunodeficiency disease. Allergy Asthma Clin Immunol. 2015;11:27.
49. Jolles S, Orange JS, Gardulf A, et al. Current treatment options with immunoglobulin G for the individualization of care in patients with primary immunodeficiency disease. Clin Exp Immunol. 2015;179:146–60.
50. Gardulf A, Nicolay U, Math D, et al. Children and adults with primary antibody deficiencies gain quality of life by subcutaneous IgG self-infusions at home. J Allergy Clin Immunol. 2004;114:936–42.
51. Misbah S, Sturzenegger MH, Borte M, et al. Subcutaneous immunoglobulin: opportunities and outlook. Clin Exp Immunol. 2009;158(Suppl 1):51–9.
52. Bourdin A, Berger J, Früh A, Spertini F, Bugnon O. Subcutaneous immunoglobulin and support program: what level of interest of patients? Rev Med Suisse. 2015;11:831–5.
53. Soler-Palacín P, Gasó-Gago I, Fernández-Polo A, et al. Intravenous and subcutaneous immunoglobulin replacement: a two-way road. Optimizing healthcare quality in patients with primary immunodeficiencies. J Clin Immunol. 2014;34:1015–7.
54. Chinen J, Anmuth D, Franklin AR, Shearer WT. Long-term follow-up of patients with primary immunodeficiencies. J Allergy Clin Immunol. 2007;120: 795–7.
55. Bonilla FA, Bernstein IL, Khan DA, et al. Practice parameter for the diagnosis and management of primary immunodeficiency. Ann Allergy Asthma Immunol. 2005;94:S1–63.
56. Tarzi MD, Grigoriadou S, Carr SB, Kuitert LM, Longhurst HJ. Clinical immunology review series: an approach to the management of pulmonary disease in primary antibody deficiency. Clin Exp Immunol. 2009;155:147–55.
57. Jolles S, Sánchez-Ramón S, Quinti I, et al. Screening protocols to monitor respiratory status in primary immunodeficiency disease: findings from a European survey and subclinical infection working group. Clin Exp Immunol. 2017;190:226–34.

21

Role of SOD3 in silica-related lung fibrosis and pulmonary vascular remodeling

Igor N. Zelko[1,2*], Jianxin Zhu[1] and Jesse Roman[1,3,4]

Abstract

Background: Work-place exposure to silica dust may lead to progressive lung inflammation culminating in the development of silicosis, an irreversible condition that can be complicated by onset of pulmonary hypertension (PH). The molecular mechanisms leading to the development of PH and lung fibrosis in response to silica are not well understood. Oxidant/antioxidant imbalance in the lung may promote fibroproliferation and vascular smooth muscle proliferation, ultimately leading to the development of PH. Herein, we analyze the development of PH and lung fibrosis in mice deficient in extracellular superoxide dismutase (SOD3), an enzyme with anti-oxidant activity.

Methods: PH and silicosis were induced in wild-type and Sod3$^{-/-}$ mice through intratracheal injection of crystalline silica at dose 0.4 g/kg. Pulmonary hypertension and lung fibrosis were characterized by changes in right ventricular systolic pressure (RVSP) and collagen deposition 28 days following silica injections. Vascular remodeling was analyzed using immunohistochemistry and morphometric analysis. The expression of genes were analyzed using qRT-PCR and Western blot.

Results: C57BL6 mice exposed to silica showed attenuated expression of Sod3 in the lung suggesting a protective role for Sod3. Consistent with this, Sod3$^{-/-}$ mice developed more severe fibrotic inflammatory nodules with increased collagen deposition. Furthermore, the expression of genes involved in tissue remodeling (Timp1), fibrotic lesion formation (Fsp1) and inflammatory response (Mcp1) were significantly elevated in Sod3$^{-/-}$ mice compared to Sod3$^{+/+}$ mice treated with silica. Infiltration of neutrophils and activated macrophages into affected lung was significantly higher in Sod3 deficient mice. In addition, silica produced more profound effects on elevation of RVSP in Sod3$^{-/-}$ compared to wild-type littermate. Increase in RVSP was concomitant with hypertrophy of pulmonary arteries located in silicotic nodules of both mouse strains, however, vascular remodeling in unaffected areas of lung was detected only in Sod3$^{-/-}$ mice.

Conclusions: Our data suggest that Sod3 and extracellular oxidative stress may play an important role in the development of pneumoconiosis and pulmonary vascular remodeling following exposure to environmental and occupational silica.

Keywords: Oxidative stress, Transcription, Expression, Crystalline silica, Pulmonary hypertension, Lung fibrosis, Silicosis, Pneumoconiosis

Introduction

The occupational exposure to crystalline silica during coal mining, sand blasting, volcanic eruption and wind erosion remains a significant hazard worldwide. Crystalline silica inhalation results in the development of silicosis and pulmonary fibrosis, which eventually results in reduced lung function and other health related issues [1, 2]. In addition to silicosis, the chronic inhalation of crystalline silica promotes the development of chronic obstructive pulmonary diseases (COPD) and lung cancer [3, 4]. Several animal models were developed to investigate the effect of silica dust on inflammatory responses in the lung and to elucidate the molecular mechanisms responsible for the pro-fibrotic effects of silica crystals [5, 6]. Crystalline silica trapped in lung alveoli induces inflammatory responses that eventually lead to fibronodular parenchymal lung disease characterized by

* Correspondence: igor.zelko@louisville.edu
[1]Department of Medicine, Division of Pulmonary, Critical Care, and Sleep Medicine, University of Louisville, 505 S. Hancock Street, CTR Bldg., room 524, Louisville, KY 40202, USA
[2]Department of Biochemistry and Molecular Genetics, University of Louisville, 505 S. Hancock Street, CTR Bldg., room 524, Louisville, KY 40202, USA
Full list of author information is available at the end of the article

excessive deposition of extracellular matrix proteins and accumulation of fibroblasts, epithelioid inflammatory cells, and cellular fragments [7, 8]. Epidemiological data indicate that patients with silicosis and other parenchymal lung diseases are frequently diagnosed with elevated pulmonary pressure [9, 10]. Moreover, increased pulmonary pressure above 25 mmHg is a strong indicator of worst outcome in patients with silicosis and other underlying interstitial lung diseases [11, 12].

The pathogenesis of interstitial lung diseases and pulmonary hypertension is incompletely understood, although recent literature points to the important role of an oxidant/antioxidant imbalance in the development of these serious disorders. Since crystalline silica is a strong promoter of inflammatory responses in pulmonary cells, mostly through the induction of a burst of reactive oxygen species in affected areas of the lung, we decided to explore the role of an antioxidant enzyme in the development of lung fibrosis and pulmonary vascular remodeling leading to pulmonary hypertension in mice treated with silica [13]. One of the most abundant antioxidant enzymes in the pulmonary vasculature is extracellular superoxide dismutase (SOD3). In the human vessel wall, SOD3 is expressed at the highest level, comprising more than half of the total vascular SOD, with activity levels ~ 10-fold higher than in other tissues [14, 15]. Vascular SOD3 interacts with heparin and other extracellular matrix proteins on the surface of endothelial and smooth muscle cells and is involved in the regulation of vascular tone under physiological conditions and during oxidative stress. It has been shown that SOD3 preserves endothelium-dependent relaxation and reduces angiotensin-induced blood pressure [16, 17]. Moreover, genetic manipulation of SOD3 expression affects the development of pulmonary hypertension in mice exposed to bleomycin or chronic hypoxia [18–20]. SOD3 activities and expression are also dysregulated during development and progression of atherosclerosis [21] and hypertension [22, 23].

In this study, we investigated the protective role of SOD3 in silica-induced lung fibrosis and in pulmonary vascular remodeling and development of pulmonary hypertension. We found that silica exposed $Sod3^{-/-}$ mice developed more lung fibrosis, increased thickening of vascular walls in remodeled pulmonary vessels, and higher right ventricular pressure (RVSP) when compared to wild-type littermate.

Material and methods

Experimental animals and animal care

C57BL/6 J mice were obtained from Jackson Laboratory (Bar Harbor, ME). The Institutional Animal Care and Use Committee of the University of Louisville approved the research protocol #15129, and the care and handling of the animals were in accordance with the National Institutes of Health guidelines.

Animal model

SOD3 knockout mice ($Sod3^{-/-}$) in the C57BL/6 J background were described previously [24]. Littermate wild-type C57BL/6 J were used as control. Adult male $Sod3^{+/+}$ and $Sod3^{-/-}$ mice (10 weeks of age) were separated into 3 experimental groups with 5 animals per group. Animals were anesthetized and placed in the supine position. Using sterile technique, the trachea was exposed via midline neck incision followed by instillation of silica or saline as described previously [25]. Crystalline silica was sterilized at 200 °C for 2 h to inactivate endotoxin contamination. Silica suspension in sterile 0.9% NaCl was prepared by vigorous vortexing immediately prior to intratracheal administration. Using a 27-gauge needle attached to a microliter syringe, 0.4 g/kg of crystalline silica suspension or the equivalent volume of saline was instilled into the trachea. The incision was then closed using surgical clips, and animals were allowed to recover. Twenty-eight days after intratracheal instillation of silica, RSVP parameters were measured and lung tissue were harvested for morphological, biochemical, and histochemical analyses. Tissue was immediately processed or quick-frozen in liquid nitrogen.

Reagents

Primers and probes for real-time PCR were obtained from Integrated DNA Technologies (Coralville, IA) and ThermoFisher Scientific (Waltham, MA). All other chemicals and enzymes were from Sigma Chemical Co. (St. Louis, MO), or Invitrogen (Carlsbad, CA).

Hemodynamic measurements

RVSP was determined with a 1F pressure transducer catheter (Millar Instruments). Briefly, the 1F pressure transducer was inserted through the right external jugular vein of anesthetized mice (100 mg ketamine/5 mg xylazine/kg of body weight, i.p.). Mice were placed on thermal plates to keep body temperature constant at 37 °C. Then, a pressure catheter was threaded into the right ventricle and RVSP was recorded using PowerLab 4/35 (ADInstruments) and analyzed using LabChart 8 software.

Lung histology and Histomorphometric analysis

Lungs were flushed with PBS and inflated and fixed with 10% formalin overnight, then embedded in paraffin, sectioned at a thickness of 5 μm, and stained with Mason's trichrome to visualize lung morphology and fibrosis. Images of lung sections were acquired using a high-resolution digital camera connected to a light microscope. Histomorphometric analysis of collagen deposition in silicotic nodules was performed using image analysis. At least six images per slide were captured at 400x magnification. The color deconvolution ImageJ software was used to evaluate the percentage of blue stained collagen in the image area. This software recognizes the image colors and decomposes them in three basic colors: blue (collagen), red, and purple. The morphometric analysis, corresponding to the blue color, was measured as the percentage of the total pixels in each image using the "threshold color" (ImageJ software), as described previously [26]. Collagen quantification was performed by an investigator blinded to treatment groups.

Immunohistochemical staining of mouse lungs for smooth muscle, von Willebrand factor (vWF), and LY-6B

Longitudinal sections (5 μm) of left lung lobe were hydrated and antigen retrieval was first performed by incubating with 0.1% pronase for 5 min at 37 °C and then heating the slides in 10 mM sodium citrate (pH 6.0) plus 0.05% Tween 20 at 98 °C for 10 min. Sections were stained with anti-smooth muscle actin-alpha antibodies clone 1A4 (Sigma) at concentration 23 ng/μl, anti-vWF antibodies H-300 (Sigma) and anti-LY-6B antibodies (Bio-Rad) at concentration 10 ng/μl. After washing, the slides were incubated with secondary antibodies labeled with either AlexaFluor 488 or AlexaFluor 594. To determine the specificity of staining, lung sections were incubated with control, non-immune IgG. Slides were analyzed with fluorescent microscopy.

Measurement of medial wall thickness

The hypertrophy of medial wall was measured in small muscularized arteries (< 200 μm) and expressed as a ratio of α-SMA stained area to perpendicular lumen radius. The measurements were performed using ImageJ (National Institutes of Health, Bethesda, MA). Pulmonary arteries were defined as vessels that accompanied airways (veins are interlobular). Five to ten pulmonary vessels were measured for each mouse. The analysis was performed by an investigator blinded to treatment groups.

Quantitative RT-PCR

Total RNA was prepared from lung using RNAqueous-Micro Kit (Applied Biosystems, Foster City, CA). The synthesis of single stranded DNA from RNA was performed using SuperScript First-Strand Synthesis System for RT-PCR and random hexamers (Invitrogen, Carlsbad, CA), according to the protocol provided by manufacturer. To quantitate the abundance of gene-specific mRNAs, quantitative PCR was undertaken using the StepOnePlus Real-Time PCR Detection System (Applied Biosystems, Foster City, CA) and an SYBR® Green Master Mix. The PCR cycles were 95 °C for 3 min, then 40 cycles of 95 °C for 15 s, 60 °C for 1 min. PCR assays were run in triplicate, and gene expression was normalized to β-Actin mRNA levels. The mouse Monocyte Chemotactic Protein 1 (Mcp1) primers were forward (5′- GAA GGA ATG GGT CCA GAC AT -3′) and reverse (5′-ACG GGT CAA CTT CAC ATT CA-3′), mouse Fibroblast-specific Protein 1 (Fsp1) primers were forward (5′-AGG AGC TAC TGA CCA GGG AGC T-3′) and reverse (5′-TCA TTG TCC CTG TTG CTG TCC-3′), mouse Sod3 primers were forward (5′-GGC AAC TCA GAG GCT CTT C-3′) and reverse (5′-GTA GCA AGC CGT AGA ACA AGA-3′), mouse endothelin 1 (ET-1) primers were forward (5′-TCT GCA CTC CAT TCT CAG C-3′) and reverse (5′-CGT GAT CTT CTC TCT GCT GTT C-3′),), mouse insulin growth factor 1 (IGF-1) primers were forward (5′-GAG ACT GGA GAT GTA CTG TGC-3′) and reverse (5′-CTC CTT TGC AGC TTC GTT TTC-3′),), mouse platelet factor 4 (PF4) primers were forward (5′-ACC ATC TCC TCT GGG ATC CAT-3′) and reverse (5′-CCA TTC TTC AGG GTG GCT ATG AG-3′), mouse platelet/endothelial cell adhesion molecule 1 (Pecam1) primers were forward (5′-AGA GAC GGT CTT GTC GCA GT-3′) and reverse (5′-TAC TGG GCT TCG AGA GCA TT-3′). PCR assays were run in triplicate, and gene expression was normalized to β-Actin mRNA levels. Primers for β-Actin were forward (5′- ACA GCT TCT TTG CAG CTC CT-3′) and reverse (5′-CCA TCA CAC CCT GGT GCC TA-3′). Analysis of Collagen Type 1 Alpha 1 chain (Col1a1), Tissue Inhibitor of Metalloproteases 1 (Timp1), Connective Tissue Growth Factor (Ctgf), Matrix Metallopeptidase 2 (Mmp2) Cu,Zn-Superoxide Dismutase (Sod1), and Mn-Superoxide Dismutase (Sod2) were performed using custom gene expression assays with FAM labeled probe obtained from Applied Biosystems. The mRNA levels for these genes were normalized for β-Actin mRNA levels that were detected with custom gene expression assay with VIC labeled probe.

Data analysis

All values are presented as means ± SEM of data from *n* independent experiments, as indicated in the figure legends. The statistical significance of differences was determined by t-test. A one-way analysis of variance (ANOVA) with Holm-Sidak post hoc test was used to compare differences between multiple treatment groups. *P*-value of < 0.05 indicated statistically significant differences.

Results

Silica exposure is associated with reduction in SOD3 expression

In order to explore the role of oxidative stress and superoxide dismutases in the development of pulmonary hypertension and silicosis, we began by analyzing the expression of three isoforms of superoxide dismutases in the lungs of control and silica-treated wild-type mice. We found that while mRNA levels of SOD1 and SOD2 did not change after exposure to silica, the expression of SOD3 gene was significantly attenuated by 27.7% in the lungs of silica-treated mice (Fig. 1a-c). Similar reductions in SOD3 protein levels were detected (Fig. 1d, e) suggesting reduced antioxidant protection in the lung 28 days after exposure to inhaled silica.

Silica exposure in the setting of SOD3 deficiency results in increased weight loss, enhanced lung lesions, and alterations in the expression of proinflammatory and tissue remodeling genes

Considering the observations in wild-type mice, we set out to evaluate the effect of silica exposure in wild-type and $Sod3^{-/-}$ mice. We found that the inhalation of crystalline silica induced an acute inflammatory response in the lung that led to the loss of body weight in affected animals. At day 2 following intratracheal silica administration (0.4 g/kg), $Sod3^{-/-}$ mice lost significantly more body weight (– 10.9 ± 5.84% for $Sod3^{+/+}$ and – 17.8 ± 1.22% for $Sod3^{-/-}$, $p < 0.05$) compared to wild-type littermates (Fig. 2a). However, the differences in body weight between $Sod3^{+/+}$ and $Sod3^{-/-}$ mice became non-significant by day 5. At day 28, both strains of mice recovered their body weight and reached the average weight of wild-type untreated animals.

To analyze the effect of intratracheal instillation of silica on lung structure, lung tissues were fixed, stained with Mason's trichrome and examined using light microscopy. Control mice showed no obvious abnormalities in lung structure, while mice challenged with silica developed noticeable fibrotic nodules with increased collagen deposition at day 28 (Fig. 2b). The quantitative analysis of fibrotic changes in the lung indicated that both $Sod3^{+/+}$ and $Sod3^{-/-}$ mice showed increased deposition of soluble collagen. The total amount of collagen in wild-type increased from 10.73 ± 1.94 μg/lobe in control mice to 31.19 ± 6.87 μg/lobe collagen in silica treated animals. $Sod3^{-/-}$ mice showed significantly higher (51.54 ± 7.62 μg/lobe) collagen accumulation in the lung (Fig. 2d). Similar results were obtained when collagen specific blue staining was analyzed in fibrotic nodules of $Sod3^{+/+}$ and $Sod3^{-/-}$ mice (Fig. 2b, c). These data suggest that expression of SOD3 might protect the lung from silica-induced accumulation of collagen and the formation of fibrotic nodules.

The development of lung lesions after exposure of lung to crystalline silica also resulted in alterations in the expression of a number of inflammatory and pro-fibrotic genes. For example, the mRNA expression of collagen type I (Col1a1) was markedly elevated in the right lobe of silica-treated lungs, coinciding with the increased levels of soluble collagen detected using Sircol Collagen Assay. However, no differences between silica-treated $Sod3^{+/+}$ and $Sod3^{-/-}$ mice were observed (Fig. 3e). On the other hand, the mRNA levels of pro-inflammatory cytokine Mcp1, pro-fibrotic fibroblast-specific Fsp1 gene and tissue-remodeling Timp1 gene were significantly upregulated in the lung of silica treated $Sod3^{-/-}$ mice, but not in $Sod3^{+/+}$ mice when compared to control (Fig. 3a-c). The differences in the upregulation of gene expression between $Sod3^{+/+}$ and

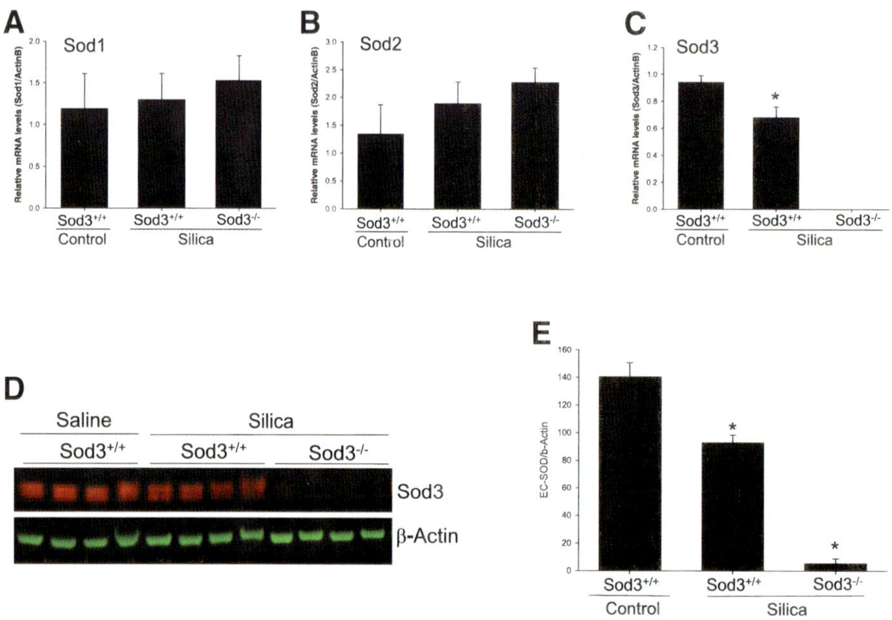

Fig. 1 Attenuation of SOD3 gene expression in the lung of silica treated mice. **a-c** Relative mRNA levels for three SOD isoforms were determined using quantitative RT-PCR and normalized to β-actin expression. **d** Western blot of lung tissues isolated from control and silica treated mice. Beta-actin was used as a control. **e** Quantitative analysis of SOD3 protein normalized to β-actin expression. The results are shown as means ± SEM, *$p < 0.05$ when compared to control lung, One Way ANOVA with Holm-Sidak post test

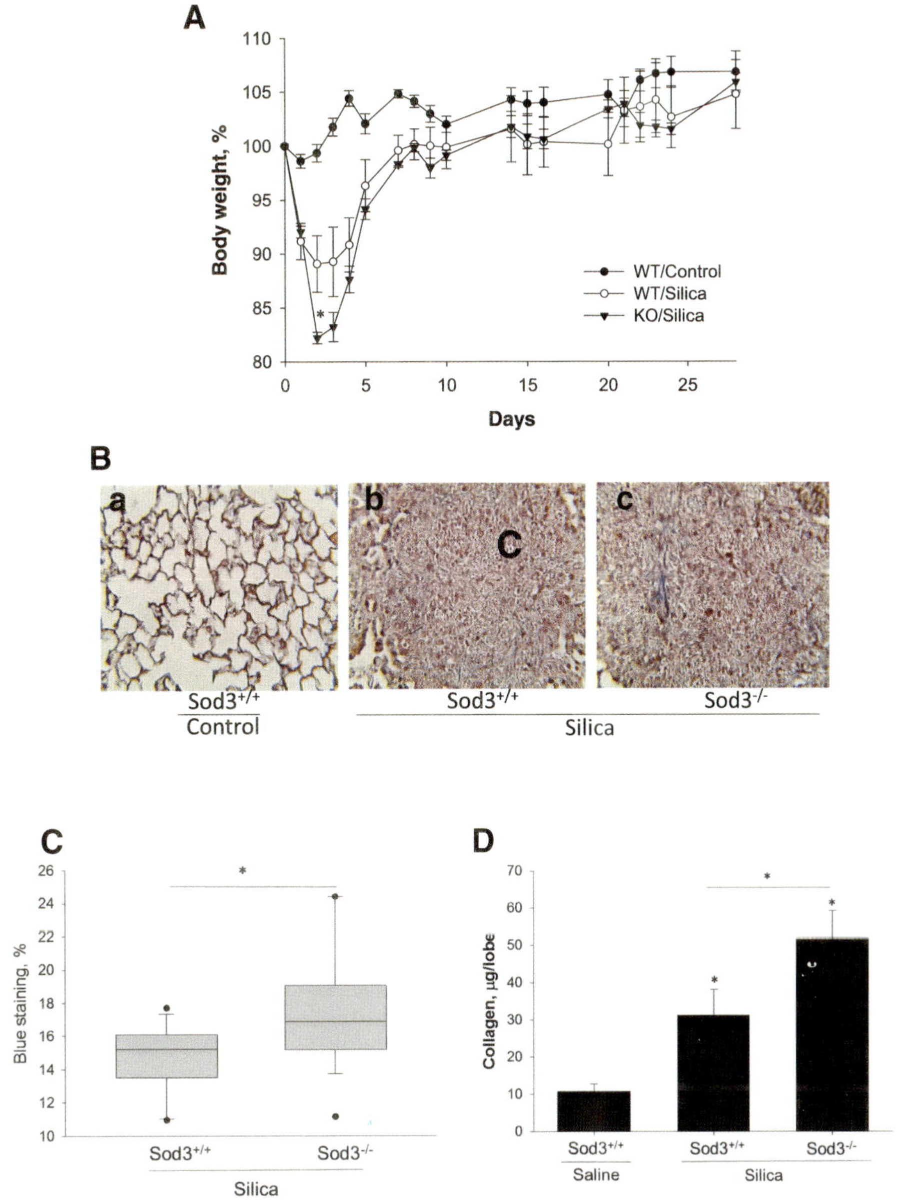

Fig. 2 Weight loss and right ventricular systolic pressure (RVSP) measurements in mice treated with silica. Deficiency of SOD3 increased body weight loss in early stage of silica-induced lung fibrosis. **a** Effect of SOD3 gene knockout on body weight loss after intratracheal injection of crystalline silica. Body weight was measured for 28 days. *$p < 0.05$ for silica-challenged Sod3$^{-/-}$ versus silica-challenged Sod3$^{+/+}$ mice. **b** Histochemical analysis of silicotic nodules in the lung of Sod3$^{+/+}$ and Sod3$^{-/-}$ mice treated with crystalline silica. 40x magnification. **c** Analysis of collagen specific blue staining. *t*-test, * < 0.05. **d** Collagen accumulation in the lung. The results are shown as mean ± SEM, *$p < 0.05$ when compared to control lung, One Way ANOVA with Holm-Sidak post test

Sod3$^{-/-}$ were observed only for Mcp1, Fsp1 and Timp1 genes (Fig. 3a-c). Surprisingly, the mRNA levels for growth factor involved in fibrotic transformation of lung (CTGF) and major extracellular matrix remodeling enzyme (Mmp2) did not change after exposure to silica in both mouse strains (Fig. 3d, f). These data suggest that loss of SOD3 expression may predispose the lung to greater inflammatory responses and enhanced pro-fibrotic signaling via distinct pathways.

Silica exposure is associated with increased neutrophil infiltration in lung, especially around pulmonary arteries

To further assess the inflammatory response in the lungs of animals, a marker of neutrophils (LY6B) was examined histologically at 4 weeks (Fig. 4a). In addition to neutrophils, Ly6B marker is expressed on the surface of macrophages polarized toward a proinflammatory phenotype [27]. Silica exposure significantly altered the recruitment of activated

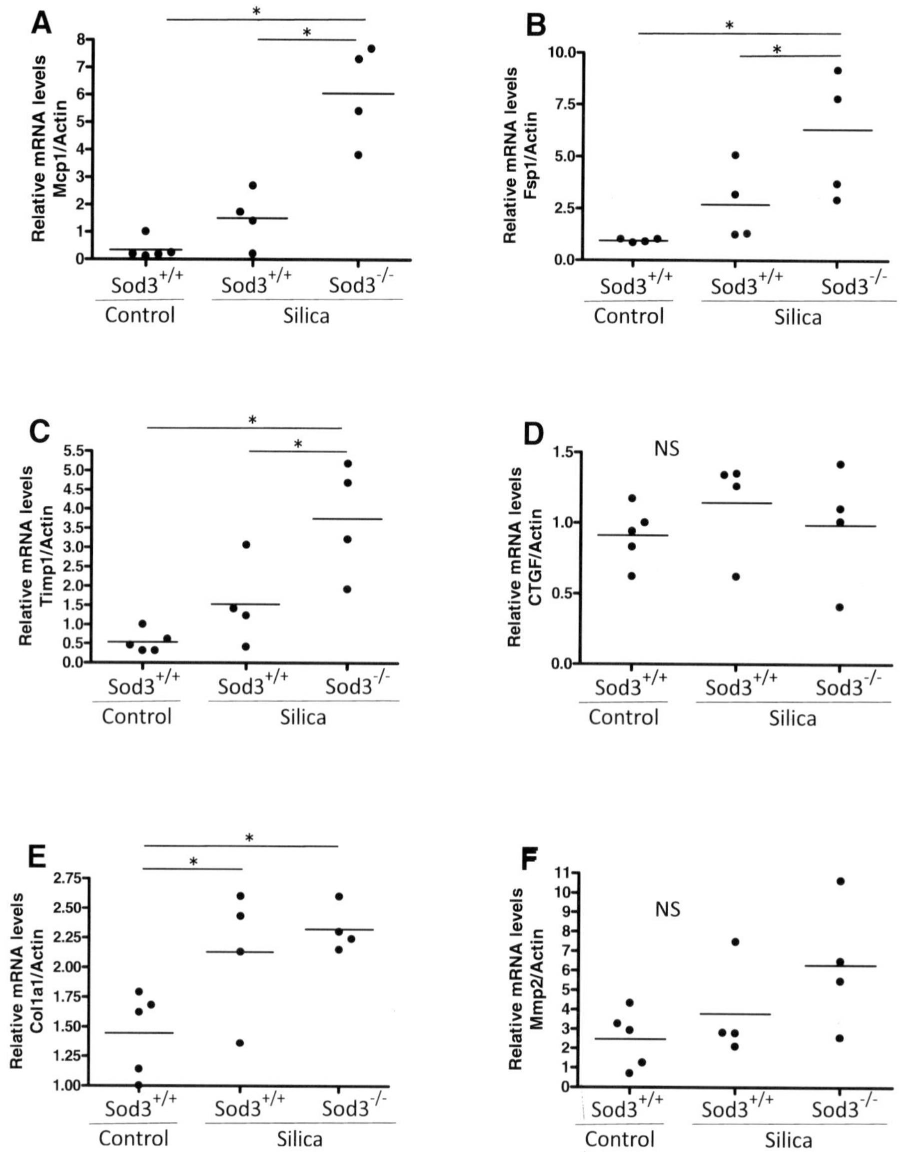

Fig. 3 Expression of pro-fibrotic and inflammatory genes in response to silica. Analysis of gene expression in the lung of silica treated mice. Whole lung mRNA levels for (**a**) monocyte chemoattractant protein-1 (Mcp1), (**b**) fibroblast-specific protein 1 (Fsp1), (**c**) tissue inhibitor of metalloproteinases 1 (Timp1), (**d**) connective tissue growth factor (Ctgf), (**e**) collagen type I, alpha 1 (Col1a1), and (**f**) matrix metalloproteinase 2 (Mmp-2) were determined using real-time PCR and normalized to beta-acting expression (β-Actin), $^{*}p < 0.05$ when compared to control lung, One Way ANOVA with Holm-Sidak post test

macrophages and neutrophils into lung areas that were free of silicotic nodules from 5.8 ± 2.6 cells per field in control mice to 9.5 ± 3.1 cells per field in silica treated mice ($p < 0.05$). However, no significant differences in inflammatory cells recruitment were observed between silica-exposed $Sod3^{+/+}$ and $Sod3^{-/-}$ mice (9.5 ± 3.1 vs 10.8 ± 3.4 cells per field). Since large clusters of LY6B positive cells were detected around pulmonary arteries, we analyzed the areas of LY6B-stained lungs in close proximity to the pulmonary vasculature. Crystalline silica inhalation caused more inflammatory cell accumulation around pulmonary vasculature in SOD3 deficient mice (6.88 ± 4.86%) compared to wild-type littermate (10.74 ± 5.94%) (Fig. 4b). Thus, while silica exposure caused the infiltration of inflammatory cells in the lung, $Sod3^{-/-}$ mice showed enhanced response specifically in the areas that are in close proximity to the pulmonary arteries. This prompted an evaluation of the pulmonary arteries.

Silica exposure is also associated with pulmonary vascular remodeling and pulmonary hypertension

Silica-related chronic lung disease has been linked to pulmonary hypertension [28]. The pulmonary hypertension and the above-described increase in perivascular infiltration

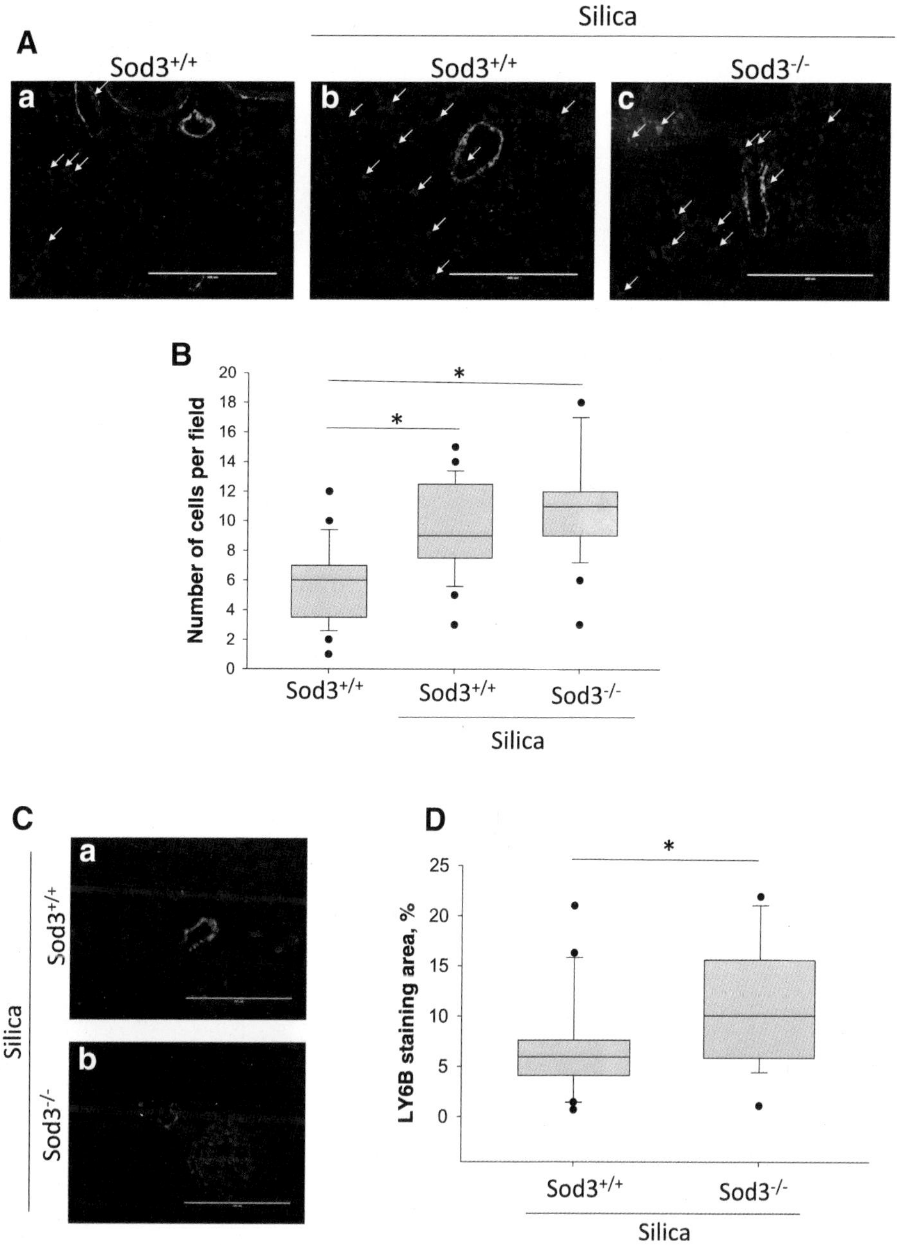

Fig. 4 Infiltration of inflammatory cells in the lung of Sod3$^{+/+}$ and Sod3$^{-/-}$ mice treated with silica. **a** Lung sections (5 μm thick) were stained with antibodies specific for macrophage- and neutrophil-specific marker LY-6B (red) and α-smooth muscle actin (green). Nuclei were stained using DAPI (blue). Images were taken using 20x objective. Representative images from unaffected areas of mouse lung from control (image a) and 0.4 mg/kg silica treated (images b and c) mice. Increased infiltration of inflammatory cells into lung found in silica treated lungs of both Sod3$^{+/+}$ and Sod3$^{-/-}$ mice (**panel b**). Bar = 200 μm. $*p < 0.05$ when compared to control lung, One Way ANOVA with Holm-Sidak post test. **c** Representative images of LY6B positive cells located in close proximity to pulmonary vessels in silicotic nodules. **d** Quantitative analysis of area in close proximity to pulmonary vessels (green) stained with LY-6B (red) specific antibodies. $*p < 0.05$, *t*-test

of activated macrophages and neutrophils detected in the lungs of Sod3$^{-/-}$ animals, justified a more in-depth look at the vascular structures. First, we analyzed the effects of silica on pulmonary blood pressure by measuring right ventricular systolic pressure (RVSP) (Fig. 5a). We found that administration of crystalline silica increased RVSP in wild-type mice from 21.4 ± 0.86 mmHg in control to 27.29 ± 2.01 mmHg in silica treated animals. Sod3$^{-/-}$ mice showed significantly higher RVSP (33.13 ± 2.17 mmHg) after silica treatment compared to Sod3$^{+/+}$ mice ($p < 0.05$) suggesting that SOD3 is protective in the setting of pulmonary hypertension secondary to silicosis.

The magnitude of structural changes in pulmonary vessels, characterized by thickening of the smooth muscle

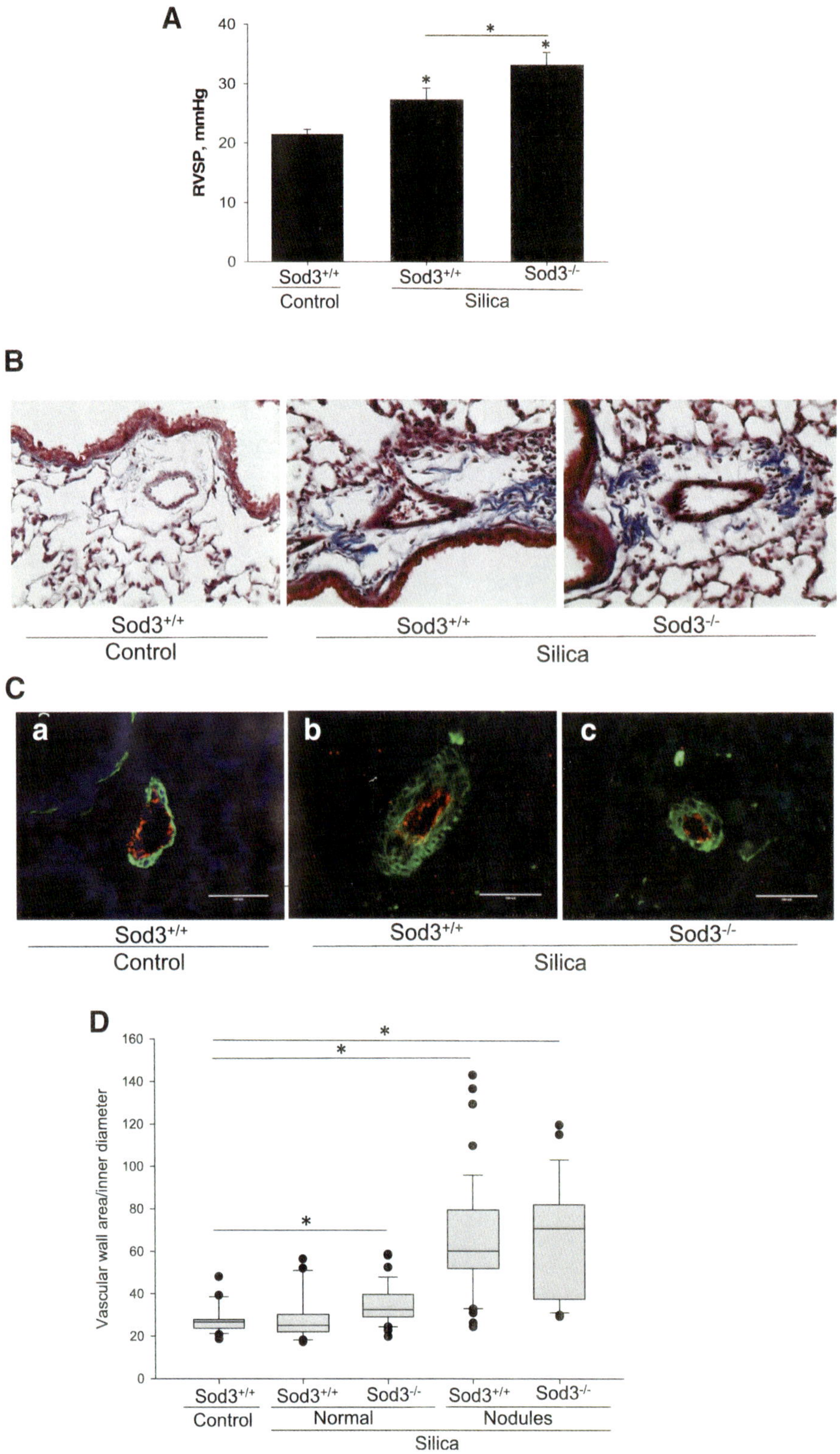

Fig. 5 (See legend on next page.)

(See figure on previous page.)
Fig. 5 Vascular remodeling in silica treated lungs. **a** Right Ventricular Systolic Pressure (RVSP) was measured using pressure catheter inserted into right ventricle through jugular vein. The results are shown as mean ± SEM, $*p < 0.05$. **b** Lung sections were stained with Mason's trichrome to visualize collagen and imaged at 400x magnification. Representative images of pulmonary arteries from control (a) and silica treated $Sod3^{+/+}$ (image b) or $Sod3^{-/-}$ (image c) mice. **c** Lung sections (5 μm thick) were stained with antibodies specific for endothelium-specific von Willebrand Factor vWF (red) and α-smooth muscle actin (green). Nuclei were stained using DAPI (blue). Images were taken using 40x objective. Panel a: representative images of pulmonary arteries from control mice. Panel b and c: images of pulmonary arteries with proliferated smooth muscle cell layer. **d** Quantitative analysis of vascular wall remodeling expressed as ratio of smooth muscle vascular wall area/inner diameter. Bar = 100 μm. $*p < 0.05$ when compared to control lung, One Way ANOVA with Holm-Sidak post test

layer, is a good measure of abnormal vascular changes. Therefore, we analyzed pulmonary artery remodeling in Mason's trichrome stained lung section following silica exposure (Fig. 5b). In addition, we stained pulmonary arteries for alpha smooth muscle actin to measure the hypertrophy of the smooth muscle layer and expressed vascular remodeling as a ratio between smooth muscle surface area divided by inner dimeter (Fig. 5c, d). Pulmonary artery remodeling was measured in the areas not affected by fibrosis and in the silicotic nodules. Interestingly, both strains of mice showed a similar increase in thickness of the vascular smooth muscle layer in structures within the silicotic nodules from 28.67 ± 6.43 in control mice to 65.63 ± 26.55 ($p < 0.001$) in $Sod3^{+/+}$ and to 64.84 ± 26.44 ($p < 0.001$) in $Sod3^{-/-}$ mice after silica exposure (Fig. 5d). However, the measurement of wall thickness in pulmonary arteries located in unaffected areas of the lung indicated remodeling of vascular walls only in $Sod3^{-/-}$ mice, but not in $Sod3^{+/+}$ mice (Fig. 5d). Thus, both hemodynamic and morphological features indicate an important role for SOD3 in development of silica-induced pulmonary hypertension.

Sod3 deficiency did not change the expression of vascular-specific genes in silicotic lungs

Treatment of $Sod3^{+/+}$ and $Sod3^{-/-}$ mice with crystalline silica for 4 weeks attenuated the expression of several endothelium- or smooth muscle-specific genes (Fig. 6). The mRNA levels for ET-1 and Pecam1 were significantly reduced in both strains of mice (Fig. 6a, d) while differences in the expression of PF4 gene between control and silica-treated mice were non-significant (Fig. 6c). Interestingly, the expression of IGF-1 was upregulated 4-fold in silica treated lungs, but no differences were detected between $Sod3^{+/+}$ and $Sod3^{-/-}$ mice (Fig. 6b). These data indicate that crystalline silica might affect the pulmonary vasculature through differential regulation of vascular- specific genes, however the lack of Sod3 in murine lungs did not change the expression of these genes in silica-injured lungs.

Discussion

Although the protective role of SOD3 in animal models of lung fibrosis has been reported previously [29, 30], its contribution to the development of pulmonary vascular remodeling associated with chronic lung diseases is not well understood. In this study, we show that SOD3 plays an important role in silica-induced lung inflammation and fibrosis. SOD3 also appears important for the development of vascular remodeling and pulmonary hypertension in this model. This work was prompted by the observation that SOD3 expression is reduced in animals exposed to crystalline silica, thereby suggesting a protective role for SOD3. Further work in SOD3-deficient animals revealed increased weight loss, lung structural changes with more pulmonary nodules, enhanced collagen deposition, and alterations in proinflammatory and profibrotic genes when compared to silica-treated wild-type animals. These changes were associated with increased inflammatory cells infiltration in the lungs of $Sod3^{-/-}$ exposed to silica. Interestingly, there was also an increase in infiltrate of activated macrophages and neutrophils in perivascular structures not noted in wild-type animals. This pointed to a role for SOD3 in vascular remodeling for which further studies were performed revealing increased RVSP in all mice exposed to crystalline silica, but an even further increase in RSVP in $Sod3^{-/-}$ animals, which was associated with increased vascular wall thickening. This is important since no previous studies indicated a role for SOD3 in silica-induced pulmonary hypertension. Interestingly, SOD3-deficient mice develop elevated pulmonary blood pressures and profound vascular wall remodeling when compared to neonatal wild-type littermates in the bleomycin model of pulmonary fibrosis [31]. However, the etiology and pathological manifestations of silica-induced changes in lung interstitium and the pulmonary vasculature are substantially different from those induced by bleomycin, thereby requiring further investigation [25]. In addition to the observed increase in RVSP in $Sod3^{-/-}$ mice, we also found differences in inflammatory cell activation and in the rate of hypertrophy of smooth muscle layer in pulmonary arteries.

Our data indicated an excessive deposition of collagen in the silicotic lungs of both strains of mice, although $Sod3^{-/-}$ mice were more susceptible to fibrosis (Fig. 2). This observation was supported by elevated expression of the collagen 1A1 and the fibroblast-specific protein 1 genes (Fig. 3). Fsp1 is related to the family of cytoplasmic

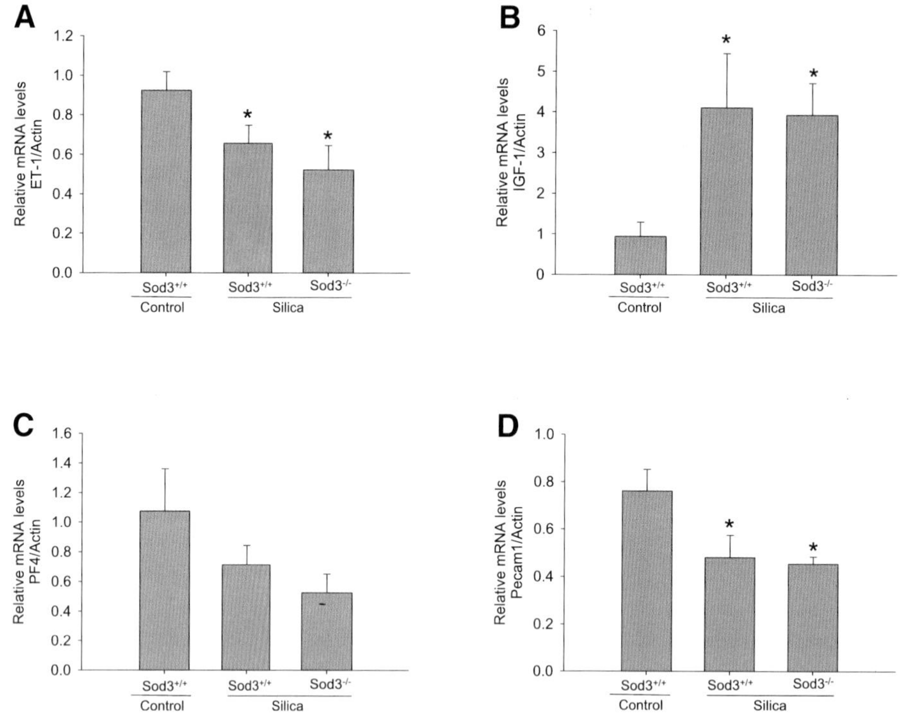

Fig. 6 Expression of vascular-specific genes. Analysis of vascular-specific gene expression in the lung of wild-type (Sod3$^{+/+}$) and Sod3 deficient (Sod3$^{-/-}$) mice. Expression of genes was analyzed 28 days following silica instillation. Whole lung mRNA levels for (**a**) endothelin 1 (ET-1), (**b**) insulin growth factor 1 (IGF-1), (**c**) platelet factor 4 (PF4), (**d**) platelet/endothelial cell adhesion molecule 1 (Pecam1) were determined using real-time PCR and normalized to beta-acting expression (Actin). The results are shown as mean ± SEM, $*p < 0.05$ when compared to control lung, One Way ANOVA with Holm-Sidak post test

calcium-binding proteins and is mostly produced by activated fibroblasts in tissues that undergo excessive remodeling [32]. The Fsp1-positive fibroblasts derived from the lung of mice treated with bleomycin are also characterized by excessive production of alpha1 procollagen. Moreover, under certain inflammatory conditions, Fsp1 is expressed by activated macrophages and other immune cells [33]. Thus, increased levels of Fsp1 in the silicotic lungs may be related to the influx and activation of fibroblasts and immune cells. Our observation of increased collagen deposition coinciding with elevated expression of fibroblast-specific genes is in good agreement with previously published literature.

Moreover, we found increased expression of TIMP-1 gene in Sod3$^{-/-}$ mice exposed to silica. The pattern of TIMP-1 gene expression was similar to MMP-2 gene expression among experimental groups, although the differences in MMP-2 expression did not reached the statistical significance. Similar small increase in Mmp-2 and 8-fold increase of TIMP-1 expression in the lung of bleomycin treated C57BL6J mice has been described previously [34]. It is possible that increase of TIMP-1 expression in Sod3$^{-/-}$ mice can be explained by increased oxidative stress in the lung of these animals [35]. In the lung, TIMP-1 produced mostly by macrophages and epithelial cells. The matrix metalloproteinases and their specific inhibitors are important elements of the tissue remodeling process. Increase in protease inhibitors would promote abnormal tissue repairing pathway resulting in scarring of pulmonary tissue and leading to pulmonary fibrosis [36]. Conversely, the pathological overproduction of MMPs would lead to tissue destruction as observed in emphysema and chronic obstructive pulmonary disease [37]. The role of TIMP-1 in development of pulmonary hypertension and vascular remodeling is controversial. Increased MMP-2 and TIMP-1 expression were identified in pulmonary artery smooth muscle cells isolated from idiopathic PAH patients [38]. Vieillard-Baron et al. reported that inhibition of MMPs activities by intratracheal delivery of TIMP-1 exacerbated pulmonary hypertension and increased muscularization and periadvetitial collagen accumulation in distal arteries of rats subjected to chronic hypoxia [39]. Other studies found evidence that ECM degradation may be essential to smooth muscle cells migration and proliferation [40]. Moreover, targeted delivery of TIMP in luminal cells inhibited neointimal formation in human saphenous veins [41]. While the reason for the discrepancy between these studies it not clear, it may be ascribable to differences in studied vascular structures. Since we investigated vascular remodeling in fibrotic lungs, it is also possible that increased hypertrophy of smooth muscle layer in pulmonary arteries can be stimulated by rise in pulmonary artery wall tension due to excessive deposition of extracellular matrix [42].

We also found increased influx of inflammatory cells in the lungs of mice challenged with silica. We used Ly6B antigen as a neutrophil marker, however, recent data suggested that Ly6B could also be expressed by specific Ly6B^{high} subset of proinflammatory macrophages. This subtype of activated macrophages exacerbate fibrotic renal injury by secreting extracellular matrix compounds including fibronectin and collagen [27]. They also produce proinflammatory cytokines and chemokines that help to recruit and differentiate additional macrophages into sites of injury creating perpetual injurious cycle. Interestingly, the number of Ly6B positive inflammatory cells in the non-affected areas of silica-exposed lungs was significantly higher in Sod3$^{-/-}$ mice suggesting an important role of SOD3 in chemotaxis of these cells into the pulmonary intersitium. Previous studies supported a role for superoxide in inflammatory cell migration [43] and a beneficial anti-inflammatory role for SOD3 in this process [44]. Moreover, acute deletion of SOD3 alone leads to massive infiltration of granulocytes, T cells, and natural killer cells in lung [45]. Crystalline silica produces its damaging effects through activation of immune cells and production of reactive oxygen species (ROS) burst [46, 47]. In turn, elevated ROS levels can lead to epithelial and vascular cell damage promoting fibrogenic remodeling of lung interstitium and proliferation of cells in the vascular media. SOD3 is a potent anti-inflammatory agent and an inhibitor of inflammatory cell influx in response to asbestos, bleomycin, hyperoxia and lipopolysaccharides [48–51]. Therefore, loss of SOD3 from the lung of genetically-modified animals may predispose pulmonary epithelial and vascular cells to ROS-induced damage due to diminishing antioxidative protection. On the other hand, infiltration of macrophages and neutrophils specifically around remodeled pulmonary vessels may deliver a new load of SOD3, thereby alleviating ROS-induced damage, while normalizing signaling pathways responsible for vascular cell proliferation and hypertrophy Interestingly, the increased influx of immune cells in Sod3$^{-/-}$ mice coincided with an elevated expression of Mcp1 gene, which is one of the key chemokines that regulate migration and infiltration of monocytes and macrophages into the lung [52]. The lack of experimental evidences supporting the role of ROS in observed exacerbation of pulmonary fibrosis and pulmonary hypertension in Sod3$^{-/-}$ mice is a major limitation of this study.

The effects of crystalline silica and other environmental and occupational particulate matter on the expression of antioxidant enzymes in the lung are not well known. We observed a decrease in the expression of SOD3 in the lungs of silica-treated mice at day 28. This attenuated expression of SOD3 is in good agreement with reduced expression of SOD3 in the lung intersitium of wild-type mice treated with bleomycin and asbestos [48, 53] and with decreased SOD3-specific staining in IPF patients [54]. On the other hand, others reported differential regulation of superoxide dismutases in the lung of silica-treated rats [55]. Kim et al. indicated that SOD3 gene expression in the lung was elevated compared to control animals starting from day 3 and up to 90 days following silica administration. This observation contrasts with ours when analyzing SOD3 expression 28 days following silica exposure in mice. There are several possible explanations for this discrepancy. First, different species of rodents (mice vs rats) were used in these studies. Second, the dosage of administered silica and differences in chemical and morphological characteristics of crystalline silica may lead to different responses. For example, it has been shown that crystalline silica with a geometric mean diameter of 1.8 μm produces more profound effects on inflammatory cell infiltration into the bronchoalveolar lavage fluid harvested from lungs when compared to silica with a diameter of 0.7 μm [56]. Further studies will be required to evaluate these differential findings and how they are relevant to the human condition.

A key finding of this work is that the fibrotic changes observed in our model were accompanied by significant vascular changes. The analysis of vascular remodeling in silica-treated animals revealed increased thickening of smooth muscle layer in the pulmonary arteries of silicotic lungs. Interestingly, no differences in smooth muscle hypertrophy were detected in the fibrotic areas between Sod3$^{+/+}$ and Sod3$^{-/-}$ mice, thereby suggesting a differential role for SOD3 in vascular and non-vascular structures. The profound remodeling of the vascular media in fibrotic areas of lung has been described previously by others and us [25, 31]. It is intriguing to note that the lack of SOD3 in these remodeled pulmonary vessels was not accompanied by changes in smooth muscle proliferation, while enhancing collagen deposition and cells infiltration. On the other hand, Sod3$^{-/-}$ mice developed significant thickening of the pulmonary artery walls located in unaffected areas of the lung when compared to wild-type littermates treated with silica. To our knowledge, this is the first description of differential vascular remodeling in non-fibrotic and fibrosing lung compartments in the setting of silica exposure.

To further investigate the potential molecular mechanisms involved in vascular remodeling, we measured the expression of several vasculature-specific genes. There were no significant differences in expression of ET-1, PECAM-1 and PF4 genes between Sod3$^{+/+}$ and Sod3$^{-/-}$ mice, although silica treatment attenuated their expression in both mouse strains. Therefore, observed exacerbation of vascular remodeling and pulmonary hypertension in Sod3 deficient mice is not associated with differential regulation of these factors after exposure to silica. In addition, we quantified mRNA levels of IGF-1 since this growth factor might be a potent mediator of vascular growth responses in settings of pulmonary hypertension. Indeed, IGF-1 was significantly elevated in silicotic lungs of both mouse strains indicating important role of IGF-1 signaling in pulmonary response to crystalline silica. Similar induction of IGF-1 expression in the lung of neonatal mice exposed to hypoxia has been described previously [57]. Although increased signaling through IGF-1 in response to silica administration is observed in this study, the other pathways triggered by EGF, FGF, and PDGF were not examined and need further investigation.

Our findings may also have a clinical relevance. The pulmonary hypertension in patients with silicosis, COPD, lung fibrosis and sarcoidosis is associated with higher mortality rate [9–11]. The elucidation of mechanisms by which silicosis may lead to elevated pulmonary pressure may provide novel therapeutic strategies. These findings further implicated important role of Sod3 in progression of silica induced lung fibrosis and pulmonary hypertension.

Conclusions

In conclusion, we report that mice lacking SOD3 developed increased RVSP and pulmonary vascular remodeling associated with enhanced collagen deposition, increased influx of inflammatory cells, and alterations in proinflammatory and profibrotic gene expression. Our results suggest that SOD3 play an important role in silica-induced lung fibrosis and vascular remodeling in the lung and provides new insight into the role of antioxidant defense mechanisms responsible for protecting the lung from the harmful effects of air pollution and occupational hazards.

Abbreviations

COPD: Chronic obstructive pulmonary disease; CTGF: Connective tissue growth factor; ET-1: Eendothelin 1; FSP-1: Fibroblast-specific protein 1; LY-6B: Lymphocyte antigen 6 complex, locus B; MCP-1: Monocyte chemoattractant protein – 1; MMP-2: Matric metallopeptidase – 2; PH: Pulmonary hypertension; RVSP: Right ventricular systolic pressure; TIMP-1: Tissue inhibitor of metalloproteinase – 1; TNF-α: Tumor necrosis factor alpha

Acknowledgments

We thank US Silica Inc. (Frederick, MD) for providing the sample of crystalline silica used in this study.

Funding

This work was supported by NIH grants R56HL128597 (Zelko) and VA Merit Review Grant BX000216 (Roman).

Authors' contributions

Conception and design: INZ; Analysis and interpretation: INZ, JXZ; Drafting the manuscript for important intellectual content: INZ, JR. All authors read and approved the final manuscript.

Competing interests

Igor Zelko research is funded by National Institutes of Health. Jesse Roman serves or has served as investigator on industry-sponsored clinical trials related to pulmonary fibrosis (Gilead, Fibrogen, Intermune, Promedia, Novartis, Boehringer Ingelheim, and Bristol-Meyers-Squibb). He also served on the boards of the American Lung Association - Midland States, the Pulmonary Fibrosis Foundation, and the American Thoracic Society. His research is funded by the National Institutes of Health and the Department of Veterans Affairs. Jian Zhu has no competing interests to disclose.

Author details

[1]Department of Medicine, Division of Pulmonary, Critical Care, and Sleep Medicine, University of Louisville, 505 S. Hancock Street, CTR Bldg., room 524, Louisville, KY 40202, USA. [2]Department of Biochemistry and Molecular Genetics, University of Louisville, 505 S. Hancock Street, CTR Bldg., room 524, Louisville, KY 40202, USA. [3]Department of Pharmacology and Toxicology, University of Louisville Health Sciences Center, Louisville, KY 40202, USA. [4]Robley Rex VA Medical Center, Louisville, KY 40202, USA.

References

1. Madl AK, Donovan EP, Gaffney SH, McKinley MA, Moody EC, Henshaw JL, Paustenbach DJ. State-of-the-science review of the occupational health hazards of crystalline silica in abrasive blasting operations and related requirements for respiratory protection. J Toxicol Environ Health B Crit Rev. 2008;11:548–608.
2. Cooper GS, Miller FW, Germolec DR. Occupational exposures and autoimmune diseases. Int Immunopharmacol. 2002;2:303–13.
3. Liu Y, Steenland K, Rong Y, Hnizdo E, Huang X, Zhang H, Shi T, Sun Y, Wu T, Chen W. Exposure-response analysis and risk assessment for lung cancer in relationship to silica exposure: a 44-year cohort study of 34,018 workers. Am J Epidemiol. 2013;178:1424–33.
4. Cullinan P. Occupation and chronic obstructive pulmonary disease (COPD). Br Med Bull. 2012;104:143–61.
5. Sellamuthu R, Umbright C, Roberts JR, Chapman R, Young SH, Richardson D, Cumpston J, McKinney W, Chen BT, Frazer D, et al. Transcriptomics analysis of lungs and peripheral blood of crystalline silica-exposed rats. Inhal Toxicol. 2012;24:570–9.
6. Davis GS, Leslie KO, Hemenway DR. Silicosis in mice: effects of dose, time, and genetic strain. J Environ Pathol Toxicol Oncol. 1998;17:81–97.
7. Huaux F. New developments in the understanding of immunology in silicosis. Curr Opin Allergy Clin Immunol. 2007;7:168–73.
8. Dostert C, Petrilli V, Van Bruggen R, Steele C, Mossman BT, Tschopp J. Innate immune activation through Nalp3 inflammasome sensing of asbestos and silica. Science. 2008;320:674–7.
9. Carlsen J, Hasseriis Andersen K, Boesgaard S, Iversen M, Steinbruchel D, Bogelund Andersen C. Pulmonary arterial lesions in explanted lungs after transplantation correlate with severity of pulmonary hypertension in chronic obstructive pulmonary disease. J Heart Lung Transplant. 2013;32:347–54.
10. Lettieri CJ, Nathan SD, Barnett SD, Ahmad S, Shorr AF. Prevalence and outcomes of pulmonary arterial hypertension in advanced idiopathic pulmonary fibrosis. Chest. 2006;129:746–52.

11. Jandova R, Widimsky J, Eisler L, Navratil M. Long-term prognosis of pulmonary hypertension in silicosis. Cor Vasa. 1980;22:221–37.
12. Takahashi K, Taniguchi H, Ando M, Sakamoto K, Kondoh Y, Watanabe N, Kimura T, Kataoka K, Suzuki A, Ito S, Hasegawa Y. Mean pulmonary arterial pressure as a prognostic indicator in connective tissue disease associated with interstitial lung disease: a retrospective cohort study. BMC Pulm Med. 2016;16:55.
13. Mossman BT, Churg A. Mechanisms in the pathogenesis of asbestosis and silicosis. Am J Respir Crit Care Med. 1998;157:1666–80.
14. Stralin P, Karlsson K, Johansson BO, Marklund SL. The interstitium of the human arterial wall contains very large amounts of extracellular superoxide dismutase. Arterioscler Thromb Vasc Biol. 1995;15:2032–6.
15. Oury TD, Day BJ, Crapo JD. Extracellular superoxide dismutase: a regulator of nitric oxide bioavailability. Lab Investig. 1996;75:617–36.
16. Abrahamsson T, Brandt U, Marklund SL, Sjoqvist PO. Vascular bound recombinant extracellular superoxide dismutase type C protects against the detrimental effects of superoxide radicals on endothelium-dependent arterial relaxation. Circ Res. 1992;70:264–71.
17. Laursen JB, Rajagopalan S, Galis Z, Tarpey M, Freeman BA, Harrison DG. Role of superoxide in angiotensin II-induced but not catecholamine-induced hypertension. Circulation. 1997;95:588–93.
18. Nozik-Grayck E, Suliman HB, Majka S, Albietz J, Van Rheen Z, Roush K, Stenmark KR. Lung EC-SOD overexpression attenuates hypoxic induction of Egr-1 and chronic hypoxic pulmonary vascular remodeling. Am J Physiol Lung Cell Mol Physiol. 2008;295:L422–30.
19. Nozik-Grayck E, Woods C, Taylor JM, Benninger RK, Johnson RD, Villegas LR, Stenmark KR, Harrison DG, Majka SM, Irwin D, Farrow KN. Selective depletion of vascular EC-SOD augments chronic hypoxic pulmonary hypertension. Am J Physiol Lung Cell Mol Physiol. 2014;307:L868–76.
20. Van Rheen Z, Fattman C, Domarski S, Majka S, Klemm D, Stenmark KR, Nozik-Grayck E. Lung extracellular superoxide dismutase overexpression lessens bleomycin-induced pulmonary hypertension and vascular remodeling. Am J Respir Cell Mol Biol. 2011;44:500–8.
21. Fukai T, Galis ZS, Meng XP, Parthasarathy S, Harrison DG. Vascular expression of extracellular superoxide dismutase in atherosclerosis. J Clin Invest. 1998; 101:2101–11.
22. Gongora MC, Qin Z, Laude K, Kim HW, McCann L, Folz JR, Dikalov S, Fukai T, Harrison DG. Role of extracellular superoxide dismutase in hypertension. Hypertension. 2006;48:473–81.
23. Fukai T, Siegfried MR, Ushio-Fukai M, Griendling KK, Harrison DG. Modulation of extracellular superoxide dismutase expression by angiotensin II and hypertension. Circ Res. 1999;85:23–8.
24. Carlsson LM, Jonsson J, Edlund T, Marklund SL. Mice lacking extracellular superoxide dismutase are more sensitive to hyperoxia. Proc Natl Acad Sci U S A. 1995;92:6264–8.
25. Zelko IN, Zhu J, Ritzenthaler JD, Roman J. Pulmonary hypertension and vascular remodeling in mice exposed to crystalline silica. Respir Res. 2016;17:160.
26. Leite SN, Jordao Junior AA, Andrade TA, Masson Ddos S, Frade MA. Experimental models of malnutrition and its effect on skin trophism. An Bras Dermatol. 2011;86:681–8.
27. Belliere J, Casemayou A, Ducasse L, Zakaroff-Girard A, Martins F, Iacovoni JS, Guilbeau-Frugier C, Buffin-Meyer B, Pipy B, Chauveau D, et al. Specific macrophage subtypes influence the progression of rhabdomyolysis-induced kidney injury. J Am Soc Nephrol. 2015;26:1363–77.
28. Rosenman KD, Zhu Z. Pneumoconiosis and associated medical conditions. Am J Ind Med. 1995;27:107–13.
29. Mouradian GC Jr, Gaurav R, Pugliese S, El Kasmi K, Hartman B, Hernandez-Lagunas L, Stenmark K, Bowler RP, Nozik-Grayck E. SOD3 R213G SNP blocks murine Bleomycin-induced fibrosis and promotes resolution of inflammation. Am J Respir Cell Mol Biol. 2016.
30. Xu D, Guo H, Xu X, Lu Z, Fassett J, Hu X, Xu Y, Tang Q, Hu D, Somani A, et al. Exacerbated pulmonary arterial hypertension and right ventricular hypertrophy in animals with loss of function of extracellular superoxide dismutase. Hypertension. 2011;58:303–9.
31. Delaney C, Wright RH, Tang JR, Woods C, Villegas L, Sherlock L, Savani RC, Abman SH, Nozik-Grayck E. Lack of EC-SOD worsens alveolar and vascular development in a neonatal mouse model of bleomycin-induced bronchopulmonary dysplasia and pulmonary hypertension. Pediatr Res. 2015;78:634–40.
32. Lawson WE, Polosukhin VV, Zoia O, Stathopoulos GT, Han W, Plieth D, Loyd JE, Neilson EG, Blackwell TS. Characterization of fibroblast-specific protein 1 in pulmonary fibrosis. Am J Respir Crit Care Med. 2005;171:899–907.
33. Osterreicher CH, Penz-Osterreicher M, Grivennikov SI, Guma M, Koltsova EK, Datz C, Sasik R, Hardiman G, Karin M, Brenner DA. Fibroblast-specific protein 1 identifies an inflammatory subpopulation of macrophages in the liver. Proc Natl Acad Sci U S A. 2011;108:308–13.
34. Manoury B, Caulet-Maugendre S, Guenon I, Lagente V, Boichot E. TIMP-1 is a key factor of fibrogenic response to bleomycin in mouse lung. Int J Immunopathol Pharmacol. 2006;19:471–87.
35. Yang ZZ, Zou AP. Homocysteine enhances TIMP-1 expression and cell proliferation associated with NADH oxidase in rat mesangial cells. Kidney Int. 2003;63:1012–20.
36. Selman M, Ruiz V, Cabrera S, Segura L, Ramirez R, Barrios R, Pardo A. TIMP-1, −2, −3, and −4 in idiopathic pulmonary fibrosis. A prevailing nondegradative lung microenvironment? Am J Physiol Lung Cell Mol Physiol. 2000;279:L562–74.
37. Beeh KM, Beier J, Kornmann O, Buhl R. Sputum matrix metalloproteinase-9, tissue inhibitor of metalloprotinease-1, and their molar ratio in patients with chronic obstructive pulmonary disease, idiopathic pulmonary fibrosis and healthy subjects. Respir Med. 2003;97:634–9.
38. Lepetit H, Eddahibi S, Fadel E, Frisdal E, Munaut C, Noel A, Humbert M, Adnot S, D'Ortho MP, Lafuma C. Smooth muscle cell matrix metalloproteinases in idiopathic pulmonary arterial hypertension. Eur Respir J. 2005;25:834–42.
39. Vieillard-Baron A, Frisdal E, Eddahibi S, Deprez I, Baker AH, Newby AC, Berger P, Levame M, Raffestin B, Adnot S, d'Ortho MP. Inhibition of matrix metalloproteinases by lung TIMP-1 gene transfer or doxycycline aggravates pulmonary hypertension in rats. Circ Res. 2000;87:418–25.
40. Zempo N, Koyama N, Kenagy RD, Lea HJ, Clowes AW. Regulation of vascular smooth muscle cell migration and proliferation in vitro and in injured rat arteries by a synthetic matrix metalloproteinase inhibitor. Arterioscler Thromb Vasc Biol. 1996;16:28–33.
41. George SJ, Baker AH, Angelini GD, Newby AC. Gene transfer of tissue inhibitor of metalloproteinase-2 inhibits metalloproteinase activity and neointima formation in human saphenous veins. Gene Ther. 1998;5:1552–60.
42. Kolpakov V, Rekhter MD, Gordon D, Wang WH, Kulik TJ. Effect of mechanical forces on growth and matrix protein synthesis in the in vitro pulmonary artery. Analysis of the role of individual cell types. Circ Res. 1995;77:823–31.
43. Gaboury JP, Anderson DC, Kubes P. Molecular mechanisms involved in superoxide-induced leukocyte-endothelial cell interactions in vivo. Am J Phys. 1994;266:H637–42.
44. Kliment CR, Tobolewski JM, Manni ML, Tan RJ, Enghild J, Oury TD. Extracellular superoxide dismutase protects against matrix degradation of heparan sulfate in the lung. Antioxid Redox Signal. 2008;10:261–8.
45. Gongora MC, Lob HE, Landmesser U, Guzik TJ, Martin WD, Ozumi K, Wall SM, Wilson DS, Murthy N, Gravanis M, et al. Loss of extracellular superoxide dismutase leads to acute lung damage in the presence of ambient air: a potential mechanism underlying adult respiratory distress syndrome. Am J Pathol. 2008;173:915–26.
46. Fubini B, Hubbard A. Reactive oxygen species (ROS) and reactive nitrogen species (RNS) generation by silica in inflammation and fibrosis. Free Radic Biol Med. 2003;34:1507–16.
47. Vallyathan V, Castranova V, Pack D, Leonard S, Shumaker J, Hubbs AF, Shoemaker DA, Ramsey DM, Pretty JR, McLaurin JL, et al. Freshly fractured quartz inhalation leads to enhanced lung injury and inflammation. Potential role of free radicals. Am J Respir Crit Care Med. 1995;152:1003–9.
48. Fattman CL, Tan RJ, Tobolewski JM, Oury TD. Increased sensitivity to asbestos-induced lung injury in mice lacking extracellular superoxide dismutase. Free Radic Biol Med. 2006;40:601–7.
49. Tan RJ, Lee JS, Manni ML, Fattman CL, Tobolewski JM, Zheng M, Kolls JK, Martin TR, Oury TD. Inflammatory cells as a source of airspace extracellular superoxide dismutase after pulmonary injury. Am J Respir Cell Mol Biol. 2006;34:226–32.
50. Ahmed MN, Suliman HB, Folz RJ, Nozik-Grayck E, Golson ML, Mason SN, Auten RL. Extracellular superoxide dismutase protects lung development in hyperoxia-exposed newborn mice. Am J Respir Crit Care Med. 2003;167:400–5.
51. Bowler RP, Nicks M, Tran K, Tanner G, Chang LY, Young SK, Worthen GS. Extracellular superoxide dismutase attenuates lipopolysaccharide-induced neutrophilic inflammation. Am J Respir Cell Mol Biol. 2004;31:432–9.
52. Loenders B, Van Mechelen E, Nicolai S, Buyssens N, Van Osselaer N, Jorens PG, Willems J, Herman AG, Slegers H. Localization of extracellular superoxide dismutase in rat lung: neutrophils and macrophages as carriers of the enzyme. Free Radic Biol Med. 1998;24:1097–106.

53. Fattman CL, Chu CT, Kulich SM, Enghild JJ, Oury TD. Altered expression of extracellular superoxide dismutase in mouse lung after bleomycin treatment. Free Radic Biol Med. 2001;31:1198–207.
54. Kinnula VL, Hodgson UA, Lakari EK, Tan RJ, Sormunen RT, Soini YM, Kakko SJ, Laitinen TH, Oury TD, Paakko PK. Extracellular superoxide dismutase has a highly specific localization in idiopathic pulmonary fibrosis/usual interstitial pneumonia. Histopathology. 2006;49:66–74.
55. Kim H, Morimoto Y, Ogami A, Nagatomo H, Hirohashi M, Oyabu T, Kawanami Y, Kuroda E, Higashi T, Tanaka I. Differential expression of EC-SOD, Mn-SOD and CuZn-SOD in rat lung exposed to crystalline silica. J Occup Health. 2007;49:242–8.
56. Kajiwara T, Ogami A, Yamato H, Oyabu T, Morimoto Y, Tanaka I. Effect of particle size of intratracheally instilled crystalline silica on pulmonary inflammation. J Occup Health. 2007;49:88–94.
57. Yang Q, Sun M, Ramchandran R, Raj JU. IGF-1 signaling in neonatal hypoxia-induced pulmonary hypertension: role of epigenetic regulation. Vasc Pharmacol. 2015;73:20–31.

22

Alterations in VASP phosphorylation and profilin1 and cofilin1 expression in hyperoxic lung injury and BPD

Mehboob Ali[1*], Kathryn Heyob[1], Trent E. Tipple[2], Gloria S. Pryhuber[3] and Lynette K. Rogers[1,4]

Abstract

Background: Hyperoxia is a frequently employed therapy for prematurely born infants, induces lung injury and contributes to development of bronchopulmonary dysplasia (BPD). BPD is characterized by decreased cellular proliferation, cellular migration, and failure of injury repair systems. Actin binding proteins (ABPs) such as VASP, cofilin1, and profilin1 regulate cell proliferation and migration via modulation of actin dynamics. Lung mesenchymal stem cells (L-MSCs) initiate repair processes by proliferating, migrating, and localizing to sites of injury. These processes have not been extensively explored in hyperoxia induced lung injury and repair.

Methods: ABPs and $CD146^{+}$ L-MSCs were analyzed by immunofluorescence in human lung autopsy tissues from infants with and without BPD and by western blot in lung tissue homogenates obtained from our murine model of newborn hyperoxic lung injury.

Results: Decreased F-actin content, ratio of $VASP^{pS157/VASPpS239}$, and profilin 1 expression were observed in human lung tissues but this same pattern was not observed in lungs from hyperoxia-exposed newborn mice. Increases in cofilin1 expression were observed in both human and mouse tissues at 7d indicating a dysregulation in actin dynamics which may be related to altered growth. CD146 levels were elevated in human and newborn mice tissues (7d).

Conclusion: Altered phosphorylation of VASP and expression of profilin 1 and cofilin 1 in human tissues indicate that the pathophysiology of BPD involves dysregulation of actin binding proteins. Lack of similar changes in a mouse model of hyperoxia exposure imply that disruption in actin binding protein expression may be linked to interventions or morbidities other than hyperoxia alone.

Keywords: Hyperoxia, BPD, Actin binding proteins, L-MSCs, CD146, VASP, $VASP^{pS157}$, $VASP^{pS239}$, Profilin1, Cofilin1

Background

Vasodilator-stimulated phosphoprotein (VASP) is one of the three mammalian Ena/VASP family members that link the cell membrane, signal transduction pathways, and the actin cytoskeleton. VASP activity is regulated by phosphorylation at serine 157 ($VASP^{pS157}$) or 239 ($VASP^{pS239}$), respectively [1–3](reviewed in [4]). VASP interacts with other actin binding proteins (ABP) such as profilin1 to promote actin polymerization [5–7] and cofilin1, to sever F-actin into ADP-actin monomers, depolymerizing F-actin and facilitating actin stabilization [5, 8–10]. Other investigations have identified differential VASP phosphorylation and its association with profilin1 and/or cofilin1 to regulate vascular remodeling and vasodilation/vasoconstriction in pulmonary vascular morbidities [11, 12] and in changes in endothelial permeability in the context of lung injury [13]. Additionally, in a lipopolysaccharide (LPS) induced acute lung injury (ALI) animal model, VASP knockout mice demonstrated greater pulmonary injury when compared to wild type animals due to decreased alveolar capillary barrier properties [14]. Moreover, airway smooth muscle cells and migrating vascular endothelial cells require $VASP^{pS157}$ for membrane or leading edge localization [15].

Improved understanding of newborn lung development and pathophysiology has led to improved neonatal

* Correspondence: mehboob.ali@nationwidechildrens.org; mehtox@hotmail.com
[1]Center for Perinatal Research, The Research Institute at Nationwide Children's Hospital, 575 Children's Cross Road, Columbus, OH, USA
Full list of author information is available at the end of the article

care over the last 20 years [16]. However, elevated oxygen tensions are still used to treat infants with Respiratory Distress Syndrome and contributes to the development of Bronchopulmonary Dysplasia (BPD) [17, 18]. Preterm infants with BPD display deficits in alveolarization, pulmonary vascular development, cellular proliferation, and suppressed injury repair [18, 19]. In response to lung injury, lung mesenchymal stem cells (L-MSCs) migrate to injury sites and accelerate repair processes [20–23]. MSCs have been investigated for their therapeutic potential in preterm infants with chronic lung disease yet the results have been mixed and concern for safety has prevented clinical trials (reviewed in [24]). Migration and proliferation of L-MSCs are likely to be regulated by alternative phosphorylation of actin binding proteins (ABPs). Moreover, MSCs can secrete nitric oxide (NO) or S-nitrosothiols (SNOs), which regulate vasculogenesis via the soluble guanyl cyclase C mediated cGMP/PKG pathway which in turn could regulate VASP phosphorylation [25, 26]. A recent clinical study found an association between increased cGMP, VASP phosphorylation at serine 239, and improved lung function in preterm infants with early symptoms of BPD, indicating a possible involvement of VASP [27].

In the present study, we utilized human neonatal lung autopsy tissue and our murine newborn hyperoxia exposure model to test the hypothesis that changes in VASP phosphorylation state and expression ABPs profilin1 and cofilin1 correlate with hyperoxic lung injury and repair and that changes in these ABPs are associated with recruitment of MSCs to the injured lung.

Materials and methods

Human lung tissues F-actin content

Human lung autopsy tissues from infants that died with BPD and infants that died at similar postnatal ages from non-pulmonary causes (control) were obtained from Dr. Gloria Pryhuber and collected as part of the BRINDL repository and Lung Map consortium [28]. Study inclusion/exlusion criteria, IRB approval and parental consent has been previously described [29]. Lung tissue sections were obtained from 16 infants, 8 infants that died with BPD and 8 infants that died of other non-pulmonary causes, (n = 8 in each group) and the clinical descriptions and co-morbidities of the infants from whom these samples were collected have been previously published [29]. F-actin content in tissue was estimated by using Alexafluor-633 tagged phalloidin (Invitrogen, Eugene, Oregon) and DAPI (Invitrogen, Carlsbad, CA) for the nucleus. Images were acquired in a blinded fashion using a confocal microscope (LSM510, Carl Zeiss, Jena, Germany) with 40X objective. Four photomicrographs were obtained from each tissue section assessed independently and averaged for each individual thus creating an n = 8 for each diagnosis. Identical confocal settings were applied to acquire all images across conditions. F-actin content/cell was quantified using NIH Image J analysis.

Human lung autopsy tissues ABPs analysis

Tissues were processed for immunofluorescence (IF) labelling using standard protocols [30]. Tissue sections were stained with primary anti-human polyclonal antibodies targeting profilin1 (catalog# 3237), cofilin1(catalog# 5175), VASP (catalog# 3112), $VASP^{pS239}$ (catalog# 3114) (Cell Signaling Technology, Inc., Danvers, MA), $VASP^{pS157}$ (catalog# sc-23,506-R) (Santa Cruz, Dallas, Texas) (dilution, 1:500), followed by secondary antibodies Alexa 488 labeled IgG (1:1000) and nuclei stained with DAPI (Invitrogen, Carlsbad, CA). Images were taken using Carl Zeiss's Axio Scope A1 Polarized Light Fluorescent Microscope (Carl Zeiss, Jena, Germany) with 40X magnification and identical settings. Four photomicrographs were obtained from each tissue section assessed independently and averaged for each individual thus creating an n = 8 for each diagnosis. Intensity of image color was quantified using NIH image J software.

Newborn hyperoxia exposure

Animal study protocols were approved by the IACUC at The Research Institute at Nationwide Children's Hospital and pregnant dams were dated as to time of delivery. C3H/HeN mice were bred and at least 2 dams were required to deliver within 12 h. Once born, the pups were randomized and equally distributed between the two dams. One dam and litter was placed in a plexiglass chamber containing 8 L/min flow of 85% O_2 while the corresponding dam and litter remained in room air (RA). The dams were switched every 24 h to prevent oxygen toxicity. The pups were removed from oxygen exposure on day 14 and allowed to recover in room air. On day of life 7 or 56 the pups were euthanized and lung tissues were snap-frozen in liquid N_2. At term, newborn mice are in the saccular stage of lung development much like a 26–36 week gestation human infant [31, 32]. Day 7 was chosen to represent acute lung injury during the course of exposure and at the time point when the inflammatory responses are greatest and alveolarization is actively taking place [33] and day 56 was chosen as point after recovery to identify any permanent changes in protein expression. Tissues from 4 mice, one from each of 4 independent litters, were used for further analyses.

Mouse lung homogenate ABPs analysis

Snap-frozen lung tissues were homogenized (10% w/v) in solution of 0.1 M Na phosphate buffer containing 5 mM EDTA (pH 7.4) using TissueLyser II (Qiagen,

Germantown, MD) and centrifuged at 12000 rpm for 20 min to prepare post mitochondrial supernatants. Protein concentrations were measured using Bio-Rad protein reagent (Bio-Rad, Hercules, CA). Equal amounts of post mitochondrial supernatants were dissolved in SDS sample buffer and proteins were separated by SDS-PAGE, transferred to nitrocellulose membranes, and probed with anti-human polyclonal antibodies targeting profilin1 (catalog# 3237), cofilin1(catalog# 5175), VASP (catalog# 3112), $VASP^{pS239}$ (catalog# 3114) (Cell Signaling Technology, Inc., Danvers, MA), $VASP^{pS157}$ (catalog# sc-23,506-R) (Santa Cruz, Dallas, Texas) (dilution, 1:500), and rabbit monoclonal antibodies targeting GAPDH (D16H11) (catalog #5174)(1:10,000) (Cell Signaling Technology, Inc., Danvers, MA). Finally, membranes were probed with horseradish peroxidase (HRP)-conjugated secondary antibody (dilution, 1:1000) (BD Pharminogen®, Franklin lakes, NJ) for 1 h at room temperature and specific bands were visualized employing Amersham™ECL™ Prime Western Blotting Detection Reagent (GE Healthcare, Buckinghamshire, UK) and the band intensity was measured by densitometry.

L-MSCs marker (CD146) analysis in human lung autopsy tissues and mouse lung homogenate

CD146 expression and levels in human lung autopsy tissues and mouse lung homogenate was assessed by IF staining and western blot analyses respectively. Human MCAM/CD146 Ab (R&D Systems, Minneapolis, MN) was used as primary antibody while HRP and Alexa 488 labeled IgG (1:1000) were used as secondary antibodies for western and IF analysis, respectively. Nuclei in lung tissue biopsy sections were stained with DAPI (Invitrogen, Carlsbad, CA) and 40X magnification images (4 from each slide) were obtained and analyzed as described previously.

Statistics

Human lung tissues ($n = 8$, each group) and mouse lung homogenate ($n = 4$, each group) were considered in present study. Statistical analyses were performed using either two-way ANOVA or Welch's unequal variances t-test (GraphPad Prism, version 7.03; GraphPad Software, Inc.) and significance is presented as "p" value or for post hoc analyses is indicated as *, $p < 0.05$.

Result

Lung tissue F-actin contents were lower in infants who die with BPD

F-actin contents were assessed by immunofluorescence in human lung autopsy tissues from infants that died with BPD and infants that died at similar postnatal ages from non-pulmonary causes (control). Lower F-actin content (Fig. 1), was observed in the tissues of infants that died with BPD than in the control group. These differences may represent an overall suppression of actin dynamics and/or cell growth.

Changes in VASP phosphorylation, and profilin 1 and cofilin 1 expression were observed in infants who died with BPD

Cofilin1, profilin1 and VASP phosphorylation were assessed by immunofluorescence. Our data did not indicate differences in total VASP fluorescence; however, we did detect lower levels of VASP phosphorylation in tissues from infants who died with BPD which created a net decrease in the ratio of $VASP^{pS157}/VASP^{pS239}$ (Fig. 2). Profilin1 immunofluorescence was lower and cofilin 1 immunofluorescence was greater in tissue sections from infants who died with BPD when compared to infants who died of non-respiratory causes (Fig. 2).

VASP phosphorylation, and profilin 1 and cofilin 1 levels in lung tissues homogenates from mouse pups exposed to hyperoxia

Western blot analyses of lung tissue homogenates from mouse pups exposed to hyperoxia for 7 days demonstrated greater expression cofilin 1 than in lungs from room air exposed controls (Fig. 3). At 56 d, $VASP^{pS239}$ protein levels were lower in lungs from mice previously exposed to hyperoxia than in mice raised in room air from birth (Fig. 1). There was a time dependent decrease in total VASP, profilin 1, and cofilin 1 between day 7 and day 56 indicating that these proteins were likely involved in lung growth and development. Alternatively, there was a time dependent increase in $VASP^{pS157}$ in both the room air and hyperoxia groups and an increase in $VASP^{pS239}$ in the room air group that was blunted by the previous hyperoxia exposure. The time dependent changes in VASP phosphorylation altered the relative ratio of $VASP^{pS157}$/ $VASP^{pS239}$ which was overall lower at day 56.

L-MSCs (CD146) in mouse lung homogenates and human lung autopsy tissues

CD146 expression was measured by immunofluorescence in lung autopsy tissues and by western blot in mouse lung homogenates. Lower levels of CD146 expression were detected in lung autopsy tissues obtained from infants who died with BPD compared to non-BPD controls (Fig. 4). CD146 levels in murine lungs tended to be higher in hyperoxia-exposed mice than in room air controls (Fig. 5) as there was an effect of both time and exposure (two-way ANOVA). The western blots (specifically in Fig. 5) possessed some small inconsistencies such as minor bubbles but these were outside the quantification area and did not affect the results as a whole and given the nature of these samples would have been

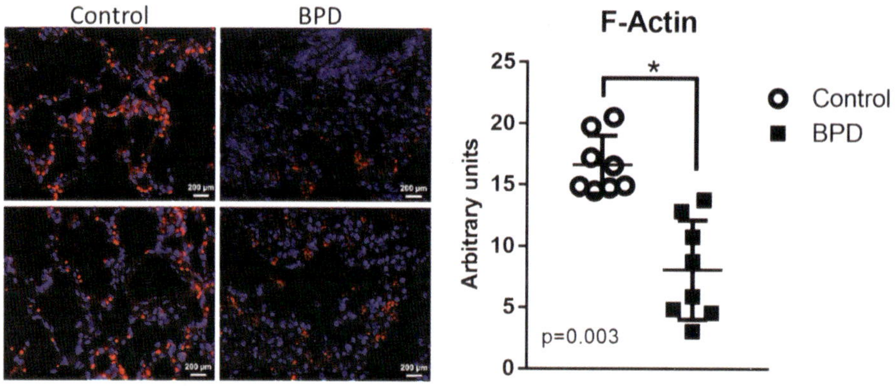

Fig. 1 Human lung autopsy tissues F-actin content. Lung tissues sections were obtained from infants that died with BPD (closed squares) or infants that died at similar ages from non-pulmonary illnesses (open circles). Phalloidin used to stain F-actin in red while nuclei stained with DAPI in blue. Confocal microscopy images at 40X magnification processed in NIH Image-J software to measure F-actin contents. Four independent images were obtained from each slide and averaged for each individual creating $n = 8$ for each group. Statistical analysis was performed using Welch's unequal variances t-test, and significance is indicated as *, $p < 0.05$; compared to controls

difficult to repeat. We also observed double bands for GAPDH on the day 7 blot, however this is consistent with many other publications of this protein [34–36] and both bands were quantified by densitometry and used for normalizing the western blot.

Discussion

The relative ratio of $VASP^{pS157}$ to $VASP^{pS239}$ represents the activity of VASP to add actin monomers and promote growth and migration. In the present study, we investigated whether alternative phosphorylation of VASP

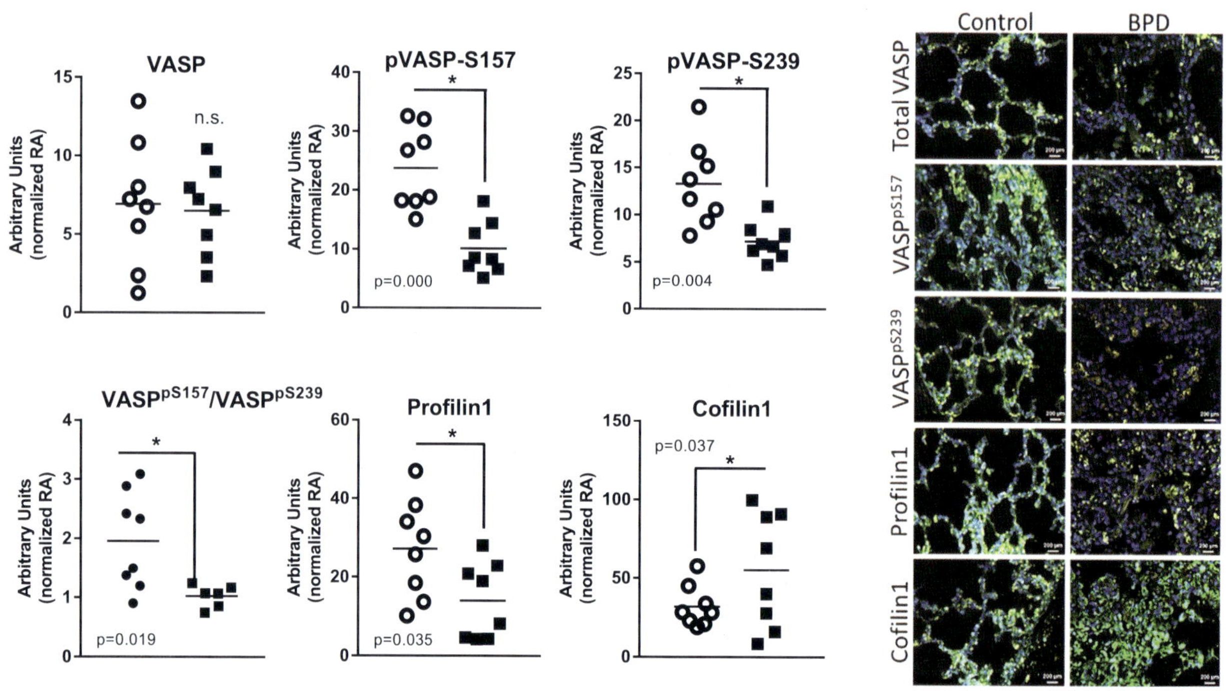

Fig. 2 VASP phosphorylation, profilin1 and cofilin1 expression in human lung autopsy tissue. Lung tissues sections were obtained from infants that died with BPD (closed squares) or infants that died at similar ages from non-pulmonary illnesses (open circles). Fluorescent microscopy followed by NIH Image J analysis was used to quantify VASP expression and differential phosphorylation, and profilin1 and cofilin1 expression in human autopsy samples. Images are 40X magnification. Green, VASP, phosphor-VASP, profilin1 and cofilin1 stained with specific antibody against each protein; red, F-actin stained with phalloidin; and blue, nuclei stained with DAPI. Four independent images were obtained from each slide and averaged for each individual creating $n = 8$ for each group. Statistical analysis was performed using Welch's unequal variances t-test, n = 8 in each group, and significance is indicated as *, $p < 0.05$; and n.s. = non significant compared to respective controls

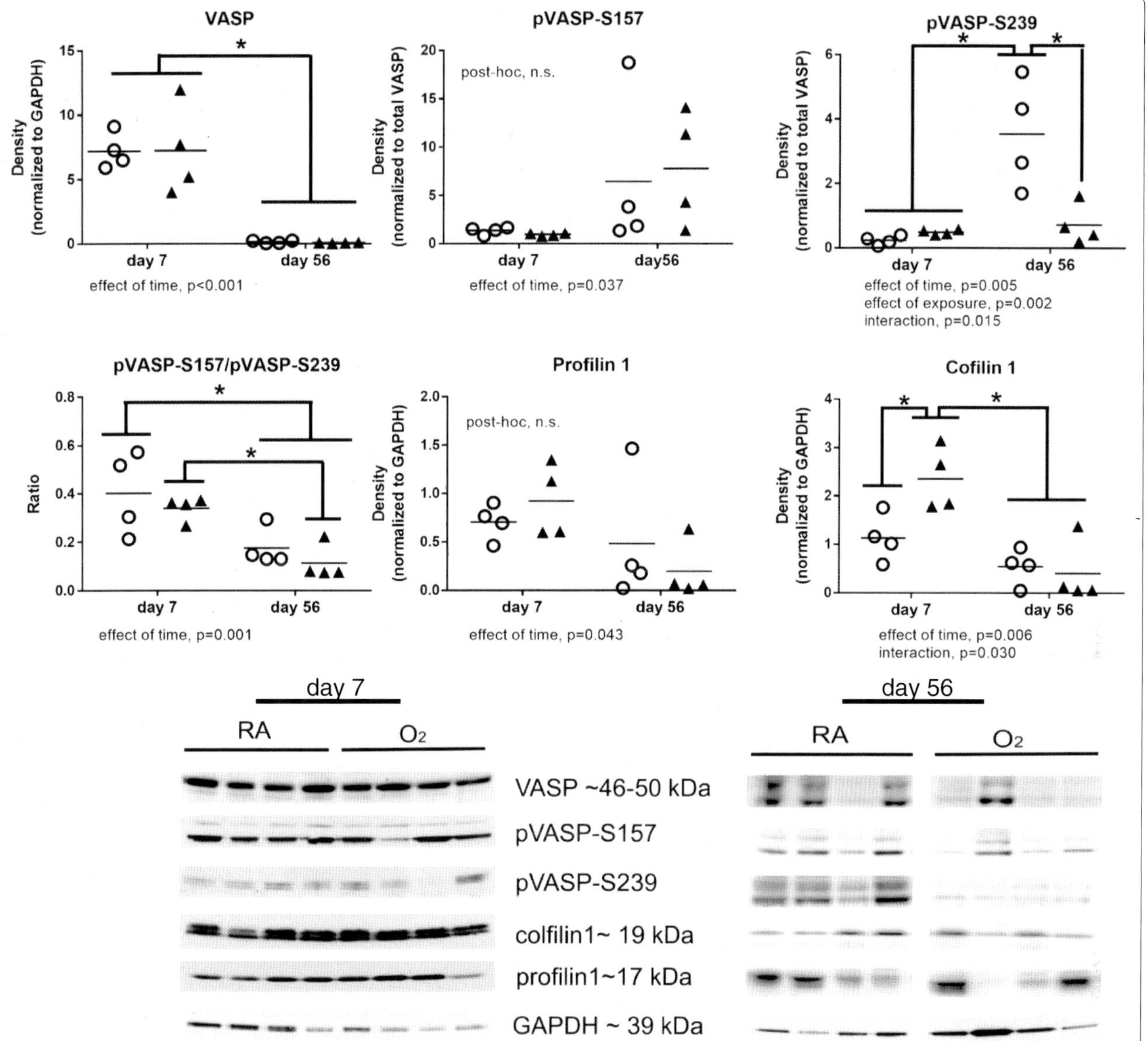

Fig. 3 VASP phosphorylation, profilin1 and cofilin1 level in lung tissue homogenates from mouse pups exposed to hyperoxia until day 7. Western blot analysis was performed on whole lung tissue homogenates obtained from mice exposed to room air (RA, open circles) or 85% O_2 (O_2, closed triangles) from birth through day 7 or at day 56 after 14 days of hyperoxia exposure and 42 days of room air recovery. Band intensity was quantified by densitometry and statistical analysis was performed using two-way ANOVA with Tukey's post hoc, $n = 4$ in each group. *, $p < 0.05$ and n.s. = non significant

or other ABPs may be associated with the deficit in lung growth and repair observed in infants that develop BPD.

To accomplish our goals, we obtained human autopsy tissues from Dr. Gloria Pryhuber for analysis and employed our murine C3H/HeN model of neonatal hyperoxia exposure [37, 38]. In human lung autopsy tissues obtained from infants who died with BPD and infants that died at similar ages with non-pulmonary morbidities (for demographic data see reference [29]), we observed less total F-actin content than in tissues from infants who died of BPD than controls (Fig. 1). This observation may be due to decreased alveolarization which, in turn, provided less tissue to analyze per microscope field or may represent a decrease in lung growth and development. Using immunofluorescence (IF) labelling, the contents of VASP, $VASP^{pS157}$, $VASP^{pS239}$, profilin1, and cofilin1 were assessed. Our data indicated overall lower levels of protein containing either sites of VASP phosphorylation and a decrease in $VASP^{pS157/VASPpS239}$ ratio in the BPD tissues compared to controls. This data indicated either lower $VASP^{pS157}$ expression and/or increased $VASP^{pS239}$ expression in infants with BPD than in control tissues (Fig. 2). Both of these interpretations could implicate an impaired tissue or cellular repair mechanism. Lower profilin1 and elevated cofilin1 levels could also be interpreted as impaired growth mechanisms

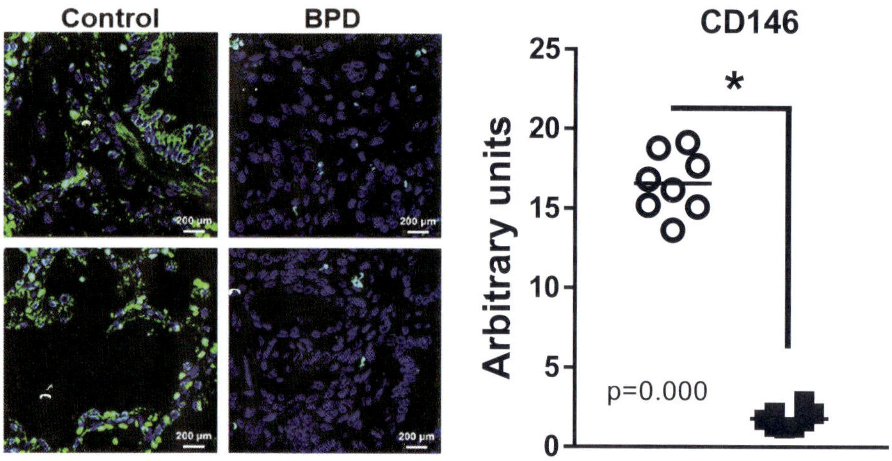

Fig. 4 L-MSCs (CD146) levels in lung tissue homogenates from mouse pups exposed to hyperoxia. Western blot analysis was performed on whole lung tissue homogenates obtained from mice exposed to room air (RA, open circles) or 85% O_2 (O_2, closed triangles) at day 7 and 56. Band intensity was quantified by densitometry and statistical analysis was performed using two = way ANOVA with Tukey's post-hoc. *, $p < 0.05$ and n.s. = non significant

as they would contribute to a decreased availability of actin monomers and increased actin end-capping.

To identity whether the changes observed in the autopsy tissues were due to acute hyperoxia exposure or to later adaptive responses, we analyzed changes in ABPs at 7d of continuous hyperoxia and at 56d, well after recovery. At 7d there were no changes in VASP expression or phosphorylation or profilin 1 expression (Fig. 3). We did however identify an increase in cofilin 1 expression in the hyperoxia-exposed mice compared to controls. At 56d of life, $VASP^{pS239}$ was lower in mice previously exposed to hyperoxia than in RA controls (Fig. 3). Expression of total VASP, $VASP^{pS157}$, profilin 1 and cofilin 1 were higher at day 7 than at day 56 and this decrease likely coincides with completion of lung development prior to day 56. Interestingly, $VASP^{pS239}$ is increased at the later time point and this increase is prevented in the mice previously exposed to hyperoxia. The relevance of this increase is uncertain but may reflect a maintenance or homeostatic effect of this particular modification that is prevented by the early exposure to hyperoxia and may reflect a later life susceptibility to disease.

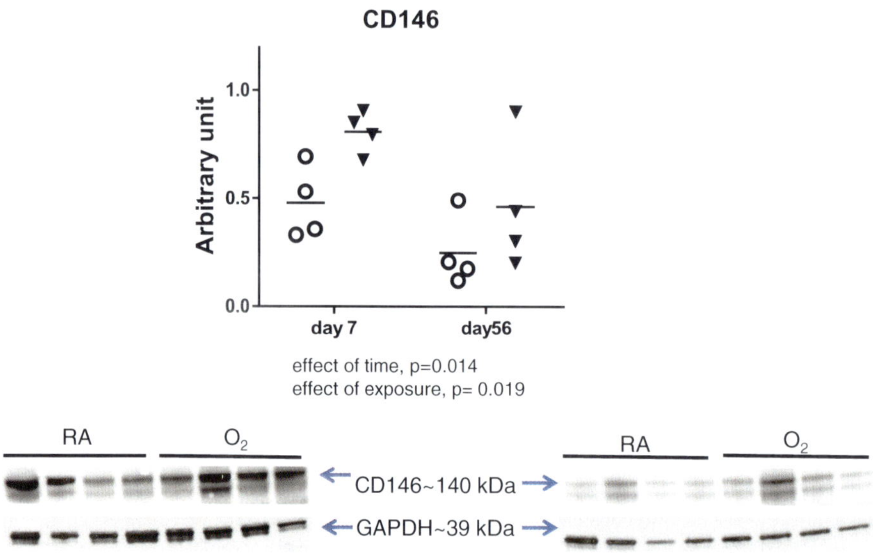

Fig. 5 L-MSCs marker (CD146) expression in human lung autopsy tissues. Lung tissues sections were obtained from infants that died with BPD (closed squares) or infants that died at similar ages from non-pulmonary illnesses (open circles). Green, CD146 stained with specific antibody; and blue, nuclei stained with DAPI. Confocal microscopy images at 40X magnification processed in NIH Image-J software. Statistical analysis was performed using Welch's unequal variances t-test, $n = 8$ in each group, and significance is indicated as ***, $p < 0.0001$; compared to controls

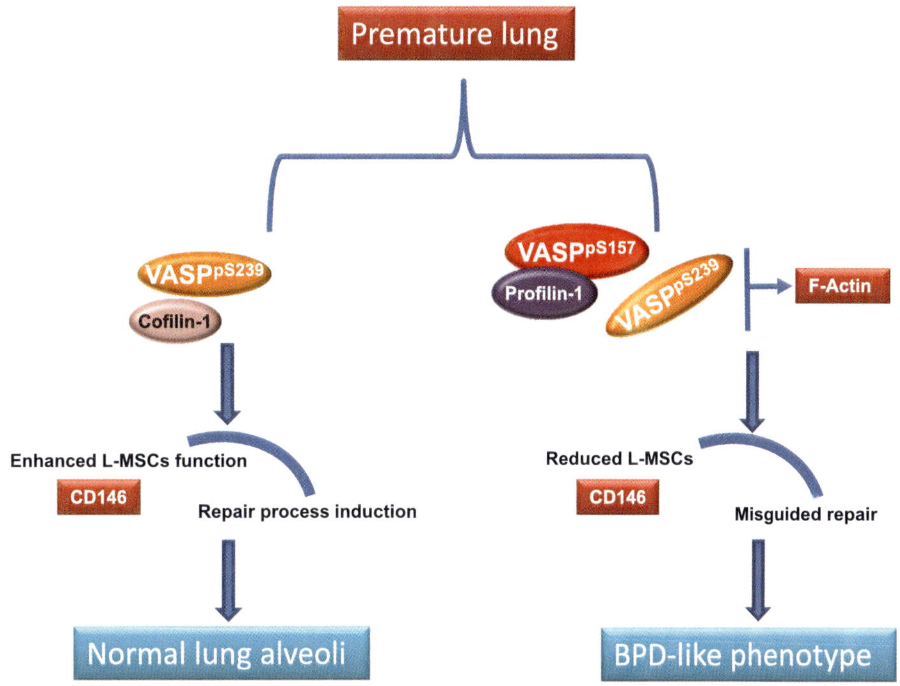

Fig. 6 Schematic representation of hypothesis. Hyperoxia exposure decreases VASP expression and phosphorylation disrupting actin dynamics in human tissues. Early responses include increases in cofilin1 in attempts to initiate repair. In later stages of injury and dysregulated repair, we observe decreases in VASP phosphorylation and profilin1 which are indicative of impaired repair. L-MSCs play a significant role in repair and proliferate in response to injury stimuli. Early increase in CD146 is indicative of enhanced L-MSCs proliferation and homing in mouse lungs, while at later stages decreased CD146 in human autopsy tissue is suggestive injury beyond repair. We speculated that disruptions in ABP dynamics may be due to interventions or morbidities other than hyperoxia alone in humans with BPD

Collectively, these data indicate that while VASP proteins and phosphorylation are likely involved in the pathology of human BPD, their dysregulation it is not likely due to hyperoxia exposure alone as in our mouse model but rather other stressors such as mechanical ventilation or potentially surfactant insufficiency. Cofilin1 levels were increased in both human tissues and 7d mouse tissues. Cofilin1 is highly regulated during development as it spatially and temporally regulates cell morphology and morphogenesis in developing tissues [7]. The aberrant increases observed in the human tissues as well as our mouse model could contribute to poor lung growth and decreases in alveolarization and should be a focus of further investigation.

Repair processes such as those initiated by hyperoxic injury, instigate proliferation of L-MSCs and migration to the site of injury [21, 23, 24, 39]. Characterization of multipotent stem cells and L-MSCs indicated that CD146 is a marker of MSCs [40, 41]. As a marker of tissue repair, we used CD146 expression in human autopsy lung tissue samples and lung tissue homogenates from our mouse model of hyperoxia injury to identify the relative amount and the localization of MSCs. We observed decreased CD146+ L-MSC expression in BPD tissues compared to control (Fig. 4) suggesting that there are fewer L-MSCs to facilitate growth and repair function. Alternatively, we observed increased CD146 expression at both day 7 and day 56 in the mouse tissue homogenates (Fig. 5). In the human tissues, injury and disease has progressed to a state that death occurred and it is likely that repair mechanisms were no longer active or had been overwhelmed by the extent of injury. At both time points in the mouse model, repair and regeneration was still taking place and the increase in L-MSCs would corroborate the role of these cells types in repair. Overall our data supports the previous findings that induction of L-MSC-mediated repair takes place in response to hyperoxia and persists but that there reaches a point in injury where repair mechanisms are no longer sufficient. Several differences were observed between mouse and human tissue measurements and these may be attributable to numerous factors. In the mouse, we measured these parameters either during acute injury (at 7d of exposure) or very late after recovery (at 56 d). In the infant lungs, there was no recovery and injury had progressed much further than observed with only 14d of hyperoxia exposure as in the mice. There are also many other confounding factors in the human tissues. For example, BPD did not exist as a single morbidity but was one of many as indicated in our previous publication [29].

Exposure to mechanical ventilation and excessive "stretch" may have created a different phenotype in the infant lungs which was not equivalent to simple hyperoxia exposure in the mouse tissues. Additionally, the human tissues were assessed by immunofluorescence and subject to subcellular expression and quenching and the mouse tissues were measured by western blot. Furthermore, the current studies did not directly investigate ABPs in L-MSCs however we speculate that the changes in ABP homeostasis is relevant to changes in L-MSCs phenotypes during lung airway injury repair.

Conclusions

These studies indicate that ABPs are affected by hyperoxia exposure during development and suggest that the alterations in VASP throughout development and/or its interaction with other ABPs are likely to contribute to diminished repair processes and may also contribute to decreased lung growth and alveolarization (Fig. 6). Further investigations are warranted to specifically evaluate alternative ABPs and their precise role in mediating lung injury and repair in the developing lung.

Abbreviations

ABPs: Actin binding proteins; BPD: Bronchopulmonary dysplasia; L-MSCs: Lung mesenchymal stem cells; O_2: Oxygen; RA: Room air; VASP: Vasodilator-stimulated phosphoprotein; $VASP^{pS157}$: VASP phosphorylation at serine 157; $VASP^{pS239}$: VASP phosphorylation at serine 239

Acknowledgements

Not Applicable

Funding

NIH funding R01HL119280 (T.E.T); and R01AT006880 and R01HD0880833 (L.K.R.).

Authors' contributions

MA conceived the ideas, designed, executed the experiments, and wrote the first draft of the manuscript and approved the final draft; KMH performed the animal studies and helped with analyses; LKR and TET helped to get materials and assisted with the design of the experiments and writing of the manuscript; GP helped to get human biopsy samples and manuscript editing. All authors read and approved the final manuscript.

Competing interests

The authors declare that they have no competing interests.

Author details

[1]Center for Perinatal Research, The Research Institute at Nationwide Children's Hospital, 575 Children's Cross Road, Columbus, OH, USA. [2]Department of Pediatrics, University of Alabama at Birmingham, Birmingham, AL, USA. [3]Department of Pediatrics, University of Rochester Medical Center, Rochester, NY, USA. [4]Department of Pediatrics, The Ohio State University, Columbus, OH, USA.

References

1. Benz PM, Blume C, Seifert S, Wilhelm S, Waschke J, Schuh K, Gertler F, Munzel T, Renne T. Differential VASP phosphorylation controls remodeling of the actin cytoskeleton. J Cell Sci. 2009;122:3954–65.
2. Aszodi A, Pfeifer A, Ahmad M, Glauner M, Zhou XH, Ny L, Andersson KE, Kehrel B, Offermanns S, Fassler R. The vasodilator-stimulated phosphoprotein (VASP) is involved in cGMP- and cAMP-mediated inhibition of agonist-induced platelet aggregation, but is dispensable for smooth muscle function. EMBO J. 1999;18:37–48.
3. Doppler H, Storz P. Regulation of VASP by phosphorylation: consequences for cell migration. Cell Adhes Migr. 2013;7:482–6.
4. Pula G, Krause M. Role of Ena/VASP proteins in homeostasis and disease. Handb Exp Pharmacol. 2008:39–65.
5. Siton O, Bernheim-Groswasser A. Reconstitution of actin-based motility by vasodilator-stimulated phosphoprotein (VASP) depends on the recruitment of F-actin seeds from the solution produced by cofilin. J Biol Chem. 2014; 289:31274–86.
6. Dominguez R. Actin filament nucleation and elongation factors--structure-function relationships. Crit Rev Biochem Mol Biol. 2009;44:351–66.
7. Ohashi K. Roles of cofilin in development and its mechanisms of regulation. Develop Growth Differ. 2015;57:275–90.
8. Pfaendtner J, De La Cruz EM, Voth GA. Actin filament remodeling by actin depolymerization factor/cofilin. Proc Natl Acad Sci U S A. 2010;107:7299–304.
9. Bamburg JR, Bernstein BW. Roles of ADF/cofilin in actin polymerization and beyond. F1000 Biol Rep. 2010;2:62.
10. Witke W. The role of profilin complexes in cell motility and other cellular processes. Trends Cell Biol. 2004;14:461–9.
11. Hassona MD, Elnakish MT, Abouelnaga ZA, Alhaj M, Wani AA, Hassanain H. The effect of selective antihypertensive drugs on the vascular remodeling-associated hypertension: insights from a profilin1 transgenic mouse model. J Cardiovasc Pharmacol. 2011;57:550–8.
12. Sartoretto JL, Jin BY, Bauer M, Gertler FB, Liao R, Michel T. Regulation of VASP phosphorylation in cardiac myocytes: differential regulation by cyclic nucleotides and modulation of protein expression in diabetic and hypertrophic heart. Am J Physiol Heart Circ Physiol. 2009;297:H1697–710.
13. Rentsendorj O, Mirzapoiazova T, Adyshev D, Servinsky LE, Renne T, Verin AD, Pearse DB. Role of vasodilator-stimulated phosphoprotein in cGMP-mediated protection of human pulmonary artery endothelial barrier function. Am J Physiol Lung Cell Mol Physiol. 2008;294:L686–97.
14. Henes J, Schmit MA, Morote-Garcia JC, Mirakaj V, Kohler D, Glover L, Eldh T, Walter U, Karhausen J, Colgan SP, Rosenberger P. Inflammation-associated repression of vasodilator-stimulated phosphoprotein (VASP) reduces alveolar-capillary barrier function during acute lung injury. FASEB J. 2009;23:4244–55.
15. Wu Y, Gunst SJ. Vasodilator-stimulated phosphoprotein (VASP) regulates actin polymerization and contraction in airway smooth muscle by a vinculin-dependent mechanism. J Biol Chem. 2015;290:11403–16.
16. Martin RJ, Fanaroff AA. The preterm lung and airway: past, present, and future. Pediatr Neonatol. 2013;54:228–34.
17. Toti P, Buonocore G, Tanganelli P, Catella AM, Palmeri ML, Vatti R, Seemayer TA. Bronchopulmonary dysplasia of the premature baby: an immunohistochemical study. Pediatr Pulmonol. 1997;24:22–8.
18. El Mazloum D, Moschino L, Bozzetto S, Baraldi E. Chronic lung disease of prematurity: long-term respiratory outcome. Neonatology. 2014;105:352–6.
19. Ramani M, Bradley WE, Dell'Italia LJ, Ambalavanan N. Early exposure to hyperoxia or hypoxia adversely impacts cardiopulmonary development. Am J Respir Cell Mol Biol. 2015;52:594–602.
20. Low AT, Medford AR, Millar AB, Tulloh RM. Lung function in pulmonary hypertension. Respir Med. 2015;109:1244–9.
21. Collins JJ, Thebaud B. Lung mesenchymal stromal cells in development and disease: to serve and protect? Antioxid Redox Signal. 2014;21:1849–62.
22. Yee M, Buczynski BW, O'Reilly MA. Neonatal hyperoxia stimulates the expansion of alveolar epithelial type II cells. Am J Respir Cell Mol Biol. 2014;50:757–66.
23. Alkhouri H, Poppinga WJ, Tania NP, Ammit A, Schuliga M. Regulation of pulmonary inflammation by mesenchymal cells. Pulm Pharmacol Ther. 2014; 29:156–65.
24. Vosdoganes P, Lim R, Moss TJ, Wallace EM. Cell therapy: a novel treatment approach for bronchopulmonary dysplasia. Pediatrics. 2012;130:727–37.

25. Bachiller PR, Cornog KH, Kato R, Buys ES, Roberts JD Jr. Soluble guanylate cyclase modulates alveolarization in the newborn lung. Am J Physiol Lung Cell Mol Physiol. 2013;305:L569–81.
26. Wagenaar GT, Hiemstra PS, Gosens R. Therapeutic potential of soluble guanylate cyclase modulators in neonatal chronic lung disease. Am J Physiol Lung Cell Mol Physiol. 2015; ajplung 00333 02015.
27. Mouchaers KT, Schalij I, Versteilen AM, Hadi AM, van Nieuw Amerongen GP, van Hinsbergh VW, Postmus PE, van der Laarse WJ, Vonk-Noordegraaf A. Endothelin receptor blockade combined with phosphodiesterase-5 inhibition increases right ventricular mitochondrial capacity in pulmonary arterial hypertension. Am J Physiol Heart Circ Physiol. 2009;297:H200–7.
28. Bhatt AJ, Pryhuber GS, Huyck H, Watkins RH, Metlay LA, Maniscalco WM. Disrupted pulmonary vasculature and decreased vascular endothelial growth factor, Flt-1, and TIE-2 in human infants dying with bronchopulmonary dysplasia. Am J Respir Crit Care Med. 2001;164:1971–80.
29. Rogers LK, Robbins M, Dakhlallah D, Yang Z, Lee LJ, Mikhail M, Nuovo G, Pryhuber GS, McGwin G, Marsh CB, Tipple TE. Attenuation of miR-17-92 cluster in bronchopulmonary dysplasia. Ann Am Thorac Soc. 2015;12:1506–13.
30. Snegovskikh V, Mutlu L, Massasa E, Taylor HS. Identification of putative fallopian tube stem cells. Reprod Sci. 2014;21:1460–4.
31. Azad MB, Moyce BL, Guillemette L, Pascoe CD, Wicklow B, McGavock JM, Halayko AJ, Dolinsky VW. Diabetes in pregnancy and lung health in offspring: developmental origins of respiratory disease. Paediatr Respir Rev. 2017;21:19–26.
32. Rackley CR, Stripp BR. Building and maintaining the epithelium of the lung. J Clin Invest. 2012;122:2724–30.
33. Rogers LK, Tipple TE, Nelin LD, Welty SE. Differential responses in the lungs of newborn mouse pups exposed to 85% or >95% oxygen. Pediatr Res. 2009;65:33–8.
34. Kanno Y, Maruyama C, Matsuda A, Ishisaki A. uPA-derived peptide, A6 is involved in the suppression of lipopolysaccaride-promoted inflammatory osteoclastogenesis and the resultant bone loss. Immun Inflamm Dis. 2017;5: 289–99.
35. Lekli I, Ray D, Mukherjee S, Gurusamy N, Ahsan MK, Juhasz B, Bak I, Tosaki A, Gherghiceanu M, Popescu LM, Das DK. Co-ordinated autophagy with resveratrol and gamma-tocotrienol confers synergetic cardioprotection. J Cell Mol Med. 2010;14:2506–18.
36. Lagares D, Ghassemi-Kakroodi P, Tremblay C, Santos A, Probst CK, Franklin A, Santos DM, Grasberger P, Ahluwalia N, Montesi SB, et al. ADAM10-mediated ephrin-B2 shedding promotes myofibroblast activation and organ fibrosis. Nat Med. 2017;23:1405–15.
37. Velten M, Britt RD Jr, Heyob KM, Tipple TE, Rogers LK. Maternal dietary docosahexaenoic acid supplementation attenuates fetal growth restriction and enhances pulmonary function in a newborn mouse model of perinatal inflammation. J Nutr. 2014;144:258–66.
38. Velten M, Britt RD Jr, Heyob KM, Welty SE, Eiberger B, Tipple TE, Rogers LK. Prenatal inflammation exacerbates hyperoxia-induced functional and structural changes in adult mice. Am J Physiol Regul Integr Comp Physiol. 2012;303:R279–90.
39. Foronjy RF, Majka SM. The potential for resident lung mesenchymal stem cells to promote functional tissue regeneration: understanding microenvironmental cues. Cells. 2012;1:874.
40. Covas DT, Panepucci RA, Fontes AM, Silva WA Jr, Orellana MD, Freitas MC, Neder L, Santos AR, Peres LC, Jamur MC, Zago MA. Multipotent mesenchymal stromal cells obtained from diverse human tissues share functional properties and gene-expression profile with CD146+ perivascular cells and fibroblasts. Exp Hematol. 2008;36:642–54.
41. Sorrentino A, Ferracin M, Castelli G, Biffoni M, Tomaselli G, Baiocchi M, Fatica A, Negrini M, Peschle C, Valtieri M. Isolation and characterization of CD146+ multipotent mesenchymal stromal cells. Exp Hematol. 2008;36:1035–46.

Permissions

All chapters in this book were first published in RR, by BioMed Central; hereby published with permission under the Creative Commons Attribution License or equivalent. Every chapter published in this book has been scrutinized by our experts. Their significance has been extensively debated. The topics covered herein carry significant findings which will fuel the growth of the discipline. They may even be implemented as practical applications or may be referred to as a beginning point for another development.

The contributors of this book come from diverse backgrounds, making this book a truly international effort. This book will bring forth new frontiers with its revolutionizing research information and detailed analysis of the nascent developments around the world.

We would like to thank all the contributing authors for lending their expertise to make the book truly unique. They have played a crucial role in the development of this book. Without their invaluable contributions this book wouldn't have been possible. They have made vital efforts to compile up to date information on the varied aspects of this subject to make this book a valuable addition to the collection of many professionals and students.

This book was conceptualized with the vision of imparting up-to-date information and advanced data in this field. To ensure the same, a matchless editorial board was set up. Every individual on the board went through rigorous rounds of assessment to prove their worth. After which they invested a large part of their time researching and compiling the most relevant data for our readers.

The editorial board has been involved in producing this book since its inception. They have spent rigorous hours researching and exploring the diverse topics which have resulted in the successful publishing of this book. They have passed on their knowledge of decades through this book. To expedite this challenging task, the publisher supported the team at every step. A small team of assistant editors was also appointed to further simplify the editing procedure and attain best results for the readers.

Apart from the editorial board, the designing team has also invested a significant amount of their time in understanding the subject and creating the most relevant covers. They scrutinized every image to scout for the most suitable representation of the subject and create an appropriate cover for the book.

The publishing team has been an ardent support to the editorial, designing and production team. Their endless efforts to recruit the best for this project, has resulted in the accomplishment of this book. They are a veteran in the field of academics and their pool of knowledge is as vast as their experience in printing. Their expertise and guidance has proved useful at every step. Their uncompromising quality standards have made this book an exceptional effort. Their encouragement from time to time has been an inspiration for everyone.

The publisher and the editorial board hope that this book will prove to be a valuable piece of knowledge for researchers, students, practitioners and scholars across the globe.

List of Contributors

Anna Winkler and Rudolf A. Jörres
Institute and Outpatient Clinic for Occupational, Social and Environmental Medicine, Comprehensive Pneumology Center Munich (CPC-M), Ludwig-Maximilians-Universität München, Munich, Germany

Kathrin Kahnert, Jürgen Behr and Nikolaus Kneidinger
Department of Internal Medicine V, University of Munich (LMU), Comprehensive Pneumology Center, Member of the German Center for Lung Research (DZL), Ziemssenstr. 1, 80336 Munich, Germany

Claus Neurohr
Robert-Bosch-Hospital, Klinik Schillerhöhe, Gerlingen, Germany

Rudolf Hatz
Department of Thoracic Surgery, University of Munich (LMU), Munich, Germany

Holger Dressel and Thomas Radtke
Epidemiology, Biostatistics and Prevention Institute, University of Zurich, Zurich, Switzerland Division of Occupational and Environmental Medicine, University of Zurich and University Hospital Zurich, Zurich, Switzerland

Lei Zhang, Yi Wang, Guorao Wu, Weining Xiong and Cong-Yi Wang
The Center for Biomedical Research, Key Laboratory of Organ Transplantation, Ministry of Education and Ministry of Health, Tongji Hospital, Tongji Medical College, Huazhong University of Science and Technology, 1095 Jiefang Avenue, Wuhan 430030, China

Weikuan Gu
Departments of Orthopaedic Surgery-Campbell Clinic, and Pathology, University of Tennessee Health Science Center (UTHSC), Memphis, TN 38163, USA

Jorge Luiz Dantas de Medeiros, Bruno Carneiro Bezerra, Thiago Anderson Brito de Araújo, Lucien Peroni Gualdi, Maria do Socorro Luna Cruz, Thaiza Teixeira Xavier Nobre and Julliane Tamara Araújo de Melo Campos
Faculdade de Ciências da Saúde do Trairi, Universidade Federal do Rio Grande do Norte, Santa Cruz, RN, Brazil

Aquiles Sales Craveiro Sarmento, Lázaro Batista de Azevedo Medeiros and Tamara Araújo de Melo Campos
Laboratório de Biologia Molecular e Genômica, Departamento de Biologia Celular e Genética, Centro de Biociências, Universidade Federal do Rio Grande do Norte, Natal, RN, Brazil

Josivan Gomes Lima
Departamento de Medicina Clínica, Hospital Universitário Onofre Lopes (HUOL)/UFRN, Natal, RN, Brazil

Miriam Barrecheguren and Marc Miravitlles
Pneumology Department, Hospital General Universitari Vall d'Hebron, CIBER de Enfermedades Respiratorias (CIBERES), P. de la Vall d'Hebron, 119-129, 08035 Barcelona, Spain

Cruz González
Pneumology Department, Hospital Clínic Universitari, Valencia, Spain

Jianjun Jin, Jiming Si, Yuanhua Liu, Huanqin Wang, Ran Ni and Jing Wang
Department of Respiratory and Critical Medicine, the First Affiliated Hospital of Zhengzhou University, No. 1, Jianshe East Road, Zhengzhou 450052, Henan Province, China

Silvia Perez-Bogerd, Alain Van Muylem
Erasme University Hospital, Chest Department, Université Libre Bruxelles, B-1060 Brussels, Belgium

Silvia Perez-Bogerd, Wim Wuyts and Veronica Barbier
University Hospitals Leuven, Department of Respiratory Diseases, B-3000 Leuven, Belgium

Heleen Demeyer, Wim Janssens and Thierry Troosters
KU Leuven, Department of Rehabilitation Sciences, B-3000 Leuven, Belgium

Wim Janssens
KU Leuven, Department of Chronic Diseases, Metabolism and Ageing, B-3000 Leuven, Belgium

Alexandra Stroda, Vincent Brandenburg, Ayham Daher, Christian Cornelissen and Michael Dreher
Department of Pneumology and Intensive Care Medicine, University Hospital Aachen, Aachen, Germany

Claudia Goettsch
Department of Cardiology, Angiology and Intensive Care Medicine, University Hospital Aachen, Würselen, Germany

Vincent Brandenburg and András Keszei
Department of Cardiology, Angiology and Intensive Care Medicine, University Hospital Aachen, Aachen, Germany

Vincent Brandenburg and Michael Dreher
Department of Cardiology and Nephrology, Rhein-Maas Klinikum Würselen, Aachen, Germany

Bruce J. Kirenga
Makerere University Lung Institute and Division of Pulmonary Medicine, Department of Medicine, Makerere University College of Health Sciences, Kampala, Uganda

Levicatus Mugenyi
Makerere University Lung Institute, Makerere University College of Health Sciences, Kampala, Uganda

Corina de Jong and Thys van der Molen
GRIAC-Primary Care, Department of General Practice and Elderly Care, University of Groningen, University Medical Center Groningen (UMCG), Groningen, The Netherlands
Groningen Research Institute for Asthma COPD (GRIAC), University of Groningen, University Medical Center Groningen (UMCG), Groningen, The Netherlands

J. Lucian Davis
Department of Epidemiology of Microbial Diseases, Yale School of Public Health, and Pulmonary, Critical Care, and Sleep Medicine Section, Yale School of Medicine, New Haven, CT, USA

Winceslaus Katagira
Makerere University Lung Institute, Makerere University College of Health Sciences, Kampala, Uganda

Moses R. Kamya
Department of Medicine, Makerere University College of Health Sciences, Kampala, Uganda

Marike Boezen
Department of Epidemiology, University of Groningen, Groningen, The Netherlands

Chen-Fang Hsu
Department of Pediatrics, Chi Mei Medical Center, Tainan, Taiwan
Taipei Medical University, Taipei, Taiwan
Kaohsiung Medical University, Kaohsiung, Taiwan
Chung Shan Medical University, Taichung, Taiwan

Chen-Hao Hsiao
Cheng Hsin General Hospital, Taipei, Taiwan
Genome and Systems Biology Degree Program, National Taiwan University and Academia Sinica, Taipei, Taiwan

Shun-Fu Tseng, Jian-Ru Chen, Yu-Jou Liao and Yi-Ping Chuang
Department and Graduate Institute of Microbiology and Immunology, National Defense edical Center, Taipei, Taiwan

Sy-Jou Chen
Department of Emergency Medicine, Tri-Service General Hospital, National Defense Medical Center, Taipei, Taiwan
Graduate Institute of Injury Prevention and Control, College of Public Health and Nutrition, Taipei Medical University, Taipei, Taiwan

Chin-Sheng Lin
Division of Cardiology, Department of Medicine, Tri-Service General Hospital, National Defense Medical Center, Taipei, Taiwan

Huey-Kang Sytwu
National Institute of Infectious Diseases and Vaccinology, National Health Research Institutes, Miaoli, Taiwan

Giovanni Sotgiu, Federica Trogu and Laura Saderi
Clinical Epidemiology and Medical Statistics Unit, Department of Clinical and Experimental Medicine, University of Sassari, Sassari, Italy

Stefano Aliberti, Andrea Gramegna, Marco Mantero, Marta Di Pasquale and Francesco Blasi
Department of Pathophysiology and Transplantation, University of Milan, Milan, Italy
Internal Medicine Department, Respiratory Unit and Cystic Fibrosis Adult Center, Fondazione IRCCS Cá Granda Ospedale Maggiore Policlinico, Milan, Italy

Maaike de Vries, Diana A van der Plaat, Judith M Vonk and H Marike Boezen
University of Groningen, University Medical Center Groningen, Department of Epidemiology, Hanzeplein 1, Groningen 9713, GZ, The Netherlands

Maaike de Vries, Diana A van der Plaat, Wierd Kooistra, Corry-Anke Brandsma, Judith M Vonk and H Marike Boezen
University of Groningen, University Medical Center Groningen, Groningen Research Institute for Asthma and COPD (GRIAC), Groningen, The Netherlands

Ivana Nedeljkovic, Najaf Amin and Cornelia M van Duijn
Department of Epidemiology, Erasmus Medical Center, Rotterdam, The Netherlands

Rikst Nynke Verkaik-Schakel
University of Groningen, University Medical Center Groningen, Department of Obstetrics and Gynaecology, Groningen, The Netherlands

Wierd Kooistra and Corry-Anke Brandsma
University of Groningen, University Medical Center Groningen, Department of Pathology and Medical Biology, Groningen, The Netherlands

Cleo C van Diemen
University of Groningen, University Medical Center Groningen, Department of Genetics, Groningen, The Netherlands

Suzy A. A. Comhair, Sara Baicker-McKee, Zeneng Wang, Jeffrey P. Hammel, Stanley L. Hazen and Serpil C. Erzurum
Cleveland Clinic, Lerner Research Institute, 9500 Euclid Avenue, NB2-40, Cleveland, OH 44195, USA

Grazyna Bochenek, Tomasz Stachura, Marek Sanak and Ewa Nizankowska-Mogilnicka
Department of Internal Medicine, Faculty of Medicine, Jagiellonian University Medical College, Krakow, Poland

Serpil C. Erzurum
Respiratory Institute, Cleveland Clinic, Cleveland, USA

Hee-Young Yoon, Sojung Park, Dong Soon Kim and Jin Woo Song
Department of Pulmonary and Critical Care Medicine, Asan Medical Centre, University of Ulsan College of Medicine, Olympic-Ro 43-Gil, Songpa-Gu, Seoul 05505, Republic of Korea

Dennis Lo, Reynold A. Panettieri Jr and Cynthia J. Koziol-White
Department of Medicine, Rutgers Institute for Translational Medicine and Science, Rutgers University, New Brunswick, NJ, USA

Joshua L. Kennedy
Department of Pediatrics, Division of Allergy and Immunology, University of Arkansas for Medical Sciences, Little Rock, AR, USA

Richard C. Kurten
Department of Physiology and Biophysics, University of Arkansas for Medical Sciences, Little Rock, AR, USA

Arezoo Mohammadipoor, Ben Antebi, Andriy I. Batchinsky and Leopoldo C. Cancio
Multi-Organ Support Technology (MOST) Task Area, US Army Institute of Surgical Research, Fort Sam Houston, TX, USA

Arezoo Mohammadipoor
Oak Ridge Institute for Science and Education, Oak Ridge, TN, USA

Andriy I. Batchinsky
The Geneva Foundation, Tacoma, WA, USA

Cheryl S. Pirozzi and Richard E. Kanner
Division of Pulmonary and Critical Care Medicine, Department of Internal Medicine, University of Utah, 26 N 1900 E, Salt Lake City, UT 84132, USA

Tian Gu
Department of Biostatistics, University of Michigan, Ann Arbor, MI, USA

Pedro M. Quibrera
Department of Biostatistics, Collaborative Studies Coordinating Center, University of North Carolina at Chapel Hill, Chapel Hill, NC, USA

A. Christenson
Department of Medicine, University of California, San Francisco, CA, USA

Nadia N. Hansel
Department of Medicine, Johns Hopkins University, Baltimore, MD, USA

R. Graham Barr
Department of Medicine, Columbia University, New York, NY, USA

Victor E. Ortega
Department of Medicine, Wake Forest University, Winston-Salem, NC, USA

Fernando J. Martinez
Department of Medicine, Weill Cornell Medical College, New York, NY, USA

Cheryl S. Pirozzi and Robert Paine III
Department of Veterans Affairs Medical Center, Salt Lake City, UT, USA

Bin Wang, Yun Zhou, Lili Xiao, Yanjun Guo, Jixuan Ma, Min Zhou, Jing Yuan and Weihong Chen
Department of Occupational and Environmental Health, School of Public Health, Tongji Medical College, Huazhong University of Science and Technology, Wuhan 430030, Hubei, China

Bin Wang, Yun Zhou, Lili Xiao, Yanjun Guo, Jixuan Ma, Min Zhou, Jing Yuan and Weihong Chen
Key Laboratory of Environment and Health, Ministry of Education and Ministry of Environmental Protection, and State Key Laboratory of Environmental Health (Incubating), School of Public Health, Tongji Medical College, Huazhong University of Science and Technology, Wuhan 430030, Hubei, China

Tingming Shi
Hubei Provincial Key Laboratory for Applied Toxicology, Hubei Provincial Center for Disease Control and Prevention, Wuhan 430079, Hubei, China

Aijun Tan
Zhuhai Center for Disease Control and Prevention, Zhuhai 519060, Guangdong, China

Carlos Machahua, Ana Montes-Worboys, Lurdes Planas-Cerezales, Raquel Buendia-Flores, Maria Molina-Molina and Vanesa Vicens-Zygmunt
Pneumology Research Group, IDIBELL, L'Hospitalet de Llobregat, Barcelona, Spain

Carlos Machahua, Ana Montes-Worboys and Maria Molina-Molina
Biomedical Research Network Centers in Respiratory Diseases (CIBERES), Barcelona, Spain

Ana Montes-Worboys, Lurdes Planas-Cerezales, Maria Molina-Molina and Vanesa Vicens-Zygmunt
Unit of Interstitial Lung Diseases, Department of Pneumology, University Hospital of Bellvitge, C. Feixa Llarga sn., 08907 L'Hospitalet de Llobregat, Barcelona, Spain

Javier Milara
Department of Pharmacology, Faculty of Medicine, Jaume I University, Castellón de la Plana, Spain

Javier Milara
Pharmacy Unit, University General Hospital Consortium, Valencia, Spain

Javier Milara, Inés Roger, Ángel Cogolludo, Esteban Morcillo and Julio Cortijo
CIBERES, Health Institute Carlos III, Valencia, Spain

Lucía Díaz-Platas
Unidade Radiofármacos PET, GALARIA, Santiago de Compostela, A Coruña, Spain

Sonia Contreras, Pilar Ribera, Beatriz Ballester, Paula Montero, Esteban Morcillo and Julio Cortijo
Department of Pharmacology, Faculty of Medicine, University of Valencia, Valencia, Spain

Ángel Cogolludo
Department of Pharmacology, School of Medicine, Universidad Complutense de Madrid, Madrid, Spain

Esteban Morcillo
Health Research Institute INCLIVA, Valencia, Spain

Julio Cortijo
Research and teaching Unit, University General Hospital Consortium, Valencia, Spain

Javier Milara
Unidad de Investigación Clínica, Consorcio Hospital General Universitario, Avenida tres cruces s/n, E-46014 Valencia, Spain

Pere Soler-Palacín
Hospital U. Vall d'Hebron, P. de la Vall d'Hebron, 119-129, 08035 Barcelona, Spain

Luis Ignacio González-Granado
Hospital U. 12 Octubre, Av. Cordoba, s/n, 28041 Madrid, Spain

Carlos Martín
Hospital U. Miguel Servet, P. Isabel la Católica, 1-3, 50009 Zaragoza, Spain

Carlos Rodríguez-Gallego
H. Son Espases, C. de Valldemossa, 79, 07120 Palma, Balearic Islands, Spain

Silvia Sánchez-Ramón
Hospital Clínico San Carlos, C. del Prof Martín Lagos, s/n, 28040 Madrid, Spain

Javier de Gracia
Hospital Universitari Vall d'Hebron - Institut de Recerca, Barcelona, Spain

Igor N. Zelko, Jianxin Zhu and Jesse Roman
Department of Medicine, Division of Pulmonary, Critical Care, and Sleep Medicine, University of Louisville, 505 S. Hancock Street, CTR Bldg., room 524, Louisville, KY 40202, USA

Igor N. Zelko
Department of Biochemistry and Molecular Genetics, University of Louisville, 505 S. Hancock Street, CTR Bldg., room 524, Louisville, KY 40202, USA

Jesse Roman
Department of Pharmacology and Toxicology, University of Louisville Health Sciences Center, Louisville, KY 40202, USA

Jesse Roman
Robley Rex VA Medical Center, Louisville, KY 40202, USA

Mehboob Ali, Kathryn Heyob and Lynette K. Rogers
Center for Perinatal Research, The Research Institute at Nationwide Children's Hospital, 575 Children's Cross Road, Columbus, OH, USA

Trent E. Tipple
Department of Pediatrics, University of Alabama at Birmingham, Birmingham, AL, USA

Gloria S. Pryhuber
Department of Pediatrics, University of Rochester Medical Center, Rochester, NY, USA

Lynette K. Rogers
Department of Pediatrics, The Ohio State University, Columbus, OH, USA

Index

A

Actin Binding Proteins, 227-228, 234

Acute Lung Injury, 13, 19-20, 141, 145, 148, 151-154, 180-181, 227-228, 234

Acute Respiratory Distress Syndrome, 15, 17, 141, 151, 181

Aerd, 112-118

Ages, 50, 71, 73, 133-134, 173-180, 228-232

Airway Hyperresponsiveness, 76, 130, 134, 137-138

Airway Obstruction, 1, 34, 41, 76, 105, 114, 155-156, 160, 162-164

Airway Smooth Muscle, 130, 133, 136-139, 145, 186, 227, 234

Alternatively Activated Macrophages, 14, 17, 19-20, 145, 151

Alveolar Macrophages, 12, 15, 17-18, 145, 148, 186

Asthma, 18-20, 39-40, 42, 69-76, 91, 94-95, 103, 110-118, 130-140, 145-148, 153, 163, 166, 172, 183, 199, 212

B

Biomarker, 48, 113-115, 117-118, 163, 173-174, 179-181, 183, 194

Bpd, 145-146, 148-150, 227-234

Bromotyrosine, 112-114, 117-118

Bronchiolitis Obliterans Syndrome, 1, 9

Bronchopulmonary Dysplasia, 141, 145-146, 150, 153, 181, 225, 227-228, 234-235

C

Cap, 90-92, 95-98, 100

Cardiovascular Disease, 67, 122, 165, 172

Cd146, 227, 229, 232-233, 235

Chemotherapy, 43-51

Chronic Obstructive Pulmonary Disease, 32, 39-42, 60, 62, 66-68, 75, 95-96, 103, 106, 111, 137, 141, 145, 151, 155-156, 163-165, 171-172, 184, 198-199, 222, 224-225

Classically Activated Macrophages, 19

Cofilin1, 227-231, 233

Conditioned Media, 132, 141-142, 151-153

Copd, 3, 30, 32-42, 52-53, 56-60, 62-68, 74-76, 94-95, 103-104, 106, 110-111, 130-132, 135-138, 141, 145-146, 148, 151, 155-156, 158, 160-167, 172, 178, 188-199, 213, 224

Corticosteroid Resistance, 182-183, 190-191, 193-194, 196-199

Crystalline Silica, 213-214, 216-219, 221, 223-226

Curdlan, 77-89

D

Diffusing Capacity, 1-6, 8-10, 53, 55, 119-120, 122-124, 128, 174, 177-178, 180, 208, 210

Dna Methylation, 103-111

E

Emphysema, 3, 10, 39, 62, 95-96, 141, 145-146, 148, 151, 153-164, 181, 222

Ewas, 103-108

Expression, 12-15, 17-19, 30, 44-51, 67, 77-78, 80-81, 87-88, 103-106, 108-110, 131, 134, 136-140, 142, 144, 146-147, 149, 178, 180-183, 185-186, 188-198, 213-218, 221-235

Extracellular Vesicles, 141-143, 151-154

F

Fibroblast Growth Factor 23, 62, 67-68

Forced Expiratory Volume, 1, 5, 9, 36, 38, 64, 67, 106, 115, 133, 137, 155, 158, 166, 168-170, 183-184, 189

H

Hap, 90-92, 96-98

Hcap, 90-92, 96-98, 100

Hiv, 69-76, 88

Hyperoxia, 145-146, 148, 223, 225, 227-229, 231-235

I

Idiopathic Pulmonary Fibrosis, 10-11, 17-19, 55, 59-61, 119, 122, 125-129, 141, 151, 173-174, 176, 180-181, 225-226

Il-17a, 77-82, 85-87

Inflammation, 2, 6, 12-13, 19-20, 48, 66, 68, 70, 113, 116, 118, 130-131, 133-138, 140, 145-147, 153, 170-172, 181-183, 186, 188, 191-193, 195-199, 211, 213, 221, 234-235

Ipf, 3, 11-18, 52, 55-56, 58-60, 119-121,
123-128, 141, 151, 173-180, 223

L

L-mscs, 227-229, 232-234

Leukotriene, 112, 117-118

Lipodystrophy, 21-22, 25-26, 28-31

Lung Disease, 1-3, 11, 13, 16, 18, 32-33, 40, 42, 60-63, 67, 76, 103, 111, 128, 136, 141, 153, 155-157, 160-162, 166, 171-172, 180, 183, 202, 204, 213, 218, 225, 228, 234-235

Lung Fibrosis, 3, 14, 17-20, 145-146, 148-149, 178, 213-214, 217, 221, 224

Lung Function, 4-5, 7, 10, 30, 32, 34-35, 37-42, 55, 59, 62-67, 70, 76, 103-106, 108, 119-121, 127-128, 134, 142, 146, 149, 156, 161, 163, 177-179, 187, 194, 205, 228, 234

Lung Tissue, 14, 66, 103-111, 146-147, 174, 182-183, 185-186, 188-189, 191-193, 195-196, 214, 227-229, 231-233

Lung Transplantation, 1, 9, 174

M

Macrophage Polarization, 11-15, 18-20

Maximal Midexpiratory Flow Rate, 155
Mep, 21-29
Mesenchymal Stem Cells, 16, 141, 143, 145, 148, 151-154, 227-228, 234-235
Metreleptin, 21-24, 26-30
Mild-moderate Disease, 32
Mip, 14, 17, 21-29, 78, 132, 137, 147-148, 151
Mrsa, 90-92, 96, 98, 100
Muc1, 182-183, 185-199

O

Oxidative Stress, 15, 30, 147, 153, 170-174, 213-215, 222

P

Parathyroid Hormone, 62-63, 65-67
Pms, 21, 24-27, 29
Pneumoconiosis, 213, 225
Prevalence, 21-22, 30, 33-34, 40-41, 69-76, 90, 94-97, 99, 103, 110-111, 118, 138, 165, 167, 169, 172, 200, 211, 224
Profilin1, 227-231, 233-234
Programmed Cell Death Ligand 1, 43, 47, 50-51
Prta, 77-89
Pulmonary Fibrosis, 10-20, 55, 59-61, 111, 119, 122, 125-129, 141, 151, 173-176, 179-181, 213, 221, 223-226
Pulmonary Function Tests, 127, 155
Pulmonary Hypertension, 20, 125, 128, 146, 152-154, 213-214, 218, 221-226

Q

Quality of Life, 31-32, 34-35, 37, 39-41, 52-53, 56, 58-60, 103, 141, 156, 209-210, 212

R

Rages, 173, 178
Respiratory Function Tests, 119
Rhinovirus, 19, 130, 132, 134, 136-140

S

Silicosis, 3, 19, 213-215, 219, 224-225
Small Cell Lung Carcinoma, 43
Spirometry, 1, 3-5, 10, 34, 40, 63, 112-113, 120, 128, 155-157, 163, 166, 172, 174, 208-209
Stewardship, 90, 101
Streptococcus Pneumoniae, 77, 88-89, 93, 99, 102, 201

T

Therapeutic Strategies, 11, 224

V

Vaspps157, 227-232, 234
Vaspps239, 227-232, 234
Ventilator-associated (VAP), 30, 90-92, 96-98